Textbook of Surgery

EDITED BY

Joe J. Tjandra
MBBS, MD, FRACS, FRCS(Eng), FRCPS, FASCRS
Colorectal Surgeon and Surgical Oncologist
Associate Professor of Surgery
Royal Melbourne Hospital and Epworth Hospital
University of Melbourne

Gordon J.A. Clunie
MB, ChB, ChM, DSc, FRCS(Eng, Edin), FRACS
Emeritus Professor of Surgery
University of Melbourne

Andrew H. Kaye
MBBS, MD, FRACS
James Stewart Professor of Surgery and Head of Department of Surgery
The University of Melbourne, The Royal Melbourne Hospital
Director of Neurosurgery and Director, The Melbourne Neuroscience Centre
The Royal Melbourne Hospital, Melbourne, Australia

Julian A. Smith
MBBS, MS, FRACS, FACS
Professor of Surgery
Head of Cardiothoracic Surgery
Monash Medical Centre
Monash University

THIRD EDITION

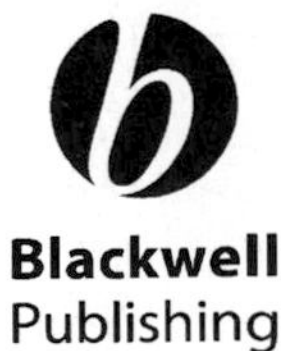

Blackwell
Publishing

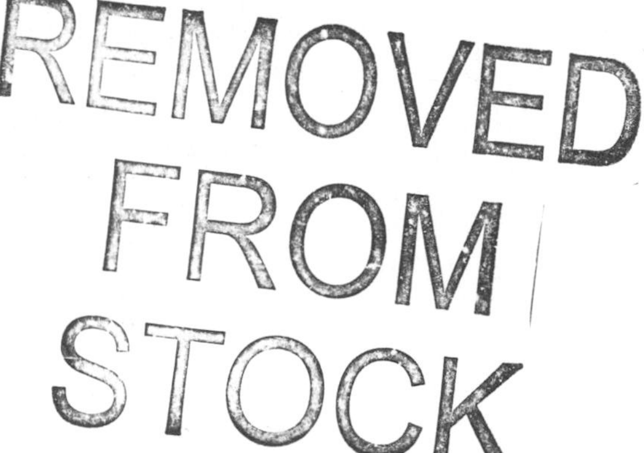

Blackwell Publishing, Inc., 350 Main Street, Malden, Massachusetts 02148-5020, USA
Blackwell Publishing Ltd, 9600 Garsington Road, Oxford OX4 2DQ, UK
Blackwell Publishing Asia Pty Ltd, 550 Swanston Street, Carlton, Victoria 3053, Australia

First published 1997
Second edition 2001
Third edition 2006

2 2008

Library of Congress Cataloging-in-Publication Data

Textbook of surgery / edited by Joe J. Tjandra . . . [et al.]. – 3rd ed.
p.; cm.
Includes index.
ISBN : 978-1-4051-2627-4
1. Surgery
[DNLM: 1. Surgical Procedures, Operative–methods. 2. Surgery–methods.
WO 500 T356 2006] I. Title: Surgery. II. Tjandra, Joe J. (Joe Janwar)

RD31.T472 2006
617—dc22

2005011599

ISBN : 978-1-4051-2627-4

A catalogue record for this title is available from the British Library

Set in 9/11.5 by TechBooks New Delhi, India
Printed and bound in Singapore by Fabulous Printers Pte Ltd.

Commissioning Editors: Fiona Goodgame & Vicki Noyes
Development Editor: Karen Moore
Production Controller: Kate Charman

For further information on Blackwell Publishing, visit our website:
http://www.blackwellpublishing.com

The publisher's policy is to use permanent paper from mills that operate a sustainable forestry policy, and which has been manufactured from pulp process using acid-free and elementary chlorine-free practices. Furthermore, the publisher ensures that the text paper and cover board used have met acceptable environmental accreditation standards.

Contents

List of Contributors

Leslie Bokey
Department of Colorectal Surgery
Concord Hospital
University of Sydney

John Cade
MD, PhD, FRACP, FANZCA, FJFICM
Director, Division of Critical Care
Royal Melbourne Hospital

Stephen Chan
MBBS, PhD, FRACS
Professor of Surgery
Western Hospital
University of Melbourne

Pierre Chapuis
DS (Qld), FRACS
Clinical Chairman
Department of Colorectal Surgery
University of Sydney
Concord Hospital

Peter Choong
MBBS, MD, FRACS, FAOrthA
Department of Orthopaedics
St Vincent's Hospital
Melbourne

Christopher Christophi
MD, FRACS, FRCS, FACS
Head of Department of Surgery
Austin Hospital
University of Melbourne

SC Sydney Chung
MD, FRCS(Edin), FRCP(Edin)
Professor of Surgery
University of Papua New Guinea

Gordon JA Clunie
MB ChB ChM DSc FRCS(Eng, Edin) FRACS
Emeritus Professor of Surgery
University of Melbourne

Neil Collier
MBMS, FRACS, FRCS
Hepatobiliary Unit
Royal Melbourne Hospital

John Collins
MBBS, FRACS
Breast Unit
Royal Melbourne Hospital

Anthony Costello
FRACS, MD
Director of Urology
Royal Melbourne Hospital

Scott D'Amours
BSc, MDCM, FRCS(C), FRACS
Department of Trauma Services
Liverpool Hospital
Sydney

Stephen Deane
FRACS, FRCS(C), FACS
Professor of Surgery
University of New Castle
New Castle

Leigh Delbridge
MD, FRACS
Professor and Head of Surgery
Department of Endocrine and Oncology Surgery
Royal North Shore Hospital
Sydney

Peter Devitt
MBBS, MS, FRCS, FRACS
Department of Surgery
Royal Adelaide Hospital

David Fletcher
MBBS (WA), MD (Melb), FRACS
Professor of Surgery
Fremantle Hospital
Perth

David Francis
BSc(Med Sci), MD, MS, FRCS(Eng), FRCS(Edin), FRACS
Surgeon
Royal Children's Hospital and St Vincent's Hospital
Melbourne

J Galbraith
OBE, MD, FRCS(Eng), FRACS, FRANZCO, FACTM, FACS
Honorary Consultant Ophthalmologist
Royal Melbourne Hospital

Frank Gardiner
MBBS, MD, FRCS, FRACS
Department of Surgery
Royal Brisbane Hospital
University of Queensalnd

Michael Grigg
MBBS, FRACS
Professor of Surgery
Box Hill Hospital
Monash University
Melbourne

John Hall
MS, DS, FRACS
Professor of Surgery
Royal Perth Hospital

John Harris
MS, FRACS, FRCS, FACS, DDU(Vascular)
Professor of Vascular Surgery
University of Sydney

Andrew G Hill
MB, CGB, MD
Department of Surgery
University of Auckland
Auckland Hospital, New Zealand

Ho Yik-Hong
MBBS Hons(Qld), MD, FRCS(Ed), FRCS(Glasg),
FRACS, FICS, FAMS
Professor and Head of Surgery
James Cook University
Townsville

Glyn Jamieson
MBBS, MS, MD, FRACS, FRCS, FACS
Dorothy Mortlock Professor of Surgery
University of Adelaide

Rodney Judson
MBBS, FRCS, FRACS
Head and Neck Surgery
Royal Melbourne Hospital

Bhadu Kavar
MBChB, FCS, FRACS
Department of Neurosurgery
Royal Melbourne Hospital

Andrew H Kaye
MBBS, MD, FRACS
James Stewart Professor of Surgery and
Head of Department of Surgery
The University of Melbourne, The Royal
Melbourne Hospital
Director of Neurosurgery and Director,
The Melbourne Neuroscience Centre
Royal Melbourne Hospital

John Laidlaw
MBBS, FRACS
Department of Neurosurgery
Royal Melbourne Hospital

Simon Law
MS, MBBChir, MA(Cantab), FCSHK, FHKAM(Surgery),
FRCS(Edin), FACS
Department of Surgery
University of Hong Kong
Queen Mary Hospital

Dean Lenz
BSc, MD
Department of Urology
Monash Medical Centre

Michael Levitt
MBBS, FRACS
Colorectal Surgeon
St John of God Healthcare
Subiaco

Iain G. Martin
MEd, MD, FRCS, FRACS
Head of School of Medicine
University of Auckland
New Zealand

Campbell Miles
MBBS, FRACS
Department of Vascular Surgery
Alfred Hospital
Melbourne

David L Morris
MBBS, MD, PhD, FRCS (Eng, Edin), FRACS
Department of Surgery
University of New South Wales
St George's Hospital

Wayne Morrison
MBBS, MD, FRACS
Department of Microsurgery
St Vincent's Hospital
Melbourne

V Muralidharan
PhD, FRACS
Department of Surgery
Austin Hospital
University of Melbourne
Melbourne

Christopher O'Brien
MB, BS, MS, FRACS
Director of Sydney Cancer Centre
Royal Prince Alfred Hospital
Sydney

Stephen O'Leary
MBBS, BMedSc, PhD, FRACS
Royal Victorian Eye and Ear Hospital
University of Melbourne

Bryan R. Parry
MBChB, MD, FRACS
Department of Surgery
University of Auckland
Auckland Hospital
New Zealand

Adrian Polglase
MB, MS, FRACS, FRCS(Eng), FRCS(Ed), FACS
Professor of Surgery
Cabrini Medical Centre
Melbourne

Jeffrey Presneill
MBBS, PhD, FRACP, FJFICM
Deputy Director, Intensive Care Unit
Royal Melbourne Hospital

Jeffrey Rosenfeld
MB, MS, FRACS, FRCS(Ed), FACS
Professor and Director of Neurosurgery
The Alfred Hospital and Monash University
Melbourne

Jonathan Serpell
MB, BS, MD, FRACS, FACS
Head of Breast, Endocrine and Surgical Oncology Unit
Frankston Hospital and Monash University
Melbourne

Julian A. Smith
MBBS, MS, FRACS, FACS
Professor of Surgery
Head of Cardiothoracic Surgery
Monash Medical Centre
Monash University

Michael Solomon
MB, BCh, BAO(Hons), MSc, LRCSI, LRCPI, FRACS
Director and Head of Surgical Outcomes Research Centre
Royal Prince Alfred Hospital Medical Centre
Sydney

James Tatoulis
MBBS, MS, FRACS
Director of Cardiothoracic Surgery and Cardiac Services
Royal Melbourne Hospital

Robert Thomas
MB, BS, FRACS, FRCS(Eng), MS
Director of Surgical Oncology
Department of Surgical Oncology
Peter MacCallum Cancer Centre
Melbourne

Joe J Tjandra
MBBS, MD, FRACS, FRCS(Eng), FRCPS, FASCRS
Colorectal Surgeon and Surgical Oncologist
Royal Melbourne Hospital

James Toouli
MBBS, PhD, FRACS, BSc(Med)
Professor of Surgery
Department of General and Digestive Surgery
Flinders Medical Center
Adelaide

Neil Vallance
MBBS, FRACS
Director, Otolaryngology, Head and Neck Surgery
Southern Health
Frankston
Melbourne

David Watters
MB, ChM, FRCS(Ed), FRACS
Professor of Surgery
Department of Clinical and Biomedical Sciences
University of Melbourne
Geelong Hospital

Daryl Williams
MBBS(Hons), FANZCA, GradDipBA
Director, Department of Anaesthesia and Pain Management
Royal Melbourne Hospital

John Wong
MBBS, PhD, FRACS, FACS(Hons)
Head of Department of Surgery
University of Hong Kong
Queen Mary Hospital
Hong Kong

Preface

Medical students and trainees must possess an understanding of basic surgical principles, knowledge of specific surgical conditions, be able to perform a few basic procedures and be part of a multidisciplinary team that manages the patient in totality. Students must also be aware of the rapid developments in technology and basic sciences and understand where these developments impinge on surgical practice.

The *Textbook of Surgery* is intended to supply this information, which is especially relevant given current surgical curriculum for undergraduates. Each topic is written by an expert in the field from his own wisdom and experience. All contributors have been carefully chosen from the Australasian region for their authoritative expertise and personal involvement in undergraduate and postgraduate teaching.

In this textbook we have approached surgery from a practical viewpoint while emphasising the relevance of basic surgical principles. We have attempted to cover most aspects of general surgery and selected topics of specialty surgery, including cardiothoracic surgery, neurosurgery, plastic surgery, orthopaedic surgery and urology. Principles that underlie the assessment, care and treatment of surgical patients are outlined, followed by sections on various surgical disorders. The final section presents a practical problem-solving approach to the diagnosis and management of common surgical conditions. In clinical practice, patients present with symptoms and signs to the surgeon who then has to formulate care plans, using such a problem-solving approach. This textbook provides a good grounding for students in surgical diseases, problems and management. Apart from forming the core curriculum for medical students, surgical trainees will also find the *Textbook of Surgery* beneficial in their studies and their practice.

With ever-expanding medical knowledge, a core amount of instructive and up-to-date information is presented in a concise fashion. Important further reading has been provided. It is our aim that this textbook will stimulate students to refer to appropriate reviews and publications for further details in specific subjects.

We have presented the textbook in an attractive and easily readable format by extensive use of tables, boxes and illustrations. We hope that this edition will continue to be valuable to undergraduate, graduate and postgraduate students of surgery, and for general practitioners and physicians as a useful summary of surgery.

Joe J Tjandra
Gordon JA Clunie
Andrew H Kaye
Julian A Smith

Melbourne
Australia

Acknowledgements

This book owes its existence to the contributions of our talented surgeons and physicians from throughout Australia, New Zealand and Asia. We are indebted to the staff of Blackwell Science Asia for their support, and to Carri Murray-Green for administrative support. We thank Associate Professor David Francis, Mr Alan Cuthbertson and Professor Robert Thomas for their assistance with previous editions which laid the foundation for this third edition.

Our patients, students, trainees and surgical mentors have all been an inspiration to us; but above all we owe a debt of gratitude to our loving families, specifically our wives Yvonne Pun-Tjandra, Jess Clunie, Judy Kaye and Sally Smith, as it was precious time spent away from them which allowed completion of this textbook. Finally the lead editor (JJT) would like to dedicate this book to his mentor, friend and colleague, Professor Victor Fazio who has contributed enormously to surgical education globally.

Principles of Surgery

1 Pre-operative management

Iain G. Martin

Introduction

This chapter covers care of the patient from the time the patient is considered for surgery through to immediately prior to operation and deals with important generic issues relating to the care of all surgical patients. Whilst individual procedures each have unique aspects to them, a sound working understanding of the common foundation of the issues involved in pre-operative care is critical to good patient outcomes.

Informed consent

Although often thought of in a purely medico-legal way, the process of ensuring that a patient is informed about the procedure that they are about to undergo is a fundamental part of good quality patient care. Informed consent is far more than the act of placing a signature on a form; that signature in itself is only meaningful if the patient has been through a reasonable process that has left them in a position to make an informed decision.

There has been much written around issues of informed consent, and the medico-legal climate has changed substantially in the past decade. It is important for any doctor to have an understanding of what is currently understood by informed consent.

Although the legal systems in Australia and New Zealand are very different with respect to medical negligence, the standards around what constitutes informed consent are very similar.

Until relatively recently, the standard applied to deciding whether the patient was given adequate and appropriate information with which to make a decision was the so-called Bolam test, that is practitioners are not negligent if they act in accordance with practice accepted by a reasonable body of medical opinion. Recent case law from both England and Australia and the standards embedded in the New Zealand's Health and Disability Commissions code of patient rights have seen a move away from the existing position. Although this area is complex, the general opinion is that a doctor has a duty to disclose to patients material risks. A risk is said to be material if 'in the circumstances of that particular case, a reasonable person in the patient's position, if warned of the risk would be likely to attach significance to it or the medical practitioner is, or should reasonably be aware that the particular patient, if warned of the risk would attach significance to it'. It is important that this standard relates to what a person in the patient's position would do and not just any reasonable person.

Important factors in considering the kinds of information to disclose to patients are:

- The nature of the potential risks: more common and more serious risks require disclosure.
- The nature of the proposed procedure: complex interventions require more information as do procedures when the patient has no illness.
- The patient's desire for information: patients who ask questions make known their desire for information and they should be told.
- The temperament and health of the patient: anxious patients and patients with health problems or other relevant circumstances that make a risk more important for them may need more information.
- The general surrounding circumstances: the information required for elective procedures might be different from that required in the emergency department.

What does this mean for a medical practitioner? Firstly, you must have an understanding of the legal framework and standards. Secondly, you must be able to document how appropriate information was given to patients – always write it down. On this point, whilst information booklets can be a very useful addition to the process of informed consent they do not remove the need to undertake open discussions with the patient.

Doctors often see the process of obtaining informed consent as difficult and complex, and this view is leant support by changing standards. However, the principles are relatively clear and not only benefit patients but their doctors as well. A fully informed patient is much more likely to adapt to the demands of a surgical intervention, and should a complication occur, they almost invariably accept such misfortune far more readily.

Pre-operative assessment

The appropriate assessment of patients prior to surgery to identify coexisting medical problems and to plan peri-operative care is of increasing importance. Modern trends towards the increasing use of day-of-surgery admission even for major procedures have increased the need for careful and systematic peri-operative assessment.

The goals of peri-operative assessment are:

- To identify important medical issues in order to
  - optimise their treatment.
  - inform the patient of the risks associated with surgery.
  - ensure care is provided in an appropriate environment.
- To identify important social issues which may have a bearing on the planned procedure and the recovery period.
- To familiarise the patient with the planned procedure and the hospital processes.

Clearly the peri-operative evaluation should include a careful history and physical examination, together with structured questions related to the planned procedure. Simple questions related to exercise tolerance (such as can you climb a flight of stairs without shortness of breath) will often yield as much useful information as complex tests of cardiorespiratory reserve. The clinical evaluation will be coupled with a number of blood and radiological tests to complete the clinical evaluation. There is considerable debate as to the value of many of the routine tests performed, and each hospital will have its own protocol for such evaluations.

On the basis of the outcomes of this consultation a number of risk stratification systems have been proposed; the only one in widespread daily use is the relatively simple ASA (American Society of Anesthesiologists) system (see Table 2.1, Chapter 2).

The pre-operative assessment and work-up will be guided by a combination of the nature of the operation proposed and the overall 'fitness' of the patient. Whilst there are a number of ways of looking at the type of surgery proposed, a simple three-way classification has much to commend it:

- Low risk: poses minimal physiological stress and risk to the patient, rarely requires blood transfusion, invasive monitoring or intensive care. Examples of such procedures would be groin hernia repair, cataract surgery, arthroscopy.
- Medium risk: moderate physiological stress (fluid shifts, cardiorespiratory effects) and risk. Usually associated with minimal blood loss. Potential for significant problems must be appreciated. Examples would be laparoscopic cholecystectomy, hysterectomy, hip replacement.
- High risk: significant peri-operative physiological stress. Often requires blood transfusion or infusion of large fluid volumes. Requires invasive monitoring and will often need intensive care. Examples would be aortic surgery, major gastrointestinal resections, thoracic surgery.

A low-risk patient (ASA I or II) will clearly require a far less intensive work-up than a high-risk patient (ASA III or IV) undergoing a high-risk operation.

Areas of specific relevance to peri-operative care are cardiac disease and respiratory disease. It is important that pre-existing cardiorespiratory disease is optimised prior to surgery to minimise the risk of complications. Patients with cardiac disease can be stratified using a number of systems (Goldman or Detsky indices) and this stratification can be used to guide work-up and interventions and provide a guide to prognosis. One of the most important respiratory factors is whether the patient is a smoker; there is now clear evidence that stopping smoking for at least 6 weeks prior to surgery significantly reduces the risk of complications.

Patient safety

Once in hospital, and particularly once under anaesthetic, patients rely upon the systems and policies of individuals and health care institutions to minimise the risk of inadvertent harm. Whilst every hospital will have slightly different policies the fundamental goals of these include:

- The correct patient gets the correct operation on the correct side or part of their body. An appropriate method of patient identification and patient marking must be in place. It must be clear to all involved in the procedure, particularly for operations on paired limbs or organs, when the incorrect side could be operated upon.

- The patient is protected from harm whilst under anaesthetic. When under a general anaesthetic the patient is vulnerable to a number of risks. Important amongst these are pressure effects upon nerves, for example those on the common peroneal nerve as it winds around the head of the fibula.
- Previous medical problems and allergies are identified and acted upon.

Prophylaxis

Infection

Infections remain a major issue for all surgical procedures and the team caring for the patient needs to be aware of relevant risks and act to minimise such risks.

Before discussing the use of prophylactic antibiotics for the prevention of peri-operative infection, it is very important that issues of basic hygiene are discussed (see Chapter 7, p. 51). Simple measures adopted by all those involved in patient care can make a real difference to reducing the risk of hospital-acquired infection. The very widespread and significant problems with antibiotic organisms such as methicillin-resistant *Staphylococcus aureus* (MRSA) have reinforced the need for such basic measures.

- Wash your hands in between seeing each and every patient.
- Wear gloves for removing/changing dressings.
- Ensure that the hospital environment is as clean as possible.

These measures, especially hand washing, should be embedded into the psyche of those involved in patient care.

In addition to the very important matters of hygiene and appropriate sterile practice, antibiotics should be used in certain circumstances to reduce the risk of peri-operative infection. Each hospital will have individual policies on which particular antibiotics to use in the prophylactic setting (see Chapter 7, p. 51). It is also important to state that whilst the use of prophylactic antibiotics can, when used appropriately, significantly reduce infectious complications, inappropriate or prolonged use can leave the patient susceptible to infection with antibiotic resistant organisms such as MRSA.

Both factors related to the patient and the planned procedure governs the appropriate use of antibiotics in the prophylactic setting.

Procedure-related factors

Table 1.1 indicates the risk of post-operative wound infections with and without the use of prophylactic antibiotics. In addition to considering the absolute risk of infection the potential consequences of infection must also be considered; for example, a patient undergoing a vascular graft (a clean procedure) must receive appropriate antibiotic cover because of the catastrophic consequences of graft infection.

Patient-related factors

Patients with immunosuppression and pre-existing implants and patients at risk for developing infective endocarditis must receive appropriate prophylaxis even when the procedure itself would not indicate their use.

Table 1.1 Risks of post-operative wound infection

Type of procedure	Definition	Wound infection rate (%) Prophylactic antibiotics	
		No	Yes
Clean	No contamination, gastrointestinal, genitourinary or respiratory tracts not breached	1–5	0–1
Clean-contaminated	Gastrointestinal or respiratory tract opened but without spillage	10	1–2
Contaminated	Acute inflammation, infected urine, bile, gross spillage from gastrointestinal tract	20–30	10
Dirty	Established infection	40–50	10

Venous thrombo-embolism

Deep vein thrombosis (DVT) is a not uncommon and potentially catastrophic complication of surgery. The risk for developing DVT ranges from a fraction of 1% to 30% or greater depending upon both patient- and procedure-related factors. Both patient- and procedure-related factors can be classified as low, medium or high risk (Table 1.2). High-risk patients undergoing high-risk operations will have a risk for DVT of up to 80% and a pulmonary embolism risk of 1–5% when prophylaxis is not used; these risks can be reduced by at least one order of magnitude with appropriate interventions.

Whilst a wide variety of agents have been trialled for the prevention of DVT, there are currently only three widely used methods:

- Graduated compression stockings: these stockings, which must be properly fitted, reduce venous pooling in the lower limbs and prevent venous stagnation.
- Heparin: this drug can be used in its conventional unfractionated form or as one of the newer fractionated low-molecular-weight derivatives. The fractionated low-molecular-weight heparins offer the convenience of once-daily dosing for the majority of patients. It must however be remembered that the anticoagulant effect of the low-molecular-weight heparins cannot easily be reversed and, where such reversal may be important, standard unfractionated heparin should be used.
- Mechanical calf compression devices: these machines work by intermittent pneumatic calf compression and thereby encourage venous return and reduce venous pooling.

The three methods are complementary and are often used in combination, depending upon the patient and operative risk factors (Table 1.2).

The systematic use of such measures is very important if the optimal benefit is to be made for the potential reduction in DVT.

Table 1.2 Prevention of deep vein thrombosis

		Operative risk factors		
		Low (e.g. hernia repair)	Medium (e.g. general abdominal surgery)	High (e.g. pelvic cancer, orthopaedic surgery)
Patient risk factors	Low (age <40, no risk factors)	No prophylaxis	Heparin	Heparin and mechanical devices
	Medium (age >40, one risk factor)	Heparin	Heparin	Heparin and mechanical devices
	High (age >40, multiple risk factors)	Heparin and mechanical devices	Heparin and mechanical devices	Higher dose heparin, mechanical devices

Pre-operative care of the acute surgical patient

A significant number of patients will present with acute conditions requiring surgical operations. Whilst the principles outlined above are still valid, a number of additional issues are raised.

Informed consent

Whilst there is still a clear need to ensure that patients are appropriately informed, there are fewer opportunities to discuss the options with the patient and their family. In addition, the disease process may have resulted in the patient being confused. The team caring for the patient needs to judge carefully the level of information required in this situation. Although it is very important that family members are kept informed, it has to be remembered that the team's primary duty is towards the patient. This sometimes puts the team in a difficult position when the views of the patient's family differ from that which the team caring for the patient hold. If such an occasion arises then careful discussion and documentation of the decision process is vital. Increasingly, patients of very advanced years are admitted acutely with a surgical problem in the setting of significant additional medical problems. It is with this group of patients that specific ethical issues around consent and appropriateness of surgery occur. It is important that as full as possible a picture of the patient's overall health and quality of life is obtained and that a full and frank discussion of the options, risks and benefits takes place.

Pre-operative resuscitation

It is important that wherever possible significant fluid deficits and electrolyte abnormalities are corrected prior to surgery. There is often a balance to be made between timely operative intervention and the degree of fluid resuscitation required. An early discussion between surgeon, anaesthetist and, when required, intensivist can help plan timing.

Pre-existing medical co-morbidities

There is clearly less time to address these issues and it may not be possible to address significant ongoing medical problems. Clearly such co-morbidities should be identified, and all involved with planning the operation should be informed. The issues are most acute for significant cardiac, respiratory, hepatic or renal disease.

Pre-operative nutrition

An awareness of the nutritional status of patients is important and such awareness should guide the decisions about nutritional support (see Chapter 5).

Before operation the malnourished patient should whenever possible be given appropriate nutritional support. There is no doubt that significant pre-operative malnutrition increases the risk of post-operative complications (>10–15% weight loss). If possible such nutrition should be given enterally, reserving parenteral nutrition for the minority of patients in whom the gastrointestinal tract is not an option. Parenteral nutrition is associated with increased costs and complications and is of proven benefit in the seriously malnourished patient only, when it should be given for at least 10 days prior to surgery for any benefits to be seen. There is increasing evidence that enteral feeds specifically formulated to boost certain immune parameters offer clinical benefits for patients about to undergo major surgery.

After operation any patient who is unable to take in normal diet for 7 or more days should receive nutritional support, which as before operation should use the enteral route whenever possible.

Specific pre-operative issues

Stomas

A number of gastrointestinal operations will require the use of a temporary or permanent stoma (see Chapter 30). Prior to operation it is important that the patient is fully informed of the likelihood/possibility of a stoma. Clearly there will be operations that result in a stoma which could not be predicted being formed but such occasions should be very rare.

The concept of having an intestinal stoma is regarded by most patients as one of the most daunting aspects of facing surgery. Prior to surgery the patient should be seen by an experienced stoma/colorectal nurse to discuss in detail the nature of the stoma, the type of appliances likely to be used and the optimal site for its placement. The nurse specialist plays a very important role both in the immediate peri-operative period and beyond.

Diabetes mellitus

Diabetes mellitus is one of the most frequently seen medical co-morbidities which complicate peri-operative care. It is clearly important that patients with diabetes mellitus are appropriately worked up for surgery.

In the weeks leading up to elective surgery the management of the diabetes should be reviewed and blood glucose control optimised. Particular attention should be paid to cardiovascular and renal co-morbidities during the pre-operative assessment.

Generally patients with diabetes should be scheduled for surgery in the morning. For patients taking oral hypoglycaemic drugs, the drugs should be stopped the night before surgery and the blood glucose monitored. Patients with insulin-dependent diabetes should be commenced on an intravenous infusion regimen. There are two approaches to this:

- Variable-rate insulin infusion. The patients blood glucose levels are monitored regularly and the rate of insulin infusion adjusted. An infusion of dextrose is continued throughout the period of insulin infusion.
- Single infusion of glucose insulin and potassium (GIK). Whilst this method has the advantage of simplicity it is not possible to adjust the rates of glucose

and insulin infusion separately and the technique can lead to the administration of excessive amounts of free water.

The variable-rate infusion is the most widespread approach and although more involved in terms of monitoring offers better glycaemic control; this in itself is associated with better patient outcomes.

MCQs

Select the single correct answer to each question.

1 Without the use of prophylaxis the risk of deep calf vein thrombosis in a patient undergoing an anterior resection for rectal cancer is likely to be at least:

a 10%
b 20%
c 30%
d 50%

2 Which of the following measures is most likely to reduce the risk of post operative wound infection with MRSA?

a 5 days of broad spectrum prophylactic antibiotics
b ensuring the patient showers with chlorhexidine wash prior to surgery
c a policy of staff handwashing between patients
d screening patients for MRSA carriage prior to surgery

3 Which of the following constitute the legal standard for the information that should be passed to a patient to meet the requirements of 'informed consent'?

a what a patient in that position would regard as reasonable
b what a reasoned body of medical opinion holds as reasonable
c a list of all possible complications contained within a patient information booklet
d all serious complications that occur in more than 1% of patients

2 Anaesthesia and pain management

Daryl Williams

Pre-operative phase

The aims of anaesthesia are fourfold: (i) no conscious awareness of pain; (ii) a still surgical field; (iii) anxiolysis, sedation or complete hypnosis; and (iv) cardiorespiratory stability. Most of the major morbidity and mortality during anaesthesia is related to inadequate pre-operative assessment or optimisation. Assessment of the patient should focus on the important risks to the patients. The seven A's of anaesthesia are critical to deduce in the pre-operative phase and these are: allergies; aspiration risk; airway assessment; aortic stenosis; apnoea, especially obstructive sleep apnoea; activity level or functional exercise tolerance; and ease of access (intravenous or invasive access).

History

Elective surgery patients are generally admitted on the day of surgery, and data collection, evaluation and patient education takes place in outpatient (pre-admission) clinics. History taking commences with review of a standard health questionnaire; positive responses can then be explored further during the personal interview. In addition to the basic information above, every patient assessment prior to elective surgery should include a history of previous anaesthetic exposure, recent illness, familial disease (including malignant hyperpyrexia), and pregnancy.

Obstructive sleep apnoea (OSA) is increasingly common in westernised society, where the incidence of obesity is increasing. Most OSA is undiagnosed and therefore routine questioning about snoring, choking feelings while sleeping, and excessive daytime somnolence are important for screening. Any elective patient thought to have OSA should be referred to a sleep physician for a sleep study pre-operatively, and also be optimised with nasal continuous positive airway pressure (CPAP) if appropriate. The long-term effects of untreated OSA are due to chronic hypoxaemia and hypercapnia and include systemic hypertension and pulmonary hypertension with right ventricular hypertrophy. These patients have significant increased risk during general anaesthesia because of difficult mask ventilation, difficult intubation and acute right heart dysfunction. More important, post-operatively OSA patients have an increased risk of respiratory obstruction because they are very sensitive to sedative/hypnotic agents. These patients should be monitored in a critical care environment if they receive any sedative/hypnotics or opioids. Patients should also be encouraged to continue to use nasal CPAP if prescribed pre-operatively.

Aspiration is more likely in patients with recent solid food intake, gastrointestinal obstruction, emergency surgery or a difficult airway. Patients are fasted prior to elective surgery, primarily to reduce the risk of aspiration of stomach contents and consequent pneumonitis. Particulate (solid matter) aspiration is the greatest risk to the patient. The volume and acidity of gastric fluid are also important, with a volume more than 25 mL or pH less than 2.5 posing greater risk to the patient. Fasting is effective in reducing the amount of gastric solids but not the volume of fluid. Inadequate preparation of the patient for direct laryngoscopy and extubation of the trachea before the return of airway protective reflexes are the main errors of anaesthetic management that may result in pulmonary aspiration.

The physical status of the patient is usually described according to the American Society of Anesthesiologists (ASA) classification (Table 2.1). Functional exercise capacity is the best and simplest measure of overall cardiorespiratory robustness and peri-operative risk. Metabolic equivalents (METs) are used to quantify activity level. An activity level of 4 METs, which is equivalent to carrying shopping bags up two flights of stairs, is generally considered adequate for most surgery. The age of the patient, ASA class, and the nature and

Table 2.1 American Society of Anesthesiologists Classification

ASA	Patient status
I	Fit for age
II	Patient has systemic disease that does not interfere with normal activity
III	Patient has systemic disease that limits normal activity
IV	Patient has systemic disease that is a constant threat to life
V	Patient not expected to survive 24 hours
E	Added to above to indicate emergency procedure

duration of the surgery are all important determinants of the choice of anaesthetic technique and the extent of patient monitoring.

Examination

The commonest fundamental mishaps in anaesthesia relate to poor airway management, and therefore a thorough assessment of the airway is critical to a good outcome. This includes ability to open the mouth, absence or presence of teeth, the size of the tongue, the ability to sublux the temporomandibular joint and the relative position of the larynx. The ability to mask ventilate the patient, intubate the patient's trachea, and access the patient trachea in the neck are all key determinates of airway management.

Valvular heart disease, especially moderate or severe aortic stenosis, poses a substantial risk for even the most basic general anaesthetic or for neuraxial regional blockade (spinal or epidural anaesthesia). A relatively fixed output through a narrow aortic valve and consequent left ventricular hypertrophy that occurs in aortic stenosis means that the oxygen supply-demand is precariously balanced. Small reductions in pre-load (end-diastolic stretch) and after-load (arterial dilation) occur commonly during anaesthesia, and the reduction in cardiac output and diastolic coronary perfusion can set up a cascade of events that leads to significant myocardial ischaemia that worsens the picture.

Routine investigations and patient optimisation

Pre-operative laboratory investigations are ordered only in response to the history or examination findings, not as a routine. However, in patients more than 50 years of age an electrocardiograph (ECG) is generally routine. Full blood examination, serum electrolytes, glucose, creatinine and chest X-ray should be used selectively. Table 2.2 is a checklist for use when clerking patients prior to surgery. Optimum treatment

Table 2.2 Guide to clerking of a surgical patient: items for discussion with the anaesthetist

Previous anaesthesia	Procedures, analgesia, history of adverse events
Family history	Muscle disorders, bleeding, reactions to anaesthesia
Medications	Potential drug interactions, systemic steroids, altered coagulation, drug reactions, peri-operative instructions
Cardiovascular	Ischaemic heart disease: risk factors (angina class), cardiac failure (dyspnoea class), arrhythmias, peripheral vascular disease, valvular heart disease (especially aortic stenosis)
Central nervous system	Stroke, TIA, seizures
Respiratory	Smoking history, asthma and triggers, bronchitis, lung function tests, arterial gases, obstructive sleep apnoea
Airway examination	Mouth opening, teeth, temporomandibular subluxability, size of tongue, neck
Endocrine	Thyroid function, diabetes (type, treatment, complications), obesity
Fluid status	Pre-operative status, peri-operative requirments and balance
Haematology	Strategy for blood replacement
Gastrointestinal	Aspiration risk
Musculoskeletal	Arthritis (especially cervical spine instability) and fixed deformities

of systemic disease may alter ASA class prior to surgery and referral to other specialists is often appropriate at this time.

Preparation

Education of patients about the surgical procedure, the choices for anaesthesia and the pain management options decrease anxiety and decrease the need for premedication with drugs. Opioid analgesia is only required to relieve pre-operative pain; benzodiazepines provide a better alternative for pre-operative sedation and anxiolysis. It is important to note that gastric emptying ceases soon after treatment with any opioid drug, and generally these patients are considered to be 'at risk of aspiration'.

Oral medications may be continued up to the time of surgery if gastric emptying and absorption are normal. Antacids, histamine$_2$-receptor antagonists and proton pump inhibitors should be continued pre-operatively to limit the occurrence of acid pulmonary aspiration. There is considerable benefit for anaesthesia in continuing most antihypertensive and cardiac drugs in terms of providing peri-operative cardiovascular stability. Asthma and chronic obstructive airway disease may be treated with inhalational drugs throughout the peri-operative period. Anticoagulants such as warfarin and potent platelet inhibitors should generally be ceased prior to surgery, although the balance of risk and benefits should be discussed with the anaesthetist.

Anaesthesia techniques

The choice of regional versus general anaesthesia should be discussed with the patient prior to arrival in the operating room. There are specific complications associated with each technique, and patients will usually indicate how much they wish to know about rare, but serious, adverse events as well as the minor morbidity. Where it is possible to provide regional anaesthesia for minor surgery by direct infiltration of local anaesthetic or by peripheral nerve blocks, the risk of major morbidity or mortality from anaesthesia is avoided.

There are a few absolute contraindications to the use of major regional anaesthesia (e.g. spinal, epidural or plexus block); these are disorders of coagulation, allergy to local anaesthetic agents, sepsis (either systemic or at the site of local anaesthetic insertion) and inability to communicate with or obtain the cooperation of the patient (Table 2.3). A prior neural deficit, or possibility of neural damage due to the surgery, are relative contraindications because of the difficulty in separating these from residual effects of the local anaesthetic. Some form of general anaesthesia can usually be offered to any patient after appropriate preparation and resuscitation. The potential for a reduction in risk with the use of regional anaesthesia comes from an avoidance of some effects of the general anaesthetics; however, there is minimal evidence to support claims of improved outcome in seriously ill patients having major surgery with regional anaesthesia.

Table 2.3 Use of regional anaesthesia

Absolute contraindications	Patient refusal, uncooperative patient Full anticoagulation Infection at injection site Septicaemia (catheter insertion) Hypovolaemia (with neuraxial block) Allergy to local anaesthetic
Relative contraindications	Partial anticoagulation Pre-existing neurological deficit Back pain
Indications	Adverse reactions to general anaesthesia (e.g. muscle disease, susceptibility to malignant hyperpyrexia)
	Reduce pulmonary complication or need for post-operative intermittent positive-pressure ventilation (respiratory disease, obesity)
	Obstetrics: avoidance of foetal depression

General anaesthesia

General anaesthesia may be divided into three phases: induction, maintenance and recovery. It aims to produce rapidly reversible loss of consciousness and amnesia, with absence of response to surgical stimulation and without deleterious effects on organ function. Analgesia and muscle relaxation are important adjuncts, although often provided by separate drugs.

Induction of general anaesthesia

Induction is often achieved with a bolus intravenous (i.v.) injection of a lipid-soluble drug that will be effectively removed from the arterial blood on first passage through the brain and other organs. Initial distribution therefore reflects the distribution of cardiac output, and loss of consciousness is induced in one arm–brain circulation. Induction of anaesthesia with an anaesthetic vapour or gas depends upon the agent's having adequate potency, avoidance of airway irritation, coughing or apnoea, and ability to achieve the necessary partial pressure in the CNS rapidly. Sevoflurane is most often used for inhalational induction of anaesthesia in paediatric practice because of difficulties with i.v. access. Halothane provides a slower induction and is sometimes preferred to sevoflurane because of the lower risk of rapid induction and airway obstruction. Sevoflurane may also be used to achieve a single-breath induction as the patient inhales and holds a high concentration of sevoflurane in oxygen.

Induction of anaesthesia is associated with relaxation of the upper airway, loss of protective reflexes and reduced respiratory effort. The airway is maintained by elevation of the jaw and application of a face mask, or by insertion of a supralaryngeal airway (e.g. laryngeal mask airway) or by a laryngeal (endotracheal) tube through the larynx into the trachea. The end-point for loss of consciousness is taken as loss of the eyelash response, but a greater depth of anaesthesia is required for instrumentation of the airway.

Maintenance of general anaesthesia

Anaesthesia is maintained by inhaled anaesthetic, i.v. infusion of anaesthetic or a combination. The advantage of anaesthetic delivery via the lung is that the partial pressure of the anaesthetic gas can be accurately measured and titrated using agent monitoring. The minimum alveolar concentration (MAC_{50}) required for lack of response to surgical incision in 50% of patients is highly reproducible for each agent, so that it is possible to be very confident that a given depth of anaesthesia is achieved during surgery. The rate of infusion of an i.v. general anaesthetic may be calculated according to a pharmacokinetic model to avoid accumulation, overdosage and prolonged hangover effect. Infusion pumps programmed for anaesthetic delivery are now available and these provide an estimate of the plasma or effect-site concentration achieved (target controlled infusion).

General anaesthesia requires continual adjustment because of the changing nature of the surgical stimulus. This is often difficult to achieve with a volatile anaesthetic alone, but the provision of balanced anaesthesia with analgesia (e.g. a potent i.v. opioid) and muscle relaxation often provides a smooth anaesthetic, with fewer adverse cardiovascular responses. Blood pressure and heart rate are usually within 20% of resting values, although different limits may be set according to the nature of the surgery and the physical status of the patient. If respiration is spontaneous, it should be regular and the end-tidal carbon dioxide is kept below a predetermined limit. With muscle relaxation, ventilation is controlled.

Recovery from general anaesthesia

Recovery is a gradual process, dependent on the continued redistribution of the anaesthetic drug in the body together with elimination or metabolism. The process is timed to result in emergence from anaesthesia as close as possible to the completion of the surgery. A considerable residue of drug may remain, especially in skeletal muscle, so that secondary peaks can occur in the plasma concentration following rewarming and restoration of muscle blood flow. The slow release of the drug from muscle and fat prevents full recovery of cognitive function for many hours and will potentiate the effects of any additional sedative drugs. Although there are differences between anaesthetic drugs for the time taken to initial emergence, the duration of anaesthesia, the extent of surgery and the requirement for opioid analgesics more often determine how soon the patient can be discharged from hospital.

Supplemental oxygen is always required in the initial recovery phase because of the continued respiratory depressant action of anaesthetic drugs, increased ventilation-perfusion mismatch, and to the displacement of oxygen from the alveoli by the excretion of large volumes of nitrous oxide if this has been used as a component of the anaesthetic. Frequent complications in the recovery phase include laryngospasm (incomplete return of protective reflexes), nausea or vomiting, and shivering with increased oxygen consumption. The use of anti-emetics such as the 5HT-3 antagonists and the application of forced-air warming blankets may reduce the incidence of complications. The plan for pain management should commence prior to emergence from anaesthesia.

Regional anaesthesia

Although major surgery can be performed using multiple peripheral nerve blocks, it is likely to be difficult for both the anaesthetist and the patient and it is easy to exceed the maximum recommended dose of local anaesthetic. Regional anaesthesia is therefore focused on providing neural blockade at the level of the spinal cord, by either spinal (subarachnoid) or epidural injection. Depending on the choice of local anaesthetic and its concentration, a marked differential between sensory and motor block can be achieved. If the regional technique is continued for post-operative analgesia, this differential becomes more important, increasing mobility and cooperation with physiotherapy. Low concentration of local anaesthetic in combination with an opioid provides analgesia with minimal motor block.

Epidural injection requires approximately a 10-fold greater mass of local anaesthetic to obtain an equivalent neural block compared to spinal injection, resulting in a greater danger from accidental intravascular injection and consequent systemic toxicity. The advantage of epidural analgesia is that the dura is not punctured and there is no incidence of headache due to loss of cerebrospinal fluid (CSF). The placement of an epidural catheter enables the block to be continued with an infusion or repeated bolus doses of drug. It is desirable to match the distribution of the sensory blockade as close as possible to the surgical incision in order to reduce the total dose as well as any side effects. Epidural injections can be made at any level of the spine from the cervical region to the caudal canal.

Spinal anaesthesia is often favoured during surgery because the onset is rapid and the blockade is more complete than can be achieved with an epidural injection. This may be critical to the success of the anaesthesia, especially if the anaesthetist wishes to avoid the use of sedation or combined regional and general anaesthesia because of the physical status of the patient.

Combined regional and general anaesthesia does offer advantages in some types of surgery. The dose of general anaesthetic required is significantly reduced, but the patient may still be paralysed and ventilation controlled to facilitate surgery. The stress response to the surgery is ablated to an extent not possible even with very deep general anaesthesia. The patient emerges from the general anaesthesia with excellent analgesia which can be extended into the post-operative period if an epidural catheter is *in situ*.

Patient monitoring during anaesthesia

The purpose of patient monitoring is to ensure patient safety and patient well-being during surgery. Clinical and equipment monitoring are both important facets of anaesthesia care. Most physiologic parameters measured act as surrogate indicators of oxygen delivery, end-organ well-being or depth of anaesthesia.

Blood pressure

Arterial blood pressure measurement is an indicator of the driving pressure through global and regional vascular beds. The flow is dependent on the perfusion pressure and the resistance. Pre-operative measurement by auscultation of Korotkoff sounds establishes the baseline arterial blood presure value for an individual patient. Automated non-invasive monitoring of blood pressure usually uses an occlusive cuff and oscillometric measurement. Automated systems are preferred intraoperatively, often because access to the arm is impeded and other tasks are likely to divert the anaesthetist from taking regular measurements. There is a tendency to underestimate high pressures and overestimate low pressures, and measurement may fail with cardiac arrhythmias such as atrial fibrillation. Direct measurement via a catheter in the radial artery is accurate and gives a continuous beat-to-beat output.

When the blood pressure is anticipated to change rapidly, as in procedures with a high risk of significant blood loss, or when strict control is needed, as in neurosurgery, the benefits of direct measurement clearly outweigh the risk. Use of a small catheter (20- or 22-gauge) made of Teflon reduces the incidence of thrombosis or intimal damage.

Electrocardiograph

Electrocardiograph monitoring used during anaesthesia generally allows the simultaneous display of two leads. One should be the standard limb lead II and the other a unipolar lead in the V5 position (the anterior axillary line at the fifth intercostal space). Lead II will indicate the presence of P waves and changes in cardiac rhythm. The V5 lead detects more than 70% of myocardial ischaemia in high-risk patients having non-cardiac surgery. Automatic detection and recording of ST segment changes are provided with many monitoring systems. These have increased the anaesthetist's awareness of intraoperative changes. However, ECG artefact from poor electrode application or placement, shivering and diathermy remain a major problem.

Respiratory monitoring

Monitoring of oxygen and carbon dioxide concentrations in the patient breathing circuit and non-invasive measurement of haemoglobin (Hb) saturation (oximetry) enables continuous assessment of the adequacy of ventilation and oxygenation. The use of an oxygen analyser, a pulse oximeter and an end-tidal carbon dioxide monitor during general anaesthesia is mandatory in most countries.

Capnography is usually based on the absorption of infrared light by carbon dioxide. The initial detection of carbon dioxide in the expired gas is critical evidence that an endotracheal tube has been placed in the trachea. Breath-by-breath analysis detects sudden changes due to a disconnection of the breathing circuit, or loss of the pulmonary circulation (e.g. with air embolism). In a patient breathing spontaneously, the respiratory-depressant effects of the anaesthetic agents are monitored and respiration assisted if required.

Pulse oximetry provides continuous monitoring of arterial oxygenation using a 'pulse-added absorbance' technique. If peripheral perfusion is poor an adequate pulse may not be detected; instruments should therefore display both the peripheral pulse waveform and the percentage Hb saturation. Monitors to determine anaesthetic gas concentrations in the breathing circuit is compulsory in most countries. Output of anaesthetic from vaporisers, and the equilibration of inspired and expired concentrations can be monitored.

Depth of anaesthesia monitoring

General anaesthesia is a state of drug-induced unconsciousness where the patient has no recall or perception of senses. The depth of anaesthesia required for surgery is dependent on the patient, the drug delivered and the surgical stimulation. Information about the depth of anaesthesia may be obtained from a processed electroencephalograph (EEG) or by monitoring auditory or visual evoked potentials. The bispectral index (BIS) is a form of processed EEG incorporating three different EEG domains and derives a number between zero (deep anaesthesia) and 100 (awake patient). BIS has been validated with varying levels of drug concentrations of anaesthetic agents and at different levels of hypnotic state. Awareness is the post-operative conscious recall of events during general anaesthesia. The incidence of awareness is approximately 0.1% in the overall surgical population. However the risk of awareness is as high as 1% in certain high-risk groups such as cardiac surgery, caesarean section, trauma patients with massive blood loss, patients with poor left ventricular function, and opioid/benzodiazepine tolerant patients. Patients having relaxant general anaesthesia in this high-risk group should be considered for BIS monitoring if available .

Acute pain management

Non-opioid analgesia

Non-steroidal anti-inflammatory drugs (NSAID) are being used increasingly in the peri-operative period. They do not have respiratory-depressant effects, do not interfere with gastric motility, do not cause emesis, and are available for either parenteral or enteral administration. Although their analgesic effect has a ceiling below that of the opioids, they can often still be an effective alternative or provide a baseline analgesia to reduce opioid requirements. Newer cyclo-oxygenase type 2 (COX-2) inhibitors have an improved side-effect profile, with negligible effects on platelet function and haemostasis. These agents can be safely used in most surgery including neurosurgery and the use of flaps in plastic surgery.

Opioid analgesia

The target plasma concentration for satisfactory analgesia with any of the opioids is highly variable between patients. Therefore patient-controlled analgesia systems (PCAS) have proved the most effective for systemic opioid delivery. With PCAS the patient initiates bolus i.v. doses of the drug; the bolus size and a lockout interval between doses being predetermined by the physician. The patient is able to titrate the opioid dose to achieve the plasma concentration that just produces sufficient analgesia. The target may change during the day reflecting periods of physiotherapy or dressing changes versus periods of undisturbed rest in bed. Excessive sedation is avoided because patients will not continue to initiate further doses as they become drowsy. It is important that attendants or relatives are warned not to attempt to assist the patient by giving extra doses of analgesia.

A relatively long-acting opioid such as morphine is usually chosen for post-operative analgesia. Pethidine (meperidine) should not be used for prolonged analgesia, especially in patients with renal impairment, because of the accumulation of the toxic metabolite norpethidine. When morphine is used with PCAS, a common bolus dose is 1.0 mg with a lockout interval of 5 to 8 minutes. It is important to ensure that the entire bolus dose is rapidly administered intravenously to the patient on request. This is best achieved if the opioid infusion device is connected to a side-arm of an i.v. fluids line that includes an anti-reflux valve to prevent the opioid being pumped backwards up the i.v. line. Continuous i.v. access is favoured for post-operative analgesia because of the need for a short-dose interval or continuous infusion to keep plasma concentrations above the therapeutic threshold. Subcutaneous infusion may be a useful alternative if i.v. access is being maintained only for analgesia. In contrast, an order for intramuscular morphine every 4 hours is unlikely to provide satisfactory analgesia for more than 20% of that interval.

Tramadol has several properties that distinguish it from other opioids used in the post-operative period. In addition to opioid activity, it inhibits noradrenaline uptake and serotinin uptake and these contribute most to the analgesia. Tramadol has high bioavailability after oral administration, so that a patient may be transferred from i.v. to oral medication as early as the surgical condition permits. Most important, it has only minimal effects on respiration and may therefore be used in many situations where other opioids are contraindicated or when respiratory depression severely limits their dosage. For many groups of surgical patients analgesia with tramadol is comparable to that with morphine, but the incidence of nausea and vomiting may be higher after tramadol.

Epidural analgesia

If the epidural route is chosen, a catheter is inserted and a bolus of local anaesthetic given to establish sensory blockade. For continuous epidural infusion the concentration of local anaesthetic is reduced to minimise motor block, and a longer-acting anaesthetic such as bupivacaine is preferred. Opioids are usually added to the local anaesthetic solution to improve analgesia and reduce the concentration of local anaesthtic agent to reduce motor block. A useful combination is 0.1% bupivacaine with 2 mcg/mL of fentanyl. Epidural opioids do not produce sympathetic blockade or have significant cardiovascular effects, but they can cause problems of severe pruritus, urinary retention and respiratory depression. Lipid-soluble opioids such as fentanyl and pethidine are quickly localised around the region where they are injected; there is limited systemic absorption, and respiratory depression.

Persistent pain

Persistent pain is commonly divided into cancer and non-cancer pain, but there is a large overlap in the treatment methods used. In approximately 20% of cases of established chronic pain, surgery is implicated as the cause. Specific surgical procedures are known to be at higher risk for chronic pain development such as thoracotomy, mastectomy, limb amputation and multi-trauma. Analgesic drugs are introduced according to a 'ladder', on which the NSAID and adjuvant drugs, such as antidepressants and anticonvulsants, are used prior to increasing doses of opioids. It is important to determine a correct opioid dose that is the minimum required for adequate analgesia, because this will slow down the development of tolerance to the opioids. Unfortunately, tolerance to all side effects does not develop at the same rate as the reduction in analgesia. With chronic treatment, respiratory depression is unlikely to be a problem, but constipation is and measures to treat it should be commenced early. Tolerance to the analgesic effects of the opioids is expected and the dose is increased accordingly. It should not be confused with physical or mental dependence.

In cancer treatment there is an increasing use of a chronic spinal catheter for the delivery of morphine. Provided that the catheter and a drug reservoir are buried subcutaneously, the incidence of infection is very low. The central administration of the morphine is extremely effective and tolerance is slow to develop. It has also reduced the need for neurolytic blocks for cancer pain. These are justified only if the pain is well localised and there is a danger of deafferentation pain, which is extremely difficult to treat, occurring some months later.

There is a considerable body of evidence suggesting that chronic pain becomes an individual disease entity irrespective of the underlying cause of pain. It is known that changes occur in the nervous system in early persistent pain, such as spontaneous firing of damaged neurons, neuro-anatomical reorganisation of the dorsal horn under the control of growth factors, death of inhibitory neurons, and reorganisation of central (brain) representation of 'painful areas'. It is therefore important that specific chronic pain strategies are utilised as distinct from disease-specific strategies. Patients with chronic pain suffer from multifaceted problems, requiring a multidisciplinary approach. Assessment of the physical, psychological and environmental factors by a team of health professionals is essential to avoid such issues as unnecessary surgery, excessive use of medications, multiple and repeated investigations, drug toxicity, and physical and mental conditioning.

Patient safety

The craft of anaesthesia has led the field in patient safety in the medical arena. The dynamic environment in the operating suite has many work practices similar to industries such as aviation and nuclear power generation. Anaesthetists have adapted many of the principles of human peformance analysis from these industries to investigate adverse outcomes in anaesthesia and healthcare more generally.

High-fidelity simulation (HFS) training provides an excellent opportunity to learn the knowledge, skills and attitudes of appropriate clinical resource management and to be aware of the non-technical aspects of anaesthesia delivery such as fixation error and distraction. In aviation, HFS training has been shown to effectively reduce adverse outcomes. The key advantages of high-fidelity simulation are that there is no risk to the patient, that the simulation can be frozen at any point in time, and that recording playback and critical analysis of performance can facilitate learning without the issues of patient confidentiality. HFS also allows teams to interact in complex environments and provides a unique opportunity to reflect upon one's practice. This reflective process allows one to 'learn from experience' rather than 'learn by experience', which is the more traditional approach of performing tasks and slowly modifying practice over time.

In the complex world of the operating theatre it is increasingly recognised that the good outcomes rely heavily on the performance of the entire team. Concepts such as graded assertiveness, where there is shared responsibility for all team members and a requirement for all team members to openly verbalise concerns, will increasingly become a part of operating suite practice. Team 'time outs' prior to surgical incision and at the time of surgical counts are examples of team responsibility to prevent wrong surgery or retained materials, respectively.

Further reading

Paige JT, Saak TE. Anesthesia. In: Doherty GM, Meko JB, Olson JA, Peplinski GR, Worrall NK, eds. *The Washington Manual of Surgery*. Philadelphia: Lippincott Williams & Wilkins; 1999:79–92.

MCQs

Select the single correct answer to each question.

1 The best indicator of cardiorespiratory capacity and reserve for surgery is:
- **a** transthoracic echocardiography
- **b** arterial blood gas analysis
- **c** thallium persantin nuclear imaging of the heart
- **d** functional exercise capacity
- **e** electrographic stress test

2 The commonest reason for poor outcome after anaesthesia is:
- **a** inadequate pre-operative assessment and optimisation
- **b** poor anaesthetic assistance
- **c** blood product unavailability
- **d** poor choice of anaesthetic agents
- **e** inadequate intravenous access

3 Absolute contraindications to performing neuraxial (epidural or spinal) local anaesthetic blockade include all of the following except:
- **a** coagulopathy
- **b** patient refusal
- **c** systemic sepsis
- **d** local infection at insertion site
- **e** pre-existing neurologic deficit

4 Patients with obstructive sleep apnoea are often undiagnosed. Clinical features of obstructive sleep apnoea include all of the following except:
- **a** snoring during sleep
- **b** excessive daytime somnolence
- **c** feelings of choking during sleep
- **d** pulmonary hypertension
- **e** aortic stenosis

5 Airway assessment should include all of the following except:
- **a** ability to open mouth
- **b** subluxability of the temporomandibular joint
- **c** thyro-mental distance
- **d** cervical spine mobility and stability
- **e** size of the uvula

3 Post-operative management

Peter Devitt

Introduction

Good post-operative management will have started before the procedure with appropriate counselling and preparation (see Chapter 1). This preparation will have included an assessment of fitness for the procedure and identification and management of any risk factors. The patient will have been provided with a clear explanation of the procedure (emergency or elective), the risk-benefits and the likely outcome. This will have included a description of what the patient should expect in terms of short- and long-term recovery from the procedure, possible complications and the necessity for any drains, stomas, catheters or other bits of tubing, normally alien to most of the population. The patient will have been reassured about pain control measures and, perhaps most difficult of all, the doctor will have tried to ensure that the patient's expectations match those of the health professional.

This chapter will focus on the care of the patient in the immediate post-operative period, up until the time of discharge from hospital. The immediate and short-term needs of the patient and care to be provided will depend on the magnitude and type of surgery.

Immediate management of the patient

Pain management

Pain relief is of paramount importance (see Chapter 2) and an appropriate drug regimen will have been prescribed by surgeon and/or anaesthetist by the end of the procedure. In checking the charts of the patient after the procedure, care will be taken that these and any other medications required are prescribed and administered. These may include antibiotics (prophylactic or therapeutic), sedatives, antiemetics and anticoagulants.

Monitoring

Depending on the nature of the procedure and the underlying state of health of the patient, the vital signs (blood pressure, pulse and respiratory state) will be measured and recorded regularly. If an arterial catheter has been inserted, blood pressure and pulse readings can be observed on a monitor constantly. The intensity and frequency of monitoring will be maximal in the recovery room and this level of scrutiny maintained if the patient is in an intensive care or high dependency area.

Measurement of the central venous pressure may be required for patients with poor cardiorespiratory reserve or where there have been large volumes of fluid administered or major fluid shifts are expected.

The patient chart will also record all fluid that has been given during and since the operation, together with fluid lost. Ideally, these figures will have been balanced by the end of the procedure, so that the duty of the attending doctor will be to monitor ongoing losses (digestive and urinary tracts, drains, stomas) and replace these. The normal daily fluid and electrolyte requirements will also be provided. If there has been major fluid shifts or if renal function is precarious, a urinary catheter will be inserted and regular (hourly) checks made of fluid losses. Serum electrolytes and haematological values will be checked frequently, again the frequency depending on any abnormalities present and the magnitude of any fluid and electrolyte replacement.

Mobilisation

Early mobilisation is encouraged. Unless there are specified orders to the contrary, all patients are encouraged to get up and move around as much as their underlying condition will allow. Obvious exceptions to this policy include patients with epidural catheters and those with severe multiple injuries. The aim of early mobilisation is to encourage good pulmonary ventilation and to reduce venous stasis. For those who cannot mobilise, physiotherapy should be provided to help with breathing and measures taken to either increase venous flow (pneumatic calf compression devices) or reduce risks of deep vein thrombosis (heparin). The timing of any planned heparin administration will depend on the nature of the procedure and the risks of haemorrhage from that procedure.

Communication

Most patients will seek some form of reassurance in the immediate post-operative period. They will want to know how the procedure went and how they are progressing. They will also want reassurance that all the tubes, lines and equipment to which they are attached are quite normal and not an indication of impending disaster. Any unexpected finding or complication encountered during the procedure should be discussed with the patient. The timing and detail of this discussion is a matter of fine judgement and may be best done in the presence of the patient's relatives.

Further care in the post-operative period

This covers the time from recovery from anaesthesia and initial monitoring to discharge from hospital. Wound care is discussed in Chapter 4.

Respiratory care

In the otherwise fit and healthy patient, maintenance of respiratory function is usually not a problem, particularly if there is optimal management of pain. Even with upper abdominal or thoracic procedures, most patients will require little respiratory support provided they are able to mobilise themselves and breathe unimpeded by pain. When assistance is required simple breathing exercises, with or without the help of a physiotherapist, is usually sufficient. Mechanical ventilation may be required in the early phase of recovery from a particular procedure. This can vary from prolonged endotracheal intubation, to intermittent positive pressure ventilation, to supplemental oxygenation by facemask or nasal prongs. In these instances the patient may require prolonged monitoring in an intensive care or high dependency unit with regular assessment of oxygen saturation (pulse oximetry and arterial blood gas analysis).

For less fit patients, and particularly those with chronic obstructive pulmonary disease, the risks of respiratory failure will be considerable and measures such as epidural local anaesthesia will be employed. Control of pain, attention to regular hyperinflation (inhalation spirometry and physiotherapy) and early mobilisation are the keys to preventing respiratory complications.

Fluid balance

Introduction

The three principles of management of fluid balance are:

- correct any abnormalities
- provide the daily requirements
- replace any abnormal and ongoing losses.

Ideally, any abnormalities will have been identified and corrected before or during the surgical procedure. In the calculation of a patient's fluid requirements, there is a distinction to be made between the volume required to *maintain* the body's normal functions and that required to *replace* any abnormal losses. The normal maintenance fluid requirements will vary depending on the patient's age, gender, weight and body surface area.

Basic requirements

The total body water of a 70-kg adult comprised 45–60% of the bodyweight. Lean patients have a greater percentage of their bodyweight as body water and older patients a lesser proportion. Of the total body water, two-thirds is in the intracellular compartment and the other one-third is divided between plasma water (25% of extracellular fluid) and interstitial fluid (75% of extracellular fluid). Therefore, a lean individual weighing 70 kg would have a plasma water of 3 L, an interstitial volume of 11 L and an intracellular volume of 28 L, making a total volume of 42 L.

The normal daily fluid requirement to *maintain* a healthy 70-kg adult is between 2 and 3 L. The individual will lose about 1500 mL in the urine and about 500 mL from the skin, lungs and stool. Loss from the skin will vary with the ambient temperature.

The electrolyte composition of intracellular and extracellular fluid (ECF) varies (Table 3.1). Sodium is the predominant cation in ECF and potassium predominates in the intracellular fluid (ICF). The normal daily requirements of sodium and potassium are

Table 3.1 Electrolyte concentrations

Electrolyte	Extracellular fluid (mmol/L)	Intracellular fluid (mmol/L)
Sodium	135	10
Potassium	4	150
Calcium	2.5	2.5
Magnesium	1.5	10
Chloride	100	10
Bicarbonate	27	10
Phosphate	1.5	45

100–150 mmol and 60–90 mmol, respectively. This will balance the daily loss of these two cations in the urine.

Replacement

If an otherwise healthy adult is deprived of the normal daily intake of fluid and electrolytes, suitable intravenous maintenance must be provided. One relatively simple regimen is 1 L of 0.9% saline and 1–2 L of 5% dextrose solution.

Both these solutions are isotonic with respect to plasma. The electrolyte solution contains the basic electrolyte requirements (154 mmol/L of sodium and 154 mmol/L of chloride) and the total volume can be adjusted with various amounts of dextrose solution. Potassium can be added as required. Other solutions (e.g. Ringer's lactate) may contain a more balanced make-up of electrolytes, but are rarely needed for a patient who is otherwise well and only requires intravenous fluids for a few days.

In the immediate post-operative period there is an increased secretion of antidiuretic hormone, with subsequent retention of water. In an adult of average build, maintenance fluids can be restricted to 2 L per day with no potassium supplements until a diuresis has occurred.

Fluid and electrolyte *replacement* is that required to correct abnormalities. Volume depletion and electrolyte abnormalities are relatively common in surgical patients, particularly those admitted with acute illnesses. Volume depletion usually occurs in association with an electrolyte deficit, but can occur in isolation. Reduced fluid intake, tachypnoea, fever or an increase in the ambient temperature may all lead to a unilateral volume loss. This will cause thirst and dehydration, which may progress to a tachycardia, hypotension and prostration. In severe cases there may be hypernatraemia and coma. Intravenous administration of 5% dextrose is used to correct the problem.

More often volume depletion is accompanied by an electrolyte deficit. Excessive fluid and electrolyte may be lost from the skin (e.g. sweating, burns), the renal tract (e.g. diabetic ketoacidosis) and the gastrointestinal tract (e.g. vomiting, ileus, fistula, diarrhoea). There is considerable scope for abnormal fluid losses in a surgical patient, particularly after a major abdominal procedure. There may be pooling of fluid at the operation site itself, an ileus might develop, fluid could be lost through a nasogastric tube or drains, and there might be increased cutaneous loss if there is a high fever.

The source of fluid loss will determine the type of electrolyte lost. There is considerable variation in the electrolyte content of different gastrointestinal secretions (Table 3.2). Loss from the upper digestive tract tends to be rich in acid, while loss from the lower tract is high in sodium and bicarbonate. Thus, patients with

Table 3.2 Approximate electrolyte concentrations

Secretions	Sodium (mmol/L)	Potassium (mmol/L)	Chloride (mmol/L)	Bicarbonate (mmol/L)	Hydrogen (mmol/L)
Salivary	50	20	40	50	–
Gastric	50	15	120	20	70
Duodenal	140	5	80	–	–
Biliary	140	10	100	40	–
Pancreatic	140	10	80	80	–
Jejuno-ileal	130	20	105	30	–
Faeces	80	10	100	25	–
Diarrhoea	100	30	50	60	–

severe and prolonged vomiting from gastric outlet obstruction may develop a metabolic alkalosis.

While the management of maintenance fluid requirements can often be done on a daily basis, the fluid and electrolyte replacements needs of an acutely ill surgical patient is likely to be more involved and necessitate close monitoring and adjustment. Clinical assessment and appreciation of the types of fluid loss will give an approximate guide to the scale of the problem, but regular biochemical electrolyte estimations will be required to determine the precise needs of what needs to be replaced. In most instances, measurement of plasma electrolyte concentrations will provide sufficient information, but occasionally it may be necessary to estimate the electrolyte contents of the various fluids being lost.

Drains and catheters

Drains serve a number of purposes. They may be put down to an operative site or into a wound as it is being closed to drain collections or potential collections. Drains may also be put into the chest cavity to help the lungs re-expand. They may be put into ducts and hollow organs to divert secretions or to decompress that structure. Examples of decompression include insertion of a tube into the common bile duct after duct exploration or nasogastric intubation to decompress the stomach after surgery for intestinal obstruction. Sump drains are used to irrigate sites of contamination or infection.

Drains can act as a point of access for infection, and whilst this may be of little consequence if the tube has been put in to drain an abscess cavity, all efforts are made to reduce contamination of any wound. There is increased use of closed drainage systems and dressings around drains are changed regularly. Any changes to tubes or bags on drains must be carried out using aseptic techniques. Once a drain has served its purpose, it should be removed. The longer a drain stays *in situ*, the greater the risk of infection.

The contents and volumes discharged through a drain must be recorded. Large volumes, such as those from the gastrointestinal tract, may need the equivalent amount replaced intravenously.

Gut function

Some degree of gut atony is common after abdominal surgery, particularly emergency surgery. The condition is usually self-limiting and of little clinical consequence. There are three conditions that can produce massive gut dilatation and pose serious problems for the patient:

- gastric dilatation;
- paralytic (small intestine) ileus;
- pseudo-obstruction (large intestine).

Gastric dilatation

Gastric dilatation is rare and when it occurs, tends to be associated with surgery of the upper digestive tract. It may occur suddenly 2–3 days after the operation and is associated with massive fluid secretion into the stomach, with the consequent risk of regurgitation and inhalation. Treatment is by insertion of a nasogastric tube and decompression of the stomach. Unfortunately, when gastric dilatation does occur, often the first indication of the problem is a massive vomit and inhalation after the dilatation has occurred. By then the damage is done and the value of a nasogastric tube at this stage is questionable. Traditionally, nasogastric tubes were used routinely for patients following laparotomy, particularly in the emergency setting. However, the nasogastric tube is often the patient's major source of irritation and discomfort in the post-operative period and its routine use should be abandoned.

Paralytic ileus

Paralytic ileus is less sinister and more common. In the acutely ill patient who has undergone surgical intervention for peritonitis, paralytic ileus may be present from the first post-operative day. Otherwise, it tends to make its presence felt about 5 days after operation, and the patient may have been making an apparently uneventful recovery. Abdominal distension occurs and the patient may vomit. Oral fluid restriction should be instituted and intravenous replacement may be required. Most cases resolve spontaneously. Occasionally a prokinetic agent may be considered.

Pseudo-obstruction

Classically, pseudo-obstruction occurs in the elderly patient who has recently undergone surgery for a fractured neck of femur. The condition is also often seen where there has been extensive pelvic or retroperitoneal injury and sometimes the condition appears to be more related to the use of opiate analgesia rather than the type of surgery itself. The atony, with abdominal distension and absence of bowel function, tends to occur 2–3 days after surgery (or from the time the injury was sustained). Pseudo-obstruction is often mistaken for mechanical obstruction and the dilatation of the colon and caecum can be massive. If the condition does not resolve spontaneously, colonoscopic decompression is usually successful. Occasionally, surgical intervention is required to prevent caecal perforation.

Important post-operative complications

Respiratory failure

If the patient's respiratory function deteriorates in the intermediate post-operative period, this is indicative of the development of a new problem. The important causes to consider are:

- pulmonary embolus;
- abdominal distension;
- opiate overdose.

Depending on the initial state of respiratory function and the degree of deterioration, the patient may require anything from supplemental oxygen supplied by face mask to endotracheal intubation. A $P\text{CO}_2$ above 45 mm Hg, a $P\text{O}_2$ below 60 mm Hg and a low tidal volume all indicate that mechanical ventilation will be required. Once appropriate ventilatory support has been achieved, the cause of the respiratory failure can be addressed.

Wound failure

Provided the surgical procedure has a minimal risk of infection (see Chapter 7) and has been performed in an uneventful manner in a low risk patient, then the chances of problems with the wound are minimal and most such wounds can be left undisturbed until the patient leaves hospital. If there are identifiable risks the wounds may need to be attended to regularly. The problems that are likely to occur with wounds relate to:

- Discharge of fluid
- Collection of fluid
- Disruption of the wound

Risk factors that may contribute to the above problems include those that:

- Increase the risk of infection (see Chapter 7)
- Increase the risk of wound breakdown

There are general and local factors that increase the risk of breakdown of a wound. General factors include those that interfere with wound healing, such as diabetes mellitus, immunosuppression, malignancy and malnutrition. Local factors include the adequacy of wound closure, infection and anything that might put mechanical stress on the wound. For example, abdominal wound failure is a potential problem in the obese, and those with chest infections, ascites, or ileus.

In the early stages of wound healing any abnormal fluid at the wound site is likely to discharge rather than collect. The fluid may be blood, serous fluid, serosanguinous fluid or infected fluid of varying degrees up to frank pus. As discussed elsewhere in this chapter, the discharge of blood from a wound may have all sorts of consequences for the patient, which will vary from prompt opening of the neck wound of a patient with a primary haemorrhage after a thyroidectomy to evacuation of a haematoma after a mastectomy.

Serous fluid may be of little significance and be the result of a liquefying haematoma from within the depths of the wound. However a serosanguinous discharge from an abdominal or chest wound may herald a more sinister event, particularly if it occurs between days 5–8 after the operation. The discharge may have been preceded by coughing or retching. Such a wound is in imminent danger of deep dehiscence with evisceration. Should such an event occur, the wound must be covered in sterile moist packs and arrangements made to take the patient to the operating room for formal repair of the wound.

Collections in and under a wound may be blood, pus or seroma. As mentioned above, the rapidity with which a haematoma appears and any pressure effects such a haematoma may cause will determine its treatment. Collections of pus must be drained. Depending on its proximity or distance from the skin surface, an abscess may be drained by opening the wound or inserting (under radiological control) a drain into a deeper-lying cavity. Seromas tend to occur where there has been a large area of dissection in subcutaneous tissues (e.g. mastectomy) or where lymphatics may be damaged (e.g. groin dissections). The seroma may not appear a week after the procedure. Seromas will lift the skin off the underlying tissues and impede wound healing. They also make fertile ground for infection. Seromas should be aspirated under sterile conditions and the patient warned that several aspirations may be required as the seroma may re-collect.

Confusion

Confusion in surgical patient is common and has many causes. Often the confusion is minor and transient and does not need treatment. The patient is typically elderly, has become acutely ill and in pain, is removed from the security and familiarity of their home surroundings, is subject to emergency surgery and more pain, is put in a noisy environment with strangers bustling around and is sleep-deprived. These factors alone would make many otherwise healthy individuals confused. Add to that recipe the deprivation of the patient from their regular medications (particularly alcohol), upset their body biochemistry, render them hypoxic and give them a concoction of opioids and other agents.

When a patient does become confused in the post-operative period, it is important to ensure that no easily correctable cause has been overlooked. Confusion is often secondary to hypoxia, where chest infection, over-sedation, cardiac problems and pulmonary embolism need to be considered. Other important causes to consider include sepsis, drug withdrawal, metabolic and electrolyte disturbances and medications.

The management of the confused patient will include a close study of the charts, seeking information on any co-existing disease (particularly cardiorespiratory), drug record, alcohol consumption and the progress of the patient since the operation. Current medications should be noted, together with the nursing record of the vital signs.

If possible, try to take a history and examine the patient. Ensure that the patient is in a well-lit room and give oxygen by face mask. Attention should be focussed on the cardiorespiratory system, as this may well be the site of the underlying problem. Some investigations may be required to help determine the cause of the confusion. These might include arterial blood gas analysis, haematological and biochemical screens, blood and urine cultures, a chest X-ray and an electrocardiogram.

Most patients with post-operative confusion do not require treatment other than that for the underlying cause. However, the noisy, violent patient may need individual nursing care, physical restraint or sedation. Sedation should be reserved for patients with alcohol withdrawal problems, and either haloperidol or diazepam should be considered in such circumstances. Most hospitals have clearly defined protocols for the management of patients going through alcohol withdrawal. These correlate the anxiety, visual disturbances and agitation of the patient with the degree of monitoring and sedation required.

Pyrexia

The body's normal temperature varies and has a range between 36.5 and 37.5°C. The core temperature tends to be 0.5°C warmer than the peripheral temperature. Thus an isolated reading of 37.5°C has little meaning by itself and needs to be viewed in context with the other vital signs. Changes in temperature and the pattern of change are more important. A temperature that rises and falls several degrees between readings suggests a collection of pus and intermittent pyaemia, while a persistent high-grade fever is more in keeping with a generalised infection.

Fever can be due to infection or inflammation. In determining the cause of the fever the following should be considered:

- the type of fever
- the type of procedure which the patient has undergone
- the temporal relationship between the procedure and the fever

Perhaps the most useful factor in trying to establish the cause of a patient's fever is the relationship between the time of onset of the fever and the procedure. Fever within the first 24 hours of an operation is common and may reflect little more than the body's metabolic response to injury. Atelectasis is common during this time and may produce a self-limiting low-grade fever.

A fever that is evident between 5 and 7 days after an operation is usually due to infection. While pulmonary infections tend to occur in the first few days after surgery, fever at this later stage is more likely to reflect infection of the wound, operative site or urinary tract. Cannula problems and deep vein thrombosis (DVT) should also be considered.

A fever occurring more than 7 days after a surgical procedure may be due to abscess formation. Apart from infection as a cause of fever, it is important to remember that drugs, transfusion and brainstem problems can also produce an increase in the body's temperature.

A careful history, review of the charts and physical examination will usually determine the cause of the fever. The next stage in management will depend on the state of health of the patient. The fever of a septic process, which has led to circulatory collapse, will require resuscitation of the patient before any investigation. Otherwise, appropriate investigations may include blood and urine cultures, swabs from wounds and drains, and imaging to define the site of infection.

Treatment will depend on the severity and type of infection. The moribund patient will require resuscitation and an educated guess from the surgeon on which antibiotic regimen to use. Surgical or radiological intervention (e.g. to drain an abscess) may be required before the patient improves. However, the well patient may have antimicrobial therapy deferred until an organism has been identified (e.g. Gram stain or culture).

Deep vein thrombosis

Deep vein thrombosis may occur in spite of prophylaxis (see Chapter 1). Presentation may be silent (60%) or as a clinical syndrome (40%) with calf pain and tenderness, oedema of the leg and/or pain on dorsiflexion of the foot (Homan's sign). Rarely, massive thrombosis occurs with gross swelling of the lower limbs and venous gangrene (phlegmasia caerulea dolens).

Investigations are essential to confirm the diagnosis prior to the commencement of therapy.

Ultrasonography and duplex scanning with Doppler ultrasound have a sensitivity and specificity greater than 90%. Lower limb venography is highly accurate but invasive and is rarely indicated.

Following diagnosis, urgent therapy is required, starting with heparin i.v. in a dose of 20,000–30,000 units per day. The patient is monitored by measurement of the activated partial thromboplastin time (APTT), which is kept at 1.5–2.5 times the control value. Heparin therapy is continued for 5–7 days and is replaced by oral vitamin K antagonists such as warfarin. The dose of warfarin is adjusted according to the thromboplastin time with reference to an international standard (INR). Heparin is discontinued when full anticoagulation has been achieved and the warfarin is continued for 3–6 months to minimise the risk of further thrombosis and the development of complications (see Chapters 70 and 72).

Oliguria

Oliguria is a common problem in the post-operative period and is usually due to a failure by the attending medical staff to appreciate the volume of fluid lost by the patient during the surgical procedure and in the immediate post-operative period. For example, the development of an ileus will lead to a large volume of fluid being sequestered in the gut and this 'loss' not being immediately evident. Before the apparent oliguria is put down to diminished output of urine, it is important to ensure that the patient is not in urinary retention. Such an assessment can be difficult in a patient who has just undergone an abdominal procedure. If there is any doubt, a urinary catheter must be inserted. Alternately, many wards are now equipped with ultrasonographic devices capable of providing an accurate estimation of the bladder content.

Diminished output of urine may be due to:

- poor renal perfusion (pre-renal failure: hypovolaemia and/or pump failure)
- renal failure (acute tubular necrosis)
- renal tract obstruction (post-renal failure).

In the assessment of a patient with poor urine output (<30 mL/h), these three possible causes must be considered. Major surgery with large intraoperative fluid loss and periods of hypotension during the procedure might suggest renal tissue damage (acute tubular necrosis), while severe peritonitis with large fluid shifts and no hypotension would be more in keeping with inadequate fluid replacement.

The treatment of oliguria depends on the cause. Pre-renal hypovolaemia is treated by fluid replacement, while poor output secondary to pump failure requires diuretic therapy and perhaps medications (e.g. inotropes, anti-arrhythmics) to improve cardiac function. To give a hypovolaemic patient a diuretic in an attempt to improve urine output may be counterproductive and detrimental.

In acute renal failure the oliguria will not respond to a fluid challenge. Management demands accurate matching of input to output, monitoring of electrolytes and even dialysis.

In summary, most cases of post-operative oliguria are secondary to hypovolaemia, and should be considered to be due to hypovolaemia until proven otherwise.

Hyponatraemia

Any reduction in the sodium concentration in the ECF may be absolute or secondary to water retention. Loss of the major cation from the ECF leads to a shift of water into the ICF. Any clinical manifestation will reflect the expansion of the ICF (e.g., confusion, cramps and coma secondary to cerebral oedema) or the contraction of the ECF in absolute hyponatraemia (e.g. postural hypotension, loss of skin turgor).

Hyponatraemia due to a decreased total body deficiency of sodium is an unusual scenario in the post-operative surgical patient. Any hyponatraemia that occurs tends to be due to dilution and is caused by the administration of an excessive amount of water. While this is a fairly frequent biochemical finding, it rarely leads to any clinically significant problem.

Any hyponatraemia secondary to dilution may also occur with inappropriate antidiuretic hormone (ADH) secretion. The trauma of major surgery will produce an increase in ADH secretion and intravenous fluid must be administered judiciously in the immediate post-operative period. A safe rule of thumb is to restrict the patient to 2 L per day of maintenance fluid until a diuresis has been established. Hyponatraemia can usually be corrected by the administration of the appropriate requirements of isotonic saline. If the patient has a severe hyponatraemia and associated mental changes; an infusion of hypertonic sodium solution may be required.

Hypernatraemia

Hypernatraemia in the post-operative patient is a less common problem that hyponatraemia. Any hypernatraemia is usually relative rather than absolute and occurs secondary to diminished water intake. Patients with severe burns or high fever may also develop hypernatraemia. An increase in the plasma sodium concentration will lead to a loss of ECF volume and relative intracellular desiccation. The first clinical manifestation is thirst and if the hypernatraemia is allowed to persist, neurological problems (e.g. confusion, convulsions, coma) may ensue. Treatment is by administration of water by mouth or intravenous 5% dextrose.

Hyperkalaemia

With normal renal function, severe and life-threatening hyperkalaemia is rare. High concentrations of potassium in the ECF can be associated with cardiac rhythm disturbances and asystole. Hyperkalaemia may occur in severe trauma, sepsis and acidosis. Emergency treatment of arrhythmia-inducing hyperkalaemia consists of rapid infusion of a 1 L solution of 10% glucose with 25 units of soluble insulin. The insulin will help drive potassium into the cells and the glucose will help counteract the hypoglycaemic effect of the insulin. At the same time 20 mmol of calcium gluconate can be given to help stabilise cardiac membranes. If an arrhythmia has already developed the calcium gluconate should be given before the dextrose and insulin. Sodium bicarbonate (20–50 mmol) can be given if the patient is acidotic. If the level of potassium is not too high, an ion-exchange resin (resonium) can be given. These resins can be given by enema and they exchange potassium for calcium or sodium. Alternatively, the patient may be dialysed (peritoneal or haemodialysis). In the management of hyperkalaemia it is obviously as important to treat the cause as it is to treat the effect.

Hypokalaemia

Low levels of potassium in post-operative patients are common but hypokalaemia is rarely so severe as to produce muscle weakness, ileus or arrhythmias. Patients with large and continuous fluid loss from the gastrointestinal tract are prone to develop hypokalaemia. If potassium supplements are required they may be given either orally or intravenously. If by the latter route, the rate of infusion should not exceed 10 mmol/h. Faster rates may precipitate arrhythmias and should only be undertaken on a unit where the patient can be monitored for any ECG changes.

Haemorrhage

The management of haemorrhage in the post-operative period may be approached in several ways. In broad terms, bleeding may be classified as either localised or generalised. If the former, it may be classified as follows:

- primary (bleeding which occurs during the operation)
- reactionary (bleeding within the first 24 hours of the operation)
- secondary (bleeding occurring at 7–10 days after the operation)

If localised, the bleeding is usually related to the operative site and/or the wound. Occasionally, the bleeding may be at a point removed from both these areas, for example gastrointestinal haemorrhage from a stress-related gastric erosion. Bleeding from the wound site is usually indicative of a mechanical problem or local sepsis. Generalised bleeding may reflect a coagulation disorder and may be manifest by the oozing of fresh and unclotted blood from wound edges and with bleeding from sites of cannula insertion.

Most cases of reactionary (and primary) haemorrhage are from a poorly ligated vessel or one that has been missed, and are not secondary to any coagulation disorder. The bleeding point may go unnoticed during the operation if there is any hypotension, and makes itself known only when the patient's circulating volume and blood pressure have been restored to normal. The bleeding in secondary haemorrhage is due to erosion of a vessel from spreading infection. Secondary haemorrhage is most often seen when a heavily contaminated wound is closed primarily, and can usually be prevented by adopting the principle of delayed wound closure.

Post-operative haemorrhage can also be classified according to its clinical presentation. The most common forms are wound bleeding, concealed intraperitoneal bleeding, gastrointestinal haemorrhage and the diffused ooze of disordered haemostasis.

The approach to management will depend on the overall condition of the patient and the assessment of the type of bleed. A stable patient with a localised blood-soaked dressing will be managed differently from a hypotensive patient with 2 L of fresh blood in a chest drain, who in turn will be managed differently from a patient with a platelet count of 15×10^9 L^{-1} and fresh blood oozing from all raw areas.

In the first case the tendency might be to apply another dressing in an attempt to achieve control by pressure. A more positive approach is to remove the dressing and inspect the wound. In most instances, a single bleeding point can be identified and controlled. In the next case, the patient has a major bleed and this is probably from a bleeding vessel within the operative site. Return to the operating room and formal re-exploration must be seriously considered. In the third case, the prime problem is one of an anticoagulation defect requiring urgent correction.

The diagnosis of post-operative haemorrhage is a clinical one, based on knowledge of the surgical procedure, the post-operative progress and an assessment of the patient's vital signs. The blood loss may not always be visible and could be concealed at the operative site or within the digestive tract. The treatment of post-operative haemorrhage depends on the severity of the bleed and the underlying cause. Hypovolaemia and circulatory failure will demand urgent fluid replacement and consideration of the likely cause and site of bleeding. Careful consideration must be given to control of localised haemorrhage and whether re-operation is warranted.

Vomiting

The causes of vomiting after surgery are many, and can be best determined by establishing the relationship between onset of vomiting and the time of the operation. The two most common causes of post-operative vomiting are drug-induced and gut atony.

Vomiting that occurs in the immediate post-operative period is usually drug related. If it is due to the effects of anaesthesia, vomiting will usually settle within 24 hours. Current anaesthetic techniques and modern anti-emetics have rendered nausea and vomiting a relatively minor post-operative problem for most patients.

Vomiting that occurs several days after operation may still be drug related, but in this instance is usually due to an opiate rather than an anaesthetic agent. Vomiting may be secondary to gut stasis, and this atony is usually self-limiting. If prolonged, a prokinetic agent can be effective.

If vomiting starts 7 days or so after abdominal surgery, a mechanical cause for the problem should be considered.

MCQs

Select the single correct answer to each question.

1 A 78-year-old woman develops an arrhythmia 2 days after a laparotomy for perforated diverticular disease. The ECG shows a bradycardia of 30 beats/min and spiked T waves. The only biochemical abnormalities are a potassium level of 6.3 mmol/L (normal range 3.8–5.2) and a creatinine level of 0.2 mmol/L (normal range 0.05–0.12). Her monitored vital signs (including ECG) are normal. What should be your first course of action?

- **a** give a rapid intravenous infusion of 1 L of 10% dextrose containing 25 units of soluble insulin
- **b** give an intravenous infusion of 20 mL of calcium gluconate
- **c** start the patient on haemodialysis
- **d** administer an enema of calcium resonium
- **e** give an intravenous infusion of 30 mmol of sodium bicarbonate

2 A 40-year-old man is confused and restless the second day after upper abdominal surgery and repair of a hiatus hernia. The *most probable* cause of his condition is:

- **a** pulmonary embolism
- **b** narcotic overdose
- **c** pulmonary atelectasis
- **d** electrolyte imbalance
- **e** starvation ketosis

3 You are asked to see a patient in your ward, 7 days following a left hemicolectomy. The patient has a discharging wound. The discharge oozes freely between the sutures and is profuse, watery and blood-stained. There are no signs of inflammation. What is the most likely diagnosis:

- **a** dehiscence of the wound
- **b** an anastomotic leak

c discharge from a wound haematoma
d wound infection
e a seroma

4 You have been asked to see a 68-year-old woman who has developed abdominal distension 5 days after a total hip replacement. Her abdomen is distended but soft. There is no localised tenderness, and rectal examination is unremarkable. A few scattered bowel sounds can be heard. The plain abdominal film shows gas all the way to the rectum and a dilated caecum and ascending colon. The radiological diameter of the caecum measures 14 cm. What will you do as immediate management of this patient?
a arrange decompression of the caecum by a caecostomy
b arrange a contrast (gastrografin) enema to exclude mechanical obstruction
c prepare the patient for laparotomy and right hemicolectomy
d arrange for decompression by colonoscopy
e insert a rectal flatus tube

5 A previously fit 55-year-old man has undergone an emergency right hemicolectomy for a perforated caecal carcinoma. Two days after the operation you note the following on his fluid balance sheet – intravenous input 2 L, nasogastric aspirate 2 L, drain losses 700 mL, urine output 500 mL. Biochemistry shows [Na^+] 135 mmol/L, [K^+] 3.0 mmol/L, [Cl^-] 100 mmol/L, [HCO_3^-] 27 mmol/L. Which of the fluid balance regimens below would you order for the next 24-hour period?
a 2 L *N* saline + 3 L dextrose 5% + 50 meq KCl
b 2 L *N* saline + 1 L dextrose 5% + 50 meq KCl
c 1 L *N* saline + 3 L dextrose 5% + 100 meq KCl
d 3 L *N* saline + 2 L dextrose 5% + 100 meq KCl
e 1 L *N* saline + 1 L dextrose 5% + 100 meq KCl

4 Surgical techniques

David M. A. Francis

Introduction

This chapter reviews techniques used in surgical practice and invasive procedures.

The operating room

The operating room is a dedicated area for surgical procedures and must be conducive to performing surgery to the highest standards of safety for patients and staff. The principal purpose of such a dedicated area is to reduce the risk of infection of patients. The operating room must be large enough for complex procedures to be undertaken, for storage of appropriate equipment, movement of staff, as well as the maintenance of a sterile area around the operative field. By changing the operating room air 20–25 times each hour at positive pressure relative to outside the room, low concentrations of airborne bacteria and particulate matter can be maintained. The number of people in the room and their movement should be minimised. Ambience should be calm and professional, and the air temperature such that inadvertent patient hypothermia does not occur. The operative field must be well illuminated by direct bright light, and surgeons sometimes wear a head light for procedures in body cavities which cannot be illuminated easily by standard operating room lights.

The surgeon's assistant has the important role of assisting and supporting the surgeon in the smooth conduct of operations. It is important to concentrate on the task at hand, to carry out the surgeon's instructions with speed and accuracy, to have a sense of anticipation, and to notify the surgeon of any potential hazard during the operation.

A face mask which covers the nose and mouth prevents droplet spread of bacteria, is worn for any invasive procedure and is changed after each case. Eye protection in the form of plain plastic glasses or a visor attached to the face mask must be worn to protect against droplet spray of infected body fluids. Gloves are worn if there is a possibility of coming into contact with patients' body fluids. Clean theatre attire, dedicated theatre shoes, and a disposable hair cover are worn while in the operating suite.

Aseptic techniques

Aseptic techniques are clinical practices which aim to prevent infection occuring in the patient as a result of the surgical procedure by:

- Preparation and cleaning the patient's skin with antiseptic fluid before it is cut or punctured.
- Use of sterilised instruments, equipment or surgical materials which might come into contact with the operative field and surgical wound.

Personnel involved directly in the operative procedure (surgeon, surgical assistant and 'scrub' nurse) wash their hands and forearms with antiseptic soap for 5 minutes before the first operation of the day and for 3 minutes before each subsequent case to reduce skin flora. Hands are dried with sterile towels, and a moisture-impermeable sterile gown is worn. One or two pairs of sterile gloves prevent transfer of bacteria from the surgeon's hands to the patient and also protect the surgeon from infected blood and body fluids from the patient.

The patient should shower or bathe with an antiseptic soap before going to the operating room. After induction of anaesthesia, hair is removed from the operative site by shaving with a razor or electric clippers. The skin is cleansed with an antiseptic solution starting at the site where the incision will be made and working away from the area, so that approximately 10–20 cm of skin around the incision site is prepared. The patient is covered with sterile linen or impermeable drapes, leaving exposed only the cleansed area around the incision site, which may be covered by a sterile adhesive plastic drape.

Surgical antiseptics

The commonest source of bacterial contamination in the operating room is from the patient. Therefore, topical antiseptic agents are used to reduce the number of skin organisms prior to any skin incision or puncture, and include:

- Aqueous chlorhexidine (0.5%) is used to disinfect mucous membranes and parts of the body adjacent to structures which would be adversely affected by more stringent antiseptics (e.g. the skin around the eyes). Aqueous chlorhexidine is bactericidal and has low tissue toxicity.
- Cetrimide (2%) is bactericidal.
- Iodine-based antiseptics (e.g. povidone iodine (10%) [Betadine], alcoholic iodine solution) destroy a wide range of bacteria, especially staphylococci, by iodisation of microbial proteins.
- Alcohol-based (70%) antiseptics kill bacteria by evaporation.

Sterility

Anything that comes into contact with the surgical wound must be sterile. The method of sterilisation depends on the item being sterilised (Box 4.1).

Box 4.1 Methods of sterilisation

Autoclave
Uses superheated steam at high pressure to reach a temperature of 121 degrees. Sterilisation is achieved when droplets of superheated water evaporate immediately upon reduction of pressure, thus destroying micro-organisms and leaving instruments dry. Most surgical instruments and linen drapes are sterilised by autoclaving.

Dry heat
Items which tolerate heat but not moisture can be sterilised by dry heat, but it is less efficient and takes longer than autoclaving.

Ethylene oxide gas
Takes several hours and is used for heat-sensitive items such as endoscopes, electrical and optical equipment and some plastics.

Glutaraldehyde
A 2% solution is used to sterilise equipment which can tolerate moisture but not heat, such as urological catheters, plastics and rubber.

Ionising radiation
Uses gamma rays and is particularly useful for sterilising single-use disposables such as plastics, dressings, scalpel blades and synthetic conduits.

Universal precautions

The risk of transmission of infectious agents from patients to staff (and *vice versa*) is reduced by practising universal precautions. Thus, it is assumed that all patients harbour potentially dangerous pathogens (e.g. hepatitis C, HIV) no matter how innocuous they appear, because carrier status cannot definitely be excluded without repeated, expensive and time consuming investigations. The principle of universal precautions is to establish a physical barrier between the patient and the carer to prevent direct contact with any potentially infected body fluid or tissue in either direction (Box 4.2).

Hazards

In addition to infection, there are many potential sources of hazard in the operating environment. Hazards, other than those intrinsic to the anaesthetic and surgical operation, are organisational, or related to operating room equipment or the transfer and positioning of the patient on the operating table.

Organisational hazards

Organisational hazards should be entirely preventable. A full history and examination of the patient must be made before surgery, including the past medical history, drug history and allergies, so that elementary errors are not made (e.g. unwittingly operating on a patient with a pacemaker or who is anticoagulated, or prescribing a drug to which the patient is allergic). Before surgery commences, the reason for and nature of the operation, together with its potential common and serious complications, and the reasonable expectations from the procedure, are discussed with the patient and family

> **Box 4.2 Universal precautions**
>
> **Barrier protection**
> Appropriate protective barriers are used during invasive procedures and handling contaminated materials – gloves, face mask, eye shield, impermeable gown, shoe covers, hair cover.
>
> **Minimising potential exposure**
> Decrease the risk of spreading potentially infected body fluids by avoiding spillages, careful disposal of materials and equipment contaminated by body fluids, having only essential personnel present during invasive procedures, excluding personnel with open wounds or abrasions, using impermeable dressings to cover wounds, using closed rather than open drains.
>
> **Elimination of needle stick injuries**
> Do not handle uncapped needles, never re-sheath used needles, and never remove a used needle from a syringe. Use needles as little as possible. Immediately dispose of used needles in a designated 'sharps' disposal container which has a one-way opening.
>
> **Elimination of other penetrating injuries**
> Sharp objects (e.g. scalpels, needles) are transferred between operating personnel in sharps dish, not from hand to hand. Hand-held needles are not used. Blunt suture needles are used where possible. Sharp instruments are not placed on the operative field or anywhere on the patient. Alert personnel to the presence of any sharp object in the operative field.

who are free to ask any questions. A consent or request for treatment form, which states the nature of the operation and the side on which the operation is to be performed if the operation is a unilateral procedure, is signed by the patient and the surgeon or deputy.

Once in the operating suite, a check is made that the patient is the correct one for that procedure, that the correct side or limb is identified and marked with an indelible pen, and that the lesion or lump is similarly marked to ensure that there is no confusion after the patient has been anaesthetised. All relevant case notes, investigation results and X-rays must be available in the operating room.

Equipment

Diathermy is used universally in surgical practice. High frequency alternating current passes from a small point of contact (active electrode) through the patient to a large contact site (indifferent electrode or diathermy plate) to produce localised heat which coagulates protein. Diathermy produces either (a) coagulation – haemostasis with a small amount of adjacent tissue damage, (b) cutting – tissue cutting with minimal tissue damage, or (c) fulgaration – haemostatsis with considerable tissue necrosis. Potential hazards include electrocution, inadvertent burn to the patient at a remote site and to the surgeon, fire associated with pooled alcohol-based antiseptics, explosion of flammable anaesthetic gases, and interference with the function of cardiac pacemakers.

A variety of lasers with different wavelengths and effects on cells and tissues are used in surgical practice for highly accurate tissue destruction (e.g. mucosal surgery, CNS tumours, dermatological lesions, aerodigestive tumours), coagulating blood vessels (e.g. gastrointestinal tract, retinal photocoagulation), and for photo-activation of intra-tumour haematoporphyrin for malignant tumour destruction (photodynamic therapy). Hazards include eye damage, explosion of anaesthetic gases, and shattering and destruction of other equipment.

Limb torniquets are used to provide a blood-less field in which to operate. The limb is elevated and exsanguinated by a rubber bandage or compressive sleeve, and the proximal torniquet inflated to 50 mm Hg (upper limb) or 100 mm Hg (lower limb) above systolic blood pressure. A torniquet should not be kept inflated for more than 60–90 minutes. Hazards include arterial thrombosis, distal ischaemia, nerve compression and skin traction.

Positioning of the patient

The patient is positioned on the operating table in such a way that the procedure is facilitated and the airway can be protected. Pressure points are padded, and limbs are positioned so that peripheral nerves, major blood vessels, joints and ligaments are not stretched or compressed. The anaesthetised patient must be in a stable position on the operating table and may need to be strapped on with broad adhesive tape. There must be no contact between the skin and any metallic surface because of the risk of diathermy burn and pressure necrosis. Sections of the operating table can be angled so that the patient is optimally positioned for the particular procedure (e.g. flexed while lying supine or on one side, head-down, head-up).

Endoscopy

Endoscopy is performed by inserting a fibre-optic telescope containing a light source and instrument channels into the gastrointestinal, respiratory and urinary tracts. The operator undertakes the procedure by manipulating the endoscope while viewing a video screen or looking down the eye piece of the instrument.

Gastrointestinal endoscopy

Endoscopy of the gastrointestinal tract allows the endoscopist to view the lumen of the oesophagus, stomach and proximal half of the duodenum (oesophagogastroduodenoscopy), colon (colonoscopy), and rectum and distal sigmod colon (sigmoidoscopy), and distal rectum and anal canal (proctoscopy). It is usually performed under sedation. Intestinal endoscopy can also be performed at laparotomy (enteroscopy) by making a small incision in the intestine and the surgeon passes the endoscope along the intestinal lumen. Procedures, such as dilatation of strictures, biospy and diathermy ablation of polyps, injection of adrenaline around bleeding gastric and duodenal ulcers, cholangio-pancreatography, removal of common bile duct calculi, injection of haemorrhoids, and tumour phototherapy can be performed using fibre-optic endoscopes.

Bronchoscopy

The upper airway, trachea and proximal bronchi can be inspected by bronchoscopy, which may be performed under local or general anaesthesia. Bronchoscopy is used for diagnosis (e.g. inspection and biopsy of lung tumours) or therapy (e.g. removal of foreign bodies, aspiration of secretions). Anaesthetists ocassionally use the fibre-optic bronchoscope to facilitate difficult endotracheal intubation. (see also Chapter 58, p. 539).

Urological endoscopy

The urethra (urethroscopy), bladder (cystoscopy), and ureters (ureteroscopy) can be inspected for diagnostic purposes. Extensive therapeutic procedures (e.g. resection of the prostate, diathermy and excision of bladder tumours, extraction of calculi) can be performed safely with far less morbidity than the equivalent open procedures.

Endoscopic surgery

Endoscopic surgery is performed by inserting a microchip video camera with a light source and specially crafted long-handled surgical instruments into a body cavity by way of small incisions. The surgeon undertakes the procedure by manipulating the instruments while viewing a video screen.

The advantages of endoscopic or 'closed' surgery are reduced post-operative pain and analgesic requirements, earlier discharge from hospital, and earlier return to normal function. However, many surgical procedures either cannot be undertaken endoscopically because of their very nature, or cannot be completed endoscopically because of difficulty or patient safety, in which case the operation is converted to an 'open' procedure. Some procedures use endoscopic techniques to assist with the procedure and an incision is made to either complete the operation or deliver the resected specimen (e.g. bowel resection, nephrectomy, splenectomy). The range of endoscopically performed operations in many surgical specialties has increased enormously over the last 10–15 years.

Abdominal surgery

Laparoscopy refers to the technique of insufflating the peritoneal cavity with gas, inserting a camera through a 10–15-mm sub-umbilical incision and inspecting the abdominal contents. Usually, three additional ports are inserted through 5–10-mm incisions in the abdominal wall and instruments (e.g. scissors, grasping devices, retractors, staplers, needle holders) are introduced and manipulated by the surgeon to perform the operation. Procedures such as cholecystectomy, gastric fundoplication, hiatus hernia repair, division of adhesions, appendicectomy, splenectomy, adrenalectomy, nephrectomy, oophorectomy, tubal ligation, and hernia repair can be undertaken laparoscopically with less morbidity than if undertaken as an open or conventional operation. Endoscopic surgery has allowed some procedures to be undertaken as day cases, whereas the same procedure performed as an open operation would require an inpatient stay of several days (e.g. cholecystectomy, hernia repair).

Thoracic surgery

Thorascopy involves inserting a camera with a light source and instruments into the thoracic cavity. The technique is used diagnostically and therapeutically for procedures such as drainage of the thoracic cavity (haemothorax, pleural effusion and empyema), lung biopsy, pleurodesis, and excision of lung bullae. The mediastinum can be inspected and mediastinal lymph nodes can be biopsied by mediastinoscopy, which may prevent the need for an exploratory thoracotomy.

Orthopaedic surgery

Large joints (e.g. knee, hip, ankle, shoulder, wrist) can be inspected by arthroscopy. Therapeutic procedures include removal of bone chips, cartilage excision and removal, and ligament repair. Arthroscopic surgery has been enormously beneficial for orthopaedic patients and has allowed far more rapid return to function.

Open surgery

Open surgery is the traditional or conventional method of operating. In general terms, open surgery involves making a surgical wound, dissecting tissues to gain access to and mobility of the structure or organ of interest, completing the therapeutic procedure, ensuring haemostasis is complete, and then closing the wound with sutures. Open surgey is performed more with the hands and direct touch than endoscopic procedures, and fingers may be used for 'blunt' dissection. The surgical wound accounts for much of the morbidity of open surgery, particularly the cutting of muscle. The range of open operations is extremely wide, as evidenced by the procedures described throughout this book.

Surgical methods

Surgical operations are performed by well worked out, standardised steps which progress in logical sequence. An operative plan is worked out by the surgeon for every operation.

Surgical instruments

There are literally thousands of surgical instruments, some simple and others extremely complex, but each designed for a specific function. The surgical incison is made with a scalpel which consists of a re-usable handle and a disposable blade. Scissors are used to cut other tissues and sutures, and for blunt dissection with the blades closed. Diathermy is used for haemostasis and to cut through tissue layers beneath the skin. Tissues are held with dissecting or tissue grasping forceps rather than the fingers. Hand-held forceps either have teeth which tend to dig into and damage tissues, or are non-toothed with poorer grasping ability. Needle holders are used to grasp needles for suturing and eliminate the need for hand-held needles, and are therefore safer. They have a ratchet so that the needle can be contained securely in the holder while not in the surgeon's hand. Retractors allow the surgeon to operate in an adequately exposed field. Self-retaining retractors keep the wound edges apart without the aid of an assistant. Retractors held by the assistant provide tissue retraction in awkward parts of the wound and in situations where retraction of specific tissues is required so that intricate parts of the operation can be performed. A sucker is used to aspirate blood and body fluids from the operative field and to remove smoke created by the diathermy. There are many instruments designed specifically for surgical specialties and procedures.

Incisions

Surgical incisions are made so that:

- The operation can be undertaken with adequate exposure of the area or structure of interest.
- The procedure can be performed and completed safely and expeditiously.
- The wound heals satisfactorily with a cosmetically acceptable scar.

Thus, incisions are to be of adequate but not excessive length and, if possible, placed in skin creases, particularly when operating on exposed areas of the body such as the face, neck and breast. Parallel skin incisions (tram tracking) and V- or T-shaped incisions are avoided because of ischaemia of intervening tissue and pointed flaps.

Tissue dissection

Ideally, surgical dissection should be performed along tissue planes which tend to be relatively avascular. The aim is to isolate (mobilise) the structure(s) of interest from surrounding connective tissue and other structures with the least amount of trauma and bleeding. Tissues should be handled with great care and respect and as little as possible. Dissection is undertaken by using a scalpel or scissor (sharp dissection), a finger, closed scissor, gauze pledget, or scalpel handle (blunt dissection), or the diathermy. Gentle counter traction on tissues by the assistant facilitates the dissection.

Haemostasis

Surgical haemostasis refers to stopping bleeding which occurs with transection of blood vessels. The majority of cases of operative and post-operative bleeding are due to inadequate surgical haemostasis rather than disorders of clotting and coagulation. Haemostasis is essential in order to prevent blood loss during surgery and haematoma formation post-operatively. Methods of surgical haemostasis include:

- Application of a haemostatic clamp to a blood vessel and then ligation with a surgical ligature (see Chapter 6, p. 45).
- Suture ligation of a vessel – under-running a bleeding vessel with a figure-of-8 suture which is tied firmly.
- Diathermy coagulation (see Chapter 2, p. 9).
- Localised pressure for several minutes to allow coagulation to occur naturally.
- Application of surgical materials (e.g. oxidised cellulose, Surgicell) which promote coagulation.
- Application of topical agents to promote vasoconstriction (e.g. adrenaline) or coagulation (e.g. thrombin).
- Packing of a bleeding cavity with gauze packs as a temporary measure until definitive haemostasis can be achieved.

Sutures

Sutures have been used to close surgical wounds for thousands of years, and initially were made from human or animal hair, animal sinews, and plant material. Today, a wide variety of material is available for suturing and ligating tissues (Box 4.3).

Sutures are selected for use according to the required function. For example, arteries are sutured

Box 4.3 Sutures

Substance	Description*	Duration+	Trade name	Uses
Plain catgut	Nat, Multi, Ab	1–2 weeks	–	Subcutaneous fat
Chromic catgut	Nat, Multi, Ab	2–3 weeks	–	Subcutaneous fat, gastrointestinal and urinary tract anastomoses
Silk and linen	Nat, Multi, Non	Prolonged	–	Skin and cardiac sutures, ligatures
Stainless steel	Nat, Mono, Non	Prolonged	–	Sternum, skin and gastrointestinal staples, orthopaedic wire,
Polyglycolic acid	Syn, Multi, Ab	3–4 weeks	Dexon	Gastrointestinal and urinary tracts, muscle, fascia, subcutaneous fat
Polyglactin	Syn, Multi, Ab	4–6 weeks	Vicryl	Gastrointestinal and urinary tracts, muscle, fascia, subcutaneous fat
Polypropylene	Syn, Mono, Non	Indefinite	Prolene	Ophthalmology, vascular sutures, abdominal closure, neurosurgery, fascia, skin
Polyamide	Syn, Mono, Non	Years	Nylon	Abdominal and skin closure, hernia repair
Polytetrafluoroethylene (PTFE)	Syn, Mono, Non	Indefinite	Gortex	Vascular anastomoses, hernia repair

*Synthetic (Syn), Natural (Nat), Monofilament (Mono), Multifilament (Multi), Absorbable (Ab), Non-absorbable (Non).
+Time during which tensile strength is maintained.

together with non-absorbable polypropylene or polytetrafluoroethylene (PTFE) sutures which are non-thrombogenic, cause virtually no tissue reaction, and maintain their instrinsic strength indefinitely so that the anastomotic scar (which is under constant arterial pressure) does not stretch and become aneurysmal. Skin wounds, for example, are sutured with either non-absorbable sutures, which are removed after several days (see Chapter 6, p. 45), or absorbable sutures hidden within the skin (subcuticular sutures) and which are not removed surgically but are absorbed after several weeks.

Sutures are available in diameters ranging from 0.02–0.50 mm. The minimum calibre of suture should be used, compatible with its function. Non-absorbable sutures are avoided for suturing the luminal aspects of the gastrointestinal and urinary tracts because substances within the contained fluids (e.g. bile, urine) may precipitate on persisting sutures and produce calculi.

The requirements of suture material are:

- Tensile strength – the suture must be strong enough to hold tissues in apposition for as long as required.
- Durability – the suture must remain until either healing is advanced or indefinitely if the healed tissue is under constant pressure.
- Reactivity – tissue reaction (i.e. an inflammatory response) allows absorbable sutures to be removed by phagocytosis but results in chronic inflammation if non-absorbable sutures remain *in situ*.
- Handling characteristics – sutures must be easy to grasp, handle and tie.
- Knot security – sutures must be able to be tied effectively so that knots do not come undone or slip.

Sutures are classified as:

- Absorbable or non-absorbable. The rate of absorption of absorbable sutures depends on what they are made of and their thickness. Disappearance of the suture occurs through inflammatory reaction, hydrolysis or enzymatic degradation.
- Synthetic or natural material. Sutures of natural (animal) origin are being phased out of surgical practice because of the very minimal risk of disease transmission. A wide variety of synthetic suture materials are available.
- Monofilament or multifilament. Monofilament sutures pass through tissues easily, are generally less reactive, and are more difficult to handle and knot securely. Multifilament sutures are braided or twisted thread, and are easier to handle and knot, but are more likely to harbour micro-organisms within the suture.

Surgical knots

Knots are tied to ensure that ligatures and sutures remain in place and do not slip or unravel. The ability to tie a secure knot is a fundamental technique in surgery, and patients' lives literally depend on knot security (e.g. the knot in a ligature used to tie off an artery). Knot security depends on friction between the throws of the ligature material, the number of throws used to tie the knot, the strength of the ligature material, and the tightness of the knot. Usually, multiple throws are used to secure the knot (e.g. two reef knots, one on the other).

Suturing

The technique of suturing depends on the tissue and wound being sutured. Sutures may be either continuous (e.g. subcuticular skin sutures, abdominal closure, vascular anastomosis), or interrupted (e.g. skin sutures, sternal wires). The function of sutures is to hold the adjacent edges of sutured tissues in apposition and to immobilise them in that position so that wound healing (i.e. neovascularisation, connective tissue ingrowth and collagen formation) is facilitated. It is essential that sutures are not tied so tightly that the tissues encompassed by them become ischaemic. Skin sutures may be supported by adhesive paper tapes.

Retention sutures (incorrectly referred to as *tension sutures*) are used to close abdominal incisions which are thought to be at increased risk of dehiscence, and are inserted to encompass a large amount of fascial tissue and are placed 3–5 cm apart.

Within the last two decades, stainless steel staples have been used to close skin wounds and to perform gastrointestinal anastomoses. Staples are quicker to use than sutures, but are relatively expensive and produce a worse cosmetic result for skin closure than subcuticular absorbable sutures.

Suture removal

Sutures are removed as early as possible to minimise the risk of infection and scarring, so long as tissue healing is sufficently advanced that the wound will not open when the sutures are removed. Sutures are therefore removed at different times, depending on tissue and general patient factors (Box 4.4). For

Box 4.4 Timing of suture removal

Site	Time of removal (days)
Face	3–5
Neck (skin crease)	5–7
Scalp	7–10
Abdomen	10
Extremity	10–14
Amputation stump	21

example, sutures are left *in situ* for a longer time in patients who are immunosuppressed, malnourished, jaundiced, or undergoing chemotherapy; who have renal failure, and in tissues judged to be relatively ischaemic, subject to increased stress and tension, and which have been irradiated.

Surgical drains

Drains are used widely in surgical practice to

- Remove blood or serous fluid, which would otherwise accumulate in the operative area (e.g. wound drain).
- Provide a track or line of minimal resistance so that potentially harmful fluids can drain away from a particular site (e.g. drain placed into an intra-abdominal abscess cavity).

Several different methods of drainage may be used depending on the required function.

- Open drainage – a drain tube or strip of soft flexible latex rubber is placed so secretions or pus can drain along the track of the drain into gauze or other dressing covering the external end of the drain tube (e.g. drain placed in an abscess cavity, drain placed prohylactically near a bowel anastomosis in case of subsequent anastomotic leak).
- Closed drainage – a tube is placed into an area or viscus to drain fluid contents into a collecting bag so that there is no contamination of the drained area from outside the system (e.g. chest drain, urinary catheter, cholecystostomy drain).
- Closed suction drain – the drain tube is connected to a bottle at negative atmospheric pressure so that fluid is sucked out of the area (e.g. wound drain, drain under skin flaps).

It is important to note both the amount and the type of fluid which drains. Large volumes of fluid drainage may need to be replaced as intravenous fluids (e.g. duodenal fistula fluid). Depending on the particular situation, it may be necessary to culture drain fluid or send it for estimation of haemoglobin, creatinine, electrolytes, amylase or protein. A radiological contrast study may be performed along the drain tube, for example to estimate the size of a cavity being drained.

Drain tubes are removed when they are no longer required, for example when there is minimal fluid being drained, or when a cavity being drained has contracted and is small. Drains are removed simply by cutting the suture which anchors them to the skin and withdrawing the tube from the patient.

Venepuncture

Venepuncture involves removing blood from a superficial vein, usually in the antecubital fossa or dorsum of the hand, by inserting a needle attached to a syringe or collection tube at negative pressure (vacutainer system). A venous torniquet is applied around the arm, which is hung in a dependent position; the patient vigorously opens and closes the hand, and the vein is gently patted to encourage venous dilatation. The skin is cleansed with antiseptic and the needle is inserted through the skin into the dilated vein at an angle of 30–45 degrees. Only the required volume is aspirated, the torniquet is released, the needle is withdrawn, the puncture site is immediately covered with a cotton wool swab, and light pressure is applied for 1–2 minutes. The site is covered with an adhesive dressing. Complications include bruising, haematoma, and rarely, infection and damage to deeper structures. Inadvertent needlestick injury to the venepuncturist is avoided by careful technique.

Intravenous cannulation

Intravenous (i.v.) cannulation is used commonly for administration of fluids and drugs. Superficial veins on the forearms and dorsum of the hands are used for i.v. cannulation. Antecubital fossa veins are best avoided for cannulation because the elbow has to be kept extended to avoid kinking of the cannula. Leg veins may have to be used in the absence of useable upper limb veins. Cannulas have a soft outer Teflon sheath attached to a hub, and a central hollow needle attached to a small chamber.

A suitable vein is identified as for venepuncture. Local anaesthetic cream is applied to the skin overlying the vein or local anaesthetic (1% lignocaine without adrenaline) is injected intradermally next to the vein after cleansing the skin with antiseptic. The cannula (needle and sheath) is inserted through the skin into the vein at an angle of 10–30 degrees and advanced into the vein in the same movement. The needle is removed from the sheath and a closed three-way tap or i.v. giving set is joined to the hub of the sheath. The cannula is secured to the skin with adhesive tape.

Intravenous infusion is painful when the infusate is cold or contains irritants (e.g. potassium, calcium, drugs of low or high pH), or if the cannula pierces the vein wall and fluid extravasates subcutaneously. Thrombophlebitis develops at the insertion site after about three days, and i.v. cannulas should be re-sited if infusions are required for longer periods.

Central venous catheterisation

Percutaneous catheterisation of a central vein is used for

- Short- or long-term venous access when peripheral veins are unsuitable or cannot be used (e.g. prolonged fluid infusion, total parenteral nutrition, ultrafiltration, haemodialysis, plasma exchange, chemotherapy).
- Short-term monitoring of central venous pressure

A central venous catheter (CVC) may be inserted into the internal or external jugular vein or the subclavian vein. Temporary CVCs are made of semi-rigid Teflon, are approximately 25 cm in length and, depending on their function, are between 1 and 4 mm in diameter and have one, two or three lumens. Long-term CVCs are made of barium-impregnated silastic and are quite flexible. They have a Dacron cuff bonded to the part of the catheter which lies subcutaneously and becomes incorporated by fibrous tissue after several weeks so that organisms cannot track along the catheter from the skin into the circulation.

Some long-term single lumen CVCs are available with a small volume chamber attached to the extravenous end of the catheter (Portacath, Infusaport). The chamber is implanted subcutaneously after the vein is catheterised and can be accessed for chemotherapy or blood sampling by inserting a needle into it through the skin.

CVC insertion is best performed in an operating theatre, under local or general anaesthesia, and with ultrasound localisation of the central vein. The patient is placed in a supine, slightly head-down position, and the surface anatomy of the vein is marked. Aseptic technique is essential. A hollow wide-bore needle is inserted into the vein, a guidewire is passed down the needle and the needle is removed. The guidewire position is checked radiologically. A plastic dilator is passed over the guidewire to dilate a track for the catheter and is removed, and the CVC is passed over the guide wire which is removed after the CVC is in place. A chest X-ray is performed to check the final position of the CVC and also to ensure that a pneumo- or haemothorax has not occurred due to inadvertent puncture of the pleura or lung. The catheter is sutured to the skin to prevent dislodgement and the exit site is dressed with an adhesive dressing.

Further reading

Keen G, Farndon JR, eds. *Operative Surgery and Management*. 3rd ed. Oxford: Butterworth-Heinemann; 1994.

MCQs

Select the single correct answer to each question.

1 Universal precautions:
- **a** protect operating theatre staff from electric shocks
- **b** prevent polluted air from entering the operating theatre
- **c** impose a physical barrier between patients and carers
- **d** are only to be used when operating on patients
- **e** protect only against bacterial pathogens

2 Endoscopic surgery:
- **a** has a very limited role in general surgical practice
- **b** is inherently unsafe because the surgeon cannot touch the structures being operated on
- **c** is associated with greater post-operative pain and immobility
- **d** enables cholecystectomy to be performed as day case surgery in some patients
- **e** can only be used for part of an operation

3 Sutures:

a should be left in the skin for a minimum of 2 weeks
b often need to be removed with local anaesthetic
c must be tied tightly so that arterial inflow into tissues is not possible
d made of catgut lose tensile strength within 3 weeks
e of all types must eventually be removed

4 Surgical drains:

a are removed when they are no longer necessary
b should always be removed the day after surgery
c are removed under general anaesthesia
d are not necessary with modern surgical techniques
e are required after the majority of general surgery procedures

5 Nutrition and the surgical patient

Bryan R. Parry and Andrew G. Hill

Introduction

There have been many improvements in the treatment of surgical patients during the 20th and early 21st century, leading to better safety, survival and scope of operative procedures. These improvements include anaesthesia, asepsis, blood transfusion, antibiotics, ventilatory support and parenteral nutrition. Nutritional advances have developed in parallel with a growing understanding of the metabolic response in injury and sepsis. This research field has recently been energised by new discoveries and techniques in molecular biology. The discovery that cytokines have effects as biological response modifiers, in addition to their immunologic mediatory role, the putative role of oxygen free radicals, and the identification of other mediators of the inflammatory response have been central to these developments. Knowledge of metabolism and expertise in nutrition are increasingly part of the stock-in-trade of the modern surgeon.

Nutrition features low in the body's homeostatic economy. Its priorities are oxygen delivery, regulation of acid–base balance and maintenance of fluid compartments. Threats to oxygen delivery are dealt with almost instantaneously by changes in minute ventilatory volume, alterations of cardiac output, and better efficiency in oxygen uptake and extraction by tissues. Acid–base abnormalities take longer to adjust, with both acute (buffering) and chronic (excretion) mechanisms. Changes in extracellular (including intravascular) and intracellular compartment volumes occur even more slowly, with the temporising expedient of intercompartmental fluxes.

The body's adjustments to starvation are slow, perhaps understandably, because they are not immediately life threatening. Nevertheless these changes are profound and critical to survival. Defective responses to nutritional deprivation are a major cause of morbidity and mortality in the surgical setting, complicated as it often is by sepsis and the response to injury. These subtle and drawn-out events can be overlooked by the clinician, resulting in a more protracted, and even jeopardised, surgical convalescence.

Body composition

The energy stores and body composition of an average 40-year-old man weighing 73 kg are shown in Table 5.1.

Fat represents a high-energy source and can be hydrolysed to free fatty acids and glycerol. The metabolism of fat produces 9.4 kcal of energy per gram. Forty-five per cent of body protein is structural and not available for metabolic interchange, while the remaining 55% is contained in cells and circulating proteins. If this protein is lost it leads to loss of function, including muscle weakness and immune deficiency. The body's stores of carbohydrate are low and act as a rapid-response provider of glucose, particularly in stress situations. The ratio of the fat-free mass (total bodyweight minus fat) to total body water (fat-free body hydration) is remarkably constant in a healthy person, but varies markedly in illness states.

Table 5.1 Energy stores and body composition in a 40-year-old 73-kg male

	Mass (kg)	Available energy (kcal)
Water	42	0
Fat	15	110 000
Protein	12	25 000
Glycogen	0.6	2 500
Minerals	3.4	0

Nutritional syndromes

Malnutrition and its complications are common but often unrecognised in surgical patients. Severe malnutrition can be defined as measured weight being greater than 20% less than recalled 'well' weight. Approximately 5% of patients coming to surgery are severely malnourished, and malnutrition is present to varying degrees in up to 50% of patients who have undergone surgery.

Studies of malnourished children, particularly in the context of developing countries, have recognised two broad syndromes of malnutrition that can be usefully transposed to the adult surgical setting. The first is marasmus, due to inadequate intake of an otherwise balanced diet (Table 5.2). In the adult this is manifested as cachexia and is commonly termed protein–energy malnutrition (PEM).

The second entity is kwashiorkor, which results from an inadequate as well as unbalanced diet containing relatively more calories than protein (Table 5.2). There is characteristic fluid retention, which may mask the commonly seen and often rapid erosion of muscle and fat stores. In the adult this is seen accompanying sepsis and after trauma.

Pathogenesis of metabolic events

In starvation, glycogen is initially broken down to produce glucose, to maintain brain function. However, glycogen is rapidly exhausted and in marasmus the body undergoes an important change, over several days, to use ketone bodies (keto-adaptation) from fat as brain fuel. This important adaptation preserves muscle protein. In sepsis and trauma, however, this does not occur and protein is catabolised to provide gluconeogenic precursors (glutamine and alanine), which in turn produce the glucose needed for the glucose-obligate tissues (including a healing wound). Accompanying this is a decrease in protein anabolism, and accelerated fat breakdown. In severe sepsis and burns this protein catabolism is even more marked and energy expenditure massively increases, fuelled by intense free fatty acid oxidation.

The metabolic response to injury is complex and was first described more than 60 years ago. However, in the past 15 years an explosion in knowledge of this field has led to important new therapeutic possibilities.

Initially it was thought that the metabolic response to injury was a neuroendocrine response, as within a few minutes of beginning an operation the level of counter-regulatory hormones (cortisol, glucagon and catecholamines) rises. In uncomplicated surgery these act only to initiate protein catabolism, as the endocrine response is relatively short-lived (lasting 24–48 hours). However protein catabolism continues for up to 1 month after major surgery. This has perplexed investigators, but recently, with advances in molecular biology, it has become clear that proinflammatory cytokines (e.g. tumour necrosis factor–alpha (TNF-α), interleukin (IL)-1, IL-6, IL-8) are important mediators of ongoing protein catabolism in injury and sepsis. These probably act locally, at the site of injury, and indirectly (via the bloodstream and in the central nervous system). Imbalances between pro- and anti-inflammatory cytokines also probably play a role

Table 5.2 Comparisons between marasmus and kwashiorkor

	Marasmus	Kwashiorkor
Nutritional defect	Impaired delivery	Impaired utilisation
Protein catabolism	Compensated	Uncompensated
Aetiology	No food	Sepsis
	No appetite	Major trauma
	Gut blocked, short, inflamed or fistulated	Burns
Metabolic rate	Normal or reduced	Increased
Prognosis if untreated	Months	Weeks
Principles of treatment	Replenish with standard nutrition	Resuscitate and support
	Use simplest available route	Control sepsis
	Treat underlying illnesses, if any	Provide non-standard nutritional regimens
Clinical course	Straightforward	Complicated

in anorexia, pyrexia, fatigue, and fat catabolism. Arachidonic acid metabolites, oxygen free radicals and nitric oxide are also important mediators.

Contributions of the disease

The disease itself may play an important role in malnutrition associated with surgical illness. Gastrointestinal disease can produce obstruction, malabsorption and fistulas. Inflammatory mediators associated with the inflammatory phlegmon may secondarily lead to PEM and worsen fluid and electrolyte disturbances. AIDS leads to severe cachexia, similar to that seen in cancer. This is probably mediated by cytokines such as TNF-α and is complicated by chronic infection and malignancies. In cancer there is a rise in resting energy expenditure and the tumour avidly retains nitrogen as well as operating at a glucose-wasteful, high rate of anaerobic metabolism. Unlike the situation in experimental animal models, these tumour effects are unlikely to explain the degree of cachexia often seen in humans. Cancer-induced anorexia and host cytokine production are probably involved.

Complications of the metabolic response to injury and malnutrition

Malnutrition is complicated by immune incompetence and decreased wound healing ability. Protein–energy metabolism may be accompanied by physiological changes such as poor muscle function, manifest as physical weakness and poor respiratory muscle function. These changes increase the likelihood of postoperative pneumonia and difficulty in weaning from ventilators.

Fatigue is a common concomitant of surgical illness and is characterised by prolonged mental and physical tiredness. After surgery it is most pronounced at 1 week, and slowly improves for up to 3 months. It is worse in the elderly, in patients who were tired prior to surgery, and in patients with cancer. It appears to have an important psychological component because it only occurs in humans.

Nutritional assessment

There is no single clinical or laboratory test that defines nutritional status exactly (Box 5.1). The aim of nutritional assessment is to define how much the patient has lost from his or her body stores of protein and fat and, as a corollary, how much remains. Some sort of assessment of physiological impairment is important, as it has been found that the PEM is clinically significant only when associated with impairment of physiological function.

Box 5.1 Some nutritional markers for nutritional assessment

- Clinical history
- Dietary history
- Skinfold thickness: biceps, triceps, subscapular
- Mid-arm muscle circumference
- Skin recall antigens
- Total lymphocyte count
- Serum albumin

Nutritional assessment begins with a careful clinical evaluation. Important features of the history are weight loss greater than 10% during the past 3 months and a change in exercise tolerance. Physical examination may reveal non-healing wounds, oedema and fistulas.

Body composition is assessed by simple clinical tests and a standard blood test. Loss of body fat is often apparent from observations of the patient but is also assessed by palpating the triceps' and biceps' skinfolds. If the dermis can be felt between finger and thumb then it is likely that the body mass is composed of less than 10% fat.

Protein stores are assessed by observation and palpation of the temporalis, deltoids, suprascapular and infrascapular muscles, the bellies of biceps and triceps and the interossei of the hands. If the tendons are palpable or the bony shoulder girdle is sharply outlined (tendon–bone test) then the patient is likely to have lost more than 30% of total body protein stores.

Plasma albumin levels are of assistance in determining the type of PEM. In kwashiorkor, the albumin may be low, reflecting the expansion of the extracellular fluid space, and this may manifest clinically as pitting oedema.

Assessment of physiological function is of vital importance because weight loss without evidence of physiological abnormality is probably of no consequence. Function is observed while performing a physical examination and then by watching the patient's activity on the ward. Grip strength is assessed and respiratory muscle strength is assessed by asking the patient to

Table 5.3 A standard nutritional impairment record

Energy and protein balance		Normal/mild	Moderate	Severe
Weight loss (degree and pattern) (for 3 months)		<10%	>10–20%	>20%
Meal size, frequency and type (for 3 months)			2/3 size	1/3 size
Output (vomiting, diarrhoea, stoma)				
Summary				
Body composition		Normal/mild	Moderate	Severe
Fat store depletion (finger–thumb test)				
Protein store depletion (tendon–bone test)				
Oedema				
Albumin		35–47 g/L	<35 g/L	<30 g/L
Summary				
Physiologic function		Normal/Mild	Moderate	Severe
Exercise tolerance/watching the patient's activity				
Grip strength (squeeze examiner's fingers)				
Respiratory function (blow a strip of paper)				
Shortness of breath, respiratory excursion				
Wound healing: unhealed wounds, scratches or sores, and infection				
Summary				
Metabolic stress		Normal/Mild	Moderate	Severe
Temperature >38°C in past 24 hours	( )	Pulse rate 100/min in past 24 hours		( )
WCC 12 000 or 3000 in past 24 hours	( )	Respiratory rate 30/min in past 24 hours		( )
Positive blood culture	( )	Surgery, trauma and sepsis		( )
Defined focus of infection	( )	Active inflammatory bowel disease		( )
Summary				
Type of protein energy malnutrition				
Normal ( ) Marasmus ( ) Marasmus/Kwashiorkor ( ) Kwashiorkor ( )				
Severity of protein energy malnutrition				
Normal/Mild ( ) Moderate ( ) Severe ( )				
Nutritional metabolic goal				

blow hard holding a strip of paper 10 cm from the lips. Severe impairment is present when the paper fails to move.

Metabolic stress will be revealed by history and examination. It is present if the patient has had major surgery or trauma in the preceding week and where there is evidence of sepsis or ongoing inflammation, such as inflammatory bowel disease.

These findings are recorded on a standard form (an example is shown in Table 5.3) and an assessment of the type of nutritional impairment is made. Marasmic patients will have weight loss greater than 10% and normal albumin, and will resemble a 'walking skeleton'. Patients with kwashiorkor have suffered from major trauma or serious sepsis and are not eating. There will be clear signs of major metabolic stress, albumin will be low and oedema is likely to be present. They may have near-normal stores of muscle and fat but this will not last for long if the situation persists. A mixture of the two conditions is termed marasmic kwashiorkor.

Determining the intensity and type of malnutrition is of great importance in setting nutritional goals. When PEM is severe and affects physiological function, post-operative complications are more common and post-operative stay is prolonged. The identification of metabolic stress is also important; because the extracellular water is expanded the response to standard nutritional intervention is impaired and the type of malnutrition is predictable.

Nutritional intervention

The principles of nutritional intervention are summarised in Box 5.2.

Box 5.2 Principles of nutritional intervention

- Pre-operative nutrition is indicated in severely malnourished patients.
- Post-operative total parenteral nutrition is provided if a normal intake has not been established within 5–7 days for a depleted patient and 7–10 days for a normal patient.
- When possible, enteral nutrition is preferred over parenteral nutrition.
- A variety of metabolic modulators are under development.

Indications for nutritional intervention

Nutritional intervention is indicated prior to surgery only in severely malnourished patients with physiological impairment. Nutritional support is required in patients who cannot eat, in whom intake is insufficient for their needs, in whom the gastrointestinal tract cannot be used, and in those with accelerated losses (Table 5.4).

There are six components of adequate nutrition: protein, water, energy (as fat and carbohydrate), electrolytes, minerals and vitamins (Table 5.5).

The requirements for these different components vary according to the patient and the clinical condition. A detailed discussion regarding this complex topic is beyond this text and interested readers are referred to the recommended reading list.

Intravenous nutrition

Intravenous nutrition (also known as total parenteral nutrition (TPN) is useful if the gut is obstructed, too short, fistulated, inflamed or simply cannot cope, such as in post-operative ileus. Total parenteral nutrition is administered by a dedicated central venous catheter inserted under sterile conditions. Central venous catheter infection is potentially life threatening and therefore care must be meticulous. Approximately 50 kcal/kg bodyweight per day and 0.3 g of nitrogen as amino acids per kilogram per day is required to achieve gain in body protein. Use of nutritional intervention must be preceded by correction of anaemia, hypoalbuminaemia, fluid and electrolyte abnormalities, and deficits in trace metals. Vitamins must be dealt with by appropriate infusions so that administered nutrients will be used efficiently.

In certain situations, intravenous nutrition can be administered by peripheral infusion. This is not common because it is not possible to provide full energy intake using this technique and it requires frequent intravenous catheter changes.

Enteral nutrition

In circumstances where the gut is functional, enteral nutrition should be used. Enteral nutrition may be important in maintaining gut barrier function, demonstrated to be of critical importance in laboratory models. Enteral nutrition is administered by mouth if possible (as high-energy nutritional supplements), but may also be delivered by a fine-bore feeding tube introduced under fluoroscopic control or using an endoscope. Fine tubes can also be placed into the jejunum at surgery and feeding can begin in the recovery room after the operation is complete. If prolonged enteral feeding is anticipated, a gastrostomy should be created, usually via the percutaneous endoscopic route.

Table 5.4 Indications for nutritional intervention in surgical patients

Indications for pre-operative nutrition	Indications for total parenteral nutrition	Indications for enteral nutrition
Severe malnutrition with physiological impairment	Gut is obstructed Gut is short Gut is fistulated Gut is inflamed Gut cannot cope	Malnutrition with a functioning gut Post-operative feeding

Table 5.5 Components of a nutrition regimen for 25- to 55-year-olds per day

Component	Requirement in health	Requirement after major surgery
Protein	1.0–1.5 g/kg	1.5–2.0 g/kg
Water	40 mL/kg	Variable according to losses
Energy	40 kcal/kg	40 kcal/kg
Electrolytes	75 mmol sodium 50 mmol potassium	Variable according to losses
Minerals	15 mEq calcium 40 mmol phosphate 10 mEq magnesium	Variable according to losses
Vitamins	B group, C, fat soluble	Some vitamins may be of benefit in surgical illness

Metabolic response modification

Although provision of adequate nutrition to patients, both pre-operatively and post-operatively, has been of immense benefit, it has proven difficult for the injured patient to gain nitrogen. Several advances in the past few years have made this goal achievable and there have been important improvements in patient recovery.

With the recognition of the importance of glutamine, several studies have demonstrated that it is beneficial to include this amino acid in solutions administered to patients. Other amino acids have important roles in particular states, such as liver and renal failure. The role of growth hormone may be shown to be important in the future, and recently its usefulness in enabling patients to become anabolic earlier has been demonstrated. Anticytokine therapy awaits a better understanding of cytokine biology, and single-agent trials have so far been disappointing. This probably relates to the complexity of cytokine production and function, and the sites of action of cytokines in injury and sepsis.

Several recent studies from Europe have shown that specialised immune-enhancing formulas improve immune function, modulate cytokine production, decrease wound infections, and improve patient recovery in patients undergoing major surgery.

Epidural anaesthesia blocks much of the early stress response to surgery and this has been postulated to be of critical importance in slowing protein loss. What may be of more importance is the mobility that epidural anaesthesia permits the surgical patient in the immediate post-operative period and the ability of the epidural block to limit post-operative ileus.

Non-steroidal anti-inflammatory drugs (NSAID) may be important in preventing arachidonic acid mediated tissue damage, as may nitric oxide inhibition and antioxidants in limiting free oxygen radical damage. These await further evaluation in clinically relevant models.

The current trend toward minimally invasive surgical interventions has led, in many cases, to early recovery from surgery and faster return to work. When these techniques are combined with other modulators, the improvements in post-operative outcome are likely to be quite profound.

Results of nutritional intervention

Short-term pre-operative nutritional intervention in severely compromised patients decreases post-operative complications. The effect is not nearly as apparent in patients with mild to moderate malnutrition. Post-operative nutritional support is one of the most important developments in modern surgery and has allowed surgeons much greater leeway in the management of surgical complications such as fistulas and bowel obstruction.

Recent work has demonstrated that outcome is improved by growth hormone, glutamine-enriched nutrition and epidural anaesthesia. Growth hormone improves post-operative fatigue, and enhances recovery in children with burns. Similarly, minimally invasive surgery results in a faster recovery from surgery and a marked improvement in post-operative fatigue.

In combination, minimally invasive surgery, early mobilisation, NSAID, epidural anaesthesia and early enteral feeding produce dramatic post-operative recovery and return to useful activity.

MCQs

Select the single correct answer to each question.

1 Nutritional markers include the following *except*:
- **a** skin fold thickness
- **b** mid-arm muscle circumference
- **c** total leucocyte count
- **d** serum albumin
- **e** skin recall antigens

2 The requirement for intravenous nutrition per day is:
- **a** 20 kcal/kg body weight
- **b** 30 kcal/kg body weight
- **c** 40 kcal/kg body weight
- **d** 50 kcal/kg body weight
- **e** 60 kcal/kg body weight

3 Marasmus is characterised by the following characteristics *except*:
- **a** inadequate intake of an otherwise balanced diet
- **b** cachexia in the adult
- **c** fluid retention
- **d** decreased metabolic rate
- **e** easy correction with standard nutrition

6 Care of the critically ill patient

Jeffrey J. Presneill and John F. Cade

Introduction to critical illness

Intensive care for complex and potentially life-threatening illness is required by about 2.5% of patients admitted to major Australian hospitals. Intensive care units (ICUs) have been widely available for approximately 30 years, but now there are about 200 ICUs in Australia, of which about 60% are level 3 or the most sophisticated. Intensive care has permitted the survival from many types of hitherto fatal illness or injury, with the interesting consequence that pathophysiological responses are now seen which could never have originally been adaptive and which may in turn lead to new therapeutic opportunities.

Intensive care is inevitably expensive, but about 85% of patients survive, most with good quality, long-term outcomes (Figure 6.1). Coexistent medical conditions substantially influence patient outcome. Prognosis is obviously worsened when there is coexistent ischaemic heart disease, diabetes, peripheral vascular disease, severe chronic obstructive airways disease or malignancy. In the absence of these co-morbidities, advanced age is not a major independent factor in short-term prognosis. Reliable prediction of patient outcome would greatly assist patient selection, clinical management and resource allocation, but models of mortality prediction based statistically on scoring systems for critical illness are suitable so far only for group comparisons and not for individual patient assessment.

Causes of critical illness

The chief categories of causes of critical illness and thus admission to ICU are shown in the figure.

Severe infection remains the most common and concerning problem in the care of seriously ill patients in hospital. It provides the most important link between either underlying or complicating illness and serious conditions such as circulatory failure, respiratory failure and organ failure. The definitions of infection and related phenomena such as sepsis and septic shock are shown in Figure 6.1. Clinically suspected sepsis occurs in approximately 10% of ICU admissions and has a mortality of 5% to 20%. Severe sepsis and septic shock has a mortality of 35% to 65% despite antimicrobial therapy and intensive life support. Survivors of severe sepsis commonly require prolonged hospitalisation due to post-sepsis multiple organ dysfunction.

The incidence of sepsis is thought to be so high because of continually emerging antibiotic resistance of micro-organisms and because of the complex and invasive procedures on increasingly sick patients that characterise modern hospital practice. The most commonly isolated organisms are *Staphylococcus aureus*, *Staphylococcus epidermidis*, *Streptococcus pneumoniae*, *Streptococcus pyogenes*, various enterococci, Gram-negative bacilli and *Candida* spp. When sepsis is suspected but the site remains unknown despite an appropriately thorough clinical investigation, the abdomen and lungs are the two most likely sites, together with intravascular catheters if such are in place.

The bodily responses to sepsis are indistinguishable from those due to non-infective inflammation or indeed to severe injury itself. The systemic response to injury in general is referred to as the systemic inflammatory response syndrome (SIRS) (Table 6.1). The definition of SIRS describes a widespread inflammatory response to a variety of clinical insults, not all of which necessarily involve bacterial infection. The constellation of clinical, haematological, and biochemical signs typically found in the presence of infection can often be observed in the absence of any identifiable infection, as with pancreatitis, trauma, burns, rhabdomyolysis, necrotic tissue and cardiopulmonary bypass.

Over the last 10 years, detailed study of the timing and associations of elevated levels of cytokines,

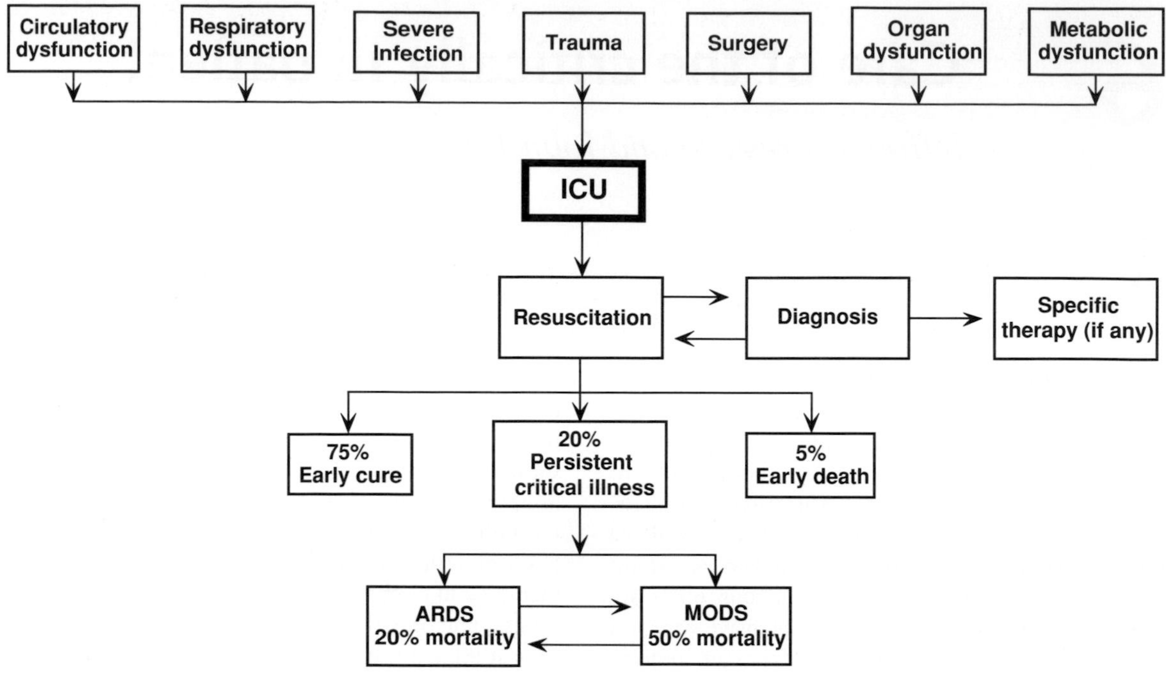

Fig. 6.1 Pathways of critical illness.

eicosanoids, oxygen radicals, proteases and autacoids in the plasma of patients with septic shock has advanced our understanding of this complex and potentially lethal clinical state, which may represent an imbalance among the various host responses to tissue injury. Experimental investigations have shown that interruption of the complex inflammatory mediator cascade can lead to striking benefits in a wide variety of animal models of infection or uncontrolled inflammation. However, until recently it has been a recurrent finding from Phase III human studies that these apparent benefits are either not confirmed or are sufficiently modest in magnitude that clinical application of the therapeutic strategy is not worthwhile. The first agent to convincingly overcome this therapeutic barrier may be the biopharmaceutical agent drotrecogin alfa (activated) [recombinant human activated protein C]. This very expensive therapy has been associated with a 20% relative reduction in mortality from severe sepsis.

Resuscitation

The key to resuscitation is that it must be prompt and complete, with restoration and maintenance of an adequate circulating blood volume (i.e., treatment of hypovolaemia). This is a fundamental requirement in all seriously ill patients. Without adequate blood volume expansion, inotropes and other therapies are less likely to be effective, and organ function is compromised. The choice of fluids for acute resuscitation is less important and remains controversial, with no universal recommendation able to be made except that replacement of losses should usually reflect the major deficit caused by the underlying disease process. Both crystalloids (e.g. 0.9% sodium chloride, compound sodium lactate or Hartmann's solution) and colloids (e.g. 4% albumin, polygeline) are available, as well as hypertonic saline (3%) and blood products. Saline 0.9% or albumin 4% in saline 0.9% have been demonstrated to result in equivalent patient outcomes from critical illness, although the overall ratio of the volume of albumin to the volume of saline administered was approximately 1 : 1.4.

Fluid resuscitation may need to be substantial because, in addition to obvious losses and to anticipated third-space needs, there is often extra volume required due to vasodilatation, capillary leak and blood flow maldistribution. Fluid resuscitation is complete if blood flow is restored (i.e. the haemodynamic goal) or

Table 6.1 Definitions in sepsis*

Infection	A microbial phenomenon characterised by an inflammatory response to the presence of microorganisms or the invasion of normally sterile host tissue by those organisms.
Bacteremia	The presence of viable bacteria in the blood.
	Similarly, for other classes of microorganisms including fungi, viruses, parasites and protozoa.
SIRS	Systemic Inflammatory Response Syndrome
	Consisting of two or more of the following: temperature >38°C or <36°C, heart rate >90 beats/min, respiratory rate >20 breaths/min or $Paco_2$ <32 mm Hg, leukocyte count >12 000 cells/mm^3 to <4000 cells/mm^3, or >10% immature (band) forms.
Sepsis	SIRS as a result infection.
	Infection is often clinically diagnosed and the absence of positive cultures does not exclude the diagnosis.
Severe sepsis	Sepsis associated with organ dysfunction, such as coagulation abnormalities, altered mental status, or oliguria
Shock	Hypotension, defined as a systolic blood pressure <90 mm Hg or a reduction of >40 mm Hg from baseline in the absence of other causes for hypotension (such as anaesthesia or antihypertensive medication).
	Studies may require this condition to be present for a definite period, often >1 h.
Septic shock	*Sepsis* with *shock*, despite adequate fluid resuscitation, along with the presence of organ dysfunction and perfusion abnormalities that may include, but are not limited to, lactic acidosis, oliguria, or an acute alteration in mental status. An adequate fluid challenge was not defined, but many studies have specified an intravenous infusion of isotonic fluid, colloid, or blood products to restore the effective circulating blood volume. Other studies nominate a volume of 500 mL to satisfy this criterion. Patients who are receiving inotropic or vasopressor agents may not be hypotensive at the time that perfusion abnormalities are measured.

* Septicaemia is no longer a recommended term as it was thought to be ambiguous (for practical purposes it was a synonym of sepsis).

if cardiac filling pressures are maximised, whichever is first. If a satisfactory haemodynamic goal has not been achieved despite maximised cardiac filling pressures and thus repair of hypovolaemia, inotrope therapy is required if myocardial contractility is impaired and/or vasopressor therapy is required if blood pressure is inadequate (e.g. in the low systemic vascular resistance syndrome). In complex situations, sophisticated haemodynamic monitoring is used to ensure that normovolaemia is achieved and maintained and to guide added pharmacological therapy.

Organ dysfunction and failure

Current functional assessment of organ damage emphasises a continuum of progressively worsening organ dysfunction rather than an arbitrary division between normality and failure. Thus, older terms such as 'multiple organ failure' (MOF) or 'multiple system organ failure' (MSOF) have been replaced by the broader term 'multiple organ dysfunction syndrome' (MODS). Except for the acute respiratory distress syndrome (ARDS), which is the pulmonary manifestation of MODS and which has precise (though still arbitrary) definitions set by international consensus, MODS has no universally agreed set of definitions. These definitional difficulties arise primarily because of incomplete understanding of the complex pathogenesis of MODS.

The incidence of MODS varies greatly with the patient group being considered. In uncomplicated surgery, it is rare. In serious and complicated surgical conditions, such as trauma, haemorrhage, sepsis, necrosis or shock, it is 5% to 10%. In uncontrolled sepsis, it is much higher. Available prophylaxis only halves its incidence in the patient groups at risk.

In humans, the organs most affected histologically are in descending order: the lungs, liver, kidney, heart, gut, brain, pancreas and adrenals, though it is likely that most if not all of the tissues and organs of the body are similarly affected. If the blood is considered an 'organ', it too undergoes profound change with the process of disseminated intravascular coagulation. If the endothelial cells are considered together, they bear much of the brunt of the systemic process, with microcirculatory dysfunction and consequent capillary leak, interstitial oedema and even haemorrhage, and later cellular infiltration.

The clinical manifestations are sequentially the systemic inflammatory response syndrome, a hyperdynamic circulatory state and hypermetabolic state, and then, after a latent period, respiratory dysfunction (within 48 h), liver and kidney dysfunction (within 1 week), persistent coma, gut dysfunction (with not only ileus and stress ulceration but also loss of barrier function and thus bacterial translocation), and nosocomial infection (initially respiratory, urinary and wound colonization and later bacteraemia and intravascular catheter infection).

The clinical picture of MODS thus progresses over about 3 weeks, by which time about half the patients will have died. Clearly, the earlier the underlying causative process is controlled, the earlier the clinical course can be aborted and the better the prognosis. Wound healing is sometimes said to give a partial guide to the progress of concomitant organ repair. The average mortality is about 50%, with most deaths occurring by 3 to 4 weeks. The mortality is higher (60%) if septic shock is present; it also increases by about 10% for each additional organ in clinical failure.

However, MODS is potentially reversible, although at the cost of complex, expensive and prolonged treatment. The average ICU stay is about a month and survivors have an average time to full rehabilitation of about 1 year.

Management of the critically ill

The detailed management of the critically ill patient is the subject of a vast literature and of many textbooks, some of them huge. But the general principles are straightforward, although their implementation can be complex and sophisticated.

- Resuscitation and maintenance of an optimal blood volume is just as much a continuing priority as it is an initial goal in the treatment of the critically ill (as discussed previously). The maintenance of an adequate circulatory state is an ongoing task.
- Treatment of respiratory impairment, together with circulatory management, comprise the twin pillars of life support in the ICU. Abnormalities of gas exchange and of pulmonary mechanics are common and are often severe. Specialised and sophisticated mechanical ventilation is the ultimate mainstay of respiratory support.
- After initial resuscitation, and while circulatory and respiratory support are in train, early diagnosis and specific therapy (if any) are required. In particular, early and complete source control is essential.
- There is much emphasis on the treatment of initial sepsis and on the prevention and treatment of complicating infections.
- Metabolic support is essential, because malnutrition can develop rapidly and is a covariable in mortality and because adequate nutrition is required for tissue repair. Enteral nutrition is preferred if technically feasible.
- Renal support may require renal replacement therapy (most commonly nowadays with extracorporeal continuous venovenous haemodiafiltration (CVVHDF).
- Psychosocial support is important both for the patient and the family. The patient needs analgesia, anxiolysis, comfort and dignity, and the family needs access, information and support.
- Intensive care requires continuous patient management by a highly skilled multidisciplinary team in a specialised environment. Meticulous attention to detail is necessary to identify problems and therapeutic opportunities as early as possible. In general, much of the care of the critically ill is founded on complex physiological support, which buys time for healing to occur.

Further reading

Dellinger RP, Carlet JM, Masur H, et al. Surviving sepsis campaign guidelines for the management of severe sepsis and septic shock. *Crit Care Med.* March 2004; 32(3): 858–873. Erratum in: Crit Care Med 2004 Jun; 32(6):1448. Correction of dosage error in text.

Bersten AD, Soni N, Oh TE, eds. *Oh's Intensive Care Manual.* 5th ed. Edinburgh: Butterworth-Heinemann; 2003.

Irwin RS, Rippe JM, eds. *Irwin and Rippe's Intensive Care Medicine.* 5th ed. Philadelphia: Lippincott Williams & Wilkins; 2003.

MCQs

Select the single correct answer to each question.

1 Treatment of critically ill patients in an intensive care unit:
  a increases the cost of care but does not improve the prognosis
  b is associated with a 50% survival rate overall
  c is associated with a 15% death rate overall
  d is required for 25% of all hospital patients at some point in their illness
  e is not indicated for any patient over 80 years of age

2 Infection in critical illness is:
  a almost always followed by dysfunction in multiple organ systems
  b only able to be diagnosed in the presence of septic shock
  c rarely associated with septic shock
  d rarely caused by common bacteria
  e often found in the lungs or abdomen

3 The systemic inflammatory response syndrome:
  a consists of at least two from a list of four categories of physiological and haematological abnormality
  b nearly always implies the presence of invasive bacterial or fungal infection
  c rarely occurs after cardiopulmonary bypass procedures
  d helps in the clinical differential diagnosis between infection types
  e is associated with more than a 50% mortality rate

4 Intravenous fluid resuscitation of hypotensive, hypovolaemic critically ill patients should be:
  a slow and gentle using only colloids
  b rapid and partial using crystalloids only
  c slow and complete using colloids only
  d rapid and complete using crystalloids or colloids or both
  e composed mostly of a solution of 4% albumin

5 Commonly applied critical care organ support involves all except one of the following:
  a mechanical ventilation for hypercarbia
  b vasopressor infusions for low cardiac output states
  c haemodiafiltration for uraemia
  d platelet transfusion for thrombocytopaenia
  e inotropic infusions for low cardiac output states

7 Surgical infections

John C. Hall

Introduction

Infection is the main enemy of the surgeon. There are a number of reasons for this:

- cosmetic and functional outcomes after surgery are compromised by infection
- trauma often results in infection due to the contamination and devitalisation of tissues
- deep infections in mesothelial cavities are life threatening
- lives can be ruined by careless exposure to blood-borne viruses.

Those who care for surgical patients can never be complacent in their efforts to diminish the risk of infection. The main ways of achieving this are:

- the washing of hands
- adherence to antiseptic and asepsis rituals
- aggressive attention to basic surgical principles
- compliance with antibiotic guidelines
- patiently accepting the measures that are necessary to prevent the spread of resistant organisms
- the adoption of universal precautions to prevent diseases due to blood-borne viruses.

In this chapter, particular emphasis is placed upon the prevention and management of infections related to surgical procedures.

Acute infection

Surgical infections occur because of a breakdown of the equilibrium that exists between organisms and the host. This may be due to a breach in a protective surface, changes in host resistance, or particular characteristics of the organism. The possible outcomes are resolution, abscess formation, extensive local spread with or without tissue death, and distant spread.

Host defence mechanisms

Areas of the body that are in contact with an external environment are protected by elaborate barrier mechanisms. Parts of these barriers are mechanical in nature, such as the keratinised layer of skin. Such physical barriers are augmented by powerful innate immune mechanisms (e.g. the low pH and fatty acid content of normal skin inhibits bacterial growth). An additional factor is that all mucous membranes are protected by lymphocyte-mediated events that result in the secretion of immunoglobulin A (IgA) antibodies. In the gut, the rapid turnover of the mucosal cells along the crypto–villus axis has a protective function because enteropathogens must adhere to enterocytes in order to cause clinical problems.

Tissue injury stimulates a cascade of events that lead to the formation of granulation tissue and eventual healing. However, extensive tissue damage inhibits the inflammatory response (e.g. the low oxygen tensions in poorly vascularised tissues impairs the oxidative killing of microbes by phagocytes). Damaged tissue also forms a nidus for bacterial growth. These factors explain the need to debride wounds in order to avoid infection.

The response of the body to microbes can be affected by immunodeficiencies of genetic origin (which are rare) or by acquired deficiencies (e.g. protein-energy undernutrition; diseases such as diabetes, cancer and AIDS; or by the administration of immunosuppressive or cytotoxic drugs). Infections often arise in immunocompromised individuals with microbes that are not usually regarded as pathogens (e.g. opportunistic infections caused by *Candida albicans* and fungi).

The organisms

The pathogenicity of microbes is determined by their capacity to adhere to and damage host cells, and then to produce and release a variety of enzymes and exotoxins. *Staphylococcus* has surface receptors that allow it to bind to host cells and extracellular matrix proteins, especially those covered by protein A molecules, which bind to the Fc portion of antibodies. *Streptococcus* and *Haemophilus* secrete proteases that degrade antibodies, and other enzymes such as haemolysins and kinases that assist in the spread of infection in the form of cellulitis or erysipelas. *Escherichia coli* carries K-antigen, which prevents the activation of complement via the alternate pathway.

Foreign bodies increase the pathogenicity of microbes by impairing local defence mechanisms. It is important to explore deep wounds adequately in order to remove foreign bodies and devitalised tissues. This is a critical issue because the use of antibiotics is no substitute for poor surgical technique. It should also be appreciated that although prosthetic materials are made of 'inert materials' they are still foreign bodies, and it is difficult to control associated infections without removing the offending prosthesis. Examples of this range from infected central venous lines to infected vascular grafts and orthopaedic implants.

Cellulitis

Cellulitis is a spreading inflammation of connective tissues that is often due to β-haemolytic *Streptococcus*. The invasiveness of this organism is due to the production of hyaluronidase (dissolution of the intercellular matrix) and streptokinase (dissolution of the fibrin inflammatory barrier). Cellulitis may be accompanied by obvious inflammation of the draining lymphatics (lymphangitis) and the draining lymph nodes (lymphadenitis). There may also be associated septicaemia. The treatment is immobilisation with elevation, antibiotic therapy, and drainage of any residual abscesses.

There is a group of patients who present with cellulitis of the lower limb complicating lymphoedema from any cause. There is usually no obvious entry site for bacteria, the cellulitis tends to be low grade and brawny in nature, and it is usually slow to recover to antibiotic therapy. Compression stockings are a useful long-term measure, but recurrence is common.

Abscesses

An abscess is a localised collection of pus. Abscesses start as inflammatory lesions, which then soften and become fluctuant because of the presence of liquefied tissues and the remnants of the inflammatory response. The only effective treatment for abscesses is drainage. In the absence of therapeutic drainage, abscesses may discharge spontaneously onto the surface or into an adjacent viscus or body cavity (e.g. a colo-vesical fistula as a result of a peridiverticular abscess in the sigmoid colon). Deep abscesses can often be localised and drained under the guidance of ultrasound. Antibiotic therapy is appropriate if there is clinical evidence of sepsis. However, failure to drain an abscess in the presence of inappropriate and prolonged antibiotic therapy can result in a troublesome chronic 'smouldering' abscess.

Bacteraemia and septicaemia

Spread of organisms into the bloodstream may be either as a transient bacteraemia, which is asymptomatic, or as septicaemia with symptoms such as fever and chills (sepsis). It should be noted that critically ill patients may exhibit a systemic response, due to cytokines and other biologically active molecules, in the absence of positive blood cultures (Systemic Inflammatory Response Syndrome). The failure of multiple organs in the presence of sepsis is referred to as 'severe sepsis'.

It is advisable to administer antibiotics when draining an abscess because of the associated sepsis and the risk of metastatic infection, especially if the patient has a prosthetic device *in situ* or a damaged heart valve. Other examples of metastatic infection include portal pyaemia with liver abscesses secondary to suppurative appendicitis and a localised staphylococcal infection, such as an infected hair follicle (a boil or furuncle), spreading to multiple systemic sites (e.g. osteomyelitis, brain abscess, perinephric abscess).

Nosocomial infections

Nosocomial infections are infections that are acquired while a patient is in hospital. More than 10% of patients admitted to the surgical wards of large hospitals develop a clinically significant infection. Hence, there is a special need for stringent precautions against cross-infection when caring for debilitated patients undergoing major surgery. Surgical wounds are classified into categories to aid the monitoring and interpretation of wound infection rates (Box 7.1).

Box 7.1 Classification of wounds

- **Clean**: No contamination from exogenous or endogenous sources (the gastrointestinal, urinary, respiratory or genital tracts are not entered). The wound infection rate should be less than 2%.
- **Clean-contaminated**: The gastrointestinal, urinary, respiratory or genital tracts are entered under controlled conditions. The wound infection rate should be less than 5%.
- **Contaminated**: There is either gross intraoperative soiling, or an emergency procedure involves entry into an unprepared gastrointestinal tract. The wound infection rate may be as high as 30%.
- **Dirty**: The presence of gross soiling prior to surgery (e.g. heavily contaminated wound, faecal peritonitis). The wound infection rate may exceed 30%.

The commonest organisms isolated from hospital-acquired infections are *Staphylococcus aureus* and a range of Gram-negative bacilli. Multiple antibiotic resistance is a particular problem. Besides multi-drug-resistant *Staphylococcus aureus*, Gram-negative organisms may become resistant to many of the antibiotics in common use. Cross-infection can occur by many routes, but of particular concern are those caused by the inappropriate activity of the attending medical staff. The main problems are failure to wash hands between attending patients (which is the single most important preventative measure), not employing antiseptic and asepsis techniques when performing ward procedures, and the careless management of infected wounds.

Wound infections

Wound infection is usually defined as the discharge of either pus or serous fluid containing pathogens. However, on occasions, cellulitis can cause considerable morbidity, such as after breast surgery. The main factors associated with wound infection are the extent of intraoperative soiling (as discussed in the classification of wounds), the presence of pre-existing co-morbidity (diseases and situations associated with immunodeficiency), age (the risk escalates when patients are over 70 years of age), and the performance of major surgery. A useful global measure of co-morbidity is the American Society of Anesthesia (ASA) classification, which is routinely recorded by many anaesthetists (see Chapter 2).

The prevention of wound infection relates to the avoidance of contamination and the judicious use of antibiotics. Strict adherence to aseptic techniques is essential, but it is now appreciated that aggressive 'scrubbing up' is counterproductive because it results in bacteria being brought to the surface of the skin. In addition, unless performed immediately prior to surgery, removing hair by razor causes skin abrasions that become colonised with bacteria leading to an increased incidence of wound infection. Post-operative dressings should be left in place for at least 24 hours after surgery; after this time wounds are relatively impervious to external contamination.

Wound infections need to be adequately drained, and this often means that it is necessary to open part of the wound. It is inappropriate to try to drain a large subcutaneous collection of pus or infected fluid through a small opening in the skin. Antibiotic usage should be in accord with the principles that apply to other abscesses.

Urinary tract infection

Urinary tract infections can occur after either instrumentation of the urinary tract or the insertion of a urethral catheter. Urinary catheters are foreign bodies that irritate the urethral mucosa and predispose to the colonisation of urine with bacteria. They must only be used for a good reason and then removed as soon as possible. Urinary tract infections may present as a pyrexia of unknown origin during the post-operative period, and the temperature may be in excess of 38°C; a characteristic that only tends to be shared with atelectasis and phlebitis. Many patients experience transitory dysuria after the removal of a urethral catheter and resolution of this problem may be aided by the induction of a mild diuresis.

Phlebitis

Intravenous cannulae, especially those used for the infusion of hypertonic nutrients and drugs, are particularly prone to infection. It is important to observe strict asepsis when inserting intravenous cannulae because it has been reported that one-third of them can become colonised with bacteria within 48 hours. The risk of phlebitis increases in an exponential manner after cannulae are left *in situ* for more than 72 hours.

Intravenous cannulae, as with other indwelling devices, are foreign bodies and should be removed as soon as possible. If removal is not possible then they should be changed to another site within 72 hours; this is only possible if the time of their insertion has been carefully documented.

Enterocolitis

The normal flora of the gut is altered by the use of broad-spectrum antibiotics, the stasis that accompanies a lack of peristalsis after abdominal surgery, and the acquisition of organisms that are prevalent within hospitals. These factors increase the likelihood of overgrowth by enteropathogens such as *Clostridium difficile* (so named because of the difficulty of growing it in culture), which secretes toxins responsible for symptoms that range from mild watery diarrhoea to profound diarrhoea associated with a florid colitis. The latter is characterised by the presence of creamy fibrinous plaques that coalesce to form a pseudomembrane (pseudomembranous colitis). Treatment includes the cessation of broad-spectrum antibiotic therapy and the introduction of either oral metronidazole or oral vancomycin. It is essential that stool cultures and toxin assays are performed on all patients with profuse diarrhoea after surgery.

Post-operative pulmonary complications

The vast majority of post-operative pulmonary complications are due to atelectasis, which is usually transitory and self-limiting. This is a mechanical event and antibiotics are contraindicated unless there is objective evidence of infection (e.g. the production of purulent sputum or radiographic evidence of pneumonia).

Antimicrobial therapy

It should be evident that the most important weapons against infection are compliance with infection control measures, adherence to basic surgical principles (debridement of dead tissue, removal of foreign bodies, drainage of pus), and the judicious use of antibiotics. A major step towards the appropriate use of antibiotics is adherence to institutional antibiotic guidelines and, in particular, drawing a clear distinction between prophylaxis and treatment.

Box 7.2 Principles of antibiotic prophylaxis

- The antibiotic should be active against the likely pathogens.
- The antibiotic should be administered so that there are adequate tissue levels at the time of contamination (i.e. before the start of the operation).
- Single-dose prophylaxis is adequate in most settings and prophylaxis should rarely exceed 24 hours.
- The chosen antibiotic should ideally be cheap and with few side effects.

Prophylaxis

Antibiotic prophylaxis is appropriate whenever its benefits outweighs its disadvantages. For example, it is difficult to justify the side effects and costs of administering prophylactic antibiotics for healthy patients undergoing the excision of a skin lesion. In contrast, it would be negligent not to provide antibiotic prophylaxis for a patient undergoing any form of gastrointestinal surgery; afterall, no ethics committee would now agree to an antibiotic trial in such patients that included a 'no treatment' control group. Antibiotic prophylaxis is particularly important if the infection of prosthetic material would be extremely adverse (e.g. joint replacements, vascular prostheses, revisional breast surgery with insertion of an implant). The principles of antibiotic prophylaxis are given in Box 7.2.

Treatment

Treatment courses of antibiotics are used to manage specific infections, but they may also be employed after surgery if there is residual infection (e.g. purulent peritonitis) or if gross contamination occurred at the time of surgery (e.g. spillage of liquid bowel contents).

As a general principle, antibiotic therapy should cease after 5 days when there is no clinical evidence of infection, the patient has been afebrile for 48 hours, and there is a normal polymorphonuclear neutrophil count. The most extreme form of antibiotic therapy relates to 'salvage therapy' within ICUs using powerful broad-spectrum agents, such as imipenum, while waiting for specific culture and sensitivity results. The factors influencing the choice of antibiotic are given in Box 7.3.

Box 7.3 Factors influencing the choice of antibiotic

- The most likely pathogens
- The pharmacology of the candidate agents
- The presence of known allergies or side effects
- The prevalence of antibiotic resistance
- The results of culture and sensitivity tests
- The costs

Resistant microbes

The resistance of Gram-positive and Gram-negative bacteria to antimicrobial agents is a major problem. This is especially so when multi-resistant pathogens cause an outbreak of infection within a hospital. Microbes have evolved elaborate mechanisms to ensure their survival, and resistance strains emerge regardless of innovations in the mechanism of action of new antibiotics. Hence, it is important for surgical staff to be fully compliant with antibiotic guidelines and infection control measures. Antibiotics should never be regarded as 'golden bullets'.

Blood-borne viral infections

The blood-borne viruses that raise special concerns are human immunodeficiency virus (HIV), hepatitis B virus, and hepatitis C virus. They all have the properties of chronicity, transmission via body fluids, and long-term health consequences. The main route of infection in health-care workers is by percutaneous inoculation. There is no evidence of transmission of any of the common blood-borne viruses by the air-borne route or from occupational or social contact that does not involve exposure to body fluids. History suggests that it is wise to presume that other blood-borne viruses will present similar problems in the future.

Universal precautions

It is crucial that all health-care workers recognise how to reduce the risks of exposure to blood-borne viruses. It must be appreciated that it is neither cost-effective nor reliable to embark on routine screening of patients for blood-borne viruses. The concept of universal precautions is based on the reality that it is impossible to identify all patients with a nosocomial virus infection and it is therefore prudent to adopt policies that regard all patients as being potentially infectious. Because percutaneous inoculation is the major route of infection, care must be taken when handling sharp instruments. Sharp instruments should only be passed to others when they are in a rigid container such as a kidney dish and never passed by hand. All sharps should be disposed of into dedicated 'sharps containers', and needles should never be resheathed. Cuts and abrasions should be covered with waterproof dressings, and disposable gloves should be worn if there is a risk of contamination of the hands with blood or any other body fluid. Protective eye-wear and a mask should be worn if there is a risk of splashing with blood or any other body fluid. It is particularly important not to abandon universal precautions during emergencies; this is the time when junior staff are at the greatest risk.

Vaccination

It is important that all health-care workers maintain their immunisation when appropriate vaccines are available. Active immunisation against hepatitis B is available but as yet there is no active immunisation against hepatitis C or HIV.

Exposure

Advice should be sought immediately after exposure to blood or any other body fluid. It is important to commence post-exposure prophylactic drugs for HIV without delay, and ideally within 1 hour of exposure. Most hospitals have an infection control manual that outlines specific requirements and policies relating to blood-borne infections.

MCQs

Select the single correct answer to each question.

1 The best prophylaxis against infection in dirty wounds is achieved by:
- a avoiding the use of local anaesthesia
- b inserting a drain into the wound
- c administering a large dose of an appropriate antibiotic
- d administering tetanus antitoxin
- e removing foreign bodies and devitalised tissues

2 Opportunistic infections caused by *Candida albicans* and fungi are not associated with:
- **a** cancer
- **b** amyloid sclerosis
- **c** diabetes
- **d** the administration of cytotoxic drugs
- **e** the use of immunosuppressant drugs after cardiac transplantation

3 Which of the following is not an example of metastatic infection?
- **a** colo-vesical fistula due to diverticular disease of the colon
- **b** liver abscess after portal pyaemia
- **c** infection in a prosthetic heart valve
- **d** brain abscess secondary to a furuncle
- **e** staphylococcal osteomyelitis in the absence of trauma

4 Appendisectomy wounds are classified as being:
- **a** clean
- **b** clean-contaminated
- **c** contaminated
- **d** contaminated-dirty
- **e** dirty

5 The concept of *Universal Precautions* is based on:
- **a** the 'barrier nursing' of all patients with a nosocomial virus infection
- **b** the resheathing of all used needles
- **c** the need to regard all patients as being potentially infectious
- **d** the importance of taking a detailed social history from every patient
- **e** the routine screening of patients for blood-borne viruses

8 Transplantation surgery

David M. A. Francis

Introduction

Transplantation is the replacement of a diseased organ with a healthy one. The concept of transplantation as a means of treating end-stage organ failure has intrigued surgeons for centuries, but has become a therapeutic reality only within the last 50 years. During that time, enormous advances have been made, including the discovery of powerful immunosuppressive drugs, identification of the molecular and cellular events involved in the rejection response, development of organ preservation methods, advances in patient care and management, and evolution of complex surgical techniques for replacement of a wide variety of organs and tissues. Today, transplant operations are fairly routine procedures. The impact of successful transplantation on the lives of recipients is immense and extremely gratifying for those involved in their care.

Allograft rejection

Allograft rejection is the recipient's normal immune response to an organ or tissue transplanted from another individual (an allograft). It results in damage to the graft and is an inevitable consequence of allotransplantation, unless either the recipient becomes tolerant to the transplanted organ or immunosuppressive therapy prevents the process. Rejection is a highly complex series of sequential and closely interrelated events involving immune cells, cytokines, antibodies, and self-regulatory mechanisms.

Clinical patterns of rejection

Several patterns of rejection are recognised on clinical and histopathological grounds. All are characterised by deterioration of graft function.

Hyperacute rejection

Hyperacute rejection occurs within minutes of restoring blood flow to the transplanted organ in the recipient. It is due to pre-formed specific cytotoxic antibodies in the recipient interacting with antigens expressed on the surface of vascular endothelium in the allograft, with subsequent activation of complement and intravascular thrombosis. It is irreversible and results in immediate graft loss. Potential recipients are screened before transplantation for the presence of such antibodies by a dye-exclusion cytotoxic cross-match test in which lymphocytes from the donor are reacted with recipient serum in the presence of a vital dye.

Accelerated acute rejection

Accelerated acute rejection occurs within 2–4 days of transplantation in patients already sensitised to donor antigens (e.g. by previous pregnancy or blood transfusion), and probably involves both cellular and humoral anamnestic responses. It may be reversible with anti-rejection treatment.

Acute rejection

Acute rejection is primarily cell-mediated rejection that is first manifest 5–7 days after transplantation in unsensitised recipients. It may occur subsequently at any time (e.g. if immunosuppressive therapy is stopped many months after transplantation). It is usually reversible with anti-rejection treatment.

Chronic rejection

Chronic rejection occurs months or years after transplantation. Deterioration in graft function is slow. Histological features include progressive obliterative arteritis and interstitial cellular infiltration and fibrosis.

The pathogenesis is poorly understood and there is no specific treatment. It is the most common type of rejection leading to loss of organ transplants.

Immunosuppression

Immunosuppressive drugs were first used in clinical transplantation in the late 1950s, and are used to prevent and treat acute rejection. Different immunosuppressive strategies and agents are used depending on the transplanted organ, occurrence of side effects, strength of the rejection response, and experience and preference of the treating clinicians. Currently, flexible combinations of prednisolone, mycophenolate, and cyclosporine or tacrolimus are the most widely used maintenance immunosuppressive regimens in solid organ transplantation. In addition, some transplant programs use anti–T cell monoclonal antibodies as 'induction therapy' for the first few days after transplantation. Acute rejection is treated with high-dose prednisolone, monoclonal antibodies or switching to a different immunosuppressive regime. Suppression of the immune system to the extent that allograft rejection is prevented has two major consequences: infection and malignant disease.

Infection

Infection is the commonest complication of immunosuppression and the commonest cause of morbidity and mortality after transplantation. Immunosuppressed patients are particularly at risk for infections that normally are eliminated by cell-mediated immune mechanisms. Within the first few weeks after transplantation, most infections are related to the surgical procedure and are usually bacterial in nature (e.g. infections of the chest, wound, intravenous lines, drain sites, urinary tract). After 1–2 months, infections are most frequently opportunistic, and can be viral (cytomegalic, herpes simplex, varicella zoster, Epstein-Barr), fungal (candida, aspergillus, cryptococcus), protozoal (*Pneumocystis carinii*, toxoplasmosis) or bacterial (*Listeria*, *Mycobacterium*, *Legionella*, *Nocardia*).

Malignant disease

Nearly all types of cancer are more common in immunosuppressed transplant recipients. Although not elucidated fully, the reasons include reduced immune surveillance of potentially neoplastic cells, infection with oncogenic viruses, prolonged antigenic stimulation of the lymphoreticular system by the allograft and, very rarely, transfer of malignant cells with the allograft. The risk for developing cancer after transplantation increases with time, especially in cancers related to environmental factors, and the overall lifetime relative risk (RR) of a transplant recipient developing cancer is approximately three times that of the general population. The most frequently observed common cancers in long-standing kidney transplant recipients are non-pigmented skin cancers (RR = 200), non-Hodgkin's lymphoma (RR = 20), cancers of the urinary tract (RR = 5), and carcinoma of the female genital tract (RR = 3). Cancers which are unusual in the general population but have a high RR in renal transplant patients include Kaposi's sarcoma (RR = 1000), lymphoma of the central nervous system (RR = 1000), thyroid cancer (RR = 300), and carcinoma of the vulva and vagina (RR = 35). Generally, malignant diseases in transplant recipients appear earlier, grow more rapidly, and metastasise earlier than in the general population.

Organ donation

Transplantation is entirely dependent on organs either donated by living donors or obtained from deceased donors with the permission of the next of kin.

Living donors

A person may donate an organ to another individual with end-stage organ failure if the donor and recipient blood groups are compatible, the recipient does not have cytotoxic antibodies directed against donor MHC antigens, and the donor is medically and psychologically suitable. Living donors are the only source of transplant organs in countries where cadaver organ donation is not accepted. Use of living donors has increased considerably over the last 10 years because of the great shortage of deceased donor organs. Live organ donation is restricted largely to kidneys and bone marrow, although recently living donor liver, pancreas, small intestine, and even lung transplants have been performed.

Organs may be obtained from three groups of living donors.

- Living related donor – donor and recipient are biologically related (e.g. parent to offspring). Such

donations currently account for 38% of kidney transplants performed in Australia.
- Living unrelated, altruistic donor – donation to a genetically unrelated but legally or emotionally related individual for altruistic reasons (e.g. husband to wife, friend to friend). About 4% of transplanted kidneys in Australia come from this source.
- Living unrelated, paid donor – donation of an organ for material gain (e.g. selling a kidney to someone with renal failure through an organ broker). Paid organ donation is regarded as unethical in many developed nations (including Australia), but is practised illegally in some developing countries where other maintenance treatments for end-stage organ failure are unavailable. In such cases, both donor and recipient may be subject to gross exploitation.

Potential live organ donors require extensive investigation to ensure that they are medically fit, that the organ to be donated is healthy, and that the donor will not suffer long-term medical or psychological consequences as a result of donating. Living donor transplant procedures are performed electively, with the donor and recipient operations performed concurrently.

Deceased donors

Although a severe worldwide shortage exists of cadaver donors with respect to the number of patients requiring organ transplants, deceased donors provide the majority of organs transplanted in developed nations. Organ donation rates in Australia and New Zealand are amongst the lowest in the developed world, with approximately 10 donors per million population (pmp) annually, while Spain has the highest rate (33 pmp). Cadaver organ donation is not practised in some countries because of the absence of brain death legislation (see below) and for cultural reasons.

The process of deceased donor organ donation

If vital organs are to be removed for transplantation, two criteria must be fulfilled.
- Death of the donor must be diagnosed with certainty.
- Transplanted organs must be in good condition so that they can sustain life within the recipient. This means that, although dead, the donor must have a circulation so that organs to be donated receive an adequate oxygen supply up to the time they are removed.

In practice, deceased donors are 'brain stem dead'; that is, the vital parts of the brain have died, there is irreversible loss of the capacity for consciousness, and the brain as a whole is incapable of functioning and sustaining life; although other organs (e.g. heart, liver, kidneys) may still function for some time after the brain is dead because the cadaver still has a circulation. Key components of the brain stem and their functions are shown in Table 8.1.

Table 8.1 Functional components of the brainstem

Structure	Function
Reticular activating system	Activation of the cerebral cortex
Respiratory centre	Respiration
Vasomotor centre	Control of heart rate and blood pressure
Cortico-spinal tracts	Transmission of all motor output from the brain
Spino-thalamic tracts and medial lemnisci	Transmission of all sensory input into the brain except sight and smell
Cranial nerve nuclei	Activity of cranial nerves

Patients admitted to intensive care units in deep coma and requiring ventilatory support because of serious brain injury should be considered as potential organ donors until proven otherwise. The precise cause of coma is determined and treated, and the neurological status is assessed repeatedly. If there is no improvement, brain stem function is assessed formally by performing simple clinical tests at the patient's bedside. The criteria for brain stem death are shown in Box 8.1. Death is defined by law in Australia, and the law requires (i) the condition of any patient who satisfies the criteria for brain stem death is demonstrably irreversible, and (ii) there is certainty of cessation of brain function. Causes of death amongst deceased organ donors are shown in Table 8.2.

After certification of death, the cadaver is assessed to determine if contraindications exist to organ donation (e.g. systemic or localised infection, extracerebral malignancy, risk of HIV infection, disease of donor organs). Maintenance of the circulation, ventilation, fluid and electrolyte balance, supportive therapy and nursing care are continued. The next of kin are asked for permission to remove specific organs and tissues for clinical transplantation and/or research purposes. If permission is refused (approximately 35% of requests),

Box 8.1 Clinical criteria for brainstem death

Apnoea
Absent respiratory movement during disconnection from the ventilator with the $Pa{CO_2}$ greater than 50 mmHg or 6.65 kPa.

No pupillary response (3rd cranial nerve nucleus)
No movement of the pupils in response to bright light.

No corneal reflex (5th and 7th cranial nerve nuclei)
No blinking in response to touching the cornea with a sterile throat swab.

No vestibulo-ocular reflex (3rd, 6th and 8th cranial nerve nuclei)
No eye movement or deviation of the eyes towards the ear into which ice-cold water is instilled.

No motor response within the cranial nerve distribution (5th and 7th cranial nerve nuclei)
No facial muscular response to painful stimuli applied either to the trigeminal nerve area or the limbs.

No gag reflex (9th and 10th cranial nerve nuclei)
No gagging movement with stimulation of the posterior pharyngeal wall with the endotracheal tube or to bronchial stimulation with a bronchial suction catheter passed into the trachea.

further treatment is discontinued. If permission is given, contact is made with the nearest transplant hospital and the transplant coordinator arranges the organ donation. Full supportive treatment is continued. Tissue typing and viral serology, including HIV status, are determined. The coroner's permission is sought when death is suspicious or traumatic. The corpse, still being ventilated, is taken to the operating theatre, and the donated organs are removed by transplant surgeons with the same care, dignity and attention to detail as in any surgical operation. Approximately 80% of cadaver organ donors are multi-organ donors. Organs are allocated to recipients according to strict and well defined criteria.

Almost all cadaver organ donors die suddenly and unexpectly, a situation which increases the enormous grief and stress experienced by their next of kin. For many families, organ donation allows some good to come from what is otherwise a disastrous and shattering event, as they realise that their loved one's donation may mean a new life for the organ recipients. Organ donation is indeed a unique 'gift of life' to recipients.

Table 8.2 Causes of death amongst Australian cadaver organ donors (ANZDATA Registry 2003 Report)

Cause of death	%
Cerebro-vascular accident	48
Road trauma	26
Other trauma	12
Hypoxia	9
Cardiac arrest	3
Cerebral tumour	2

Organ preservation

If organs are to function immediately and sustain life in recipients after transplantation, they must be removed expertly from the donor and treated to minimise ischaemic damage. In deceased donors, the organs are mobilised and surrounded with sterile ice, and their arteries are perfused with cold (4–6°C) preservation solution (*in situ* perfusion), and again after removal (extracorporeal perfusion). Only extracorporeal perfusion is used in living donor operations.

The perfusion fluid
- Rapidly cools the organs, thereby reducing their metabloism and oxygen requirement.
- Flushes out blood and prevents intra-organ thrombosis.
- Reduces the impact of ischaemic damage.

Preservation solutions contain
- Electrolytes – usually high potassium and low sodium.
- Buffer – e.g. citrate, phosphate, potassium lactobionate.
- Impermeants to reduce cellular oedema and swelling – e.g. mannitol, raffinose.
- Agents designed to reduce ischaemic damage and reperfusion injury – anti-oxidants, enzymatic inhibitors, calcium channel blockers, anti-inflammatories.

After removal from the donor, the organs are placed in sterile plastic bags, which are sealed, placed in a coolbox and surrounded by ice. Organs may be transported to other hospitals, perhaps interstate. Maximum storage times are 30–36 hours for kidneys, 12–20 hours for livers, 10–20 hours for the pancreas, and 4–6 hours for hearts and lungs.

Kidney transplantation

Kidney transplantation was the first clinical transplant discipline and became established with the advent of immunosuppressive therapy in the early 1960s. The kidney is the most frequently transplanted solid organ. Approximately half of the 9,000 patients maintained currently on dialysis in Australia and New Zealand are suitable for kidney transplantation, the remainder being excluded largely because of other serious medical conditions, particularly cardiac and respiratory disease. The need for kidney transplantation is estimated at approximately 40 pmp per year, about four times that of the deceased donor organ donation rate. The current rate of kidney transplants in Australia and New Zealand is 31 pmp.

Living donor nephrectomy is performed usually through a loin incision, or with laparoscopic assistance and a lower abdominal incision. The deceased donor operation involves removal of both kidneys and proximal ureters, together with the abdominal aorta and inferior vena cava. The kidney is transplanted into an iliac fossa, close to the bladder. The renal artery and vein are anastomosed to the respective iliac vessels and the ureter is anastomosed to the side of the bladder (uretero-neocystostomy).

Post-operatively, particular attention is paid to the recipient's urine output, blood pressure, fluid status, renal function and immunosuppression. As with all immunosuppressed patients, infection is a particular concern. Average hospital stay is 7–10 days.

Potential complications

Complications are infrequent but potentially serious because recipients may have had long periods of chronic illness and debility before transplantation and are immunosuppressed. Potential complications include:

- General complications of any operation – wound problems (infection, haematoma, dehiscence, hernia), infections (chest, urine, drip sites), deep vein thrombosis.
- Vascular – transplant renal artery and vein thrombosis, anastomotic bleeding, peri-transplant haematoma, transplant renal artery stenosis.
- Lymphatic – lymphocele.
- Urological – ureteric ischaemia, necrosis, stenosis and obstruction, and urinary fistula.
- Scrotal – oedema, epididymo-orchitis, hydrocele.
- Neurological – damage to ilio-inguinal, genito-femoral and femoral nerves.
- Allograft rejection.
- Recurrent disease in the transplant – diabetic nephropathy, focal segmental hyalinosis, metabolic causes of renal failure.

Results

One- and 5-year patient and kidney survival rates are shown in Table 8.3. Of 16,270 kidney transplants performed in Australia and New Zealand during the

Table 8.3 Patient and graft survival after transplantation

	Patient survival (%)		Graft survival (%)	
Organ	1 year	5 year	1 year	5 year
Heart	90	80	90	80
Lung	80	50	80	50
Heart–lung	65	40	65	40
Liver	87	84	87	84
Deceased donor kidney	94	85	91	76
Living donor kidney	98	92	94	86
Pancreas	95	90	75	70
Isolated intestine	55	10	55	10
Combined intestine and liver	65	30	65	30
Multi-visceral	40	10	40	10

40-year period 1963–2002, 6854 (42%) are still functioning. Graft survival is significantly better for recipients of living rather than deceased donor renal transplants. The commonest cause of transplant failure is chronic rejection.

As with other successful solid organ transplants, most renal transplant recipients experience vastly improved health and vitality, are well rehabilitated, and are fit for full-time work. Particular benefits to paediatric recipients are social and developmental rehabilitation and 'catch-up' growth in those with growth retardation. Renal transplantation is also the most cost-effective treatment for chronic renal failure.

Liver transplantation

Unlike end-stage renal, pancreatic or intestinal failure, no artificial means of support exists for patients with liver failure, and so patients either die before a liver transplant becomes available or come to transplantation with advanced liver disease and its complications, including jaundice, malabsorption, malnutrition, coagulopathy, cardiomyopathy and pulmonary disease. Liver transplantation is indicated for end-stage cirrhosis (primary parenchymal, cholestatic and vascular disease), acute fulminant hepatic failure, and rare congenital metabolic disorders.

Careful pre-operative evaluation of potential recipients is essential so that the precise diagnosis, absence of malignancy, and prognosis with and without transplantation are known. Recipients and donors are matched for blood-group compatibility, liver size, and negative cytotoxic cross match. A donor liver may be reduced in size by surgical resection or even split to suit two recipients, but these procedures add considerable risk.

The recipient operation is a major undertaking and is often prolonged because of its difficult nature and often the need to perform vascular reconstruction before transplantation. Operation involves (i) establishment of veno–venous bypass via the femoral and axillary veins, (ii) excision of the recipient's liver (hepatectomy), (iii) implantation of the donor liver by anastomosing the donor supra- and infra-hepatic inferior vena cava (IVC), portal vein and hepatic artery to those of the recipient, (iv) biliary reconstruction by anastomosis of the donor common bile duct to the recipient's common bile duct or jejunum, and (v) donor cholecystectomy.

Post-operatively, patients are monitored intensively, with attention to their cardiovascular and fluid status, ventilation, liver function and coagulation, blood loss, prevention of sepsis, and immunosuppressive therapy.

Complications include primary non-function, bleeding, hepatic artery and portal vein thrombosis, and biliary tract leakage and obstruction. Primary non-function occurs in 1–5% of liver transplants and necessitates urgent re-transplantation. In spite of formidable potential complications, patient survival is approximately 85% at 1 year (Table 8.3) and 70% at 10 years, a remarkable result for an otherwise uniformly fatal condition. Liver transplantation is very demanding on hospital resources, surgical expertise and personnel, and is limited to a few centres of excellence.

Heart transplantation

Cardiac transplantation is performed for irreversible end-stage heart failure when life expectancy without transplantation is less than 50% at 1 year. Underlying disorders in adults include cardiomyopathy (42%), ischaemic heart disease (40%), valvular disease (5%), myocarditis (5%), or chronic rejection of or coronary artery disease in a previous transplant (5%).

Cardiac donors are selected with extreme care because the donor heart must function immediately after transplantation. Donor and recipient should be blood group compatible and cytotoxic cross match negative, and body weights should be within 10–15% of each other.

The recipient is placed on cardiopulmonary bypass and the diseased heart is removed (cardiectomy) by excising the ventricles but preserving the atrial septum and most of each atrium. The right and left atria of the donor heart are sutured to the respective recipient atrial remnants, and the pulmonary artery and aorta are anastomosed to their respective vessels. Cardiac rhythm is restored when the coronary arteries are reperfused with blood.

Post-operatively, cardiac pacing, careful intravascular volume loading, inotrope infusion and ventilatory support are required, in addition to intensive immunosuppression and antiviral prophylaxis. Electrocardiography and endomyocardial biopsy are performed frequently to detect cardiac rejection.

Early post-operative complications include cardiac failure, arrhythmias, haemorrhage, tamponade, and infections. Most patients experience one or more episodes of acute rejection within a few months of transplantation, often in the absence of clinical features. Accelerated transplant coronary artery disease occurs commonly after transplantation and is the leading cause of death after the third post-transplant year, and is the reason for most cases of retransplantation. One- and 5-year survival rates are shown in Table 8.3. Rehabilitation after successful transplantation is generally good, with 80% of survivors being restored to their pre-illness level of function.

Lung transplantation

Lung transplantation is undertaken for end-stage parenchymal or vascular lung disease in patients with poor life expectancy and quality when there is no alternative effective therapy.

Suitable lung donors are scarce because prolonged donor artificial ventilation often leads to pulmonary infection. Recently, living donors have been used occasionally for donation of the right or left lower lobe.

In single lung transplantation, the diseased lung is excised, and anastomoses are made between the donor and recipient left atria, pulmonary artery, and bronchus or tracheae. Double lung transplants require cardiopulmonary bypass, removal of both lungs, and anastomoses between the donor and recipient main bronchi, pulmonary arteries and left atria.

Post-operatively, patients require positive end-expiratory pressure ventilation, careful fluid management to avoid pulmonary oedema, antibiotics, anti-viral and anti-fungal prophylaxis, and intensive immunosuppression. Operative mortality is 10–15%. Subsequently, lung function is monitored closely with regular pulmonary function tests. Bronchoalveolar lavage and transbronchial biopsy are performed whenever rejection is suspected. Potential complications include airway anastomotic dehiscence, atelectasis and infections, and chronic rejection manifesting as obliterative bronchiolitis.

In spite of the poor condition of patients requiring lung transplantation, the enormity of the surgery, and the formidable potential complications, 1- and 5-year survival rates are 80% and 50% respectively for unilateral and bilateral single lung transplants (Table 8.3). The majority of patients have dramatic improvement in lung function.

Heart–lung transplantation

Heart–lung transplantation (HLT) is performed for end-stage primary pulmonary hypertension, congenital heart disease with Eisenmenger's syndrome, and lung diseases causing cor pulmonale, in patients with very limited life expectancy.

Some centres perform HLT for parenchymal lung disease and pulmonary hypertension in the presence of a healthy heart, rather than lung transplantation, which is associated with problematic bronchial anastomotic healing. In these cases, the healthy heart of the HLT recipient can be transplanted to a second recipient in need of a heart transplant (domino operation).

Survival rates (Table 8.3) reflect the severity of the surgical procedure and the potential for serious post-operative problems with the heart in addition to the lungs.

Pancreas transplantation

Pancreas transplantation provides insulin-producing islet tissue, thereby restoring physiological insulin secretion and carbohydrate metabolism, and reducing the progression of microvascular complications. It involves transplanting either a large number of islets as free grafts or the whole pancreas as a vascularised graft, and usually is performed late in the course of insulin-dependent diabetes mellitus, in long-standing diabetics who also require a kidney transplant because of diabetic nephropathy.

Islet transplantation

The advantage of islet transplantation is that only insulin-secreting tissue is transplanted, thereby eliminating a major source of post-operative morbidity associated with the unwanted exocrine pancreas. Transplantation of islets involves embolisation into the liver through the portal vein by direct injection or percutaneous catheterisation.

Islet transplantation has been hampered by inefficient islet isolation techniques, which are time-consuming and yield low islet numbers from each donor pancreas. Also, there are no clinically useful markers of vascular insufficiency or rejection other than hyperglycaemia, the appearance of which signifies loss of the whole islet graft. Recently, these problems have been tackled by using multiple donors for a single recipient and transplanting islets with other organs (kidney, liver) and assuming that islet and solid organ rejection occurs concurrently.

Vascularised pancreas transplantation

The whole pancreas, together with the second part of the duodenum (to preserve the blood supply to the head of the pancreas), an aortic patch which includes the origins of the coeliac trunk and the superior mesenteric artery, and the portal and splenic veins are removed from the deceased donor. This tissue block is transplanted into an iliac fossa; the aortic patch and portal vein are anastomosed to the respective iliac vessels, and the second part of the duodenum is joined to either the small intestine or bladder.

Graft pancreatitis, anastomotic leakage, pancreatic fistulas, arterial and venous thrombosis of the graft, and pancreatic rejection are all serious complications and are associated with considerable morbidity and even mortality. Successful transplantation has an immensely beneficial effect on the patient's quality of life but is not life saving, and established complications of diabetes are not reversed, although mild neuropathy may improve and a concomitant kidney transplant may be protected from developing diabetic nephropathy. One-year patient and graft survival rates are 95% and 75%, respectively (Table 8.3).

Intestinal transplantation

Several hundred intestinal transplants have been performed for irreversible severe intestinal failure due to short bowel syndrome or absorption and motility disorders in patients in whom parenteral nutrition is failing. An intestinal segment may be transplanted alone or in combination with the liver or other abdominal viscera. Results are generally poor (Table 8.3) due to graft rejection, sepsis and multi-organ failure.

Other tissues

Bone

Free bone autografts or allografts act as matrices within which new bone forms and are used as bone fragments to fill small bony defects or to strengthen bone fusion.

Vascularised autografts (e.g. fibula, rib, iliac crest) are used when a length of anatomically similar bone is required to replace a section of bone lost because of trauma or resection for malignant disease (e.g. jaw reconstruction with iliac crest bone). After successful anastomosis of nutrient vessels, the graft remains viable and heals to adjacent bone.

Skin

Skin autografts (skin grafting) are used as split-skin or full-thickness skin grafts to cover skin defects after trauma or surgery. Recently, skin has been taken from patients with extensive burns, cultured, and the resulting sheets of keratinocytes used as thin layers of fragile epidermis without a dermis.

Skin allografts are used rarely to provide wound cover where skin loss is so extensive that it cannot be replaced by autografting alone. The allograft allows time for healing of denuded sites, but because skin is highly immunogenic, it is usually rejected and has to be replaced with another allograft or an autograft taken from a re-epithelialised area.

Hand transplantation

A few cases of hand allotransplantation for uni- and bilateral hand amputees have been technically successful. Generally, intense immunosuppression is required, and graft survival and functional results are problematic.

Future of transplantation

Clinical organ transplantation has an exciting future and is likely to be an expanding area of surgery. Perhaps the most pressing challenge to overcome is the acute organ donor shortage, which currently is the biggest limitation to transplantation. It is imperative that medical and paramedical personnel and the wider community become aware of the need for deceased donor organs, the concept of brain death, and the enormous cost-benefits of successful organ transplantation.

Scientific advances likely to have positive impacts on clinical transplantation are:

- Encapsulated cell systems – cells (e.g. islets, hepatocytes) are encapsulated in selectively permeable membranes which prevent them from coming into contact with immune cells but allow ingress of oxygen and nutrients.
- Gene transfer – *in vivo* or *ex vivo* implantation into target cells of new genes and the sequences which

regulate their expression (e.g. induction of graft tolerance, delivery of immuno-modulating molecules to the graft or recipient, treatment of genetic inborn errors of metabolism).

- Xenotransplantation – genetic manipulation of donor animals (e.g. pigs) so that organs transplanted to humans are not rejected.
- Artificial organs – used to maintain patients until a donor organ is available or as a permannetly implanted device (e.g. left ventricular assist device, total artificial heart).
- Tissue engineering – implantation of pre-formed biomaterial constructs to treat a functional or anatomical defect (e.g. arterial conduits, breast tissue, bioartificial liver and pancreas, and tissue patches for the intestine, bladder and heart).
- Further elucidation of the immune response and development of specific immunosuppressive agents with the aim of achieving tolerance.

Further reading

Morris PJ, ed. *Kidney Transplantation: Principles and Practice*. 5th edn. Philadelphia: WB Saunders Co; 2001.

Ginns LC, Cosimi AB, Morris PJ, eds. *Transplantation.* Massachusetts: Blackwell Science; 1999.

ANZDATA Registry Report 2003, Australia and New Zealand Dialysis and Transplant Registry. Adelaide, South Australia.

Garner JP. Tissue engineering in surgery. *Surg J R Coll Surg Edinb Irel.* 2004; 2:70–78.

MCQs

Select the single correct answer to each question.

1 Immunosuppression:
 a is only required for organ transplants where the donor and recipient are unrelated
 b has the side effects of increased risk of infection and malignancy
 c aims to knockout bone marrow and stem cells
 d should be doubled if two organs are transplanted (e.g. kidney and pancreas)

2 Organ donation:
 a between husband and wife is doomed to failure
 b from deceased donors exceeds current demand for organs from deceased donors
 c requires that brain stem death criteria are fulfilled
 d in Australia is amongst the highest in the developed nations

3 Kidney transplantation:
 a has a 5-year kidney survival rate of approximately 75–85%
 b requires immunosuppression for transplantation between monozygotic twins
 c is one of the least commonly performed organ transplants
 d leads to only poor quality of life in most recipients

4 Liver transplantation:
 a is contra-indicated if jaundice is present
 b cannot be performed from live donors
 c requires no immunosuppression because of the antigen filtering system in the liver
 d can be life saving in cases of fulminant hepatic failure

5 Pancreas transplantation:
 a can be undertaken using the whole pancreas or just the islets of Langerhan
 b is used in patients with pancreatic enzyme deficiency syndromes
 c using the whole pancreas has a patient survival rate of 15% at 2 years
 d does not allow successful recipients to stop exogenous insulin

9 Principles of surgical oncology

Robert J. S. Thomas

Introduction

Surgical resection of cancers remains the cornerstone of treatment for many types of cancers. Historically, surgery was the only effective form of cancer treatment, but developments in radiation therapy and chemotherapy have demanded that surgeons work with the other disciplines of medicine in order to achieve best results for the patient with cancer.

This type of interaction between the medical disciplines together with the supportive care groups required by cancer patients is defined as multidisciplinary care. It is now widely recognised that for optimal treatment of cancer a multidisciplinary team with the surgeon as part of this team is essential.

Surgery is effective treatment for cancer if the disease is localised. Defining the extent of the cancer before surgery has become much more accurate with modern imaging methods including computed tomography (CT), positron emission tomography (PET) scanning and high resolution ultrasound. The exploratory operation to determine the extent of disease, or attempting a 'curative' resection when the disease has already spread beyond the bounds of a 'surgical' cure, is not part of the modern surgical treatment of cancer. Oncological trained surgeons are now distinguished from more general surgeons because of the particular needs of the cancer patients.

Clinical trials are required to evaluate new treatments and treatment combinations. The struggle against the scourge of cancer has seen an explosion in basic research directed towards cancer. This academic element to cancer care is a constant feature as all those involved in cancer care endeavour to advance the understanding of the management of cancer patients.

These preceding paragraphs define the discipline of surgical oncology. In summary, surgical oncology is the involvement of a specialty trained surgeon as part of a multidisciplinary team program, the use of appropriate surgery in an adequately staged patient and the involvement of the surgeon in academic programs particularly involved with clinical trials.

The use of effective techniques in the operating theatre, the careful management of the patient undergoing surgery and supportive post-operative care are similar requirements to those of all other disciplines of surgery.

Communication with the patient and family, the obtaining of informed consent and the careful honest, realistic but where possible optimistic explanation of the results of surgery, are all matters of high importance to all surgical practice. However, the ability to talk sympathetically to cancer patients and their family is particularly important in the field of surgical oncology.

Multidisciplinary care

Surgeons need to understand the principles and practical consequences of the treatment offered by radiation oncologists, medical oncologists and the paramedical disciplines in order to be able to work in a team to treat cancer patients.

Radiation oncology

Ionising radiation is usually delivered to tumours as external beam therapy. This is generated by linear accelerators. Radiation kills living cells both by direct DNA damage and by the formation of free oxygen radicals in the cells. Free radical formation is the predominant effect and depends upon the level of oxygenation of the cell. Hypoxic areas of tumours are thus protected from the effects of radiation and large necrotic tumours will not respond well to this form of treatment.

When a linear accelerator is used to supply external beam therapy to a tumour, the patient goes through a series of planning exercises to accurately delineate the tumour and direct the radiation as accurately as possible to the tumour to minimise the impact on normal tissues. The linear accelerator is usually located in a large concrete bunker, often underground to provide protection to staff and patients.

An alternative method of administration of radiation is by using a local radiation source applied close to the tumour. This is known as brachytherapy. It is a highly effective form of therapy in tumours such as cervical cancer, other gynaecological cancers and prostate cancer.

Both normal and neoplastic cells are affected by radiation, so the dose which can be given in any situation is limited by the tolerance of the surrounding normal tissues. Tissues particularly at risk include the bone marrow and gastrointestinal tract, which contain rapidly dividing cells. The spinal cord is also at risk as it does not have repair mechanisms able to manage radiation-induced injury. However damage to DNA in cells from radiation can be repaired by a complex series of intracellular mechanisms. The normal tissues thus can recover from radiation provided the dose is not extreme, but malignant cells can also repair such damage. The actual dose of radiation (unit of measurement is a Grey) required to kill a particular tumour varies. Some cancers, for example Hodgkin's disease and cancer of cervix and some breast cancers, can be sterilised completely with acceptable degrees of damage to the surrounding tissues. Other cancers, for example melanoma and sarcoma, can rarely be eradicated using acceptable doses.

Fractionation of the dose of radiation over a period of time, by utilising daily low doses does provide better tumour response and less damage to normal structures than a single large dose.

The use of more modern methods of imaging and computerised dose planning allows for far more effective delivery of radiotherapy than in the past. The calculation of optimal doses and the delivery through new techniques, such as intensity modulated radiotherapy, has improved results and minimised side effects from radiotherapy.

The effectiveness of radiation treatment can be enhanced by the use of a radiation sensitiser. A commonly used sensitiser is 5 Fluorouracil® given by intravenous (i.v.) injection or by i.v. infusion.

Radiation may be delivered with curative intent, for example in treatment of seminoma of testis or as palliation for advanced or metastatic disease. A common use of radiation in this setting is for treatment of painful bony metastases, seen for example in lung cancer and prostate cancer. Effective symptom relief is often achieved with the use of radiation therapy.

Radiation therapy, often combined with chemotherapy, so called chemoradiation, may be used preoperatively (neoadjuvant therapy) or post-operatively (adjuvant therapy).

Neoadjuvant therapy prior to surgery is designed to reduce the bulk of a large primary tumour in order to improve the likelihood of successful surgical resection. This is now the standard of care in the management of locally advanced rectal cancers. Neoadjuvant therapy in this situation has been demonstrated to reduce the likelihood of local recurrence after surgery.

Post-operative adjuvant radiotherapy is also used when pre-operative therapy has not been given. As an example, this has also been shown to reduce post-operative rectal cancer recurrence particularly when positive glands are removed at the time of resection of the rectum.

There are particular benefits to giving the radiation therapy before surgery. These include the fact that the normal tissue planes allow better oxygenation of tissues without the post-operative damage where scarring and potentially hypoxic areas are left behind following surgery. It is also easier to define and localise the tumour to be irradiated without this scarring. This is associated with less damage to the normal tissues as the radiation can be applied very accurately to the tumour. Again, using the example of rectal cancer, pre-operative localisation of the rectal cancer with MRI allows for accurate radiation doses to be given to the rectal tumour. Post-operatively however, the small bowel becomes adherent in the pelvis and thus can receive a significant degree of radiation damage because of its fixed position. Pre-operative treatment is better as the patient can be postured to remove the small bowel out of the pelvis, thus reducing small-intestinal radiation exposure.

Medical oncology

Medical oncologists use cytotoxic agents to modify tumour growth. The drugs interfere with cell division by a variety of methods and can be classified according to the site of action on the cell division process. Recently new classes of drugs have been developed as advances have occurred in the understanding of the molecular and genetic factors involved in cancer. Examples include angiogenesis inhibitors, EGF receptor blockers and most dramatic and widely used Imatinib (Glivec®), a Bcr-Abl protein kinase antagonist which blocks the binding site for ATP. It inhibits the growth of certain tumours, including gastrointestinal stromal tumour, and chronic myeloid leukaemia, with sometimes drastic effects.

Some cancers can be cured with chemotherapy alone. Testicular tumours and Hodgkin's disease are such examples. These are the exceptions however and for most solid tumours chemotherapy treatment produces a limited complete response or partial response.

Many randomised controlled clinical trials have demonstrated survival benefit from the use of chemotherapy even when cure cannot be obtained. Like radiation therapy, chemotherapy is given either as neoadjuvant therapy (i.e. pre-operatively), or post-operatively (adjuvant therapy), where it is used after a surgical resection. Post-operative adjuvant therapy is given where a complete resection has occurred but the potential for metastatic disease remains. Breast cancer and colon cancer are two cancers where landmark clinical trials have demonstrated significant improvement in survival with the use of a course of adjuvant chemotherapy after resection of the primary tumour and adjacent lymph nodes.

Chemotherapy does have significant side effects, particularly haematological and gastrointestinal, as the rapidly dividing cells in these areas are susceptible to the drugs. Neutropenia, thrombocytopenia, and diarrhoea and other gastrointestinal upsets are common side effects. Many of these symptoms can be ameliorated by medication.

Chemotherapy is usually given in cycles to reduce side effects and to improve tumour response by catching new clones of resistant cells as they redevelop after the initial cell kill in the primary tumour.

Supportive care

The holistic approach to the care of the cancer patient encompasses a range of supportive and coordinating services through the management phase of the illness. This is often delivered by a range of nursing and allied health professionals. Psychosocial support includes investigation and treatment of cancer patients by suitably trained nursing staff, social workers, psychologists and psychiatrists. Each discipline can offer some support depending on the problem faced by the cancer patient. A nurse coordinator often aids in the management of the patient. The use of such professionals has been shown to improve outcomes for cancer patients. The most extensively studied model is the breast care nurse who acts as a facilitator and informant for breast cancer patients. This type of support is likely to spread to the management of other cancer patients.

Surgeons treating cancer patients learn to recognise that they are members of a team rather than the sole arbiters of the patients' treatment programs.

Palliative care services

Modern palliative care programs are part of the services offered to cancer patients. These services include ambulatory and hospice programs for management of the end stages of life when attempts to cure or actively treat the cancer have ceased. Physical and psychological symptom control is an important part of modern multidisciplinary care. Palliative care physicians also help in pain control and symptom control in the earlier stages of the illness and thus broaden their influence in the journey of the patient with cancer.

Principles of surgery for malignant disease

The principles involve screening and diagnosis, assessment of the patient, staging of the extent of cancer, decision about treatment by multidisciplinary team, principles of operative surgical oncology, rehabilitation and follow-up. Each of these will be dealt with in turn.

Screening and diagnosis of malignant disease

Screening

Surgical resection has the potential to cure early or localised cancers which have not metastasised. In general early cancers equate with curability. For example, a malignant polyp in the colon is usually curable by surgery. However, this does not always hold true. Small breast cancers may metastasise early with cure not inevitable from surgical excision alone. However the principle of early diagnosis, or an early asymptomatic cancer, is accepted as the most effective way of reducing the mortality from cancer. Screening for cancer to detect early asymptomatic cancers is now commonplace.

For screening to be effective, the test must be able to detect a common cancer at a stage when it can be cured by treatment. The test must be sensitive, specific and acceptable to the public. It must also be offered to the population age at risk. For screening to be effective it must be introduced on a population basis. Screening of individuals by a doctor is known as case finding.

Controlled clinical trials of population screening have been carried out and do show survival benefit in a number of diseases. The most effective screening program has been cervical screening where, since its introduction, there has been a substantial fall in mortality from cervical cancer in all age groups. Similar less dramatic effect is seen with breast cancer screening by mammography, colon cancer screening using faecal occult blood testing and follow-up colonoscopy. Cancer of the stomach is screened for in Japan but the disease is now of low incidence in Western countries making screening not cost effective. Barrett's mucosa is common in Western countries but the incidence is not sufficient to make endoscopic screening for this condition effective. Lung cancer in high risk groups (heavy smokers), although an apparently attractive group for screening, has not been used in a general population program because it is not cost-effective or clinically useful using current technologies.

Surgeons are involved in screening programs performing endoscopies and biopsies (e.g. abnormal Barrett's mucosa), excising polyps from the colons at colonoscopy and biopsying mammographically detected breast lesions.

Diagnosis

A tissue diagnosis is essential prior to the creation of any management plan for a cancer patient. The consequences of many cancer treatments are so severe that only rarely can treatment be commenced without a pathological diagnosis. Tissue is obtained by fine needle aspiration, core biopsy or by excisional biopsy.

FINE NEEDLE ASPIRATION CYTOLOGY

Fine needle aspiration cytology (FNAC) and core biopsy can be done on an outpatient basis and provides a rapid diagnosis of accessible lesions such as breast lumps, head and neck lymph nodes and thyroid swellings. For less accessible lesions ultrasound guidance for the biopsy needle is necessary and commonly used. Core biopsies (Trucut®) can give a definite tissue specimen and can be performed in the clinic as well as by radiologists using ultrasound or CT radiological guidance. Internal lesions in for example the lung, peritoneal cavity or any solid organ can also be accessed by these methods.

Lymph glands or masses in the neck are a particular situation where a FNAC diagnosis allows for treatment planning which may involve a major neck dissection to remove the entire lymph node field. An incisional biopsy is not recommended as it may compromise the chance to achieve a satisfactory clearance of lymph nodes at a later date.

All of these techniques rely on the expertise of the pathologist to make a definite diagnosis on the basis of either the cytological characteristics of the tumour or more advanced pathological techniques, for example immunohistochemistry.

EXCISIONAL BIOPSY

Where a local mass or skin lesion can be completely excised without significant morbidity, excisional biopsy is the treatment of choice, removing the problem at the same time as making the diagnosis.

This technique is commonly used for skin lesions, particularly suspected squamous cell carcinoma, basal cell carcinoma and melanoma. Usually the procedure can be carried out under local anaesthetic in an outpatient theatre setting with minimal morbidity and discomfort.

HISTOPATHOLOGY

At times the histopathologist cannot accurately define the tissue of origin of a tumour deposit after excision. Many advanced histological techniques are now available to distinguish tumours from one another. For example, monoclonal antibodies against leucocyte antigen may help differentiate carcinoma from lymphomas. S100 antibody staining can distinguish melanoma from anaplastic carcinoma. More recently genomic techniques including array studies have been used to clarify the histological diagnosis of various tumours. Rarely a definite diagnosis cannot be made, particularly of the site of an anaplastic carcinoma. Clinical examinations and investigation have then to be performed to try and define the primary diagnosis, as the therapeutic plan will differ for different primary organ sites.

Assessment of the patient

An important early part of the assessment of a patient with cancer is to determine the health and fitness of the patient. Many cancer treatments are demanding on the physical and psychological resources of the patient. An idea of the 'health' of the patient can be gained from a simple clinical assessment, the Eastern Cooperative Oncology Group (ECOG) status. Patients who are ECOG 3 or lower will usually have a poor outcome from any treatment including major surgery.

All patients undergoing major surgery need assessment of the clinical status including, where appropriate, tests of cardiac function, for example scans and angiography if indicated, respiratory status by lung function tests and renal function tests including creatinine clearance.

Modern surgical oncology is required to be precise and accurate in resecting tumours where appropriate and be conducted with minimal morbidity and mortality. Pre-operative testing of the physical status of the patient is mandatory to obtain good results from major cancer surgery.

Staging of malignant disease

Accurate staging of the extent of disease is of great importance in formulating a treatment plan. Clinical stage is that defined by clinical examination and imaging of the patient. It is often not accurate but with the use of high quality CT and PET scanning the accuracy is improved. Pathological staging is that defined after excisional surgery by the anatomical pathologist. It is accurate in defining the extent of disease associated with a primary tumour. Small-volume or micrometastatic disease is not easily detected by any method of examination. The most commonly used staging system used is the TNM (tumour, nodes, metastases) system. The AJCC booklet describes the TNM staging system for all cancers. Suffixes to the T, N, and M indicate the size of the tumour and presence or absence of nodal disease or metastases. For example, T2 N1 M0 indicates the stage of a tumour e.g. carcinoma of the colon where the tumour has spread into the muscularis propria but not through the wall of the colon where there are adjacent lymph nodes involved (N1) but no metastases detected (M0). The staging system is varied according to the primary site of the tumour.

Rectal cancers have a long-standing clinical and pathological staging system known as the Cuthbert-Dukes staging system. Dukes A is local disease in the rectum not invading muscularis propria; Dukes B, the tumour has extended through the wall of the bowel; and Dukes C, where there is lymph node involvement. Dukes D is when distant metastases are present. The Dukes system is commonly used alongside the TNM system.

Methods of clinical staging include radiological methods such as CT, MRI and ultrasound. Within the area of nuclear medicine are PET scanning and nuclear scanning generally (e.g. bone scanning). For intra-abdominal tumours laparoscopy is an added staging method which detects occult disease.

Decision about treatment at the multidisciplinary conference

Armed with information about the diagnosis of the cancer, the extent of the disease, that is the clinical stage of the disease and the fitness of the patient, decisions can be made about the most appropriate treatment program. Ideally consultation with a multidisciplinary team occurs at this stage, however if the decision regarding surgery is straightforward, the multidisciplinary conference usually occurs after the surgery when a pathological stage has been determined. However many cancers require down-staging with radiotherapy or chemotherapy prior to surgery, and multidisciplinary consultations early are important to facilitate this process.

The provision of written information to the patient and family, with careful and repeated discussions, is necessary to ensure that the patient can give informed consent to any treatment plan offered. Patients have the right to refuse all or some of the treatment plan and they are encouraged to be part of the decision making process.

At this stage discussions regarding involvement in research projects, use of resected tissues and involvement in clinical trials need to be commenced.

Principles of operative surgical oncology

The technical issues in surgical oncology are not different from other surgical intervention. Open surgery, laparoscopic surgery, robotic surgery, ablative interventions and other technical interventions all have a place in modern surgical oncology. However some important oncological principles exist which must be followed by the surgeon for a satisfactory outcome.

Definition of curative surgery

Despite modern staging methods, occult tumour spread is still discovered by the surgeon, for example small-volume peritoneal disease or unsuspected nodal disease. Frozen section examination of the disease is necessary to confirm the diagnosis. So-called curative surgery is only performed when a total excision of all the tumour is possible. The primary tumour and the associated lymph node drainage fields are excised in continuity. A measure of the adequacy of the oncological surgical operation is demonstrated by the findings on pathological examination of the specimen. The operative specimens need to be correctly orientated by the surgeon to allow the pathologist to carefully examine and interpret the specimen given to him. The key issues are:

- whether the margins of the specimen removed are clear of tumour
- the total number of lymph nodes excised together with the number of involved lymph nodes.

Standards exist for the adequacy of the surgical excision to be assessed in many tumours.

Palliative surgery

Here the operation is performed to overcome some symptom-producing consequence of the tumour either by resection or bypass. This is to remove a potentially symptomatic lesion even though a cure is known to be impossible. Examples include the following:

- In case of pyloric obstruction from an advanced cancer of the stomach, a gastrojejunostomy will provide good palliation of vomiting.
- Resection of a bleeding cancer of the colon is justified even in the presence of metastases.

Many other examples exist. 'Tailoring' this type of surgery to the needs of the patient without undue morbidity or loss of quality of life is an important role for an oncological surgeon.

Margins of surgical excision

The degree to which normal tissues should be removed with the primary tumour is a subject constantly being researched. A universal rule is not possible to formulate. In general a margin of 2–5 cm is suggested. Particular examples follow:

- For excision of melanomas the depth of excision is more important than the extent of surrounding skin. A margin of 2 cm usually suffices in contrast to the 5 cm previously practiced.
- However for oesophageal resection the majority of the oesophagus needs to be resected because the tumour does spread up and down in the submucosal plane.
- Soft tissue sarcomas may spread along aponeurotic planes so that complete excision requires the resection of the entire muscle group and fascial compartment to encompass this type of spread.
- The recognition that spread of rectal cancer occurs into perirectal tissues has led to the use of the total mesorectal excision of the rectum to improve the completeness of resection.

The principle of complete local excision with an adequate margin is paramount in surgical oncology and it needs to be achieved in different ways depending on the type of tumour being resected.

Lymph node resection

Traditionally the draining lymph nodes from a primary tumour are excised with the local lesion. The main benefit of this removal is increased staging information, which will affect the decisions regarding post-operative adjuvant therapy. In some situations there may be a survival benefit from removal of early-involved lymph nodes. However prophylactic excision of uninvolved nodes does not provide a survival advantage to the patient and exposes the patient to increased morbidity from the node removal. An example is the prophylactic removal of groin lymph nodes (radical groin dissection), when these glands are not involved. This operation is nowadays not performed when the glands are clinically not involved as randomised controlled trials have shown that survival rates have not improved but the morbidity from the operation is significant. Poor skin healing and swelling of the affected leg are two such complications.

Rehabilitation

It is necessary to undertake rehabilitation of the cancer patient who has undergone major resectional surgery. This usually involves the allied health disciplines, part of the oncology team. The type and duration of the process will vary according to the type of tumour and surgery performed. Some examples are as follows.

- Post head and neck surgery, for example laryngectomy, voice production can be learned by

development of oesophageal speech. Resection of part of the tongue will require re-education of speech.
- Gastric cancer resection involving partial gastrectomy produces a major impact on the nutritional status of the patient. Dietetic support is required to re-educate the patient to a new balanced regular eating program.
- Removal of large muscle groups or amputation will require physiotherapy and orthotic involvement to enable the patient to learn to live with the defect and walk or move as best possible.

The ability to adequately rehabilitate patients who have suffered significant disability as a result of the presence of the cancer and need for resection is critical in understanding the quality of life issues affecting cancer patients. As outcomes research becomes more common in assessing results of cancer treatment, there will be a better understanding of this important issue.

Follow-up of patient after initial treatment program

A program of follow-up is required for cancer patients after their initial treatment. This is for two main reasons. This is to observe the patient and investigate when appropriate to detect recurrent disease, which can then be treated effectively. By definition this is only likely to be useful to the patient when strong effective post-operative therapies are available which will have a real impact on the control of cancer. Where no such therapy exists intensive follow-up is not recommended.
- One example of this is the early detection of liver metastases after colorectal cancer treatment. Survival gains are possible when appropriately staged patients with liver metastases are successfully resected.
- Breast cancer follow-up is also intense because of the variety of therapies which are available to control disease. However strong proof from intensive follow-up of cancer patients impacting on survival is lacking for breast cancer as for most tumours.
- Detection of asymptomatic but untreatable recurrent cancer does not do the patient any favour.
- Regular follow-up provides the opportunity to manage the adjuvant therapy programs which are offered to many patients for 6–12 months following the initial treatment for the cancer.

Secondly the follow-up provides an opportunity to support the patient through the psychological upsets which accompany the diagnosis and treatment of cancer. Increasingly it is recognised that severe psychological morbidity exists in cancer patients who have been treated. This exists even if the cancer is apparently cured. This has led to a developing interest in the concept of survivorship, that is understanding the needs of the 'cured' cancer patients. Psychosocial support is essential for many cancer patients and is best delivered in the setting of multidisciplinary care.

Clinical trials and research

Clinical research is essential to evaluate the new and previously untested treatments. Surgeons are involved in a number of ways:
- Provision of tissue for tissue banking. This is a fast growing program throughout the world. The provision of fresh tissues for genetic studies is of paramount importance to the understanding of malignant disease. Highly organised tissue banking programs are now being put in place. These involve the collection and storage of tissues under standardised conditions, the collection of other material, for example blood and bone marrow, and most important and perhaps most difficult, the collection of accurate clinical data to be evaluated alongside the laboratory data. Surgeons provide the tissues and have the chance to be involved in the projects that interest them and so should keep a careful watch on the ethical issues which abound in this complex area of clinical and laboratory research.
- Surgeons are involved in clinical trials. Surgeons recruit patients for clinical trials which allocate patients to treatment programs directed towards the first stages of treatment of cancer. The recruiter for randomised clinical trials must be able to demonstrate equipoise in relation to the arms of the study and be able to assure the patient that there is no reason why he or she should not enter the trial, as current knowledge suggests that both treatment arms, although different from each other, have equal efficacy.

Patients involved in clinical trials are generally thought to receive better care than those outside the trial. This relates to the level of care and attention given to the patient, which is engendered by the demands of the trial. An increase in the clinical trials recruitment is a major ambition of the surgical oncology movement.

Conclusion

The principles of surgical oncology can be applied to many of the systemic practices of surgery. In simple terms the surgeon operating on cancer patients in the 21st century must have some understanding of the malignant process, be prepared to work as part of a team and offer multidisciplinary care, communicate well with a very concerned sometimes desperate group of patients, operate with a high level of skill and perform an adequate cancer operation, help the patient rehabilitate from the treatment and finally be prepared to be involved in the advancing area of surgical science as applied to cancer patients. As God knows, surgeons cannot cure all cancers on their own.

MCQs

Select the single correct answer to each question.

1 Ionising radiation is particularly effective in treatment *except* in:
- **a** Hodgkins disease
- **b** Carcinoma of the breast
- **c** Cancer of the rectum
- **d** Cancer of the uterine cervix
- **e** Cutaneous melanoma

2 Screening for malignant disease is effective in the following situations except:
- **a** Where a tumour is detected at a stage where it can be cured by treatment
- **b** Screening is undertaken on an individual patient basis
- **c** There is high public acceptance of the process
- **d** Specificity of screening is high
- **e** Sensitivity of screening is high

3 The following statements in relation to simultaneous regional lymph node dissection at the time of primary tumour excision are true *except*:
- **a** Allows more accurate tumour staging
- **b** Allows provision of appropriate prognosis to the patient
- **c** Can be undertaken with little morbidity
- **d** Allows appropriate adjuvant treatment to be undertaken
- **e** May confer a survival advantage

Upper Gastrointestinal Surgery

10 Gastro-oesophageal reflux

Glyn G. Jamieson

Introduction

The reflux of gastric contents into the oesophagus probably occurs intermittently in everyone, particularly after eating. However, the oesophagus usually reacts to this by initiating a peristaltic wave that clears its contents back into the stomach. We are not aware of this happening. It is when we become aware of it, usually because of symptoms of burning retrosternal pain (heartburn) and/or regurgitation of the contents into the mouth (water brash), that we call the condition gastro-oesophageal reflux and think of it as a medical disorder. In fact, gastro-oesophageal reflux is a very common disorder in societies living a Western lifestyle, with symptoms occurring once or twice a month in about one-third of the community, and symptoms occurring daily in approximately 5% of the community.

Aetiology/pathogenesis

The reason why gastro-oesophageal reflux develops is unknown, but it certainly appears to be a disease associated with the Western lifestyle, and most clinicians believe that such things as overeating (and its consequence of obesity), alcohol and smoking are important factors that are strongly associated with the problem. Factors that normally prevent gastro-oesophageal reflux have all been implicated in its pathogenesis.

Lower oesophageal sphincter

This is a high-pressure zone interposed between the positive pressure environment of the abdomen, and the negative pressure of the thorax. This sphincter relaxes when a peristaltic wave approaches it with a bolus, and then contracts again when the bolus has passed through into the stomach. In patients with severe gastro-oesophageal reflux disease, the lower sphincter often has no recordable tone, and thus appears to be patulous. However, many patients with reflux disease have normal tone in their lower oesophageal sphincter, and a loss of tone may be a consequence of damage from the acid and other gastric contents that are contained in the refluxate. Even if low tone is not an initiating factor of abnormal reflux, it is certainly a perpetuating factor.

Oesophageal peristaltic activity

Many patients with gastro-oesophageal reflux disease have disordered motility in the oesophagus and consequently clear refluxed material poorly. However, once again this may be a consequence, and a perpetuating factor, of reflux rather than an initial cause of reflux damage.

Hiatus hernia and loss of normal anatomy

In the general population, hiatus hernia has captured the imagination, perhaps because it is alliterative and therefore easy to say, and it is a suitably harmless condition, so that a multitude of what are really dietary indiscretions can be ascribed to the hernia! There is undoubtedly a strong association between hiatus hernia and gastro-oesophageal reflux; a majority of (but not all) patients with severe reflux disease have a sliding hiatus hernia. Conversely, there are many more patients who are shown to have a hiatus hernia on barium meal examination than there are patients with symptomatic reflux disease. Hiatus hernia is considered in more detail later in this chapter.

Refluxed material

Gastric contents usually contain gastric juice and food and sometimes duodenal content. Although much has been written about bile in refluxate (pancreatic juice has been all but ignored), its actual role remains uncertain. What has been shown is that if gastric acid is eliminated, the great majority of patients lose their symptoms, so it seems that acid is by far the most important constituent of the refluxate.

Surgical pathology

Most patients with gastro-oesophageal reflux have a normal oesophageal mucosa. However, in severe forms of the disease erosions occur, leading to ulceration that can become confluent. As with any inflammatory process, healing is associated with the development of fibrous tissue, and if enough fibrous tissue forms, like any scar, it will contract, leading to narrowing and foreshortening of the oesophagus (so-called stricture formation).

In a small proportion of patients, the oesophageal mucosa takes protective measures into its own hands and replaces the squamous mucosa with gastric (columnar) mucosa. This is often called Barrett's oesophagus, after the Australian-born surgeon Norman Barrett who first described it. Patients who develop Barrett's oesophagus often lose their symptoms, so this might be thought a particularly successful ploy on the part of the oesophagus. Unfortunately, the columnar mucosa is unstable and is regarded as a premalignant condition. Indeed, the incidence of adenocarcinoma in the region of the gastro-oesophageal junction is steadily increasing in Western countries and it is thought that this is through the mechanism of Barrett's oesophagus.

Very occasionally, a gastric ulcer can develop in the gastric mucosa of the oesophagus and it is then called a Barrett's ulcer, to distinguish it from ulcers that occur in inflamed squamous mucosa. Although adenocarcinoma occurring in a Barrett's oesophagus and, to a lesser extent, stricture formation, are the two most important complications of gastro-oesophageal reflux, probably the most common complication is chronic blood loss leading to iron-deficiency anaemia. This is seen most frequently in a hospital setting in bed-bound patients. Respiratory problems such as chronic infections (common in children) and asthma, occasionally may also be complications of gastro-oesophageal reflux disease.

Hiatus hernia

Although a hiatus hernia can exist without gastro-oesophageal reflux, and vice versa, it is nevertheless common to consider the two entities together. The reason for this is the strong association between reflux and the most common type of hiatus hernia (i.e. a sliding hiatus hernia). A sliding hiatus hernia (Fig. 10.1) is so called because it fulfils the definition of a sliding hernia (i.e. the viscus forms part of the wall of the hernial sac). This is because there is an unperitonealised area (bare area) at the back of the stomach. Thus, when the gastro-oesophageal junction passes up through the hiatus, there is a sac of peritoneum on the front and sides of the hernia, but not posteriorly. The loss of the acute angle of entry of the oesophagus into the stomach removes one of the anatomical barriers to reflux, and clearly makes reflux more likely to occur. However, it probably requires some measure of deficiency in other antireflux mechanisms of the lower oesophagus before reflux occurs with hiatus hernia. Why a sliding hiatus hernia occurs is unknown, but it is probably some

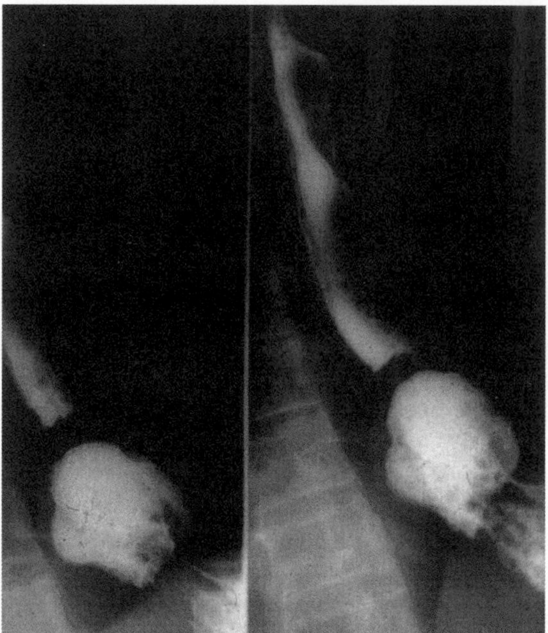

Fig. 10.1 Barium swallow and meal demonstrating a sliding hiatus hernia. This oesophagus is 'shortened' and the stomach is drawn up into the chest.

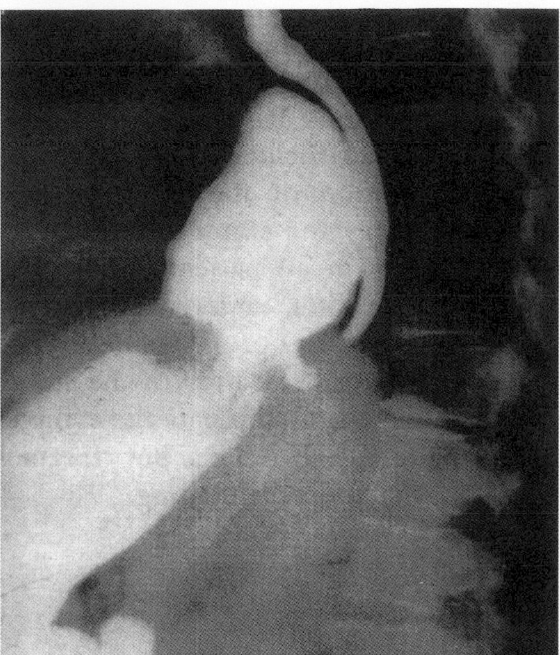

Fig. 10.2 X-ray demonstrating a barium-filled fundus of stomach in the chest and alongside the oesophagus. This is a para-oesophageal or rolling hiatus hernia.

combination of attenuation of hiatal attachments combined with the upwards pull of the longitudinal muscle of the oesophagus. A sliding hiatus hernia, as such, probably never causes symptoms; any symptoms are almost certainly the result of associated gastro-oesophageal reflux.

A para-oesophageal hiatus hernia (Fig. 10.2) occurs when the gastro-oesophageal junction remains in its normal position, but part of the anterior wall of the stomach rolls up alongside the oesophagus and into the mediastinum (it is sometimes called a rolling hiatus hernia). Such a hernia has a complete peritoneal sac. These hernias can sometimes be huge and involve virtually all of the stomach, so that the gastro-oesophageal junction and the pylorus lie alongside each other. In spite of their size, these hernias are, somewhat surprisingly, occasionally asymptomatic. Symptoms associated with them include pain and discomfort after meals, and episodes of more acute pain that are probably associated with intermittent twisting of the stomach. Patients sometimes present as an acute emergency, with strangulation of the hernia. If the condition is discovered coincidentally (often by a chest X-ray that shows a fluid level in the mediastinum behind the heart), provided the hernia is asymptomatic, then it seems reasonable to leave it, instructing the patient to seek urgent medical attention if pain and/or vomiting should develop. However, it should be noted that some clinicians believe all hernias should be repaired, if the patient is regarded as fit for surgery. In reality, a para-oesophageal hernia alone is quite uncommon, because usually the gastro-oesophageal junction also slides up into the chest. The condition is then called a mixed hiatus hernia and the patient is likely to have some symptoms, usually gastro-oesophageal reflux.

The type of operation carried out for hiatus hernia varies with the type of hernia. Sliding hiatus hernia, when gastro-oesophageal reflux is the problem, is treated by bringing the gastro-oesophageal junction back into the abdomen, narrowing the hiatus with sutures by approximating the muscle pillars of the hiatus posterior to the oesophagus, and performing an antireflux operation, usually a fundoplication. With para-oesophageal hiatus hernia, the contents of the sac are reduced, the hiatus is narrowed, as described above, and the fundus of the stomach is fixed with sutures to the diaphragm. If reflux is thought to be a problem, an antireflux procedure is carried out. Some surgeons advocate an antireflux procedure in all circumstances. Today, all of these procedures are usually undertaken laparoscopically.

Clinical presentation

The majority of patients present with retrosternal burning pain occurring after eating, and more particularly after eating certain foods. For example, many patients find such things as pastries, sweet biscuits, tomato sauce and fatty foods as likely to cause heartburn. Certain types of activity also sometimes bring on heartburn (e.g. stooping while gardening or lifting heavy objects). Heartburn is nearly always temporarily relieved by taking antacids. Some patients find that their heartburn is worse when they are lying down, and they then tend to wake with the problem during the night. Many patients are also aware that if they overeat or indulge in more alcohol than is their custom, then their problem is worse. Regurgitation of either gastric contents, or sour or bitter fluid into the mouth, is a symptom in some patients and occasionally such patients wake at night coughing and spluttering, having inhaled a small amount of the refluxate. Although unusual, some patients present with the complications of their reflux disease, having never experienced heartburn or regurgitation, or at least only having experienced it in a very mild way. Most often in this setting the presentation is difficulty in swallowing, but other presentations may be tiredness from iron-deficiency anaemia, recurrent respiratory infections, hoarseness of voice, halitosis and loss of enamel on the teeth.

Investigations

The great majority of patients with reflux either never go to the doctor with their problem at all, or are relatively simply treated with antacids and changes to their lifestyle, such as weight reduction, reducing alcohol intake and avoiding foods that exacerbate the problem. In some patients, the addition of intermittently administered acid-lowering drugs, such as H_2 receptor blockers, also ameliorates their symptoms.

Which patients should be investigated further? Patients with typical heartburn that can be treated easily with occasional antacids do not require further investigation. Patients with atypical symptoms, or patients in whom high-level therapy such as proton-pump inhibitors are required to control symptoms, should first undergo an endoscopy. If erosive oesophagitis is found, further investigation is not warranted. If the patient has a normal oesophagus on endoscopy, then monitoring of the oesophagus over a prolonged time, usually 24 hours, is indicated in order to obtain a pH profile, which can then be correlated with the patient's symptoms. If an abnormality is seen on endoscopy, then it is biopsied and sent for histology.

Treatment

Simple treatment has already been described and is well known to most people. High-level therapy consists of either the prolonged taking of proton-pump inhibitors (e.g. omeprazole, lanzoprazole) or antireflux surgery. The advantage of drug therapy is its low morbidity, while its disadvantages are the need to take the therapy lifelong, and therefore its cost and the unknown effect of chronic administration of the drug over a long period. If regurgitation is a major problem, proton-pump inhibitors are less effective because they do not stop gastro-oesophageal reflux occurring, but merely reduce the acid in the refluxed material.

The advantage of operative therapy is that it cures the problem, while its disadvantages are the morbidity of the operation itself and the fact that it usually leaves the patient unable to belch effectively. This leads to a feeling of being bloated after eating, and patients sometimes have to modify their eating habits to a degree (usually to smaller meals). In fact, patients who are trying to lose weight sometimes see this as a positive outcome from their operation.

Operative management

It is important to realise, when discussing high-level management such as lifelong proton-pump inhibition or surgery, that we are referring only to the small group of patients who are at the severe end of the reflux spectrum. The indications for surgery are really dictated by the patient's problems from the reflux. When the patient suffers complications such as severe dysphagia from stricture formation or recurrent respiratory problems from spillover into the larynx, then the balance is strongly tilted towards surgery. However, such complications occur in a small minority of patients. The majority of patients at the severe end of the reflux spectrum have reflux symptoms that are spoiling their enjoyment of life and they then have a choice of drug therapy to control their symptoms, or surgery.

In the past, the pain associated with surgery and the prolonged period away from normal activity afterwards tended to put people off having an operation. However, the advent of laparoscopic surgery has changed this. Nevertheless, laparoscopic antireflux surgery is not without problems, so it should still only be offered to patients at the severe end of the reflux spectrum. Furthermore, it is only suitable in patients with reasonably straightforward disease and is best avoided in patients with shortened oesophagus (relatively rare), and in patients who have had previous upper abdominal operations in the area of the oesophagus and stomach. Patients undergoing laparoscopic antireflux surgery should also be aware that there is approximately a 2% conversion rate to open operation because of difficulties that may be encountered during the laparoscopic procedure. Open operation can be undertaken via either the abdominal or the thoracic route. Most operations today are undertaken abdominally

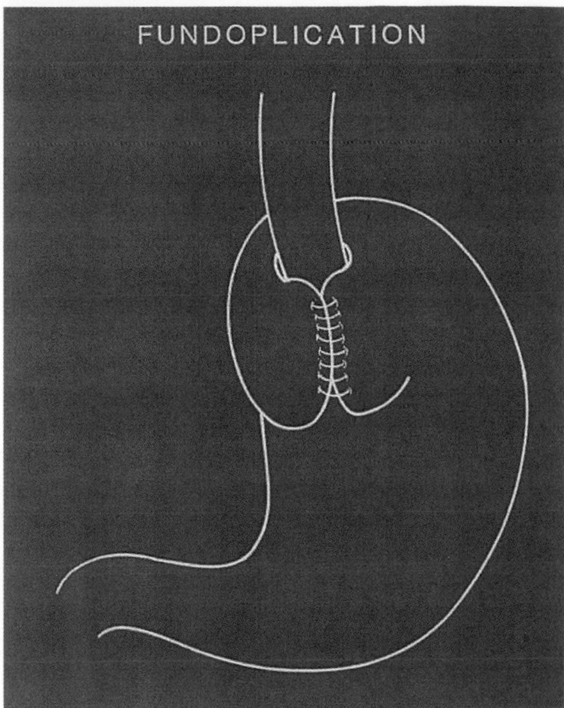

Fig. 10.3 Fundoplication: The stomach is wrapped around the lower oesophagus and controls acid reflux.

because the morbidity from the procedure is substantially less through this route.

The most common operation performed is one where the fundus of the stomach is drawn around behind the oesophagus and then stitched to itself in front of the oesophagus. This is called a fundoplication (Fig. 10.3) and although the way in which it works is not entirely clear, it is known that this wrapping of the oesophagus is extremely effective in its antireflux action. As already mentioned, it is so effective that it holds gas in the stomach as well as other stomach contents. Furthermore, even with the vigorous antiperistalsis of vomiting, it usually prevents retropulsion of gastric contents into the oesophagus.

Complications specific to antireflux surgery are usually related to dysphagia, which occurs if the wrap is too tight, the oesophageal hiatus is made too narrow, the gastro-oesophageal junction is pulled through the wrap, or para-oesophageal herniation occurs alongside the wrap. In some patients, the wrap seems to break down with time and the incidence of recurrent reflux is about 15% over many years. It is possible to undertake further antireflux surgery in such circumstances, although surgery is usually more difficult the second time around.

Post-operative management is relatively standard, with oral fluids being commenced immediately, and a soft diet introduced when the patient is able to tolerate it. Discharge usually occurs 6–8 days after open surgery or 2–3 days after laparoscopic surgery. Because patients feel so well after laparoscopic surgery, they have to be advised to not do anything that raises their intra-abdominal pressure to high levels (such as heavy lifting) for about 8 weeks, to allow the hiatus to adequately seal with fibrous tissue. Otherwise there is a tendency for an early para-oesophageal hiatus hernia to occur.

Further reading

Richter JE. Long-term management of gastroesophageal reflux disease and its complications. *Am J Gastroenterol.* 1997; 92(Suppl. 4):30S–34S.

Jamieson GG. *Surgery of the Oesophagus.* Edinburgh: Churchill Livingstone; 1988.

Siewert JR. Gastro-esophageal reflux disease: Surgical point of view – introduction. *World J Surg.* 1991; 16:287.

MCQs

Select the single correct answer to each question.

1 In gastro-oesophageal reflux, the following statements are true *except*

- **a** alcohol consumption and smoking are important aggravating factors
- **b** is often associated with disordered oesophageal motility
- **c** a hiatus hernia is invariably present
- **d** barretts oesophagus may develop
- **e** iron deficiency anaemia may occur as a result of chronic blood loss

2 The following statements on the management of gastro-oesophageal reflux are correct *except*

- **a** 24-hour oesophageal manometry and pH monitoring is mandatory in the presence of oesophagitis demonstrated endoscopically
- **b** a proton pump inhibitor is an effective treatment
- **c** laryngeal spill-over is an indication for surgery
- **d** the most appropriate operation is a laparoscopic fundoplication
- **e** dysphagia may complicate anti-reflux surgery

11 Tumours of the oesophagus

Simon Law and John Wong

Benign tumours of the oesophagus

Benign tumours of the oesophagus account for less than 1% of all oesophageal neoplasms. Leiomyomas are the most common; rarer entities include papillomas, fibrovascular polyps, granular cell tumours, adenomas, haemangiomas, neurofibromas, and lipomas.

Leiomyomas are smooth-muscle tumours arising in the oesophageal wall. They are usually solitary, well encapsulated with an intact overlying mucosa, and grow slowly. Most small (<5 cm) leiomyomas are asymptomatic and are incidental finding on barium study (see Fig. 11.1A). Diagnosis is made from the typical appearance on imaging, and endoscopy reveals intact mucosa. Sometimes leiomyomas can grow as an annular lesion producing dysphagia. There is no good evidence that they undergo malignant transformation to leiomyosarcoma.

Small, asymptomatic leiomyomas can be observed. Surgical removal is warranted for symptomatic or large leiomyomas (>5 cm). Simple enucleation is performed. Oesophageal resection is occasionally necessary for large or annular tumours.

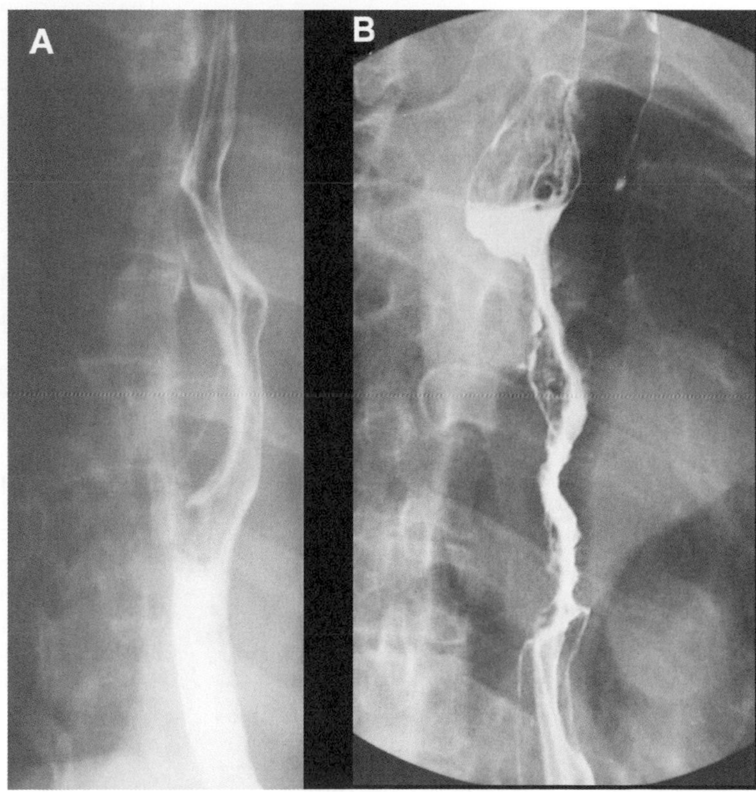

Fig. 11.1 (**A**) Barium contrast study showing the typical features of a leiomyoma of the oesophagus with a smooth semilunar defect in the contour of the oesophageal lumen and an intact mucosa, clear borders and a sharp angle between the tumour and the normal wall. (**B**) Barium contrast study showing a stenotic cancer of the mid-oesophagus with irregular mucosa, stenosis, proximal dilatation and 'shouldering'.

Malignant tumours of the oesophagus

Epidemiology

Oesophageal cancer is the ninth most common cancer and the sixth most frequent cause of cancer death worldwide. Squamous cell cancer is the most common. There is marked geographical variation in the incidence of oesophageal cancer. Countries in the so-called 'Asian oesophageal cancer belt', which stretches from eastern Turkey and east of the Caspian Sea through northern Iran, northern Afghanistan and southern areas of the former Soviet Union, such as Turkmenistan, Uzbekistan and Tajikistan, to northern China and India, have high incidence rates. The disease is also common in the Transkei province of South Africa, and Kenya. In high incidence areas, the occurrence of oesophageal cancer is 50- to 100-fold higher than in the rest of the world, for instance the incidence rate is over 160 per 100 000 population in Henan Province of China and is only 2 to 3 per 100 000 population in North America, Australia, and most areas of Europe.

Smoking and alcohol intake are the main aetiological agents, though in certain areas, other dietary factors are implicated (see Table 11.1). Patients with other aerodigestive malignancies have a 5–8% risk of developing synchronous or metachronous oesophageal squamous tumours, probably because of exposure to the same environmental carcinogens and the phenomenon of 'field cancerization'.

In western countries, the most striking change in epidemiology in the past three decades was the increase in incidence of adenocarcinomas of the lower oesophagus and gastric cardia. In the United States, the rate of adenocarcinoma has risen by more than 350% since 1970, surpassing squamous cell cancer around 1990. This shift in cell type is not apparent in Asian or African countries. The phenomenon is believed to be related to gastro-oesophageal reflux disease, obesity, and the pre-malignant condition of Barrett's oesophagus. Barrett's oesophagus is a condition in which the squamous epithelium of the distal oesophagus is replaced by a columnar epithelium characterized by the presence of specialized intestinal metaplasia. Diagnosis used to rely on endoscopic finding of a length of columnar epithelium of more than 3 cm, but current definition centres on histological identification rather than absolute length. The prevalence of adenocarcinoma in patients with Barrett's oesophagus averages about 13%, equivalent to at least a 30-fold increase in the risk of cancer compared to the general population. The Barrett's epithelium progresses through low-grade to high-grade dysplasia to invasive cancer. It is also suggested that the high prevalence of *Helicobacter pylori* infection in the East has a protective role against reflux, and hence Barrett's oesophagus and cancer. This hypothesis remains controversial.

Table 11.1 Factors associated with pathogenesis of oesophageal cancer

Environmental factors	Specific conditions
Smoking	History of aerodigestive tract malignancy*
Alcohol consumption Hot beverages* N-nitroso compounds*	Achalasia* Lye corrosive stricture* Plummer vinson (paterson kelley) syndrome*
Betel nut chewing*	
Deficiencies of*: Green vegetables Vitamins A, C and E Niacin Riboflavin Beta-carotene Zinc Molybdenum	Tylosis* Barrett's oesophagus†
History of radiation to mediastinum (e.g. ca breast)	
Low socio-economic class* Obesity† Fungal toxin or viral infection	

* Predisposes to squamous cell cancers.
† Predisposes to adenocarcinomas.

Surgical pathology

Squamous cell cancers and adenocarcinomas constitute the majority, together accounting for over 95% of all cancers. Other tumours, all of which are uncommon, include muco-epidermoid carcinoma, small cell carcinoma, adenoid cystic carcinoma, adenosquamous carcinoma, basaloid squamous cell carcinoma, sarcomas, lymphoma and melanoma. In countries where increase in adenocarcinomas is not observed, the majority of squamous cell cancers are located in the middle or lower portions of the oesophagus, while adenocarcinomas are mostly gastric cardia in position. This is in contrast to the West, where most adenocarcinomas are found in the lower oesophagus and gastric cardia.

In patients with Barrett's oesophagus, the premalignant dysplastic stages allow endoscopic surveillance to be carried out; however the optimal interval, benefits and cost-effectiveness are uncertain since most patients with oesophageal carcinoma present without a history of Barrett's oesophagus. Endoscopic ablation of Barrett's mucosa by laser, photodynamic therapy or other means followed by intensive acid suppressive therapy or fundoplication has been advocated in order to revert the epithelium to a squamous type. Whether such strategies can halt the progression to cancer is still under investigation.

The oesophagus has a rich plexus of intramural and submucosal lymphatics. Lymphatic spread tends to spread early and longitudinally, even to the neck and abdomen. Multi-centric tumours and submucosal spread should be searched for when a diagnosis of oesophageal cancer is made.

Clinical features

Oesophageal tumours are generally described with respect to their location in the oesophagus. The cervical oesophagus extends from the cricopharyngeus muscle at C6 level to the thoracic inlet (approximately 18 cm from the upper incisor teeth). The upper third of the intrathoracic oesophagus extends from the thoracic inlet to the tracheal bifurcation (24 cm), the middle third includes the proximal half of the oesophagus between the tracheal bifurcation to the diaphragmatic hiatus, the lower third being the distal half of this segment, and a short segment of abdominal oesophagus remains. The junction between the middle and lower thirds corresponds to approximately 32 cm from the upper incisor teeth, and the gastro-oesophageal junction ends at 40 cm.

Increasing incidence of adenocarcinomas of the lower oesophagus and cardia has prompted a classification of adenocarcinomas around the gastro-oesophageal junction, which includes adenocarcinomas found within a distance of 5 cm proximal and distal to the gastro-oesophageal junction (Fig. 11.2). Depending on the bulk and epicentre of the tumours, type I tumours are lower oesophageal (many are Barrett's) adenocarcinomas, type II centres at the

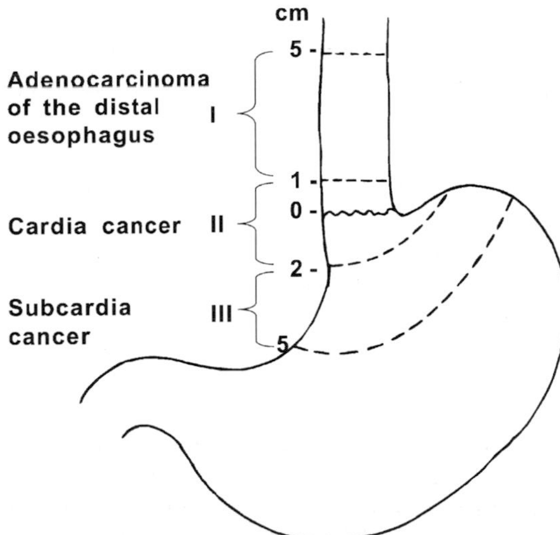

Fig. 11.2 Classification of adenocarcinomas around the gastro-oesophageal junction.

cardia, and type III are subcardiac cancers. It is suggested that the three types differ in pathologic and clinical features.

Most patients are more than 50 years of age, with a male predominance. Dysphagia is the most common symptom, and is rapid in onset, progressing from difficulty in swallowing solid food and later to liquid within a matter of weeks. Symptom of dysphagia is usually not felt until the tumour is advanced. The site of the 'hold-up' sensation has only a modest correspondence to the location of the tumour; it is usually located above, but not below, the actual site of obstruction.

Regurgitation, loss of weight, and substernal pain or discomfort are common. Hoarseness signifies recurrent laryngeal nerve palsy from direct tumour infiltration or from lymphatic spread and is thus a poor prognostic sign. Coughing or choking on eating may be due to aspiration, predisposed by the presence of vocal cord palsy if present, or the development of an oesophageal-respiratory fistula. Squamous cell cancers of the oesophagus rarely bleed. Patients with dysphagia and also evidence of gastrointestinal bleeding are more likely to have adenocarcinomas of the gastro-oesophageal junction. Exsanguinating haemorrhage from an oesophageal-aortic fistula is rare. Cervical lymph nodes should be searched for. Haematogenous spread to the lungs, liver, bones and other visceral organs, as well as hypercalcaemia from bone metastases or as a paraneoplastic phenomenon, are not infrequent.

Investigations

A barium swallow identifies the location and length of oesophageal narrowing, mucosal irregularity, dilatation of the proximal oesophagus, and the 'shouldering' impression made by the upper border of the tumour (see Fig. 11.1B). Features suggestive of advanced disease include deformity of the oesophageal axis, and sinuses that extend into the mediastinum or frank fistulation into the respiratory track. Most tumours present at an advanced stage, so diagnosis is not problematic. In earlier lesions, biopsies together with brush cytology improve the diagnostic accuracy. The application of Lugol's iodine stain helps direct biopsies to dysplastic or early mucosal lesions, since only normal oesophageal mucosa is stained brown, and the interested areas will remain unstained.

Staging methods

Accurate pre-operative staging allows selection of the most appropriate treatment. Current TNM staging classifications are shown in Table 11.2. Bronchoscopic examination is mandatory for tumours in close proximity to the tracheo-bronchial tree. Direct tumour infiltration precludes surgical resection. Vocal cord paralysis suggests recurrent laryngeal nerve involvement. A pan-endoscopy also serves to examine the rest of the

Table 11.2 Stage groupings for oesophageal cancer

T: Primary tumour
- Tx Tumour cannot be assessed
- Tis *In situ* carcinoma
- T1 Tumour invading lamina propria or the submucosa, does not breach submucosa
- T2 Tumour invading into but not beyond the muscularis propria
- T3 Tumour invades the adventitia but not the adjacent structure
- T4 Tumour invades the adjacent structure

N: Regional lymph nodes*
- NX Regional nodal status cannot be assessed
- N0 No regional lymph node involvement
- N1 Regional lymph node involved

M: Distant metastases
- Mx Distant metastases cannot be assessed
- M0 No distant metastasis
- M1a Upper thoracic oesophagus with metastases to cervical nodes
  Lower thoracic oesophagus with metastases to coeliac nodes
- M1b Upper thoracic oesophagus with metastases to other non-regional nodes or other distant sites
  Lower thoracic oesophagus with metastases to other non-regional nodes or other distant sites
  Middle thoracic oesophagus with metastases to cervical, coeliac, other non-regional nodes or other distant sites

Stage	T	N	M
Stage 0	Tis	N0	M0
Stage I	T1	N0	M0
Stage IIa	T2	N0	M0
	T3	N0	M0
Stage IIb	T1	N1	M0
	T2	N1	M0
Stage III	T3	N1	M0
	T4	N0–N1	M0
Stage IVa	Any T	Any N	M1a
Stage IVb	Any T	Any N	M1b

* For cervical oesophageal cancer, regional nodes are the cervical nodes. For intrathoracic cancers, the mediastinal and peri-gastric nodes (excluding coeliac nodes), are considered regional.

upper aerodigestive tract to look for other synchronous tumours. The use of computed tomography (CT) scans to assess the depth of oesophageal wall penetration, the degree of contiguous mediastinal structures and regional lymph node involvement are not sufficiently accurate except in overtly advanced cases. The obliteration of a 'fat plane' around the oesophagus may suggest extra-oesophageal infiltration although the paucity of fat especially in patients who have substantial weight loss makes this inaccurate. CT scans are more useful to detect distant metastases.

Endoscopic ultrasonography (EUS) is best in T-stage and regional nodal (N) staging, the accuracy of determining T-stage ranges between 85% and 90%, while N-staging accuracy approximates 70% to 90%. Recent advances also allow EUS-guided fine needle aspiration cytology of suspicious lymph nodes to be carried out.

Positron-emission tomography (PET) with 18-F-fluoro-deoxy-D-glucose (FDG) is increasingly used, and is of particular value in picking up distant nodal or systemic metastases. Sensitivity, specificity and accuracy rates for the detection of distant metastases of 88%, 93% and 91% respectively are reported, but local-regional staging of N_1 disease seems inferior to EUS. Laparoscopic and thoracoscopic staging are practised in selected centres. The former may be useful for lower oesophageal or cardiac tumours, the latter is more invasive, and its use is unlikely to gain widespread support.

Principles of treatment

A simplied therapeutic algorithm is shown in Figure 11.3. Patients with obvious disseminated disease should be palliated by non-surgical means. Those with

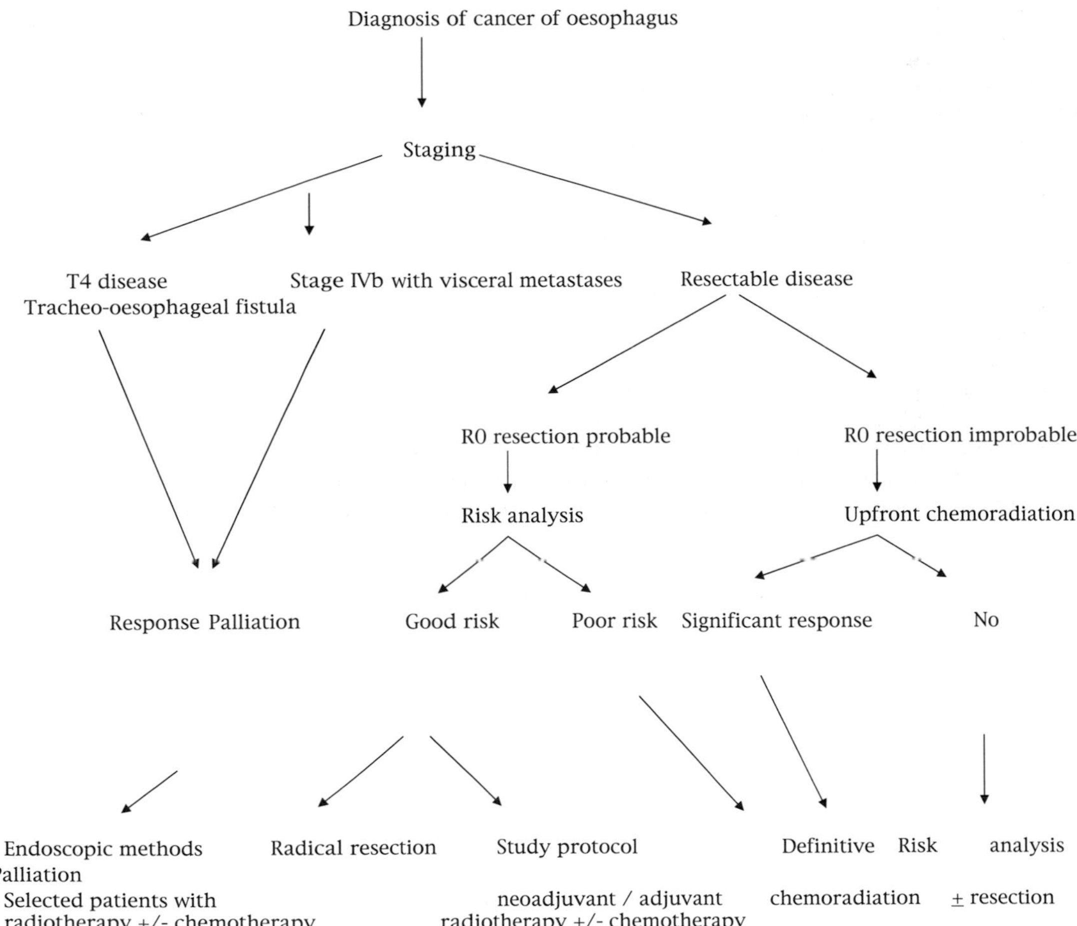

Fig. 11.3 Management protocol for patients with oesophageal cancer.

early disease generally do well with surgical resection, provided an R0 resection (curative procedure with macroscopic and microscopic clear margins) can be performed. In patients with local-regional advanced disease, upfront combined treatments including chemotherapy and radiotherapy are often used, and subsequent surgical resection depending on response. There is, however, no clear evidence that this gives superior result to surgical resection alone.

Operative treatment

Contraindications against surgical resection include presence of distal visceral or nodal metastases, direct infiltration of the tracheo-bronchial tree or aorta, although sometimes accurate diagnosis of the latter may be established pre-operatively. The indication for palliative surgery has lessened, while other effective options are available.

Potential surgical candidates should have a careful risk assessment especially with regards to cardiopulmonary status. Smoking should be stopped and active chest physiotherapy instituted. Pre-operative enteral nutrition or parenteral nutrition may be beneficial.

For tumours of the middle and lower third of the oesophagus, the most often performed operation is the Lewis-Tanner (Ivor Lewis) operation (see Fig. 11.4A). The stomach, the blood supply of which is based on the right gastric and right gastroepiploic vessels, is mobilised via laparotomy. A pyloroplasty or pyloromyotomy is performed to enhance gastric drainage. The oesophagus is then resected through a right thoracotomy. The stomach is delivered up into the thorax via the diaphragmatic hiatus to anastomose with the divided oesophagus near the apex of the thoracic cavity.

In type II and III tumours around the gastro-oesophageal junction, an extended total gastrectomy with a distal oesophageal resection is often performed, although some surgeons advocate a proximal gastric and distal oesophageal resection. Both can be accomplished via the abdomen or with an additional thoracotomy.

In tumours of the upper thoracic oesophagus, oesophagectomy can be performed through a right thoracotomy, then by simultaneous left cervical and abdominal incisions the stomach can be prepared and delivered up to the neck for anastomosis (McKeown's procedure; see Fig. 11. 4B).

In transhiatal oesophagectomy, the oesophagus is 'shelled' out by the surgeon's hand introduced in the posterior mediastinum via the diaphragmatic hiatus and the neck without a thoracotomy. This partly blind procedure may lead to injury to mediastinal structures, such as the membranous trachea, and has also been criticised as an inadequate cancer operation. In experienced hands however, it is safe, and its proponents claim similar survival to the transthoracic approach. Various minimal-access methods including combinations of thoracoscopy, laparoscopy and mediastinostomy have been attempted. The myriad of surgical methods implies a lack of consensus to which is the best. Proof of their superiority over conventional techniques is not forthcoming.

Most surgeons perform lymphadenectomy of the upper abdomen and mediastinum (two-field dissection). Some surgeons, especially in Japan, advocate the addition of bilateral neck dissection (three-field dissection) because of the high incidence of positive cervical lymph nodes found when neck dissection is carried out (up to 30%), and better cure rate is claimed. Again the optimal extent of lymph node dissection is a controversial subject.

The stomach is most commonly used for oesophageal substitution. In patients with previous gastric surgery, other substitutes like the colon or jejunum can be used. In cases where the substitute is brought to the neck for anastomosis, the posterior mediastinum (orthotopic), retrosternal route or subcutaneous space are alternatives.

Tumours of the cervical oesophagus require the resection of the larynx and pharynx, and the stomach is usually used to restore continuity (pharyngo–laryngo–oesophagectomy). A terminal tracheostome is performed and alternative voice rehabilitation is required. For tumours limited to the postcricoid region, resection need not involve the thoracic oesophagus and a free jejunal graft can be placed in the neck to restore intestinal continuity after pharyngo-laryngectomy. For these tumours, in order to preserve the larynx, often non-operative treatment such as chemoradiation therapy is used as an alternative to surgical resection.

Complications of surgery

Pulmonary complications are the most common, followed by cardiac problems (see Table 11.3). Cessation of smoking, peri-operative chest physiotherapy, care to avoid fluid overload, and regular bronchoscopic

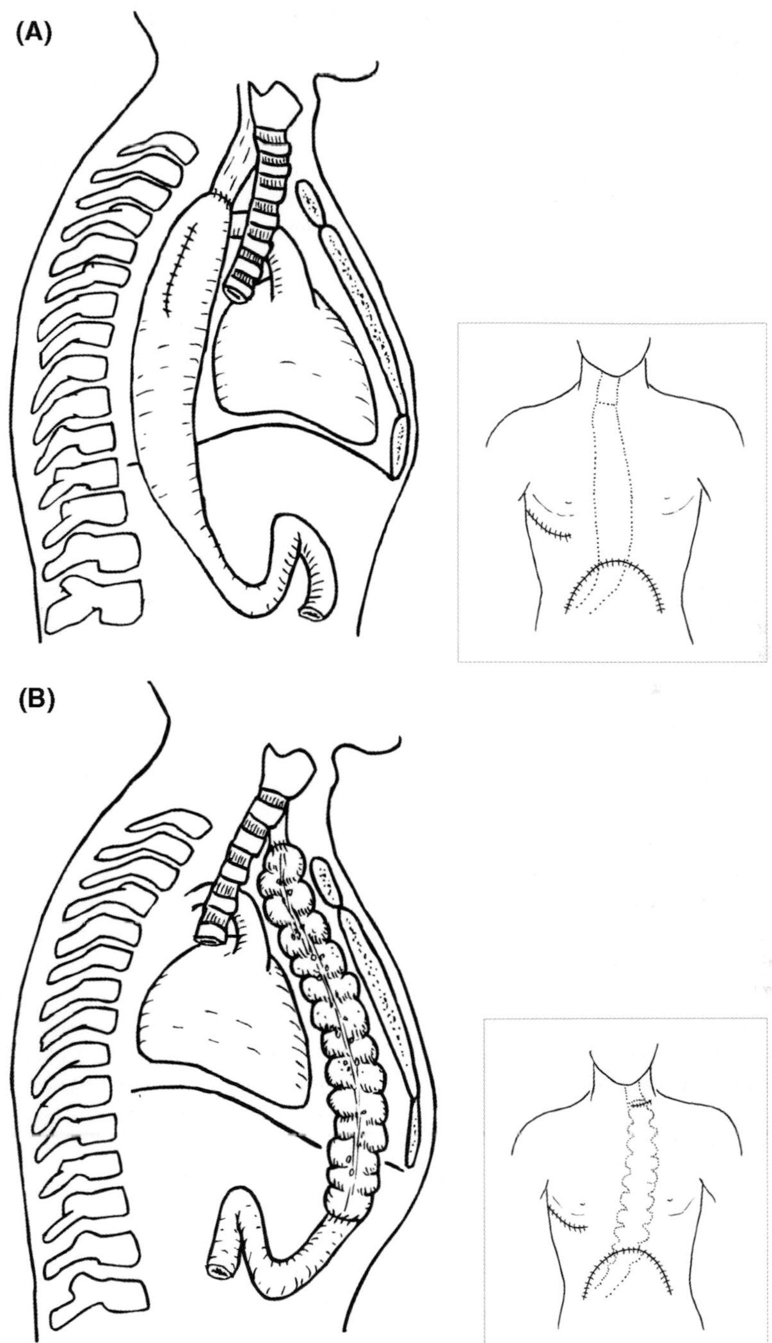

Fig. 11.4 (**A**) A Lewis–Tanner (Ivor Lewis) oesophagectomy with intra-thoracic esophago-gastrostomy. (**B**) A three-phase oesophagectomy. The colon is placed in the retrosternal route in this example with anastomosis in the neck.

Table 11.3 Complications after oesophagectomy

Medical	Surgical
Cardiac • Atrial arrhythmia* • Myocardial infarction • Cardiac failure Pulmonary • Atelectesis* • Pneumothorax • Bronchopneumonia with or without aspiration* • Sputum retention* • Pleural effusion* • Pulmonary embolism • Respiratory failure Other medical† • Renal failure • Hepatic failure • Stroke	• Intra-operative or post-operative haemorrhage • Tracheo-bronchial tree injury • Recurrent laryngeal nerve injury • Anastomotic leakage • Gangrene of conduit • Intra-thoracic gastric outlet obstruction or gastric stasis • Herniation of bowel through diaphragmatic hiatus • Chylothorax • Empyema • Wound infection

Note: Surgical complications are technique- and operator-dependent, thus incidences can vary.
* Relatively common occurrence.
† Should be all uncommon.

clearance of retained sputum are beneficial. Early tracheostomy in patients who have poor cough effort, especially in those who have vocal cord paralysis, is invaluable for facilitation of sputum suction. Atrial arrhythmia is also common; most are benign and are controlled with appropriate medication. It is important, however, to look for an underlying cause since it may be indicative of pulmonary or surgical septic pathologies.

Surgical complications are mostly related to faulty techniques. Anastomotic leak, which was once a common event, should now be rare in specialised centres (<5%). Treatment principle involves adequate drainage, antibiotics and nutritional support. Convincing evidence exists that demonstrates a hospital-volume and surgeon-volume outcome relationship with complex surgery like oesophagectomy. Mortality rate in dedicated centres is below 5%.

Non-operative treatments

Chemotherapy and radiotherapy

In the past, external-beam radiation has been used as the main alternative to surgery. Relief of dysphagia is however less effective, and radiation strictures may develop. Chemoradiation therapy gives superior result to radiation alone in the treatment of oesophageal cancer, both in terms of response rate, local control, and long-term survival. Radiotherapy alone has thus mostly a palliative role in patients who cannot tolerate the addition of chemotherapy. Brachytherapy, or intraluminal radiotherapy, whereby radioactivity is delivered in close proximity to the tumour via a tube placed inside the oesophagus, can also produce good palliation.

As neo-adjuvant or adjuvant therapy with surgery, neither radiotherapy and/or chemotherapy has been conclusively demonstrated to improve overall survival compared to surgical resection alone. Only patients with good response tend to benefit. All these treatments have potential disadvantages, such as prolonging treatment time and toxicities and increasing peri-operative morbidity.

Most commonly used conventional drugs used for oesophageal cancer are cisplatin and flurouracil. New drugs are being explored. Search for reliable markers for prediction of response to chemoradiation is important, so that potentially toxic treatments are not given to those unlikely to respond. Various serological, histological, and molecular markers are being examined; metabolic imaging by PET scan, with its measurement of 'tumour activity', shows some promise in predicting response early in the course of treatment.

Other treatment options

For early mucosal lesions, endoscopic mucosectomy can be performed. The mucosal cancer is 'raised' by injecting saline in the submucosal plane; it is then snared by an electrocautery loop as in polypectomy.

Placement of a prosthetic tube across the tumour stenosis may be indicated in patients not otherwise suitable for other treatment to palliate the symptom of dysphagia. Traditional tubes placed by laparotomy (e.g. Celestin tube, Mousseau–Barbin tube) or oesophagoscopy under sedation (e.g. Atkinson tube, Souttar tube) are now rarely used since they have been superseded by a variety of self-expanding metallic stents (see Fig. 11.5). Placement of these stents is less traumatic and immediate complications are less.

Laser therapy (Neodymium:yttrium aluminium garnet [Nd:YAG] laser) vaporises the tumour to restore luminal patency. Recannulation often requires repeated treatment sessions, and the effect is temporary.

Other less commonly used non-surgical options include injection of the tumour with alcohol or chemotherapeutic agents, photodynamic therapy, and use of a bicap heater probe. The choice of therapy depends on availability, cost and consideration of efficacy.

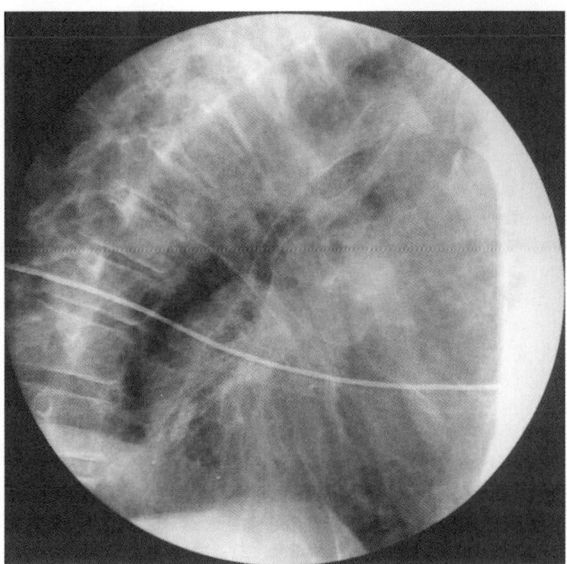

Fig. 11.5 A self-expanding metallic oesophageal stent *in situ*.

Prognosis

Overall prognosis remains poor with oesophageal cancer because of late disease presentation. At the authors' institution, in patients with squamous cell carcinomas and who undergo surgical resection alone, 5-year survival of patients with stage I, II, III and IV disease are 83%, 32%, 13% and 7% respectively. The figures were 31% and 8% for R0 and R1/2 resections, and were 35% and 15% for those with node negative and positive disease respectively. In large Western series, it has been suggested that overall survival in patients with adenocarcinomas is better that those with squamous cell cancers.

Surgery remains the mainstay treatment for oesophageal cancer, offering the most complete and lasting restoration of swallowing ability and a chance of cure. In specialised centres oesophageal surgery can be performed safely on a wide spectrum of patients. For centres with less experience, more restrictive patient selection is essential. How to integrate various combined multimodality treatment programmes of chemotherapy and radiotherapy deserves more study, and their impact on long-term prognosis should be evaluated in well-conducted clinical trials.

MCQs

Select the single correct answer to each question.

1 For patients suffering from oesophageal cancer, which of the following symptoms indicates the WORST prognosis?

a hoarseness of voice
b weight loss of more than 10% of usual body weight
c dysphagia to solid and semi-solid food
d regurgitation of swallowed food
e odynophagia

2 A 75-year-old man complains of progressive dysphagia for 2 months. He has loss of 10 lb in weight and can only tolerate a liquid diet. Oesophageal cancer is suspected. Which of the following investigations is MOST likely to detect evidence of distant metastases from his cancer?

a upper endoscopy
b endoscopic ultrasonography
c positron emission tomography
d ultrasound +/− fine needle aspiration of neck
e CT scan

3 Out of the following, the MOST LIKELY risk factor for the development of a squamous cell cancer of the oesophagus is:
- **a** smoking
- **b** alcohol intake
- **c** obesity
- **d** history of cancer of the larynx
- **e** achalasia

4 The most common benign tumour of the oesophagus is:
- **a** adenosquamous carcinoma
- **b** fibrovascular polyp
- **c** leiomyoma
- **d** haemangioma
- **e** neurofibroma

5 The diagnosis of chylous leak after oesophagectomy is NOT helped by:
- **a** analysis of chylomicrons in the chest tube output
- **b** lymphangiogram
- **c** milk challenge
- **d** gastrografin contrast swallow
- **e** test for triglyceride in chest tube output

12 Peptic ulcer disease

S. C. Sydney Chung

Introduction

Peptic ulcer is a common condition. Ten per cent of the population suffer from it at some time or another. The incidence and severity of peptic ulcer disease are decreasing in the Western world but they are increasing in developing countries. Because of the widespread use of non-steroidal anti-inflammatory drugs (NSAID), the incidence of ulcer disease in the elderly is increasing.

Aetiology

Peptic ulcers occur when the balance between acid-pepsin digestion and the defence mechanism of the mucosa is disturbed. Classical sites for peptic ulcers are the first part of the duodenum, the angula incisura and the antrum of the stomach, the lower end of the oesophagus in patients with gastro-oesophageal reflux, the efferent limb of a gastroenterostomy, and inside a Meckel's diverticulum if there is ectopic gastric mucosa.

Acid hypersecretion was thought to be the most important factor in the causation of ulcers, in particular duodenal ulcers. The classical example of the effect of increased acid production is the Zollinger–Ellison syndrome. Gastrin produced by the pancreatic or duodenal adenoma causes maximal stimulation of the parietal cell mass, producing massive amounts of acid and resulting in a particularly aggressive form of peptic ulcer disease. Recent evidence, however, indicates that *Helicobacter pylori*, a Gram-negative organism that resides in the mucus layer of the antrum, is the real culprit in the majority of cases. The organism is found in more than 90% of patients with duodenal ulcers and about 70% of patients with gastric ulcers. The exact mechanism through which the bacteria cause peptic ulceration is still conjectural, but eradication of the bacteria heals the ulcer and prevents recurrence. Such a discovery has completely revolutionised the understanding of the pathogenesis and management of peptic ulcers.

Mucosal defence against acid-pepsin digestion consists of the mucous layer on the mucosa serving as a barrier between the lumen and the epithelial surface, the secretion of bicarbonate and the rapid turnover of mucosal cells. Helicobacter infection, NSAID intake, reflux of bile into the stomach and by mucosal ischaemia are factors that can weaken the mucosal defence and contribute to the development of ulcers.

'Stress ulcers' are common in severely ill patients, particularly those treated in intensive care units. Cushing's ulcers and Curling's ulcers are stress ulcers occurring after head injuries and severe burns, respectively. These ulcers are caused by increased acid production in stressed patients, and mucosal ischaemia as a result of splanchnic hypoperfusion.

Duodenal ulcer

Practically all duodenal ulcers occur in the duodenal bulb. This part of the duodenum is in the direct path of the acid contents of the stomach. Alkaline pancreatic juice and bile, which enter the duodenum in the second part, have not yet had an opportunity to neutralise the gastric acid. Duodenal ulcers are more common than gastric ulcers. They tend to occur in younger patients and are more common in men than in women. There is also a genetic predisposition; the disease is more common in family members of index cases, patients with blood group O, non-secretors of blood group antigens in the saliva, and those with high circulating pepsinogen.

Clinical features

The cardinal symptom of duodenal ulcer is pain. The pain is typically localised to the epigastrium, is dull or burning in character, starts several hours after a meal, wakes the patient at night and is relieved by food or antacids. Nausea and vomiting may be present during acute exacerbation but are not prominent features. In contrast to patients with non-ulcer dyspepsia, ulcer patients localise the pain to the epigastrium with one finger. Apart from mild tenderness in the epigastrium, patients with uncomplicated ulcer disease do not have physical signs.

The course of duodenal ulcer disease is one of relapses and remissions. The patient complains of episodes of severe pain lasting for weeks, interspersed by months of remission, the pattern repeating itself over several years. The disease may burn itself out after 10–15 years.

Diagnosis

It is difficult to differentiate duodenal ulcer from other causes of dyspepsia (gastric ulcer, non-ulcer dyspepsia, reflux oesophagitis, gastric cancer, gallstone) with confidence on clinical grounds alone. Barium meal may show an ulcer crater. However, it may be difficult to differentiate active ulceration from scarring. Flexible endoscopy is the most accurate diagnostic method. The oesophagus, stomach and the first and second part of the duodenum can be clearly seen using this technique.

Helicobacter pylori can be demonstrated by serology, by the urea breath test, or in antral biopsies using microscopy or the rapid urease test. Culture of organisms is difficult and rarely performed in clinical practice. Serology detects past as well as current infection and is simple to conduct as only a drop of blood is necessary. The accuracy of the commercially available test kits have improved but their validity must be confirmed for each country as there are geographical differences in the genetic makeup of the bacteria. Serology cannot be reliably used to assess the success of eradication therapy, as antibody levels can remain raised for prolonged periods even after successful eradication In the urea breath test, urea labelled with a non-radioactive (C13) or radioactive (C14) carbon isotope is given by mouth. Helicobacter produces urease, which split the urea into ammonia and carbon dioxide. If C13 or C14 is detected in the exhaled breath the presence of Helicobacter is confirmed. The urea breath test is a reliable non-invasive way of confirming the success of eradication therapy. In patients who have undergone endoscopy, a convenient test is the rapid urease test. Antral biopsies are embedded into a gel containing urea and an indicator dye (neutral red). The ammonia produced as a result of urease is alkaline and changes the indicator dye to a red colour. This gives a rapid result – often within an hour – and is cheaper than histology. The use of proton pump inhibitors such as omeprazole lead to a suppression of organism numbers in the gastric mucosa. This can lead to false negative results in patients undergoing urea breath test, urease test and even histology. It is recommended that patients on proton pump inhibitors have these ceased at least 2 weeks prior to urea breath testing or, if testing is to be performed at endoscopy, that biopsies are taken for histology from both antrum and body of stomach to increase the yield.

Treatment

The aim of treatment is to alleviate the ulcer pain, to heal the ulcer, to prevent recurrence and to forestall complications. With powerful anti-secretory drugs and effective regimens to eradicate Helicobacter, these aims can be achieved by medical therapy in the great majority of patients. Apart from giving up smoking and avoiding, if possible, ulcerogenic drugs, lifestyle modification such as a change in diet or avoidance of stress is not necessary. Such changes are difficult to make and there is little evidence that they accelerate ulcer healing. Nowadays, elective surgery for uncomplicated ulcer disease is rarely, if ever, indicated. Nearly all ulcer surgery is performed as an emergency procedure for complications.

Commonly used drugs

ANTACIDS

Antacids may be in tablet or liquid form. They are either magnesium based (liable to cause diarrhoea) or aluminium based (may cause constipation). Antacids give rapid relief of ulcer pain but do not heal ulcers unless taken in very high doses.

HISTAMINE-2 RECEPTOR ANTAGONISTS

Histamine-2 receptor antagonists (H_2 blockers) are the first group of drugs that can effectively block gastric acid secretion. Examples are cimetidine, ranitidine and famotidine. Relief of pain occurs after a few days and up to 90% of ulcers heal after a 6-week course. Once the drug is stopped, however, acid production returns to normal and ulcer recurrence is highly likely.

PROTON PUMP INHIBITORS

Proton pump inhibitors such as omeprazole or lansoprazole leads to complete inhibition of gastric acid production. Symptomatic relief and ulcer healing is even more impressive than H_2 blockers. However, once the drug is stopped ulcer recurrence is common. Proton pump inhibitors have been shown to both prevent and heal ulcers associated with NSAID use.

SUCRALFATE

Sucralfate is a drug that is not absorbed but exerts its action by physically covering the ulcer base. Ulcer healing rates are similar to H_2 blockers.

ERADICATION OF *Helicobacter pylori*

Eradication of *H. pylori* is now the cornerstone of ulcer treatment. It is also the main reason why elective surgery for peptic ulcer disease is now very rare. The bacteria dwells in, and is protected by, the mucous layer of the gastric pits and are difficult to eradicate. Multiple drugs need to be administered simultaneously. Effective combinations should result in eradication in more than 90% of patients, if patient compliance is satisfactory. Examples of such combinations are 1–2 weeks of triple therapy using bismuth, tetracycline and metronidazole. Side effects, especially gastrointestinal upsets, are common. Combinations of a proton pump inhibitor and two other antibiotics (e.g. amoxycillin and clarithromycin) taken for 1 week are equally effective and have fewer side effects. This combination has become first line therapy in most countries.

Surgery

The classical operations for duodenal ulcer disease are designed to reduce gastric acid production (Table 12.1).

Table 12.1 Operations for duodenal ulcers

(%)	Mortality	Side effects	Recurrence rate (%)
Pólya's gastrectomy	2–5	+++	5
Vagotomy and drainage	1	+	5–10
Highly selective vagotomy	<0.5	±	15
Vagotomy and antrectomy	2–5	++	1

Nowadays their use is almost entirely confined to the management of ulcer complications. Essentially one can remove the acid-producing part of the stomach or sever the vagus nerve, which controls acid secretion.

PÓLYA'S GASTRECTOMY

Acid is secreted by parietal cells in the body and the fundus of the stomach. In order to ensure adequate reduction of acid output, at least two-thirds of the stomach needs to be resected. Patients who have had this operation are unable to tolerate large meals. Weight loss, malnutrition and anaemia are common. The rapid entry of food into the intestine leads to 'dumping syndromes'; the patient feels faint or unwell after a meal. This may be due to transudation of fluid in response to an osmotic load in the gut (early dumping, occurring 10 minutes after a meal) or rapid absorption of glucose, leading to insulin release and rebound hypoglycaemia (late dumping, occurring 2–3 hours after a meal).

TRUNCAL VAGOTOMY AND DRAINAGE

Gastric acid production may also be decreased by dividing the vagus nerve, thus removing the nervous stimulation of the parietal cell mass. If the whole vagal trunk is cut, delay in gastric emptying occurs in a significant number of patients because the motor supply to the antrum is also severed. A drainage operation, either a pyloroplasty or gastro-enterostomy, is necessary. These operations are relatively easy to perform and are useful in emergency situations. Between 5 and 10% of patients complain of diarrhoea, due to rapid transit of food through the gut.

HIGHLY SELECTIVE VAGOTOMY

This operation aims to divide the vagal fibres supplying the parietal cell mass but leave the innervation of the antrum (the nerve of Laterget) intact. The operation is technically demanding and time-consuming. Side effects are almost non-existent but the recurrence rate is higher than other procedures.

VAGOTOMY AND ANTRECTOMY

In this operation the vagal trunks are divided to remove the vagal stimulation of acid production and the antrum is resected to remove the source of gastrin, another potent stimulator of gastric acid secretion. Continuity of the gastrointestinal tract is restored by gastroduodenal anastomosis. The main attraction of this operation is the very low ulcer recurrence rate.

Gastric ulcer

Gastric ulcers are less common than duodenal ulcers. They affect the older age group. Gastric ulcers are more common in patients from lower socioeconomic groups. Non-steroidal anti-inflammatory drugs are a common cause of gastric ulcers.

Clinical features

As in duodenal ulceration the usual presentation is epigastric pain. The pain is typically exacerbated by food; nausea, unremitting pain and weight loss are common. Differentiation from duodenal ulcer (and gastric cancer) is unreliable.

Diagnosis

In double-contrast barium meal examination the stomach wall is coated with a thin layer of barium and effervescent drink is given to distend the stomach with gas. Benign gastric ulcers appear as craters, penetrating beyond the expected stomach contour, with mucosal folds radiating from the ulcer like spokes of a wheel. Irregular ulcer edges, a crater protruding into the lumen of the stomach, irregular mucosal folds with no peristalsis, and ulcers located at sites other than the lesser curvature and the antrum, suggest malignancy. All demonstrated gastric ulcers must be investigated by endoscopy and biopsy.

Through the endoscope a benign gastric ulcer has smooth, regular margins. The most common site is the angular incisura, followed by the lesser curvature and the antrum. An ulcer seen outside these locations should be presumed malignant. Malignant ulcers are irregular with raised, rolled-up edges. With potent acid suppression, even malignant ulcers may completely heal over temporarily, leaving an area of mucosal irregularity. All gastric ulcers must have multiple biopsies taken from all four quadrants of the ulcer. After a course of therapy, repeat endoscopy to assess healing and repeat biopsy are mandatory.

Treatment

Although acid output is normal or low in patients with gastric ulcers, ulcer pain is controlled and the ulcer heals with acid suppression. H_2 blockers or omeprazole may be used. Because gastric ulcers are larger than duodenal ulcers they generally take longer to heal. Some 70% of gastric ulcers are associated with *H. pylori*. Eradication of the bacteria is indicated in such patients to reduce the recurrence rate. Other gastric ulcers are caused by NSAID. If it is not possible for the patient to stop taking NSAID, a proton pump inhibitor taken concurrently confers a degree of protection.

Gastric cancer may masquerade as a gastric ulcer. If complete healing of the ulcer is not achieved with two or three courses of medical therapy, surgical resection of the ulcer is indicated.

The aim of surgical treatment is to resect the ulcer-bearing part of the stomach. The operation of choice for gastric ulcers is Billroth I gastrectomy, in which the distal half of the stomach is removed and gastroduodenal continuity restored. In elderly, frail patients, and in those with an ulcer high on the lesser curvature where resection would entail removal of most of the stomach, excision of the ulcer with vagotomy and pyloroplasty may be an alternative.

Complications of ulcer disease

Complications of duodenal ulcers include bleeding, perforation and gastric outlet obstruction.

Bleeding

Peptic ulcer bleeds occur when the ulcer erodes an artery in the ulcer base. Classical textbook cases of posterior duodenal ulcers eroding the gastroduodenal artery and gastric ulcers eroding the left gastric artery are rarely seen. Most cases of ulcer bleeding result from erosion of medium-sized arteries in the submucosa.

Peptic ulcer bleeding is the most common cause of upper gastrointestinal haemorrhage and is a frequent cause of emergency hospital admission. The mortality is about 10% and has remained constant despite advances in diagnosis and treatment. This is due to an increase in the number of elderly people presenting with this condition.

About 85% of bleeding ulcers stop bleeding spontaneously and do not require specific measures to stop the haemorrhage. The mortality in those who continue to bleed or develop rebleeding while in hospital is 10-fold higher. The likelihood of rebleeding may be predicted on clinical grounds and the appearance of the ulcer on endoscopy. Haematemesis and shock on admission suggest a large initial bleed and are associated with a higher risk of recurrent haemorrhage. Ulcers with stigmata of recent haemorrhage, such as a visible vessel or an adherent blood clot seen on endoscopy, are also more likely to rebleed. On the other hand, if a clean-based ulcer is seen on endoscopy the risk of rebleeding is very low. The risk of rebleeding decreases with time after the initial bleed. If rebleeding does not occur within the first 72 hours it is unlikely to occur.

Clinical features

The patient may vomit fresh blood and clots (indicating torrential bleeding) or coffee-ground material (acid-haematin resulting from the action of gastric acid on haemoglobin). More commonly the patient passes melaena (semi-liquid, tarry stool with a characteristic sickly smell). The consistency and colour of the melaena may give some clue to the rapidity of the bleeding; the redder and less well formed the stool, the brisker the haemorrhage. There may be a background of long-standing peptic ulcer disease, and history of another episode of bleeding in the past. In 30% of patients there is a history of recent intake of NSAID or aspirin. The patient may complain of dizziness or faint on getting up from a supine position or after going to the toilet.

Apart from melaena on rectal examination, patients with a mild to moderate amount of blood loss show little abnormality on examination. A postural drop of blood pressure is the first clinically detectable sign of hypovolaemia. Tachycardia, sweaty palms, hypotension, anxiety and agitation are signs of shock and call for urgent blood volume replacement.

Treatment

RESUSCITATION

All patients who have had a significant gastrointestinal bleed within the past 48 hours should be admitted to hospital. A large-bore intravenous cannula should be inserted and blood drawn for baseline tests and cross-matching. In the acute stage, the haemoglobin level is a poor guide to the need for transfusion as haemodilution may not have occurred. The decision to replace the blood volume by plasma expanders or blood should be based on signs of hypovolaemia and the rapidity of the bleeding. In elderly patients with poor cardiac reserve, or in patients with massive bleeding, monitoring the central venous pressure by a central venous line gives a more accurate indication of the amount of fluids needed.

IDENTIFY THE BLEEDING POINT

If facilities allow, all patients admitted with upper gastrointestinal haemorrhage should undergo endoscopy within 24 hours of admission. Patients who vomit fresh blood or are in shock may have ongoing massive blood loss and should undergo endoscopy once they are resuscitated. An accurate diagnosis forms the basis of logical treatment, and the precise location of bleeding is of paramount importance should surgery be needed to control bleeding.

CONTROL BLEEDING

Ulcer bleeding stops spontaneously in about 80% of patients. Only a small percentage require specific measures to stop bleeding. In recent years endoscopic procedures have become the first-line method of controlling ulcer bleeding. The most popular methods are injection therapy using adrenaline solution and/or sclerosants, such as polidocanol, absolute alcohol or ethanolamine, contact thermal methods, such as the heater probe or multipolar electrocoagulation, or a combination of the above. Endoscopic haemostasis should be applied for ulcers with active bleeding or stigmata of recent haemorrhage predictive of high risks of rebleeding. Surgery remains the most definitive method of controlling ulcer haemorrhage, and is indicated when endoscopic haemostasis fails to control the bleeding, or when rebleeding occurs. The morbidity and mortality of emergency surgery for ulcer bleeding is high. In principle, the operation performed should be the minimum compatible with permanent haemostasis. The choice of operations is determined by the site and size of the ulcer as well as the experience and preference of the surgeon. Most bleeding duodenal ulcers may be managed by underrunning the bleeding vessel together with vagotomy and pyloroplasty. Large, deep ulcers destroying the first part of the duodenum may require a Pólya's gastrectomy. Bleeding gastric ulcers are best treated by gastrectomy. In frail, elderly patients an alternative is ulcer excision, with or without vagotomy and drainage.

Perforation

Perforation occurs when the ulcer erodes through the full thickness of the gut wall. Gastric and duodenal contents spill into the peritoneal cavity causing generalised peritonitis. The most frequent site of perforation is the anterior wall of the first part of the duodenum. Males outnumber females in a ratio of 9 to 1. The incidence of ulcer perforation in the elderly is increasing because of the increased use of NSAID.

Clinical features

The patient presents with sudden onset of severe abdominal pain. The onset of pain is so sudden that the patient can often accurately pin-point the exact moment when the perforation occurred. Approximately 10% of patients have no preceding history of dyspepsia. The physical signs in the abdomen are dramatic. There is generalised tenderness, guarding and rebound tenderness. The abdominal muscles are held rigid, giving the classical 'board-like rigidity'. Abdominal respiratory movements and bowel sounds are absent. The percussion note over the liver may be resonant because of free intraperitoneal air. In patients in whom the perforations are sealed off by adjacent organs the signs may be localised to the epigastrium. In other cases the spillage from the perforation may track down the right paracolic gutter, resulting in maximal tenderness in the right iliac fossa. This is the so-called 'right paracolic gutter syndrome' and may be mistaken for acute appendicitis.

Investigations

A plain chest radiograph with the patient in the erect position shows free gas under the diaphragm in 80% of cases.

Treatment

Once a definitive diagnosis is made, the patient should be given parenteral opiates for pain relief, intravenous fluids should be administered and a nasogastric tube passed as soon as possible to decompress the stomach to avoid ongoing contamination. Unless there is clear evidence that the ulcer has been sealed off, an operation should be performed without delay. The operation of choice is a simple patch repair. A piece of omentum is sutured over the perforation to plug it (Fig. 12.1). This is followed by a thorough lavage of the peritoneal cavity with copious amounts of warm saline to remove all the exudate and food particles.

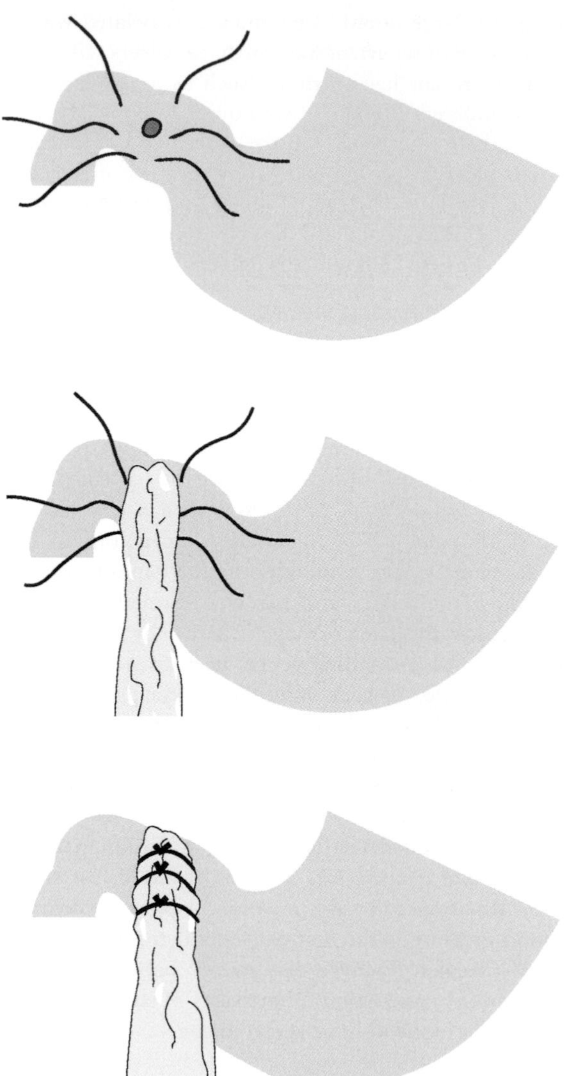

Fig. 12.1 Patch repair of perforated duodenal ulcer with a pedicle of omental plug.

If facilities and a surgeon experienced in laparoscopic surgery are available the patch repair can be performed laparoscopically, avoiding a painful wound.

The discovery that peptic ulcer disease can be cured by eradication of *H. pylori* has diminished the enthusiasm for definitive surgery at the same time as the patch repair. For patients who are Helicobacter-negative, an ulcer-curing operation (e.g. vagotomy and pyloroplasty, or highly selective vagotomy) may be considered if there has been a long history of troublesome ulcer disease with complications, provided that the condition of the patient is good and the degree of contamination of the abdomen not too severe.

Obstruction

Long-standing duodenal or prepyloric ulcers may cause gastric outlet obstruction. It may be due either to fibrosis resulting from chronic ulceration and healing or to oedema associated with acute ulceration.

Clinical features

The cardinal symptom is repeated vomiting of undigested food that is non–bile-stained. There may be weight loss and dehydration. Abdominal examination shows a dilated, distended stomach. Succussion splash (splashing noise on rocking the patient's abdomen) is present several hours after a meal.

The inability to take fluids by mouth and vomiting of gastric juice lead to severe fluid and electrolyte problems. The patient rapidly becomes dehydrated and salt depleted. Loss of acid and chloride ions in the gastric juice result in hypochloraemic alkalosis. There may be a large deficit of total body potassium. Because of the severe sodium depletion, the distal renal tubules secrete potassium and hydrogen ions in exchange for sodium ions in the glomerular filtrate. The urine is therefore acidic in severe cases of gastric outlet obstruction, although the patient is alkalotic. This is the so-called paradoxical aciduria.

A gastric cancer in the antrum or the pyloric canal causing obstruction may present in an identical manner.

Treatment

Fluid and electrolyte losses should be replaced by infusion of normal saline. Large amounts of potassium are likely to be required. Administration of potassium supplements should be guided by estimation of the serum level and acid–base balance. It should only commence when renal failure is excluded. Correction of alkalosis is not necessary. Once the fluid and electrolyte deficiencies are corrected the body's homeostatic mechanisms will restore the acid–base balance.

The stomach should be decompressed with a nasogastric tube. Food particles may block the tube. Irrigation and lavage through a wide-bore stomach tube is usually necessary. Intravenous omeprazole is given. Once the stomach is cleansed endoscopy should be carried out to confirm the diagnosis and to exclude malignancy. If the obstruction is due to oedema around an active ulcer, such measures may restore patency. In the majority of cases, operative management is required. The obstruction is either enlarged (vagotomy and pyloroplasty, pyloric dilatation with highly selective vagotomy), bypassed (vagotomy and gastroenterostomy) or resected (Pólya's gastrectomy, vagotomy and antrectomy). In elderly patients unfit for surgery, dilatation of the stenotic area using a balloon catheter under endoscopic guidance may be considered.

Zollinger–Ellison syndrome

This is a rare disease caused by overproduction of gastrin by G cell tumours of the pancreas or the duodenum. Maximal stimulation of the parietal cells leads to intractable peptic ulcerations. Ninety per cent of gastrinomas occur within the 'gastrinoma triangle' bounded by the cystic duct and bile duct, the junction of the head and neck of the pancreas, and the second and third parts of the duodenum. Two-thirds of all gastrinomas occur outside the pancreas. More than 60% of gastrinomas are malignant. Twenty per cent of patients with Zollinger–Ellison syndrome have micro-adenomatosis of the pancreas rather than discrete tumours.

Clinical features

The diagnosis should be suspected when peptic ulcers occur at unusual sites, such as the second part of the duodenum or the jejunum, or ulcers recur after adequate surgery. One-third of patients have watery diarrhoea due to high gastric output. Dehydration, and acid–base or electrolyte imbalance may occur.

Diagnosis

Measurement of gastric acid output

Because of the high circulating gastrin, the basal acid output (BAO) is high and stimulation with pentagastrin does not elicit significant increase. A BAO of more than 15 mmol/h and a BAO to maximal acid output ratio (BAO : MAO) of more than 0.6 is highly suggestive.

Gastrin assay

Gastrin can be measured by radioimmunoassay. The diagnosis is confirmed by demonstrating a high fasting gastrin level.

Treatment

The aim of treatment of Zollinger–Ellison syndrome is two-fold:

- to control the high gastric acid output and sever the ulcer diathesis
- to treat the gastrinoma

In the past a total gastrectomy was recommended to remove gastric acid production. Nowadays, the ulcer diathesis can usually be controlled by an adequate dose of omeprazole. If a single discrete tumour can be identified in the pancreas or the duodenum, surgical excision is the treatment of choice.

MCQs

Select the single correct answer to each question.

1 With a perforation of a duodenal ulcer which occurred 6 h ago, which of the following features is LEAST likely to be present?
- **a** generalised abdominal tenderness and guarding
- **b** the bowel sounds are hyperactive
- **c** percussion over the liver may demonstrate resonance
- **d** the respiration is shallow and the abdominal muscles are held rigid
- **e** plain radiograph shows free gas under the diaphragm

2 Which of the following factors is MOST likely to be associated with a significant risk of rebleeding from a duodenal ulcer?
- **a** no further bleeding within 72 hours of the initial bleed
- **b** a clean based ulcer seen on endoscopy
- **c** age less than 50 years
- **d** a visible vessel with adherent clot seen on endoscopy
- **e** the patient is female

3 The treatment of choice for a perforated duodenal ulcer in a 56-year-old man with a strong history of ulcer disease and signs of peritonitis after 12 hours is
- **a** conservative management with nasogastric suction and intravenous fluids
- **b** vagotomy and pyloroplasty
- **c** omental patch repair and peritoneal lavage
- **d** highly selective vagotomy
- **e** partial gastrectomy

13 Gastric neoplasms

Iain G. Martin

Introduction

Whilst most developed countries have seen dramatic reductions in the overall incidence of stomach cancer it remains the second commonest malignancy worldwide. Whilst adenocarcinoma account for more than 90% of all malignant stomach tumours, two other tumours should be considered, these are gastric lymphoma and gastric GI stromal tumours. The majority of this chapter will deal with adenocarcinoma.

Gastric adenocarcinoma

Fifty years ago adenocarcinoma of the stomach was the most frequently seen cancer in most countries, and whilst it has decreased rapidly in incidence it remains an important cancer in terms of cancer registrations and deaths. Gastric cancer overall has a poor prognosis in most countries outside of Japan, with overall 5 years' survival rate being around 10%.

Epidemiology

Gastric cancer is generally a disease of the elderly, with average age at presentation being 70 years and a 2 to 1 male to female predominance. The overall incidence varies from 6 per 100,000 in the USA to 70 per 100,000 in Japan.

There has been an important change in the epidemiology of adenocarcinoma of the stomach over the past 50 years. The commonest site of cancers was in the antrum of the stomach, with proximal third gastric cancers being unusual. Over the past 5 decades, antral gastric cancer has become less common whereas proximal third cancers more common – to a point where proximal cancers are now the most commonly seen in most developed countries. Whilst all the reasons behind this change are not clear some factors have been identified. The key identified aetiological factors for non-cardia gastric cancer are *Helicobacter pylori* infection, high nitrite intake, low intake of fruit and vegetables, smoking and high salt intake. Reductions in the incidence of *H. pylori* infection, higher fruit and vegetable intake and lower nitrite intakes have probably accounted for the reductions in the incidence of non-cardia gastric cancer. The reasons behind the increase in proximal gastric cancer are far from clear.

Pathogenesis

Although a simplification there are two broad histological types of gastric cancer, intestinal type cancers and diffuse type cancers (around 20–30% have a mixed picture). There is little evidence to support the two types' having different aetiological factors although the molecular pathways involved in the pathogenesis are different. The diffuse type is associated with abnormalities of the CDH1 gene, which codes for the protein e-cadherin. Mutations of this gene are responsible for the only identified hereditary form of gastric cancer, hereditary diffuse gastric cancer (HDGC).

Diagnosis

Patients with gastric cancer present with a range of symptoms including dyspepsia, upper abdominal pain, bloating and fullness, weight loss and vomiting. They can also bleed and present with anaemia; it is relatively uncommon for these tumours to present with haematemesis. There are no uniquely diagnostic symptoms and therefore a high index of suspicion is required to make the diagnosis.

Patients who have obvious physical signs on clinical examination (abdominal mass, supraclavicular lymph nodes etc.) almost invariably have incurable disease.

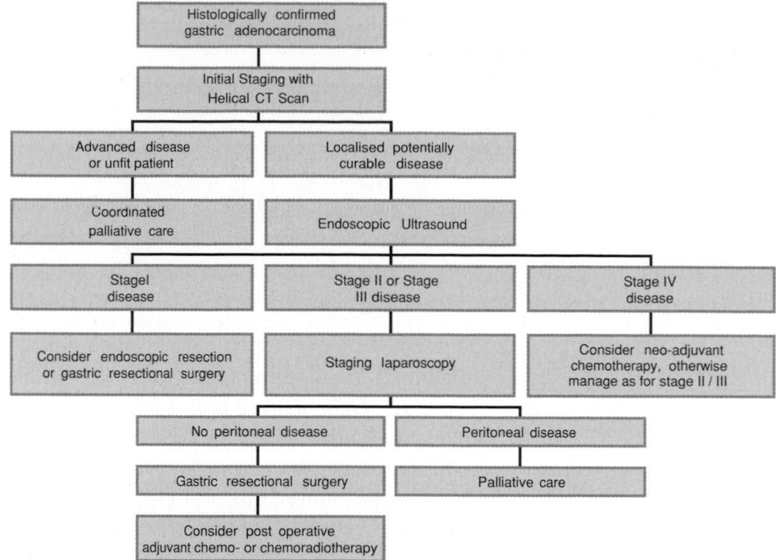

Fig. 13.1 Management of gastric adenocarcinoma.

The main diagnostic test in upper gastrointestinal endoscopy and any patient with new or changed upper gastrointestinal symptoms should have an endoscopy. Abnormalities are biopsied to confirm the diagnosis of gastric adenocarcinoma, Fig. 13.1.

In Japan with its very high incidence of gastric cancer there exists a population-based screening programme but no other country has an incidence high enough to justify such a programme.

Staging

Having established the diagnosis of malignancy the next phase of patient management is to stage the tumour. Staging coupled with an overall assessment of the patient will enable the appropriate treatment to be planned. Staging of gastric cancer is optimally carried out by a combination of helical CT scan and where available endoscopic ultrasound examination. Endoscopic ultrasound (EUS) is a relatively new modality that is complementary to gastroscopy and computed tomography (CT). The normal stomach wall has five distinct layers. Endoscopic ultrasound with a high frequency (7.5–12 MHz) transducer is relatively accurate at assessing the T stage. Its sensitivity for detecting nodal metastases is better than that of CT, but it still cannot reliably exclude nodal disease.

Computed tomography scanning is important in excluding hepatic metastases, and also in showing gross nodal involvement. It is poor at assessing the T stage of the primary tumour and frequently fails to show small-volume peritoneal disease.

The combination of CT and EUS will have an overall accuracy of 80–85% for the staging of gastric cancer; most of the inaccuracy is as a result of understaging. Laparoscopy is becoming established as an essential part of the preoperative staging of gastric cancer. In about 15% of cases small-volume hepatic or peritoneal disease is discovered laparoscopically, which was undetected by CT. The information obtained from the staging information is described using the TNM system, which for gastric cancer is detailed as follows

- T Stage
  - T1, tumour in mucosa or submucosa
  - T2, tumour into/through muscularis propria
  - T3, tumour through serosa
  - T4, tumour invading other structures
- N Stage (requires at least 15 nodes to be examined)
  - N0, no nodes involved
  - N1, 1–6 nodes involved
  - N2, 7–15 nodes involved
  - N3, more than 15 nodes involved
- M Stage
  - M0, no distant metastases
  - M1, distant metastases

The information can also be used to place the patient's tumour into a stage group, I through IV. For example a T3 N0 M0 tumour is in stage II whereas a T3 N2

M0 tumour would be stage III. There is a clear relationship between stage and survival. Five-year survival rate for stage I to IV tumours is approximately 90%, 60%, 30% and 5% respectively. Unfortunately the vast majority of gastric cancers in the Western world are stage III or IV at the time of diagnosis although in Japan with screening and aggressive diagnosis the majority of patients present with curable stage I or II disease. T1 cancer is known as 'early gastric cancer' (EGC), irrespective of the state of the lymph nodes. Early gastric cancer is subdivided according to the macroscopic appearance into protruded (type I), superficially elevated (IIa), flat (IIb), superficially depressed (IIc) and excavated (III).

Treatment

Having staged the tumour and assessed the whole patient in terms of their general fitness, the next stage is to decide on the appropriate treatment. This should involve a careful discussion with the patient regarding the diagnosis and the benefits and risks of the proposed interventions. The treatment planning should where possible involve a multi-disciplinary team of surgeon, gastroenterologist, oncologist, nurse and pathologist. The team should also include when appropriate a palliative care specialist.

Endoscopic treatment

A small number of patients will be diagnosed with early stage T1 tumours. Of these a proportion are suitable for endoscopic mucosal resection. In Japan nearly half of all cancers are treated in this way and as a consequence there are carefully derived systems for deciding which tumours are appropriate for such treatment. There are clearly considerable advantages for the patient if surgery can be appropriately and safely avoided

Surgery

The majority of patients with potentially curable disease will have a surgical resection as the mainstay of their treatment. The operation may involve resection of the distal stomach or the entire stomach. There has been very considerable debate around whether the operation should involve extensive resection of the lymph nodes draining the stomach. The Japanese with their very high incidence of gastric cancer are convinced that such a lymph node dissection adds to the chance of achieving a cure. Two large randomised controlled trials and several smaller trials carried out in Western countries have failed to show a conclusive benefit for the more radical lymph node dissections although further analysis has shown potential benefit for patients with stage II and early stage III disease. Following gastric resection intestinal continuity is usually restored with a Roux-en – Y type reconstruction that reduces the risk of bile reflux into the remaining stomach or oesophagus. There is some evidence from meta-analysis that the use of a jejunal pouch may improve the functional outcome after total gastrectomy.

When informing patients about major gastric resection it is important that they are aware that there is a 2–5% associated mortality and a 20–30% incidence of significant complications. The risk of mortality is related to the volume of operations carried out in the surgical unit and high volume units report mortality rates of 1% or less.

EARLY COMPLICATIONS

The post-operative course for a patient having a gastric resection for cancer can be stormy, especially if the patient has a total gastrectomy. Potential complications include the usual cardiac, respiratory and wound complications that may occur in any patient undergoing abdominal surgery. There is a risk of anastomotic leakage, especially after total gastrectomy and oesophagojejunal anastomosis. The suture or staple line where the duodenum has been divided may also break down. Fluid collections or abscesses are common, particularly if extensive lymph node dissection has been performed. Dissection of lymph nodes from the pancreas risks causing acute pancreatitis. Sometimes the gastric remnant does not drain well into the jejunum and the patient may have prolonged nasogastric drainage or vomiting. This may be due to a mechanical obstruction (efferent loop obstruction) or to poor motility of a partially denervated gastric remnant. Obstruction of the afferent loop can occur early in the post-operative course and lead to disruption of the duodenal stump. It can also occur late and lead to post-prandial pain and nausea commonly relieved by vomiting. Afferent loop obstruction is due to a poorly constructed afferent loop, and usually requires surgical correction.

LATE COMPLICATIONS

- Late complications are due to changes in the anatomy and the physiology of the upper gastrointestinal tract. The complications include reflux gastritis and/or oesophagitis, dumping syndromes, diarrhoea and nutritional deficiencies. Most of the problems are most marked in the few months after surgery and most fade within about one year.

- Reflux gastritis is due to loss of the pylorus and easy passage of alkaline biliary and pancreatic fluid into the stomach. There is endoscopic evidence of gastritis in most patients who have had a loop jejunostomy as a reconstruction, but only a small proportion have significant symptoms. Medical therapy is not very effective, and some patients require surgery to divert the small bowel fluid from the stomach via a Roux-en-Y gastrojejunostomy.
- Dumping refers to an array of gastrointestinal and vasomotor symptoms attributed to rapid gastric emptying. The symptoms include fullness, abdominal pain, nausea, vomiting and diarrhoea. The vasomotor symptoms are due to rapid fluid shifts into the bowel lumen, and are the typical symptoms of hypovolaemia. 'Late' dumping is due to an insulin surge soon after a meal, followed by reactive hypoglycaemia. The treatment of dumping is dietary. Patients should eat small frequent meals, try to separate dry foods from liquids, and avoid simple sugars. The severity of symptoms settles with time.
- Nutritional deficiencies may result from changes in appetite, from gastritis or dumping syndromes, or from recurrence or progression of the cancer. It is normal for patients to lose about 10% of their pre-operative weight after a total gastrectomy and 5% after distal gastrectomy.
- Anaemia is common after gastrectomy. This may be due to vitamin B12 deficiency from loss of intrinsic factor after total gastrectomy and/or poor iron absorption due to failure of conversion of iron from the ferric to the ferrous form through the absence of acid. After total gastrectomy patients require regular vitamin B12 injections.
- Both osteoporosis and osteomalacia are more common after gastrectomy. The reasons for this are not entirely clear but may result from reduced absorption of calcium and/or vitamin D.

Adjuvant therapy

Even with potentially curative surgery with removal of all visible tumour and clear resection margins most series report 5-year survival between 30 and 40%. Therefore there is a clear need to look at whether additional adjuvant therapy can offer survival benefit. The literature in this area is not clear but trends are emerging which will guide future research. There is some evidence that neo-adjuvant chemotherapy can downstage gastric cancers although the post-operative survival benefits are not yet defined. Post-operative adjuvant chemotherapy has been shown to be of benefit in several of the randomised controlled trials carried out and a meta-analysis of all trials to date has shown a significant benefit in favour of chemotherapy. However despite the meta-analysis because of the very heterogeneous nature of the trials included in the analysis such treatment is not usual in the majority of centres. A recent large multicentre study looked at the use of post-operative chemoradiotherapy following surgery for gastric cancer and showed a significant survival benefit. Whilst further studies are needed it does appear that adjuvant therapy offers some benefit for patients with gastric cancer and such treatments should be considered.

Palliation

Unfortunately the majority of patients with gastric cancer either present with advanced disease or develop recurrence following surgery. Therefore palliation is very important. Whilst not universally accepted there seems to be little benefit at all for patients with advanced gastric cancer undergoing surgery where all of the detectable tumour is not removed. The overall survival in such patients is not different from those who do not undergo resection. One of the commoner indications for palliative surgery is gastric outlet obstruction from a stenosing distal gastric cancer and even in this situation the use of expandable metal mesh stents can offer better palliation in a significant proportion. The median survival in patients with non-curable gastric cancer is 4–6 months and it is important that soon after the diagnosis is made a clear management plan is established with the palliative care team to maximise the quality of the patients remaining life.

Gastric lymphoma

Lymphoma of the stomach accounts for 2–5% of all gastric neoplasms. In general they are of B cell origin although T cell lymphomas do occur. The commonest gastric lymphoma arises from mucosa associated lymphoid tissue (MALT) rather than lymph nodes. The occurrence of MALT in the stomach is thought to be a response to chronic inflammation most frequently occurring as a result of *H. pylori* infection. There is no longer any doubt that *H. pylori* is a very important cause of gastric lymphoma. B cell lymphomas of the stomach can be classified as either low grade or high grade depending upon their histological characteristics.

Following diagnosis patients with gastric lymphoma should be appropriately staged with a combination of CT scan and endoscopic ultrasound. The treatment of low grade MALT lymphoma is eradication of Helicobacter infection if present. This results in tumour resolution in 70–100% of cases. Treatment of those patients who do not respond or those with high-grade tumours is with chemoradiotherapy. Surgery is generally reserved for the treatment of tumour or treatment related complications such as haemorrhage or bleeding.

Gastric GIST

Gastrointestinal stromal tumours were until the last decade described as leiomyomas or leiomyosarcomas and it is only with advances in molecular biology that this particular tumour has been recognised as a discrete entity. GI stromal tumours can arise anywhere in the GI tract but the stomach is the commonest site. They are mesenchymal tumours believed to originate from the interstitial cells of Cajal. They generally present as elevated submucosal swellings that ulcerate or bleed; a number are discovered as incidental findings at endoscopy. GIST's behave in a somewhat unpredictable manner with many appearing to be completely benign and others as an aggressive malignancy. Increased risk of malignant behaviour is associated with increasing size and the number of mitoses seen within pathological specimens.

GIST tend to spread through local invasion and haematogenous spread, lymph node metastases are unusual. Once diagnosed and staged through a combination of CT scanning and if available endoscopic ultrasound treatment is surgical resection. There is no role for associated lymph node dissection.

At a molecular level GIST's are characterised by an abnormality of one of several transmembrane growth factor receptors, the commonest (85–90%) being the molecule c-kit (CD117). Recently it has been demonstrated that the c-kit antagonist imatinib can produce very significant tumour regression of advanced GIST's. There is no current data to support the use of imatinib in the adjuvant setting.

MCQs

Select the single correct answer to each question.

1 Following a gastric resection for a stage III gastric cancer the patient asks whether any further therapy will improve their prognosis. Which of the following statements is true?

a chemotherapy is of no use in this setting
b chemoradiotherapy may improve outcome
c radiotherapy may improve outcome
d adjuvant chemotherapy is standard treatment

2 A 67 year old man is found to have a submucosal 5 cm tumour in the body of his stomach. The treating physician considers that this may be a gastrointestinal stromal tumour. Which one of the following statements is correct?

a this tumour has a propensity to spread to lymph nodes
b this tumour is benign and unlikely to metastasize
c it is difficult to predict how this tumour will behave
d the tumour is very aggressive and survival is normally limited

3 Following gastric resection a patient is told that they have a T2 N1 (stage II) cancer of the stomach. They ask about 5-year survival, how many patients from 100 with such a tumour would be alive at 5 years?

a 10
b 30
c 60
d 90

4 Endoscopic ultrasound is used in the staging of gastric cancer. Which of the following statements is true?

a when good quality CT scan is available, EUS adds little to staging accuracy
b CT scan is better than EUS in assessing N stage
c the availability of EUS removes the need for staging laparoscopy
d EUS is better than CT in assessing T stage

Hepatopancreaticobiliary Surgery

14 Gallstones

David Fletcher

Introduction

The gall bladder is second only to the appendix as the intra-abdominal organ most commonly requiring surgical intervention. The surgical management of the gall bladder pathology has changed because of the following developments. The first is the development of ultrasound, which allows accurate diagnosis of the presence of gallstones as well as the presence of complications such as acute cholecystitis, obstructive jaundice/cholangitis and pancreatitis. Such accurate diagnosis has allowed early surgical intervention. The second major advance has been duct imaging by endoscopic retrograde cholangiopancreatography (ERCP), allowing both diagnosis and treatment of one of the major complications of gallstones, obstructive jaundice. The third major change has been the development of laparoscopic cholecystectomy.

Aetiology and pathogenesis

Incidence

Gallstones are common; they are more common in females, with the incidence rising with age. At the age of 30 years, 5% of females and 2% of males either have or have had gallstones, with the proportion rising at 55 years to 20% and 10%, and at 70 years to 30% and 20%, respectively.

Types of stones

Gallstones are composed of two basic components, cholesterol and pigment.

Cholesterol stones

Cholesterol stones account for 80% of gallstones, either as pure cholesterol stones or more commonly as mixed stones. The process of cholesterol stone formation is summarised in Fig. 14.1. Cholesterol is delivered to the liver from the gut in chylomicrons or from other tissues in low-density lipoproteins. Plasma cholesterol is then regulated by hepatic synthesis or excretion of cholesterol. Synthesis of cholesterol can be from acetate under the influence of the enzyme HMG CoA (3-hydroxy-3-methylglutaryl coenzyme A). Cholesterol elimination occurs as a result of its secretion into bile in three ways: as cholesterol itself, as bile salt (under the influence of 7α-hydroxylase) or as cholesterol esters. Once in bile, the cholesterol is kept in solution in vesicles that are stabilised by secreted phospholipids. During fasting, and particularly if there is prolonged fasting (e.g. during intravenous alimentation), cholesterol crystals form in the supersaturated bile and, combined with gall bladder stasis, results in sludge. This process is exacerbated by mucin and inhibited by bile salts (particularly ursodeoxycholic acid), non-steroidal anti-inflammatory drugs and caffeine. This is perhaps another example of how a daily dose of aspirin (besides its effect in the cardiovascular system), perhaps

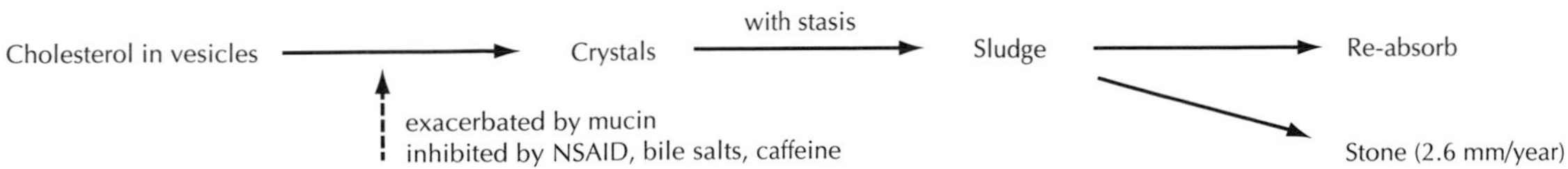

Fig. 14.1 Pathogenesis of cholesterol gallstones.

washed down by a cup of coffee, may be of value. Any factor that increases plasma, and thus bile cholesterol, also exacerbates the production of sludge, for example, increased body fat (further increased by age and female sex), high animal fat in the diet, or metabolic conditions (diabetes, cystic fibrosis, familial hyperlipidaemias, pregnancy). Stones may also occur as a result of bile salt depletion (e.g. from drugs such as clofibrate) or from malabsorption of bile salts in the distal ileum due to disease or resection.

Biliary sludge, once formed, can re-absorb or can go on to stone formation. In patients who become symptomatic, the time from stone initiation to the development of symptoms is approximately 8 years, and the time to cholecystectomy approximately 12 years.

Pigment stones

Pigment in bile is a result of bilirubin production, the bilirubin first being solubilised by conjugation to form a diglucuronide. Stones may occur as a result of three processes. First, if there is an increase in bilirubin load due to haemolytic anaemias. Second, if the bilirubin once more becomes insoluble due to glucuronidases in bile (e.g. if there is stasis or obstruction, allowing contamination with glucuronidase-containing bacteria). Third, if the patient has cirrhosis, in which there is depletion of glucuronidase inhibitors in the bile.

The deposition of this pigment in the gall bladder bile results in the formation of multiple small black stones. When this process occurs in the bile duct, it produces a primary duct stone.

Clinical diagnosis

Biliary pain is of two types, obstructive or inflammatory. Obstructive symptoms occur when the neck of the gall bladder is obstructed by a stone and gall bladder contraction continues under the influence of cholecystokinin and neural reflexes from the duodenum. The rise in tension in the gall bladder wall is detected by sparsely distributed bare nerve endings of sympathetic afferents. These fibres pass centrally via the coeliac plexus. The resultant visceral foregut pain is therefore dull, poorly localised, usually extends right across the region of the epigastrium and may radiate around to the back, most commonly via the right side, and can be felt between the scapulae. The pain will be noted to be of fairly rapid onset as the pressure in the gall bladder increases (unless the patient is woken from sleep by the pain), and is invariably associated with nausea and often vomiting. The pain usually lasts a number of hours and abates only when the stone either dislodges or, less commonly, passes through the cystic duct into the bile duct. The patient is left feeling unwell for as long as 1–2 days. The pain is not colicky because there is no cyclical peristalsis of note in the gall bladder.

Inflammation

If the stone does not become dislodged, at first a sterile inflammatory response develops and this may be followed by an infective cholecystitis. The most common organism is *Escherichia coli*, followed by a *Klebsiella* and, occasionally, *Streptococcus faecalis*. The inflammatory process extends to involve the parietal peritoneum, and involves somatic afferents of that dermatome segment, and the patient's perception of the pain will change. The pain moves to the right hypochondrium, becomes sharp and well localised, and is exacerbated by movement or deep breathing. The pain (parietal) is sharper and more localised because of the dense innervation of the peritoneum by specialised sensory nerves of the somatic nervous system. On examination of the right hypochondrium, guarding and Murphy's sign may be present. If the gall bladder is under the liver and not in contact with the parietal peritoneum, the diagnosis can be made by having the patient take a deep breath while a hand indents the right upper quadrant. As the inflamed gall bladder descends and contacts the sensitive peritoneum, sharp parietal pain occurs and muscle tone reflexly or immediately rises (involuntary guarding).

Complications

If the gall bladder remains obstructed and the inflammatory process continues, an empyema results and nearby omentum, colon and duodenum become inflamed and adherent to the gall bladder, producing a phlegmon. If the abdomen is gently examined, through the increased muscle tone a mass can usually be identified. The patient has now usually had symptoms for 2–3 days and has a high fever and hyperdynamic circulation of sepsis. If the inflammation still remains unresolved, the next development may be gall bladder gangrene and local perforation, which is indicated by the development of a swinging fever. Exceedingly rarely, the whole process may spontaneously resolve if the gall bladder develops a fistula into the associated bowel, usually the duodenum. Even more rarely, the discharged gallstone, as it passes down the bowel, may produce a small-bowel obstruction, most commonly at the duodenojejunal (DJ) flexure, or the distal ileum. A plain abdominal X-ray will show gas in the biliary tree in association with the small bowel obstruction.

Investigations

Ultrasound

Ultrasound has been a major advance in the diagnosis of gallstones. The typical appearance is of a bright echo (white), with acoustic shadowing (dark area) radiating beyond the stone (Fig. 14.2). Cholecystitis might be inferred by the demonstration of thickening of the gall bladder wall (>4 mm) with, occasionally, a decrease in density adjacent to the gall bladder wall suggesting a halo effect, which is a manifestation of surrounding oedema. Gall bladder wall thickening may also be due to fibrosis but, in this case, gall bladder volume is usually reduced. The ultrasound may also suggest the presence of duct stones by showing ductal dilation or may occasionally suggest another complication of gallstone disease, pancreatitis, as shown by altered echogenicity in the pancreas. In acute cholecystitis, the lower bile duct and the pancreas may be difficult to visualise because of gas in the duodenum.

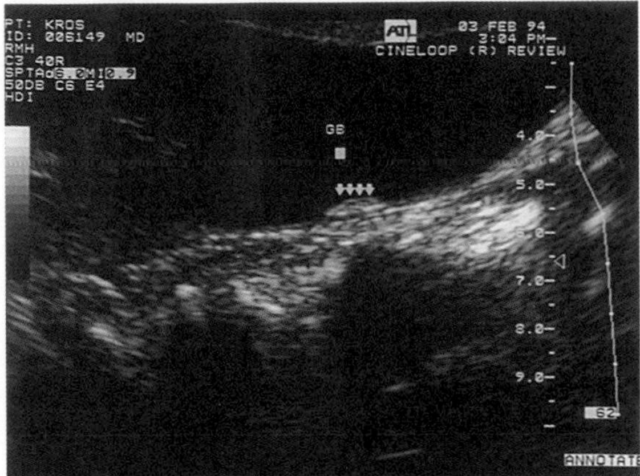

Fig. 14.2 Ultrasound of gall bladder containing gallstones, showing an echo with acoustic shadowing.

Ultrasound is particularly operator dependent and unless the entire gall bladder is visualised, stones may be missed. Biliary sludge may also be missed because it frequently does not produce an acoustic shadow. False negative examinations (i.e. missed stones) occur in approximately 5% of examinations.

Oral cholecystography

Failure of the gall bladder to concentrate orally administered contrast (i.e. failure to visualise the gall bladder) is suggestive of either cystic duct obstruction or the presence of a recent attack of acute cholecystitis. Even if the gall bladder does concentrate the contrast, small stones can be easily missed, resulting in a false negative examination rate of 5%.

Oral cholecystography is now used rarely but is of value as a follow-up to ultrasound if there is a strong clinical suspicion that the patient has stones but the ultrasound is normal. Performing the two procedures reduces the false negative rate to less than 2%, particularly if the cholecystogram is performed soon after the acute episode of pain.

Cholescintigraphy

This test is rarely used, again since the advent of ultrasound. Failure of the intravenously delivered dose of technetium-labelled hepato-iminodiacetic acid (^{99m}Tc-HIDA) to outline the gall bladder suggests cystic duct obstruction. Some suggest that the test can diagnose occult gall bladder calculus disease by showing delaying emptying in response to a fatty meal. This requires validation because many patients with chronic biliary-type pain (i.e. recurrent upper abdominal pain over a long period of time) have a normal gall bladder and are frequently shown to have irritable (spastic) bowel syndrome.

Endoscopic retrograde cholangiopancreatography

This examination is not necessary in uncomplicated gallstone disease. It is only used for sampling bile in patients with recurrent biliary-type pain or recurrent pancreatitis where gallstones are strongly suspected on history, but have not been identified by either ultrasound or oral cholecystography. The aspirated bile is examined under the microscope for cholesterol crystals and debris (microlithiasis).

Haematology and biochemistry

An elevated white cell count will confirm acute cholecystitis, but adds little to the history and examination findings of the diagnosis.

Liver function tests and serum amylase should be measured routinely because approximately 10% of patients will have concomitant common duct stones (see Chapter 39). The liver function tests will be abnormal only if the stone is currently obstructing the duct. Similarly, the amylase may be elevated for approximately 24 hours if a stone passing through the final common channel of the bile/pancreatic ducts induces an episode of pancreatitis. Because of renal secretion of amylase, plasma amylase rapidly normalises, although urine amylase frequently remains elevated for up to 5 days.

Operative treatment

The procedure is cholecystectomy with operative cholangiography (Box 14.1).

Pre-operative preparation

The procedure is performed under general anaesthesia after a minimum 4-hour fast. Prophylaxis against deep vein thrombosis is considered if the patient is older than 40 years of age. Prophylactic antibiotics are generally used, especially if the patient is more than 40 years of age, a duct stone is suspected, the patient's immune state is depressed (diabetes, steroid administration) or the patient is morbidly obese. A single dose of a second-generation cephalosporin is adequate but may be extended for 24–48 hours post-operatively in the presence of severe sepsis.

Box 14.1 Gallstones: clinical situations and recommended management

- Incidental (asymptomatic): no treatment required.
- Incidental (at laparotomy): remove if technically/ anaesthetically suitable.
- Biliary pain: elective laparoscopic cholecystectomy.
- Acute cholecystitis: urgent cholecystectomy.
- Post-endoscopic sphincterotomy for common bile duct stone: elective laparoscopic cholecystectomy if cystic duct obstructed.
- Gallstone pancreatitis: laparoscopic cholecystectomy within same admission.

Surgical technique

Open cholecystectomy

The abdomen is opened, usually by a right subcostal incision. The cystic duct and artery are carefully dissected and confirmed to arise and terminate, respectively, in the gall bladder. An intra-operative cholangiogram is then performed by passing a catheter into the cystic duct and injecting contrast to outline the biliary tree. This is done because there is approximately a 10% probability of a stone being present in the bile duct at the time of cholecystectomy; this probability rises with increasing age. Some surgeons would suggest that a cholangiogram only be performed in those in whom a bile duct stone is suspected (i.e. those with a past history of jaundice or pancreatitis, abnormal liver function tests, dilated cystic duct, common bile duct or a palpable stone in the duct). These criteria, however, underestimate the presence of duct stones (approximately 4% of patients have an unsuspected stone). If a bile duct stone is identified on the cholangiogram the duct is explored (see Chapter 15).

After the cholangiogram is confirmed to be normal, the cystic duct and artery are ligated and the gall bladder is removed from the bed of the liver. Many surgeons will place a drain to the gall bladder bed for approximately 24 hours because, occasionally, a small leak of bile may occur from small ducts that pass directly to the gall bladder from the bed. The abdomen is then closed.

Laparoscopic cholecystectomy

Laparoscopic cholecystectomy was first performed in 1987 by Mouret in France and by Uhre in Germany. It was made possible by the development of the miniature video-chip camera which, when attached to a laparoscope and handled by an assistant, allowed the surgeon to operate with both hands. A cannula is inserted in the umbilicus, through which the laparoscope is passed. Three other cannulae are inserted for grasping and exposing the gall bladder and for performing the dissection. The principles and techniques are the same as for the open procedure.

For a period after the introduction of the technique, unlike the practice in the era of open cholecystectomy, some surgeons were not using intra-operative cholangiography to diagnose concomitant duct stones. Those patients with suspected duct stones (see above) were given a pre-operative ERCP. This preliminary procedure and the associated endoscopic sphincterotomy to remove any duct stones identified was an unnecessary risk because the stones would have passed spontaneously in half to two-thirds of patients by the time of cholecystectomy. However, intra-operative cholangiography to detect duct stones and to help outline bile duct anatomy and reduce duct injury is becoming common once more.

The cholangiogram is performed either via a catheter passed through one of the cannulae or via a needle puncture in the abdominal wall. Following completion of the cholangiogram, the cystic duct and artery are clipped with small metal clips and divided. The gall bladder is removed from its bed, using electrocautery. The gall bladder bed is carefully examined for any evidence of bile leaks. The gall bladder is then removed via the umbilicus, the peritoneal cavity is washed out and the small incisions closed. Most surgeons do not use a drain to the gall bladder bed, first because evidence to suggest that it improves the outcome from bile leak is limited and, second, the drain is a major cause of post-operative pain.

Post-operative care

The post-operative management of patients who have undergone laparoscopic versus open procedures are vastly different. Following the open procedure, patients require adequate pain relief either via narcotic infusion or patient-controlled analgesia. They have nil by mouth for 24–48 hours because of the ileus resulting from intra-operative handling and thus require intravenous fluids for approximately 2 days. Because the post-operative pain leads to atelectasis, they need early mobilisation and elderly patients with pre-existing respiratory disease require active physiotherapy. Low-dose heparin needs to continue in patients at high risk of thromboembolism until they are fully ambulant. The mean post-operative stay is 5 days.

In contrast, patients undergoing laparoscopic cholecystectomy have markedly less pain and ileus. As most patients are ambulant the day of surgery, physiotherapy is rarely required. Narcotic analgesics are usually required as an occasional injection during the first 24 hours, with simple oral analgesics perhaps then required for up to 10 days after discharge. Most patients are discharged home on the second post-operative day. Return to normal activity is rapid with the laparoscopic approach: 2 weeks compared to 4 weeks for the open approach.

Significant complications

The laparoscopic approach has fewer minor complications (3% cf. 6%), less wound infection (0.5% cf. 1.5%) and fewer respiratory complications (1.9% cf. 2.5%) compared with open cholecystectomy. The early experience, however, suggests that the laparoscopic approach has had more major complications. Significant bile duct injury occurs in 0.15% of open cholecystectomies, but has reduced twofold since the introduction of laparoscopic cholecystectomy. This is partly because surgeons who were new to the technique had difficulty in identifying the cystic duct from the bile duct with a fixed, two-dimensional view of the anatomy via the laparoscope. In this regard intra-operative cholangiography is particularly helpful. Any patient with persistent pain following a laparoscopic procedure, particularly if they develop a fever, must be suspected of having a duct injury. Liver function tests must be performed immediately. If these are abnormal, then the operative cholangiogram should be reviewed in case it demonstrates a missed injury (e.g. contrast leaks or missing duct segments). An ultrasound is then used to identify a fluid collection and an ERCP is used to identify the nature of the ductal injury.

Although not a complication, persistence or recurrence of biliary-type pain may occur. A proportion of these patients will either have a retained common duct stone, sphincter of Oddi dysfunction (usually secondary to trauma from duct exploration or passage of stone) or possibly wound neuralgia due to segmental nerve injury. Many, in whom no cause for further pain can be identified, have been labelled as having post-cholecystectomy syndrome. This condition does not exist and represents those patients who did not require a cholecystectomy in the first place (i.e. their pain was not due to the gallstone and therefore the gall bladder removal has not influenced their symptomatology).

Choice of operation

With the introduction of laparoscopic cholecystectomy, the approach has been to reserve the laparoscopy for the easiest cases; that is, those patients who do not have acute cholecystitis, are not excessively overweight and do not have evidence of stone in the bile duct. As a result, operative mortality is low (0.1%). The high-risk patients, therefore, are the ones who are still having open cholecystectomy. This explains why, in the current era, patients having open cholecystectomy are having a higher complication rate and a higher operative mortality (rising sixfold from 0.3 to 1.8% in the past decade). It is this high-risk group of patients who would benefit most from the less morbid laparoscopic approach. Experienced surgeons are now offering laparoscopic cholecystectomy more often, and now more than 80% of cholecystectomies performed in Australia are being performed laparoscopically. If the biliary anatomy is too complex because of severe inflammation, the laparoscopic procedure can be converted to open cholecystectomy. Severe respiratory disease may require a lower intra-abdominal insufflation pressure, and portal hypertension (because of the risk of intra-operative bleeding) remains a relative contraindication.

Management of clinical situations

Incidental gallstone on ultrasound

Unless it is clear from the history that any symptom the patient has can be attributed to the gallstone, then the gall bladder should be left untreated, particularly if there are serious co-morbid factors. Asymptomatic gallstones become symptomatic at a cumulative rate of 1% per year (e.g. a 30-year-old with asymptomatic stones who lived to 80 years would have a 50% chance of requiring their gall bladder to be removed, while for a 60-year-old there would only be a 20% chance that they would need to have their gall bladder removed in their lifetime). The probability that the gall bladder needs to be removed reduces even further if the patient has associated medical conditions likely to shorten their life that concomitantly increase the risk of prophylactic surgery. A major complication in a patient who did not need a cholecystectomy in the first place is the biggest disaster of all. Prophylactic cholecystectomy might be considered in one limited circumstance; that is, in patients with diabetes because they tend to develop more serious cholecystitis.

Incidental gallstone at laparotomy

For some unknown reason, the incidental gallstone palpated at laparotomy performed for another procedure has a higher probability of developing future symptoms, possibly as high as 75% at 12 months. As the abdomen is already open, and provided the incision gives adequate exposure of the gall bladder and bile ducts and, further, that the patient is tolerating the anaesthetic, the addition of cholecystectomy and operative cholangiography is preferable to a subsequent procedure, which will be required in the majority.

Biliary pain

Once gallstones cause biliary pain, recurrence is inevitable; during a 5-year period all patients get further symptoms and 20% develop a complication (cholecystitis, obstructive jaundice, pancreatitis). Unless operative risk is high or survival short, elective laparoscopic cholecystectomy should be performed. The decision as to whether the pain is biliary is a clinical one.

Acute cholecystitis

In the past, patients presenting with presumed acute cholecystitis were treated with analgesics, antibiotics to deal with biliary sepsis, nil by mouth, and intravenous fluids until the episode subsided. At 6 weeks, when the inflammation was presumed to have completely settled, elective cholecystectomy was performed. The problem was that this meant the expense of two hospital admissions. In addition, in 15% of patients the inflammation did not settle and empyema or gangrene developed, forcing cholecystectomy when the anatomy was most inflamed and difficult to identify, and raising the risk of common bile duct injury. By that stage the patient was septic and catabolic, further increasing the risk of complications.

With the development of ultrasound and a confident diagnosis of acute cholecystitis, immediate cholecystectomy became the norm. If done early in the attack, the oedema of early inflammation made dissection easy. All cases have their pathology dealt with in the same admission, reducing costs. The window of opportunity to perform laparoscopic acute cholecystectomy is shorter. The procedure has to be performed before the gall bladder becomes too thick-walled or gangrenous, or the anatomy becomes too difficult to identify. Ideally, acute laparoscopic cholecystectomy should be performed within 48 hours of onset of the attack. While an operating-theatre list is obtained, analgesic is given, the patient is fasted, intravenous fluids used and antibiotics (second- or third-generation cephalosporins) given.

Post-endoscopic sphincterotomy for complicated common bile duct stone

This problem occurs particularly in the older age group. Of patients over 60 years of age presenting for the first time with biliary calculi, in nearly 50% of cases the symptoms will be because of stones in the common bile duct rather than stones in the gall bladder. If the presentation is because of a complication of that duct stone, ideal management is by endoscopic sphinctero-tomy. After successfully treating the duct stone, the dilemma is then what to do with the gallstones (i.e. what is the probability they will become symptomatic in the patient's remaining life). If the cystic duct is unob-structed at ERCP then, during a 2-year period, 30% of patients will die from other causes associated with age and only 30% overall will require gall bladder removal. If the cystic duct is obstructed at ERCP, all patients will develop complications. Therefore, if the patient has an unobstructed cystic duct and, particularly, if they have associated co-morbidity, they should be advised of the nature of gall bladder symptoms and asked to present promptly should the symptoms occur, so that the chole-cystectomy can be performed acutely. Those patients with an obstructed cystic duct should have an early elective (laparoscopic) cholecystectomy.

Gallstone pancreatitis

Gallstone pancreatitis is dealt with in Chapter 17. However, in brief, gallstones are a major cause of pan-creatitis occurring as a result of the passage of a stone through the common channel of the pancreatic and bile ducts. The advent of better diagnostic tests, including ERCP/bile sampling, has shown that more than half of the cases of pancreatitis previously thought to be idiopathic are due to gall bladder microlithiasis. All patients admitted with pancreatitis must have gall-stones as a cause excluded.

MCQs

Select the single correct answer to each question.

1 An 80-year-old woman presents with biliary pain and stones are seen in the gall bladder on ultrasound. The probability of the pain being due to a stone in the common bile duct is approximately:
a 5%
b 10%
c 20%
d 30%
e 50%

2 A 73-year-old man presents with cholangitis. He has had no previous abdominal operation. The definitive treatment should be:
a cholecystectomy and choledocholithotomy
b ERCP and sphincterotomy with stone extraction
c antibiotic therapy followed by laparoscopic cholecystectomy
d choledocholithotomy
e ERCP, sphincterotomy with stone extraction and later consideration of cholecystectomy

3 Which of the following is the appropriate investigation in a patient presenting with a recent episode of right upper quadrant pain and a normal physical examination?
a abdominal CT scan
b ERCP
c plain X-ray of the abdomen
d upper abdominal ultrasound
e cholescintigraphy

15 Benign and malignant diseases of the hepatobiliary system

Neil Collier and D. Morris

The biliary system

Introduction

Bile duct obstruction causing jaundice and cholangitis is frequently encountered in surgical practice. Most often this is due to gallstones or pancreatic malignancy.

Primary diseases of the bile duct are individually uncommon. When considered overall, they are however a significant cause of bile duct obstruction.

Anatomical and functional considerations

The biliary tree is a conduit for the passage of bile from the hepatic biliary cannaliculi to the duodenum. Because of a paucity of muscle in the bile duct wall there is little peristaltic action except in the ampullary segment. This segment controls the flow of bile into the duodenum and acts as a barrier to proximal migration of the duodenal contents.

The bile duct develops embryologically from the ventral hepatic bud of the foregut. There are numerous anatomical variants in the branching structure of the bile duct. These lead to differences in the segmental biliary anatomy, which have important surgical implications. Such variations may increase the risk of biliary injury during cholecystectomy (Fig. 15.1).

Clinical features

Abnormalities of the bile duct will produce obstructive jaundice or cholangitis or both.

Jaundice

In clinical practice, differentiation from hepatocellular jaundice due to drugs, toxins or infection is the first priority. The clinical features of biliary obstruction include pale stools, dark urine and itch, and are usually diagnostic. If jaundice is episodic or associated with pain, rigors and pyrexia, then obstruction is highly likely. Fluctuating jaundice indicates intermittent obstruction from a stone or polypoid peri-ampullary cancer. Loss of weight is a strong indication of malignancy and is a common feature of pancreatic cancer.

Biliary fistula

Biliary fistula, either external or into the peritoneal cavity, is a feature produced by biliary trauma, either iatrogenic or following penetrating injury. Collection of

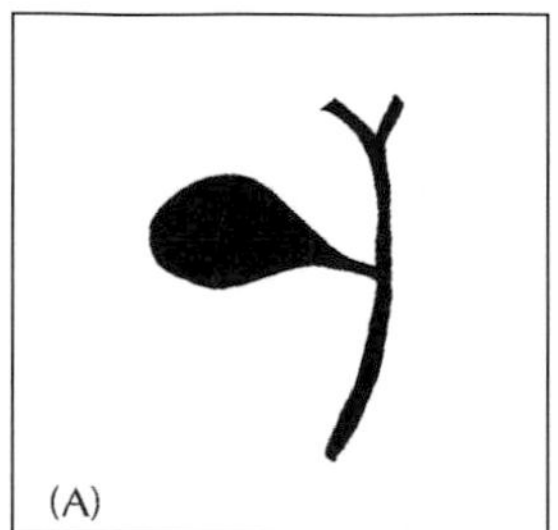

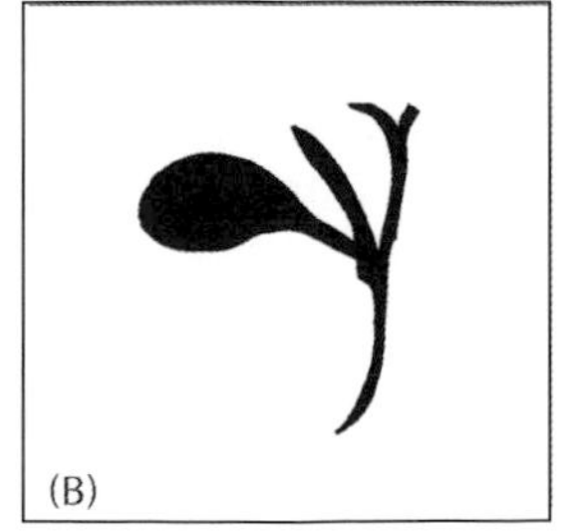

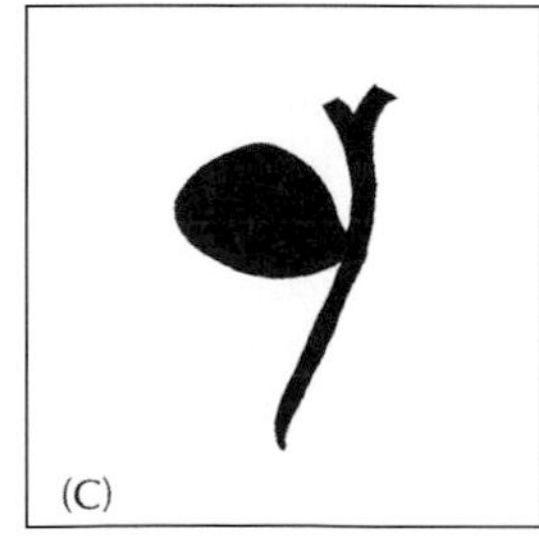

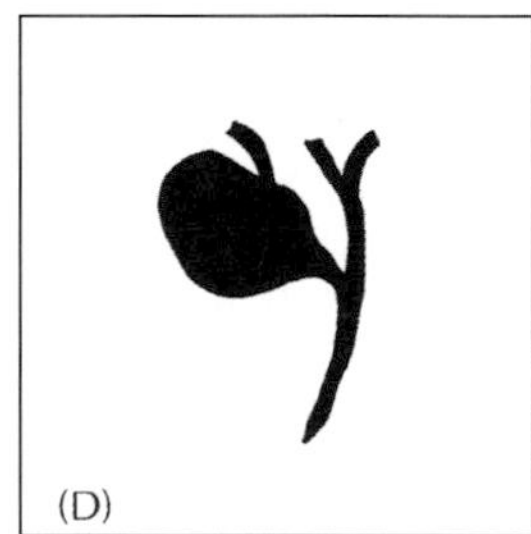

Fig. 15.1 Biliary variations increasing the risk of biliary injury: (**A**) Normal; (**B**) low-entry posterior sectoral duct; (**C**) short cystic duct and (**D**) sectoral duct drainage into gall bladder.

bile in the peritoneal cavity does not necessarily produce pain unless the bile is infected, in which case biliary peritonitis may occur. Large-volume fistulae will produce significant fluid and electrolytic loss and, when prolonged, nutritional problems from fat malabsorption. Spontaneous closure of low-volume fistulae may occur unless there is distal biliary obstruction.

Biliary disease in childhood

Congenital biliary anomalies such as atresia or choledochal cyst, usually present in early childhood. Occasionally, choledochal cysts will have a delayed presentation until adult life and rarely will present in middle age. Biliary malignancy is not seen in childhood, but gallstones are occasionally seen and are more common after major illness or injury.

Sclerosing cholangitis

Primary sclerosing cholangitis (PSC) is associated with inflammatory bowel disease. This will produce intermittent or progressive jaundice, and the biliary disease may occasionally pre-date the intestinal symptoms. Like most biliary diseases, it may also produce pancreatitis either due to bile duct stone formation or from stricturing of the ampullary segment of the bile duct. Choledochal cysts and PSC are both strongly associated with the development of cholangiocarcinoma.

Chronic obstruction

Chronic biliary obstruction associated with persistent low-grade infection may be a precursor to biliary malignancy. Biliary cirrhosis leading to liver failure and portal hypertension is a late feature of chronic obstruction.

Investigations

In the jaundiced patient, laboratory investigations should include haematological tests, clotting profile and standard liver function tests. The abnormalities of liver function demonstrate an obstructive pattern, with invariable elevation of the alkaline phosphatase and γ-glutamyl transpeptidase (GGT). If an obstructive pattern is seen, the next step is abdominal ultrasound, which is the key diagnostic test. This test will be followed by a variety of more invasive investigations, depending on the results obtained.

Ultrasound

Ultrasound is widely available, cheap, non-invasive and able to determine the presence of obstruction by demonstrating biliary dilatation. In experienced hands, it can show the level of obstruction. The detection of space-occupying lesions in the liver, porta hepatis or pancreas will depend on the body habitus of the patient and will also be affected by the amount of surrounding intestinal gas. Stones in the gall bladder are easily seen, although stone detection in the bile duct is less reliable.

Endoscopic retrograde cholangiopancreatography

Endoscopic injection of contrast into the biliary and pancreatic ducts is an accurate method of demonstrating biliary obstruction and determining its cause (Fig. 15.2). Endoscopic retrograde cholangiopancreatography (ERCP) can be combined with interventional techniques such as:

- tumour cytological brushings or biopsy
- sphincterotomy and stone extraction
- insertion of stents to overcome biliary obstruction

Percutaneous transhepatic cholangiography (PTC)

Radiological injection of contrast into the intrahepatic bile ducts is preferable to ERCP when the ampulla is inaccessible, or when previous biliary surgery has transected the bile duct. This procedure may also be combined with complex interventional techniques to overcome biliary obstruction, either temporarily or as permanent palliation for malignancy.

Computed tomography

Computed tomography (CT) is an accurate method of diagnosis for all forms of hepatobiliary disease. It can detect both intra- and extra-hepatic focal mass lesions and may be able to differentiate benign from malignant tumours. By combining CT with intravascular contrast injection, greater diagnostic accuracy can be achieved by demonstrating hepatic and portal vessels, and by increasing the difference in attenuation between lesions and the surrounding normal structures.

Computed tomographic cholangiography

More recently, with advances in computer technology, CT cholangiography has been introduced into clinical

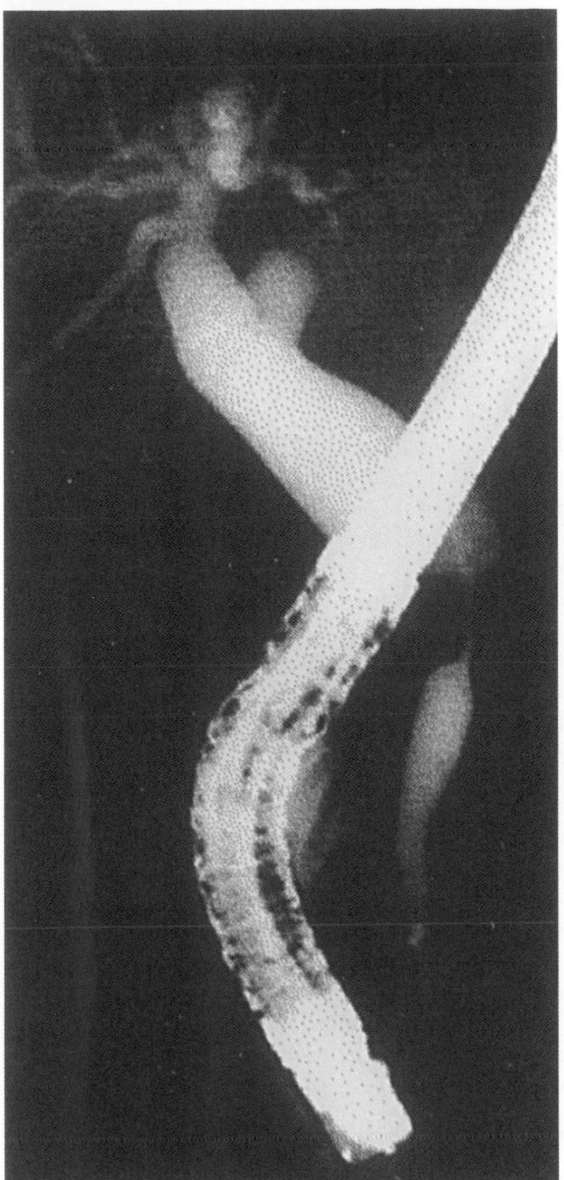

Fig. 15.2 Endoscopic retrograde cholangiopancreatography showing stricture due to biliary carcinoma.

practice. Intravenous contrast material is administered to provide non-invasive opacification of the bile duct. The limitation is that in a patient with bilirubin greater than twice the normal level, biliary opacification will not be obtained. However, this technique has largely replaced ERCP when used for purely diagnostic purposes in a non-jaundiced patient.

Magnetic resonance cholangiopancreatography (MRCP)

Magnetic resonance can provide useful imaging of the liver, particularly by outlining the vascular anatomy. Recent technical advances have occurred in which MR can now be used to accurately image the bile ducts, even in jaundiced patients. A three-dimensional biliary reconstruction is possible, which is particularly useful as a pre-operative diagnostic tool for hilar malignancies and is helpful in assessing resectability.

Operative cholangiography and choledochoscopy

Operative cholangiography and choledochoscopy are useful in selected patients during biliary surgery. Cholangiography is usually carried out by placing a catheter through the cystic duct, although direct needle puncture of a bile duct can also be used. Choledochoscopy can be performed with either rigid or flexible instruments. Some dilatation of the bile duct is necessary, however, to allow passage of these instruments.

Isotope scanning

Nuclear scanning of the liver has largely been replaced by other modalities. Using hepatobiliary agents labeled with nuclear isotopes, such as hepatobiliary 99m Tc-iminodiacetic acid (HIDA), biliary imaging can be obtained and is particularly useful for defining the site of leakage in a biliary fistula. This test is ineffective when there is significant biliary obstruction.

Specific conditions

Biliary strictures

Narrowing of the extrahepatic bile duct is most often due to malignancy in surrounding organs, with the tumour extending into or compressing the ducts. Primary malignancy of the pancreas, gall bladder, duodenum, liver or nodal disease in the porta hepatis are all more common than primary biliary malignancy (cholangiocarcinoma).

Benign strictures are most often the result of inadvertent damage to the bile duct during cholecystectomy and may occur immediately or after a delay of up to 10 years from operation. Benign strictures may also occur in PSC or in complex stone disease.

Cholangiocarcinoma

Adenocarcinoma of the bile duct is a rare tumour occurring most commonly after the age of 60 years. It can also occur in young patients and is more common in males. The tumour usually arises at the biliary confluence (Klatskin tumour). Presentation is with painless obstructive jaundice, and macroscopically the tumour is a sclerosing mass up to 4 cm in diameter. Characteristically, the tumour invades locally into surrounding blood vessels, nerves and the liver substance. Vascular occlusion is frequent and will lead to segmental or hemilobar atrophy of the liver.

Adenocarcinoma at the distal end of the bile duct is more often polypoid and is associated with a better prognosis as it is more often resectable.

Although cholangiocarcinoma can occur in patients with PSC or choledochal cyst, in Western countries no cause is usually found for this disease. It is, however, more common in Southeast Asia and this is probably due to the high prevalence of helminthic infection of the biliary tree.

Although slow growing, this tumour is highly lethal and most patients die within a few months of diagnosis. In selected patients resection is possible in specialised units and will lead to approximately 30% survival at 3 years.

When resection is not possible because of the patient's condition or the extent of the tumour, either palliative bypass surgery or endoprosthetic stent insertion is used to relieve jaundice. Stenting is more difficult than for low bile duct obstruction and results are less predictable.

Recently, radiotherapy has been used intraluminally to treat this disease. Iridium brachytherapy has been used as an adjunct to palliative surgery with encouraging results.

Benign strictures

Benign strictures most commonly result from iatrogenic damage to the bile duct at the time of cholecystectomy. Less commonly, such strictures may follow blunt external biliary trauma, usually from motor accidents. Rare causes of benign strictures include atresia of the biliary tree in neonates and PSC, a condition associated with ulcerative colitis in adults. The latter results in multiple intra- and extrahepatic strictures that may mimic carcinoma. The condition may be associated with malignant transformation.

IATROGENIC STRICTURES

Benign post-cholecystectomy strictures occur after approximately 1 in 350 cholecystectomies. The introduction of laparoscopic cholecystectomy resulted in an increase in the rate of duct injury. With greater experience, the duct injury rate has steadily declined.

Injuries to the duct occur due to misinterpretation of the biliary anatomy. They are more common in inexperienced hands and in association with acute inflammation of the gall bladder where Calot's triangle is obliterated. They tend to occur in young patients particularly when the bile ducts are of a narrow calibre.

In the surgical dissection of the cystic duct, the common bile duct is inadvertently divided and a variable segment of the common hepatic duct is often removed, leading to either high occlusion of the ducts or biliary fistula. Common presentation following such an injury is either with bile drainage through a drain tube or bile peritonitis. Large volumes of bile in the peritoneal cavity may however be painless when the bile is sterile.

Late presentation after biliary injury is with jaundice. This may occur when the initial injury is incomplete or is due to ischaemia from diathermy damage of the biliary vasculature or ducts.

TREATMENT OF BENIGN STRICTURES

In the majority of patients, benign strictures should be treated by surgical intervention. Many of these patients are young and stenting would at best produce temporary relief of obstruction. Biliary reconstruction after duct injury involves anastomosing a defunctioned limb of jejunum, that is, a Roux-en-Y loop to the proximal biliary tree. This will lead to excellent results when early intervention is undertaken in an expert centre. The complexity of the reconstruction depends both on the size of the ducts involved and the proximal extent of the duct injury. With very high injuries, results are less certain and anastomotic restricturing will occur in approximately 20% of cases. This can usually be dealt with, without resorting to further surgery by percutaneous dilatation carried out through the Roux-en-Y loop using radiological techniques.

Primary sclerosing cholangitis is a relapsing, remitting condition and treatment is often nonsurgical. Stenting and dilatation may provide initial improvement. Late surgical intervention with either bypass, dilatation or liver transplantation will be necessary in severe cases.

Biliary infections

In Western countries, biliary infection results from intestinal bacteria ascending into the bile duct secondary to biliary obstruction. In Asia, intrahepatic infection and stone formation are common, a condition called cholangiohepatitis. It is believed, although not proven, that the high incidence in Asia is due to the increased incidence of helminthic infection within the biliary tree.

Several species of liver fluke are known to infect humans. *Fasciola hepatica* is widespread but is mainly found in South America and parts of Europe. The adult worms infest cattle and sheep, and man is an accidental host infected by eating raw vegetables. The worm lives in the biliary tree and its presence produces fibrosis and, in severe cases, cholangitis and abscess.

A more common parasite is *Clonorchis sinensis*. This fluke is endemic in East Asia and infection occurs by eating raw fish. The adult worm migrates up the bile duct and usually dies there, causing obstruction, infection and stone formation. The presence of the fluke may lead to an increased incidence of cholangiocarcinoma.

Infection with *Ascaris lumbricoides* is common in Asia, Africa and Central America. Infection is via the faecal–oral route and the adult worm inhabits the small intestine. It may migrate up the bile duct causing cholangitis, pancreatitis or stone formation. The worms are large and may be seen on ultrasound or at ERCP. Worms may spontaneously migrate back into the intestine but they may also die within the bile ducts, causing obstruction.

Congenital biliary anomalies

Although considered congenital anomalies, biliary atresia and choledochal cyst may both be acquired conditions occurring or developing within the first few weeks of life.

Biliary atresia

Biliary atresia presents in the first few weeks of life. It is thought that an inflammatory process from an unknown cause affects the bile duct in the newborn infant. There is variable destruction of the extrahepatic bile ducts, causing obstructive jaundice and liver failure. Surgical correction of this abnormality before 8 weeks of age produces the best outcome.

Other anomalies associated with biliary atresia include intestinal malrotation and genitourinary anomalies. An aberrant communication between the biliary and pancreatic ducts has been reported in association with the condition, but it is not clear whether this is aetiologically important. Correction of this condition is by hepaticojejunostomy when a segment of extrahepatic duct is patent, or by porto-enterostomy for the more common severe case. In the latter operation, a jejunal Roux-en-Y loop is anastomosed to the porta hepatis after excision of the atretic duct remnants in the porta. Liver transplantation is frequently required for severe cases and atresia is the commonest indication for paediatric transplantation. Excellent long-term results are achieved with transplantation.

Choledochal cyst

Cystic dilatation of the intra- or extrahepatic ducts is a rare condition, usually presenting before the age of 16 years. In 20% of cases, presentation is in adult life. Symptoms produced by the cyst include cholangitis, pancreatitis, stone formation and jaundice. Infants may occasionally present with an abdominal mass. The cause of this condition is debated. Anomalous communication between the biliary and pancreatic ducts is frequently found, but a degree of distal biliary obstruction may also be aetilogically important in the development of the cyst.

Cysts are classified according to their site and shape, although 80% are fusiform abnormalities of the extrahepatic bile duct (Fig. 15.3). Type II cysts are extremely rare.

The preferred surgical method of treatment is complete cyst excision with biliary reconstruction, because of the risk of malignant transformation if the cyst is left *in situ*. The rate of malignant transformation may be as high as 25% for untreated cysts. When multiple intrahepatic cysts are present complete excision may not be possible and treatment consists of producing good biliary drainage by excising any extrahepatic component.

Biliary spasm

Whether motility disorders of the sphincter of Oddi can produce pain syndromes is controversial. Manometric measurements on the sphincter muscle may be carried out at the time of ERCP to demonstrate high pressure

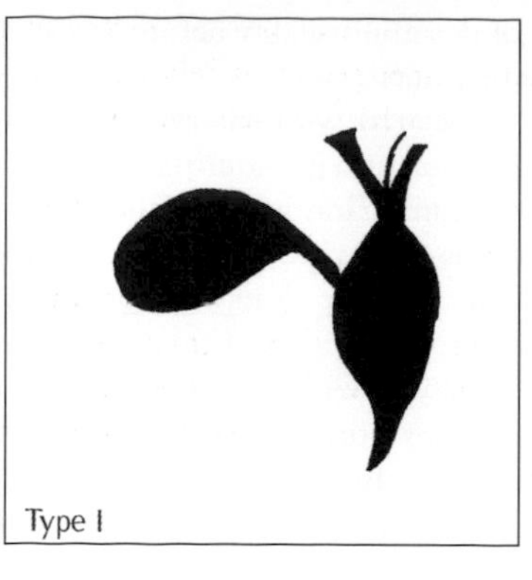

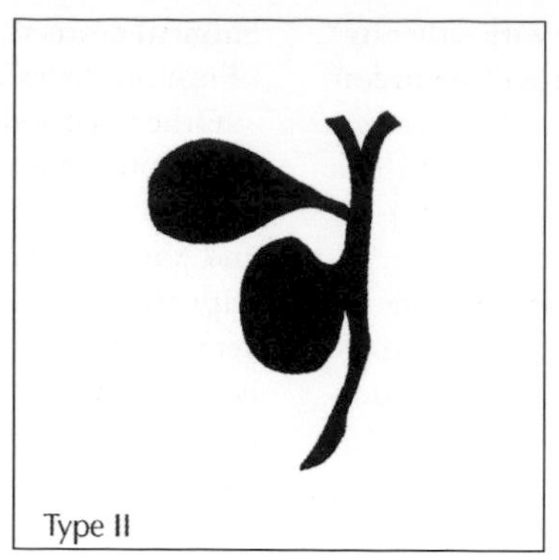

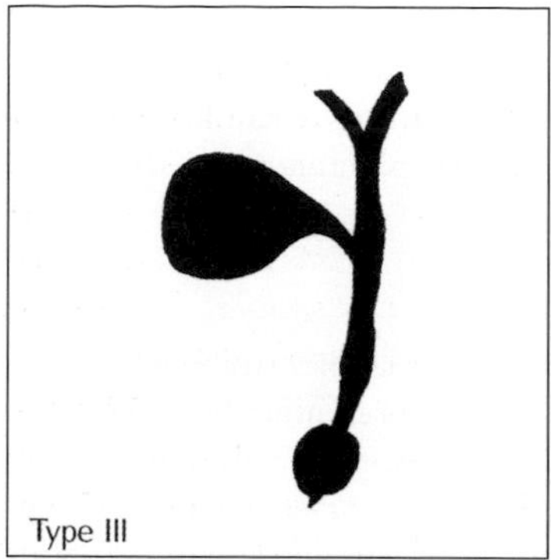

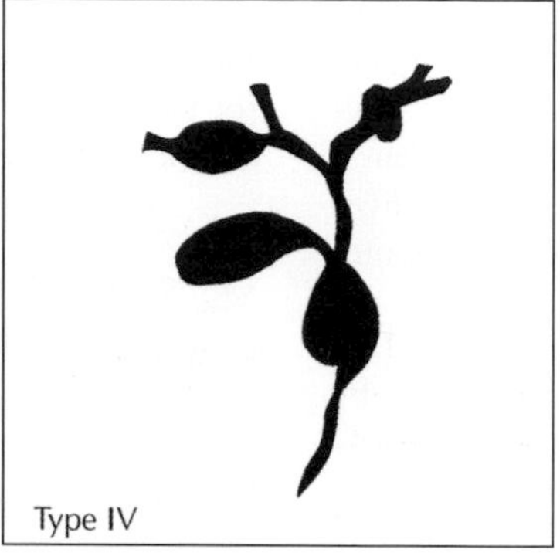

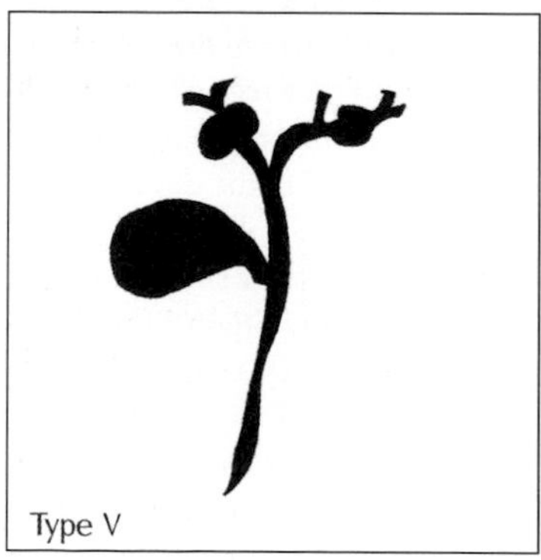

Fig. 15.3 Classification of choledochal cysts (after Todani, Alonso-Lej).

contractions and retrograde peristalsis, which may produce symptoms in susceptible individuals. This is usually seen in young women. Documentation of biliary dilatation, obstructive abnormality of liver function during attacks, and provocation of attacks with known agents causing biliary spasm will support the diagnosis.

Treatment by antispasmotics, endoscopic sphincterotomy or, occasionally, surgical sphincteroplasty, have all been used in this difficult group of patients with varying success.

Surgical treatment of biliary disease

Pre-operative preparation

Patients who are jaundiced are often coagulopathic, have increased risk of infection, and are susceptible to renal failure in the presence of hypovolaemia. Important measures in the pre-operative period include correction of any clotting disorders by administration of intravenous vitamin K or fresh frozen plasma.

Aggressive rehydration to maintain circulation and urine flow is important to reduce the risk of renal failure. Prophylactic antibiotics are essential to prevent intra- and post-operative bacteraemia. Anaesthetic monitoring during operation will include measurement of urine output and central venous pressure. In very ill patients, a Swan-Ganz catheter to measure the right heart pressure may be necessary.

Operative approaches

Accurate and complete pre-operative investigation will minimize the surgical difficulties encountered during the operative procedure. The standard approach to the bile duct is a right subcostal incision, which may be extended across the midline when access is difficult.

Exposure

The bile duct is exposed at the free edge of the lesser omentum and intra-operative cholangiography may be performed through the cystic duct after removal of the gall bladder. The bile duct is identified by needle aspiration of bile, and stay sutures are inserted before the duct is opened axially. For access to the biliary confluence, the junction of Glisson's capsule at the base of the quadrate lobe (segment IV) and the anterior peritoneum of the portal structures are divided, exposing the left hepatic duct, which always lies extrahepatically.

Exploration

Exploration of the bile duct may be performed with a variety of minimally traumatic instruments and choledochoscopy may be performed with either a rigid or a flexible endoscope. If tumours are resected, or if a distal obstruction is being bypassed, the duct is anastomosed, usually to a defunctioned loop of jejunum. In elderly patients, the bile duct may also be anastomosed to the duodenum (choledochoduodenostomy) in circumstances where there is distal biliary obstruction or concern about retained gall stones.

Post-operative care

The pre-operative risks, including coagulopathy and renal dysfunction also pertain to the post-operative period. Continued fluid balance monitoring and repeated assessment of renal function are essential. Liver function will often temporarily worsen after surgery. Patients with sepsis will need aggressive antibiotic therapy, and may need care in an intensive care unit. Wound healing in a jaundiced patient is delayed and adequate nutrition must be achieved either by parenteral or enteral feeding.

Drain tubes are almost invariably used after biliary surgery and are removed once it is clear that no biliary leakage has occurred. If a T-tube is *in situ*, a check cholangiogram is carried out approximately 1 week after surgery. Patients are often discharged with a T-tube in place, and the tube is removed on the first post-operative visit.

Endoscopic therapy

Many advances in endoscopic approaches to the bile duct have occurred in the past 30 years. Endoscopists may now perform palliative stent insertion, stricture dilatation, stone extraction or tumour biopsy, and brushings for cytology. The limitation of stents used for palliating malignant obstruction is their short period of patency, usually less than 2 months. Plastic stents were used initially but have now been largely replaced by expandable metal stents with a diameter of up to 1 cm. These are associated with a longer period of patency but cannot be removed and should not be used where surgery might later be necessary.

Endoscopic stents are the preferred choice in elderly or frail patients and in patients with extensive malignant disease.

Percutaneous approaches

All the above procedures performed endoscopically can also be carried out using a transhepatic approach by radiologists skilled in biliary interventional techniques. The transhepatic approach does carry a risk of bleeding and biliary fistula, but is more appropriate when endoscopic access is not possible or is difficult. Where obstruction is segmental or lies high within the biliary confluence, percutaneous procedures are often more accurate than those performed endoscopically because of the ability of the radiologist to select the most appropriate ductal segment for intervention.

Percutaneous approaches may be combined with surgical reconstructive procedures, where access to the biliary tree can be obtained by a puncture of the Roux-en-Y loop that has been fixed to the deep surface of the abdominal wall. Such percutaneous transjejunal cholangiography (PTJC) is particularly useful in patients with benign strictures where dilatation may be necessary repeatedly, or where stents can be placed when there is recurrence of tumour after previous biliary surgery.

Conclusion

Treatment of biliary disorders involves a multimodality approach with collaboration between the radiologist, endoscopist and surgeon. This produces the optimum outcome for the patient. For complex conditions, combined approaches are best carried out in major hepatobiliary units where all such expertise is available.

Liver tumours

Benign liver tumours

Adenoma

Adenomata are benign tumours that have a solid appearance on ultrasound or computed tomography (CT) scans and can present acutely with intraperitoneal rupture and bleeding. They have a strong association with the oral contraceptive pill and may regress following cessation of the pill. They probably have some malignant potential and if they show progressive increase in size on serial imaging studies, should be removed for this reason. Apart from the risk of malignancy, the major concern is their tendency to rupture with massive haemorrhage; therefore, this condition must be considered in young women presenting with abdominal pain, signs of hypovolaemic shock and features of haemoperitoneum. After resuscitation, the treatment is resection of the affected liver segment.

Focal nodular hyperplasia

Focal nodular hyperplasia (FNH) is not a true neoplasm but is probably due to a fibrous reaction to vessel ingrowth. Again, it is most common in young women. It has a characteristic central stellate scar on CT due to fibrous septae.

Macroscopically, it appears as a nodular firm vascular mass. Histologically, it may resemble cirrhosis with regenerating nodules and connective tissue septae. There may be symptoms of right upper quadrant pain. No specific treatment is required and the main purpose of management is to distinguish the lesion from neoplasms.

Haemangioma

Haemangioma is the most common benign liver tumour and is cavernous in nature, with fibrous septae and a well-defined capsule. The tumours may again be related to the oral contraceptive pill and may regress when the pill is stopped. They may also enlarge during pregnancy. Most are asymptomatic but they can present as a mass lesion or with spontaneous haemorrhage. Contrast CT is diagnostic with peripheral then central infilling of the tumour with contrast, giving a halo and then target appearance. Magnetic resonance imaging (MRI) is also of value, as the T_2-weighted image appearances are characteristic. These modalities now mean that biopsy is unnecessary. Biopsy can precipitate catastrophic bleeding and is strongly contraindicated.

Most haemangiomas require no treatment except radiological surveillance. Pain or enlargement may herald rupture and in these circumstances the tumour should be enucleated or the involved liver segment resected.

Focal fatty change

Focal fatty change can occur in the liver, particularly in obese patients and in those with diabetes mellitus. This is not a true tumour but can be confused with one, although a CT scan or an MRI shows a characteristic appearance.

Malignant liver tumours

Primary hepatocellular cancer or hepatoma

More than 300 cases of hepatocellular cancer (HCC) occur in Australia each year. It is a very common cause of cancer death in China and in Africa (up to 100 per 100,000 each year). In these countries the tumours have a very close relationship to hepatitis B surface antigen (HBsAG) positivity, with underlying cirrhosis, which increases the risk at least 200-fold. In Western countries, alcoholic cirrhosis is present in at least 90% of cases. It is clear that immunisation against hepatitis B virus and control of alcoholism offer a major opportunity to reduce the incidence of this highly malignant tumour. There are also associations with haemochromatosis and excessive intake of anabolic steroids. There is a slightly increased incidence with the oral contraceptive pill.

Surgical pathology

Hepatocellular cancers are adenocarcinomas that are frequently multicentric, often softer than the surrounding liver and can be difficult to distinguish from regenerative nodules in the cirrhotic liver. Spread is local to structures such as the diaphragm and distant to sites such as the lung and bone. A fibrolamellar type is seen mainly in young women and has a much better prognosis.

Clinical features

As with any cancer, HCC can present with clinical features of the primary tumour or of secondary deposits, or with the general features of malignant disease. The specific clinical features of the primary tumour can include pain, jaundice due to biliary compression or replacement of liver tissue, and haemorrhage due to oesophageal varices, sometimes precipitated by portal vein thrombosis. Intraperitoneal rupture and bleeding can occur. The diagnosis may be established before the onset of symptoms following screening for HCC using the serum α-fetoprotein (α-FP) test in cirrhotics, whether they be alcoholics or HBsAG-positive.

Investigation

Investigations for primary HCC are given in Box 15.1.

Box 15.1 Investigations for primary hepatocellular carcinoma

- Liver function tests to assess the degree of liver damage.
- Coagulation studies, particularly of prothrombin and platelet function.
- Hepatitis B surface antigen (HBsAG).
- α-Fetoprotein (α-FP). Ninety-five per cent of HCC patients demonstrate a rise in levels, although patients with small tumours may have normal values. The absolute value is not prognostic but repeated measurement is important in assessing response to treatment and follow-up.
- Ultrasound scan. The lesions are often hypoechoic compared with adjacent liver, but may be hyperechoic if the tumour contains fat.
- Computed tomography scan. With contrast this is used to assess site, size and number of primaries. Intra-arterial lipiodol, which is concentrated in most HCC, provides a sensitive test although lesions less than 1 cm in size may not be demonstrated.
- Magnetic resonance imaging is of value if ultrasound or CT scan fails to demonstrate a lesion, although its major role is with lesions greater than 2 cm in diameter.
- Percutaneous biopsy of liver if α-FP is normal.
- Laparoscopy to determine evidence of peritoneal disease.
- Dye excretion test (bromsulphthalein) is used to assess function of liver and whether the patient will tolerate resection (retention $>$30% contraindicates surgery).
- Bone scan to look for extrahepatic disease.
- Pulmonary CT scan to demonstrate lung secondaries.
- Arteriography may be useful to identify aberrant arterial anatomy in preparation for resection.

Treatment

RESECTION

Liver resection can be undertaken, provided there is no disease outside the liver, there is sufficient reserve of liver function, the lesion is less than 5 cm in diameter and a curative resection with a 1 cm margin is possible. Operative mortality of liver resection for HCC, at approximately 10%, is much greater than for liver metastases because of the reduced liver function and limited ability of the cirrhotic liver to regenerate. Postoperative liver failure is the principal risk, and bleeding and sepsis are also frequently seen. The types of liver resection are covered later.

LIVER TRANSPLANTATION

The very well differentiated variant of HCC, fibrolamellar carcinoma, is much less likely to spread outside the liver, and good results of transplantation have been described. Transplantation is also of value in small HCC with poor liver function due to their cirrhosis.

ARTERIAL CHEMO-EMBOLISATION

The ability of lipiodol (iodised poppy seed oil; an old radiological contrast agent) to be concentrated in HCC when administered through the hepatic artery can be used to treat HCC by selectively delivering a cytotoxic agent (adriamycin or cisplatin) or radiation (using ^{131}I) to the cancer. Approximately 75% of HCC take up lipiodol and, of these, more than 50% will achieve at least a tumour marker (α-FP) response. Radiological evidence of shrinkage occurs somewhat less frequently. Variations in tumour response are seen; some patients remain tumour-free for several years after this type of therapy.

ALCOHOL INJECTION

Percutaneous injection of absolute alcohol under ultrasound control can destroy small HCC. This is clearly an attractive non-operative option that may produce a cure. The best results are achieved in lesions of 2-cm diameter or less.

Prognosis

The prognosis of HCC is very poor, with a median survival of untreated symptomatic patients being approximately 3 months. For the comparatively small number of patients who are suitable for resection, 5-year survival is approximately 20%. It is hoped that this level of success will rise with more effective screening of at-risk patients.

Secondary liver cancer

The liver is frequently involved in the advanced stages of many different tumours and, while palliation of symptoms may be achieved, there are a few situations where very prolonged survival or even cure can be achieved. Specific forms of metastasis are susceptible to definitive treatment. For example, the occasional melanoma patient will have only a solitary liver metastasis that can be treated by resection. Very occasionally, patients with solitary metastases from other cancers (e.g. stomach, breast, sarcomas) have been cured by resection, but in the vast majority the possible benefit of resection is limited by the presence of disease outside the liver.

Some other types of tumour in which treatment can be of value will be considered in more detail.

Liver metastases from neuroendocrine tumours

This is one form of tumour where surgery has much to offer the patient with liver metastases. Metastases may be responsible for hormone secretion and particular syndromes (see Chapter 36), so that control of those metastases by debulking or resection can be of great benefit, although not necessarily prolonging life.

There are a number of surgical options:

- Transplantation. This can be done if there are very large numbers of lesions (melon seed liver). Results are good provided there is no disease outside the liver.
- Resection. Very extensive surgery is justified by long survival and good palliation.
- Cryotherapy. This gives encouraging results as measured by tumour markers, radiology and long-term survival.
- Embolisation. This is sometimes useful in palliation of symptoms for quite prolonged periods.

Colorectal cancer

Colorectal cancer is the most common cause of cancer death in non-smokers in most of the developed world. Liver metastases are a common cause of death but, importantly, are the only site of metastatic disease in a significant number of patients. Regular serum carcinoembryonic antigen (CEA) tests after resection of primary colorectal cancers allows early diagnosis of liver metastases. In patients with unresectable disease, treatment is palliative for symptoms such as pain. The disease is potentially curable by resection if there is no extrahepatic disease, there are fewer than four metastases and the lesions are anatomically resectable with a 1-cm resection margin.

Investigations to be carried out are largely those defined for HCC (Box 15.1), with serum CEA levels in place of α-FP. As with HCC, the investigations are directed towards assessing liver function and the presence of disease beyond the potential limits of resection.

Curative treatment of liver metastases

Resection of up to two-thirds of the healthy liver is possible and is relatively safe, with an operative mortality of well under 5%. Factors that increase operative risk include jaundice, cirrhosis, significant concomitant medical disease of the heart or lungs, very extensive hepatic resections and the need for resection of the vena cava. Age alone is not a strong risk factor. Liver resection can now be done frequently without the need for blood transfusion because of:

- a better understanding of intrahepatic vascular anatomy (Fig. 15.4)

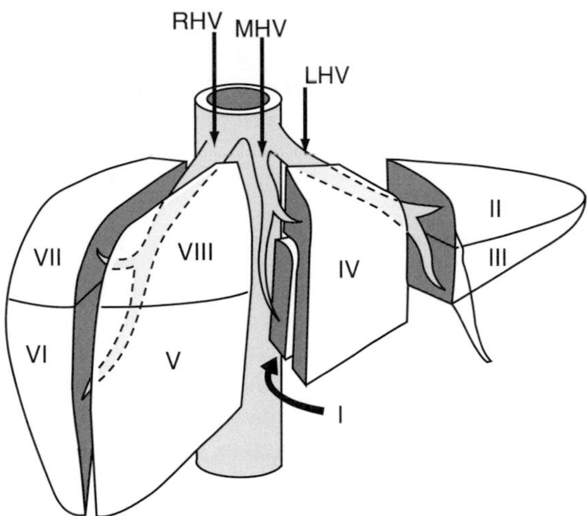

Fig. 15.4 Liver segments. RHV, right hepatic vein; MHV, middle hepatic vein; LHV, left hepatic vein.

- inflow occlusion (temporary occlusion of blood flow into the liver)
- the use of an ultrasonic aspirator (CUSA), which is a surgical instrument with a vibrating tip driven by an ultrasound transducer, used with a flow of fluid to dissect through the liver, allowing almost bloodless hepatic dissection
- intra-operative ultrasound, which allows precise identification of lesions, vessels and their relationship
- total vascular exclusion of the liver; clamping the outflow (hepatic veins) as well as the inflow allows rapid bloodless hepatic surgery.

The liver was divided into eight segments by a French anatomist, Cuinaud (Fig. 15.5). Segment I is the caudate lobe, just in front of the inferior vena cava. Segments II/III are the left lateral segment, to the left of the falciform ligament. Segment IV is also part of the left liver and is between the entry of the falciform ligament and the gall-bladder fossa. Segments V–VIII comprise the right lobe and are divided by vessels. All segments can be removed independently but the common resections are: right lobectomy V–VIII, left lobectomy II–IV, left lateral segmentectomy II, III, and extended right hepatectomy = right lobectomy + IV (Fig. 15.5).

Specific complications of liver resection include:

- *Haemorrhage*. This is usually due to a surgical cause (e.g. a clip or tie that has fallen off) and is easily corrected. Occasionally haemorrhage is secondary to coagulopathy, with many oozing sites due to inadequate liver function. Disseminated intravascular coagulation is usually a result of sepsis.

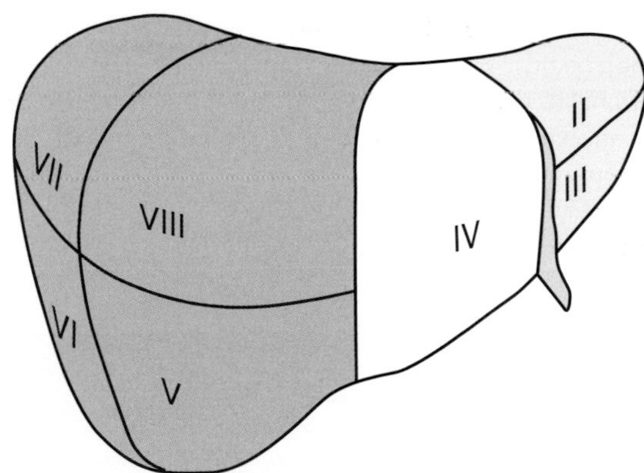

Fig. 15.5 Liver resection.

- *Sepsis*. This is usually in the form of a local abscess due to bile leak or infected haematoma, and is treated by a radiologically placed drain.

HEPATIC CRYOTHERAPY

This technique allows some patients with lesions that are unresectable to be treated and does not require excision or destruction of much normal liver. A liquid nitrogen probe device is used and freezing monitored by intra-operative ultrasound. A 5-year survival of 20% in patients with unresectable disease has been seen. Other methods of imaging-controlled destruction include percutaneous placement of laser fibres and radio frequency (RF) destruction. These less invasive techniques may offer similar results.

Palliative treatment

PAIN CONTROL

Hepatic pain is controlled by analgesia and by steroids to reduce distension of the liver capsule. Radiotherapy may halt the progression of rapidly enlarging and painful liver metastases. Systemic chemotherapy has a limited effect.

REGIONAL OR HEPATIC ARTERY CHEMOTHERAPY

There is now good evidence from controlled trials to show that chemotherapy in the form of 5-fluorouracil or 5-fluorodeoxyuridine (FUDR) administered via the hepatic artery may extend life in patients with inoperable liver metastases. Patients with extrahepatic disease do not benefit from this treatment. A small implantable catheter system is placed in the gastroduodenal artery, with the tip of the catheter in the common hepatic artery. The gall bladder is removed to prevent cytotoxic cholecystitis. The catheter is connected to either a subcutaneous port that is accessed by needle and connected to an external pump system, or a totally implantable pump.

The advantages and disadvantages of hepatic artery chemotherapy over systemic chemotherapy are given in Box 15.2.

Box 15.2 The advantages and disadvantages of hepatic artery chemotherapy over systemic chemotherapy

Advantages
- Higher response rate (approximately 75% *vs* 25%)
- Lower toxicity because chemotherapy is given at a rate to allow hepatic first-pass metabolism
- Better survival data (approximately 20 months *vs* 8 months untreated)

Disadvantages
- Operative procedure to place the catheter
- Cost, especially if an implantable pump is used (A$10,000)
- Specific complications, such as FUDR, causes dose-related cholangitis
- 5-Fluorouracil may cause arterial thrombosis or, rarely, an aneurysm that can cause major gastrointestinal bleeding
- Thrombosis of the catheter
- Infection of the catheter

HEPATIC ARTERY EMBOLISATION

Hepatic artery embolisation, using a radiologically placed catheter and gelfoam or steel coils, has been advocated for advanced liver metastases to palliate a large painful liver. This technique relies on the principle that the metastases have a predominantly arterial supply, while normal liver derives a higher proportion of its blood supply from the portal veins. Hepatic arterial embolisation will often induce considerable regression of metastasis but does not significantly affect the function of the normal liver.

SIRT (Selective internal radiotherapy)

This treatment utilises radioactive yttrium labelled particles which are given by hepatic artery injection, selectively delivered to tumour because of its principally arterial supply as opposed to the portal venous supply to the hepatic parenchyma. An injection of vasoconstructor further increases selectivity because tumour vessels do not contain smooth muscle. Although high response rates are seen, this does not control systemic disease.

Systemic chemotherapy

The value of systemic chemotherapy in metastastic CRC has dramatically changed because of the availability of new agents. As well as 5FU, the oral agent Xeloda (capecitabine) and parenteral agents irinotecan and oxaliplatin provide significant response. Biological therapies to block growth factors such as VEGF are effective in metastic CRC.

MCQs

Select the single correct answer to each question.

1 The following investigation should always be performed when investigating obstructive jaundice:
  a liver ultrasound
  b ERCP
  c CT scan
  d MRCP
  e PTC

2 Bile duct injury during laparoscopic cholecystectomy is more common:
  a in the presence of cholecystitis
  b when the surgeon is inexperienced
  c if the biliary anatomy is unusual
  d when the operation is complicated by haemorrhage
  e all of the above

3 Cholangiocarcinoma is most commonly found:
  a in the periphery of the liver
  b in the gall bladder
  c at the biliary confluence
  d in the distal bile duct
  e in the duodenum

4 Primary sclerosing cholangitis is not associated with:
  a inflammatory bowel disease
  b carcinoma of the bile duct
  c gallstones
  d multifocal biliary strictures
  e hepatocellular carcinoma

5 Primary hepato-cellular carcinoma may be caused by all of the following except:
a alcohol
b haemochromatosis
c hepatitis B virus
d steroids
e gallstones

6 Liver metastases may be treated by all of the following except:
a arterial embolisation
b cryotherapy
c laparoscopic resection
d open lobectomy
e regional chemotherapy

16 Liver infections

C. Christophi and V. Muralidharan

Introduction

Liver infections are classified according to the category of the infecting agent as viral, bacterial or parasitic. Viral infections include both primary hepatitis viruses or secondary causes where the liver is involved during systemic viral infections such as cytomegalovirus, HIV and herpes simplex. This chapter will not discuss viral infections of the liver.

Bacterial infectons

Pyogenic abscess

Aetiology

Pyogenic or bacterial abscess may be caused by several factors and is classified by the route of entry of the organisms. Infections may arise from the biliary tract, portal vein and hepatic artery or by direct extension.

- Infections arising from the *biliary tract* are the most common and result in 30% to 50% of the total number of pyogenic abscesses. The resultant cholangitis leads to liver abscesses, which are frequently multiple. Biliary obstruction is commonly present from causes such as choledocholithiasis and benign or malignant strictures. Other causes of cholangitis include iatrogenic intervention from endoscopic retrograde cholangiopancreatography (ERCP) or percutaneous transhepatic procedures.
- Another common route of entry of infection is the *portal vein*. Conditions such as complicated diverticular disease, appendicitis, peritonitis and pancreatitis may cause portal vein pyaemia, resulting in pyogenic liver abscesses.
- Septicemia from any cause may also give rise to multiple liver abscesses via dissemination from the *hepatic artery*. These account for 5 to 15% of pyogenic liver abscesses. Common causes include bacterial endocarditis, pneumonia and intravenous drug abuse.
- Other causes of liver abscesses include complicated liver trauma from blunt or penetrating causes, or by direct extension from other conditions such as empyema of the gall bladder. In a number of cases, the cause is not obvious.

The infecting organism varies according to the site of entry. In biliary or portal vein sepsis, the organisms are enteric and usually polymicrobial. *Staphylococcus aureus* is evident in 20% of cases and is confirmed predominantly from haematogenous spread.

Clinical presentation and diagnosis

The most common presenting symptoms include pyrexia and rigours associated with right upper quadrant pain, general malaise and anorexia. Examination may reveal tender hepatomegaly. A pleural effusion may be present. Occasionally, hypotension and cardiovascular collapse may be the presenting symptoms.

Investigation

Liver function tests may show hyperbilirubinemia and raised alkaline phosphatase and transaminase levels. Blood cultures are frequently positive. A leucocytosis is usually evident.

Radiological investigations include ultrasound or CT scan of the abdomen to determine the size, characteristics, number and anatomical location of the liver abscesses. A chest X-ray may show an elevated hemidiaphragm or a pleural effusion. Further tests such as an ERCP or a colonoscopy may be required to determine the cause of pyogenic liver abscesses.

Treatment

Therapeutic principles include symptomatic measures, appropriate antibiotic therapy and drainage of the liver abscess. In addition the diagnosis and eradication of the underlying cause is essential.

- Symptomatic measures include a regimen of analgesics and attention to adequate nutrition and hydration.
- Antimicrobial therapy is dependent on the underlying cause. Biliary or enteric causes involve microbial cover against Gram-negative and anaerobic organisms. Haematogenous causes usually include antibiotic cover against the staphylococcus organisms. Administration of antibiotics is usually prolonged over several weeks to eradicate infection and avoid recurrence.
- Drainage of the abscess may be achieved by percutaneous drainage under ultrasound control or by repeated percutaneous aspiration. Open surgical drainage is now rarely indicated.
- Frequent clinical, biochemical, microbial and radiological follow-up is required to assess progress and detect relapses.

Parasitic infections

Amoebic liver abscesses

Aetiology

Amoebic infestation is caused by the organism *Entamoeba histolytica*. It is rare in Australia but endemic in many areas of the tropics such as India and other parts of Asia. Transmission is by passage of cysts in the stool, the cysts then being ingested orally as a result of poor hygienic practices. The organism penetrates the mucosa of the gastrointestinal tract to gain access to the liver by the portal venous system. The resultant abscess has an "anchovy paste" appearance and may be secondarily infected, usually by enteric organisms. Risk factors include malnutrition, depressed immunity and low socioeconomic status.

Complications of amoebic abscess include rupture into the peritoneal cavity or hollow viscus such as colon or stomach. Rarely there may be pleuropulmonary involvement.

Clinical features

The onset of the disease may be sudden or gradual. Right upper quadrant pain associated with general malaise and weight loss are the most common symptoms on presentation. Pyrexia and sweating occurs in about 60% of patients. Approximately 30% of patients have diarrhoea. Signs may include tender hepatomegaly and, occasionally, jaundice.

Investigation

Full blood examination may show leukocytosis and eosinophilia. Liver function tests are frequently deranged and show a hepatocellular pattern of injury. Amoebic serology and stool cultures are usually positive. Ultrasound with needle aspiration and culture confirm the diagnosis.

Treatment

Symptomatic measures include analgesics and attention to nutrition and hydration. Antimicrobial therapy is the mainstay of treatment. This may be associated with percutaneous drainage or repeated aspiration if necessary. The antibiotic of choice is metronidazole.

Hydatid disease

There are two forms of hydatid disease, the most common being *Echinococcus granulosus*, which causes cystic hydatid disease. *Echinococcus alveolaris* is a much rarer form and is characterised by an infiltrative pattern of liver involvement.

Echinococcus granulosus

PATHOLOGY

In this disease, the human is an intermediate host. The ova are ingested by humans from the faeces of tapeworm-infected dogs. Dogs are usually infected by feeding of offal of infected sheep. The ova reach the stomach of the human, where they hatch, penetrate the wall of the intestine and pass to the liver by the portal vein. Others may pass from the liver into the lung, brain, or other organs. Development of the cyst in liver then occurs. These cysts exhibit a slow growth pattern and infection usually occurs in childhood.

The cyst has a characteristic appearance (see Fig. 16.1). There is a capsule or exocyst, which is really the compressed host tissue. The endocyst includes the laminated membrane from the parasite, which contains the germinal layer and scolices. The cyst is fluid-filled and also contains brood capsules. The natural history of hydatid cysts is that of continued growth. Apart from local compressive effects, rupture may occur into the

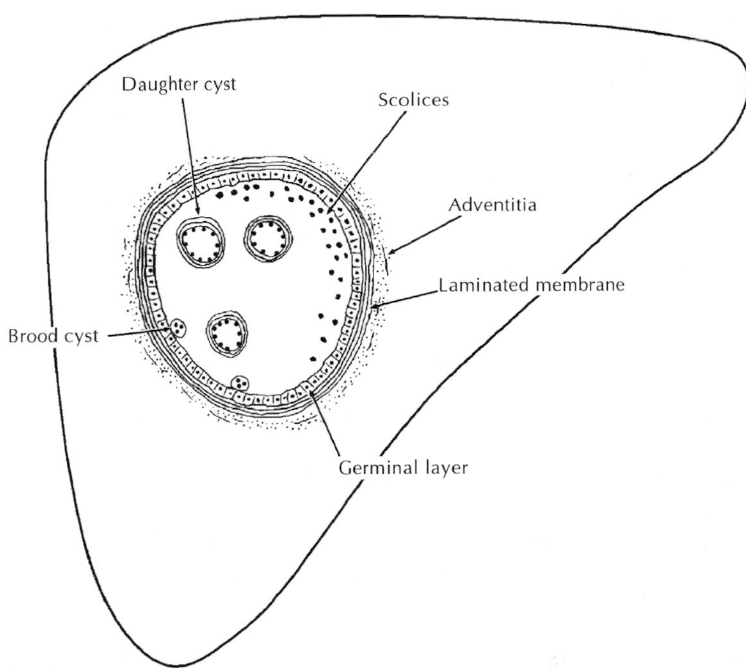

Fig. 16.1 Hydatid cyst of the liver.

biliary tree causing obstructive jaundice. Rupture into the peritoneal or thoracic cavity may also occur in addition to hematogenous spread to other organs such as lung, bone, brain and spleen. The cysts may become secondarily infected.

CLINICAL PRESENTATION

Hydatids may be symptomless and are detected as incidental findings on radiological investigations for other conditions. The most common symptoms are right upper quadrant pain, jaundice, pruritus and pyrexia. A persistent cough may indicate pulmonary involvement.

INVESTIGATION

Liver function tests may show either an obstructive or hepatocellular pattern. Full blood examination may reveal a leukocytosis or eosinophilia. There are numerous serological tests available. The most sensitive and specific test is immunoelectrophoresis, which is not only diagnostic but is an indicator of the response to treatment. Radiological tests to assess the size and location of the cyst include ultrasound and CT scan. ERCP or magnetic resonance cholangiopancreatography (MRCP) may be indicated to detect biliary connections or bronchobiliary fistulas.

TREATMENT

- *Conservative*
  Small (<2–3 cm) asymptomatic cysts, which are deep in the parenchyma, require no treatment. Complications in this group are rare. These patients however need regular follow-up.
- *Medical*
  Drug therapy may be used alone or in conjunction with surgical procedures. Mebendazole or albendazole may be used in patients with hydatid disease who are regarded as poor risk for surgery or with widely disseminated disease. It may be also be used by percutaneous injection under ultrasound localisation directly into the cyst. These drugs may also be administered either before or after definitive surgery to minimise the risk of recurrence. Prolonged courses over 6–12 weeks are usually required. Medical therapy alone is successful in 30 to 50% of cases. These drugs may be toxic to the liver and bone marrow and require careful monitoring.
- *Surgery*
  The principles of surgical management include (a) complete neutralisation and removal of the parasite components, including the germinal membrane, scolices and brood capsules; (b) prevention

of contamination or spillage to prevent anaphylaxis or recurrence and (c) management of the residual cavity.

Procedures may include liver resection, with total excision of the cyst, including the capsule (pericystectomy). This is rarely indicated and is suitable for peripheral or pedunculated cysts.

Scolicidal agents are frequently injected into the cyst prior to manipulation to destroy active components and prevent recurrence if spillage occurs. Commonly used agents include cetrimide or hypertonic saline. The contents of the cyst are then evacuated. The residual cavity may be filled with saline and closed (capittonage) or obliterated by an omental pedicle, especially in infected cysts.

Biliary communications may need to be closed and bile duct explored to remove hydatids causing biliary obstruction.

Alveolar echinococcus

PATHOLOGY

This is a rare condition caused by *Echinococcus multilocularis*, whose life cycle is different from that of *Echinococcus granulosus*. Natural hosts include foxes, rodents, dogs and cats. It is endemic in the northern hemisphere, especially Japan, China and Central Europe. Humans are an unusual and intermediate host.

It is a progressive, destructive disease. Death results from liver parenchymal destruction and liver failure. The disease may extend to the brain and lung and may be associated with severe myositis. Vesicles invade the host liver tissue by extension of the germinal layer, which remains in an active proliferative state.

CLINICAL FEATURES

Early symptoms are usually non-specific and vague. The most common initial presentation is mild right upper quadrant pain. Tender hepatomegaly or a mass may be present. As the disease progresses, jaundice, ascites and hepatic insufficiency occur.

In the early stages, a high index of suspicion in endemic areas is required. Differential diagnosis includes hepatoma, tuberculosis, hemangioma or focal nodular hyperplasia.

INVESTIGATION

Radiological investigations such as ultrasound, computed tomography (CT) scan and magnetic resonance imaging (MRI) may provide additional information. Serology may be non-conclusive in the early stages of the disease; however, it may subsequently confirm the underlying process. Occasionally, laparoscopy and biopsy may be required. Even at operation, the accuracy of diagnosis is only 50%.

TREATMENT

The only known definitive cure for *E. alveolaris* is liver resection. Transplantation has been performed on selected cases but long-term outcome is uncertain. Albendazole, although unable to eliminate the parasite, may slow progression of the disease and should be administered on an indefinite basis in conjunction with surgery.

Liver fluke disease

Infestations of clinical importance include those by *Fasciola hepatica*, *Clonorchis sinensis* and *Ascaris lumbricoides*. These parasites are trematodes and undergo both sexual (definitive host) and asexual (intermediate host) reproduction.

Fasciola hepatica

PATHOLOGY

This condition exists all over the world but is commonly seen in Middle and Western Europe, South America and the Caribbean. It is known as the common sheep fluke and is found in sheep- and cattle-rearing countries.

The parasite inhabits the gall bladder and bile ducts and passes ova in the stool. The human is an incidental host, especially those eating raw vegetables. Cysts are ingested from vegetables and subsequently penetrate the intestinal wall. They then migrate by the transperitoneal route and invade the liver capsule and enter the biliary system, where they are sometimes confused as stones.

CLINICAL FEATURES

Patients may be asymptomatic or present with acute or chronic symptoms. Acute symptoms include a sudden onset of right upper quadrant pain, pyrexia or cholangitis and symptoms of allergic reactions. Hepatosplenomegaly may be present. Chronic symptoms include intermittent biliary colic, cholecystitis, jaundice anaemia and hypoproteinaemia.

INVESTIGATION
Full blood examination may show eosinophilia. Liver function tests show features consistent with cholestasis. Stools are examined for the presence of ova. Specific serological testing usually confirms the diagnosis.

TREATMENT
The condition is treated by albendazole, praziquantel or bithional. Cholecystectomy and exploration of the common bile duct by ERCP may also be necessary.

Clonorchis sinensis

PATHOLOGY
Chlonorchis sinensis is a flat worm which inhabits the biliary tree. Cysts from infected fish are ingested and migrate from the duodenum into the bile ducts. Ova are excreted from the stools. The intermediate host is a snail, which completes the life cycle by infecting fish. Humans are infected by eating raw fish.

The biliary epithelium becomes inflamed from constant irritation, leading to cholangitis, ductal fibrosis, stricturing and stone formation. There is a high incidence of cholangiocarcinoma.

CLINICAL FEATURES
The classic symptoms associated with clonorchis infestation are recurrent pyogenic cholangitis. There are recurrent attacks of right upper quadrant pain, jaundice and pyrexia. Examination may reveal tender hepatomegaly and splenomegaly if portal hypertension exists.

INVESTIGATION
Imaging of the biliary tree by MRI or ERCP is essential to delineate the distribution of stones and strictures. Ova are demonstrated in faeces or duodenal aspirate.

TREATMENT
The drug of choice is Praziquantel. Surgery is indicated if stones or strictures are present.

Biliary ascariasis

PATHOLOGY
The roundworm *Ascaris lumbricoides* is endemic in tropical and subtropical areas. The worms inhabit the small intestine and enter the common bile duct by the duodenal ampulla of Vater.

CLINICAL FEATURES
They induce mechanical obstruction of the biliary tree. Cholangitis, empyema of the gall bladder and multiple liver abscesses may occur as a result of secondary infection.

INVESTIGATION
Stool examination commonly demonstrates the presence of worms. Ultrasound is highly accurate in delineating the worms in the biliary tree.

TREATMENT
Non-operative management is successful. Mebendazole and pyrantel pamoate are used over 3 days. ERCP may be required for patients with cholangitis and biliary stones.

MCQs

Select the single correct answer to each question.

1 Regarding pyogenic liver abscesses, which one of the following is true?
- **a** commonest source for sepsis is the small bowel
- **b** a single organism is usually causal
- **c** obstructive jaundice is a common symptom of pyogenic abscess
- **d** drainage of the abscess and appropriate antibiotic therapy are the mainstay of management
- **e** open surgical drainage of the abscess is an essential part of present treatment

2 Regarding amoebic liver absesses, which one of the following is false?
- **a** it is an uncommon disease in Australia and is endemic in South and Southeast Asia
- **b** intestinal amoebiasis, which leads to liver abscess, is transmitted by the faeco-oral route
- **c** amoebic serology is usually positive in these patients
- **d** mainstay of treatment is antimicrobial therapy
- **e** amoebic liver abscess must never be drained by percutaneous technique

3 Regarding hydatid disease, which one of the following is incorrect?
- **a** the human is an end host, which breaks the development cycle of the parasite
- **b** initial infection occurs through the alimentary tract and is asymptomatic
- **c** the natural history of a hydatid cyst in the human is one of slow progressive growth

d rupture of a hydatid cyst is a common event
e most symptoms are related to pressure effects on the liver and surrounding organs

4 Which one of the following statements regarding the management of hydatid cysts is false?
a extremely small cysts may be managed conservatively provided they are followed up to monitor growth
b medical management is successful in the majority of cases
c medical therapy is usually used to supplement surgical intervention
d the most common surgical technique is that of evacuation of the content and de-roofing of the cyst and the placement of an omental patch in the cavity
e prevention of spillage of the contents into the peritoneal cavity is of critical importance

5 The following are true of liver infestations:
a the liver fluke *Fasciola hepatica* is acquired from sheep and cattle and infests the biliary tree
b the flat worm *Clonorchis sinensis* is usually ingested by eating raw fish
c *Clonorchis sinensis* infestation leads to recurrent cholangitis and a high incidence of cholangiocarcinoma
d biliary ascariasis is caused by the migration of the common intestinal roundworm into the biliary tree
e all of the above

17 Diseases of the pancreas

James Toouli

Pancreatitis

Introduction

The classification of pancreatitis has previously been made difficult owing to the description of various combinations of acute and chronic conditions with nomenclature that attempted to relate the classification to the aetiology. It is best to regard pancreatitis as either acute or chronic. Within these two broad divisions there are patients who may have recurrent episodes of acute pancreatitis and others who have chronic pancreatitis but who, in addition, experience attacks of acute pancreatitis (i.e. acute on chronic).

Acute pancreatitis

Acute pancreatitis is an acute inflammatory process of the pancreas, with varying involvement of other regional tissues or remote organ systems. This definition of acute pancreatitis was derived at a conference held in Atlanta in 1992 with the aim of providing a clinically based classification of acute pancreatitis and its complications. The Atlanta definition does not relate to either aetiology or pathological findings, as neither of these may be obvious to a clinician on first seeing a patient with the clinical features of acute pancreatitis.

The incidence of acute pancreatitis in the developed world has been demonstrating a progressive increase and it is estimated to be approximately 100 cases per 1 million people per year. However, this incidence will vary in different regions and is dependent on aetiological factors existing in a country. In countries with a relatively high consumption of alcohol, incidence of pancreatitis may be higher compared to countries with a low consumption of alcohol. Acute pancreatitis occurs most commonly in patients in the 30- to 60-year-old age group, with alcohol-related pancreatitis being more common in males and gallstone-related pancreatitis being more common in females.

Aetiology and pathogenesis

The causes of acute pancreatitis fall into three major categories: one third of cases are due to alcohol consumption; one third are secondary to gallstones; and one third are due to a variety of conditions that includes trauma, hyperlipidaemia, hypercalcaemia, miscellaneous drugs (e.g. thiazide diuretics), infections (e.g. mumps), tumours (e.g. ampullary tumours), sphincter of Oddi dysfunction, anatomical causes (e.g. pancreas divisum) or idiopathic (unknown) causes.

It is difficult to imagine that one single mechanism would explain the pathogenesis of acute pancreatitis given the diversity of the aetiological causes. However, all of these factors have one thing in common; that is, there is a triggering of activation of pancreatic trypsinogen to trypsin that then begins the process of autodigestion seen in all forms of acute pancreatitis.

The pancreas is the major organ in the abdomen producing digestive enzymes. These enzymes in their activated form break down the complex molecular structure of proteins, lipids and carbohydrates to yield simple amino acids, mono- and diglycerides plus glucose and fructose for subsequent absorption in the small intestine. This process takes place in the upper small intestine. The pancreatic enzymes are activated in the duodenum, where their action begins.

There are a number of protective mechanisms that prevent the pancreas from autodigestion by these powerful enzymes. Trypsinogen and the other proteolytic enzymes are secreted in their inactive form and do not become activated until they reach the duodenal lumen. The enzymes are formed in the acinar cells, and stored in zymogen granules within the cell. These

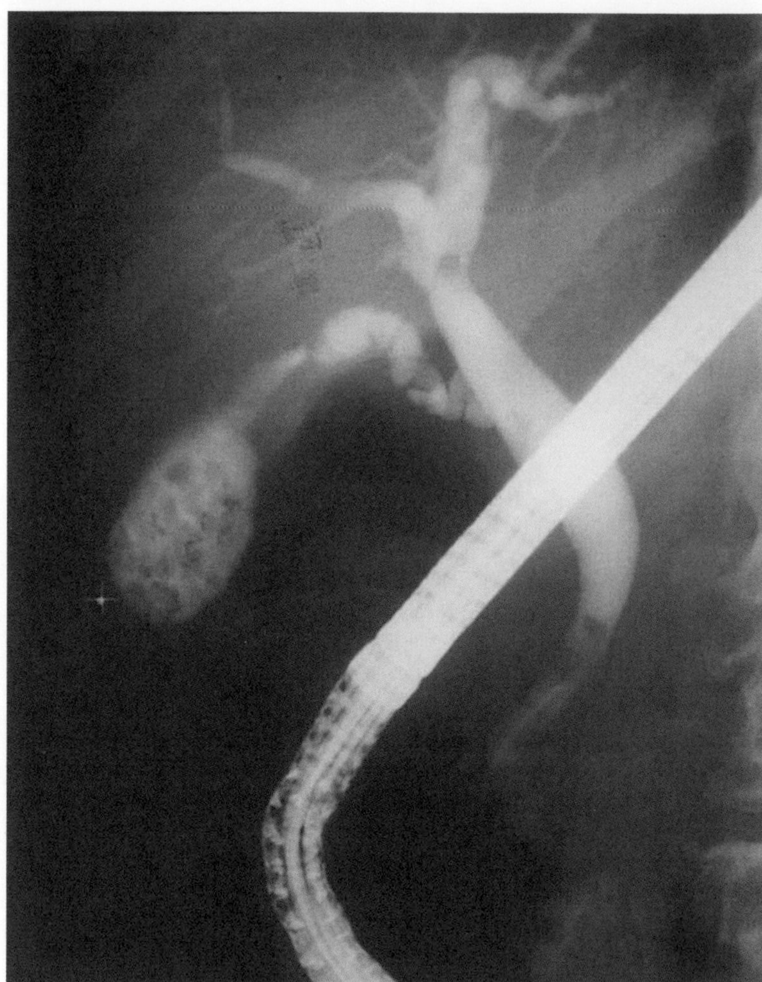

Fig. 17.1 Endoscopic retrograde cholangiogram demonstrating the biliary system in a patient who presented with gallstone pancreatitis. The cholangiogram shows multiple small gallstones in the gall bladder and bile duct. Passage of one or more of the gallstones into the duodenum induced pancreatitis.

membrane-lined granules protect the cell from any activated enzyme. Pancreatic acinar cells produce an anti-trypsin molecule that further adds to the protection by an antagonist action on trypsin. Finally, the inactivated enzymes are secreted into the pancreatic ductules, are diluted by the richly alkaline fluid secreted by the ductular epithelium, and are rapidly propelled into the main pancreatic duct to be secreted into the duodenum, where they first come into contact with their specific activating factors (e.g. protein, carbohydrate, lipid).

Inappropriate activation of trypsinogen to trypsin within the pancreatic parenchyma will give rise to trypsin autodigestion of the pancreas and result in acute pancreatitis. It has been demonstrated that alcohol produces direct chemical damage to pancreatic acinar cells, particularly the membranes of the zymogen granules, thus allowing leakage of trypsinogen into the cell cytoplasm. Consequently, activation of the enzymes may occur, resulting in activation of an inflammatory cascade. Viral infections and drugs may have a similar mode of action. Gallstones cause pancreatitis when they pass from the gall bladder to the bile duct and then through the sphincter of Oddi into the duodenum (Fig. 17.1). In some patients, there is a transient impaction of the stone at the sphincter. This may well result in abnormal motility of the sphincter, which raises the pressure within the pancreatic duct and retards flow. The elevated pancreatic duct pressure may cause some back pressure on the acinar cells, which in itself may cause their damage and re-activate trypsinogen. Another factor may be the back-flow of duodenal juice, which may be associated with sphincter dysmotility and further enhance trypsinogen activation within the pancreas.

Once trypsin has been activated, autodigestion of the pancreas begins. This injurious process sets up the normal inflammatory response, which is characterised by oedema, leucocytosis and increased vascularity. Furthermore, biologically active compounds of the cytokine system are activated and released into the circulation, resulting in effects on the heart, the surfactant of the lung and renal function.

The severity of an acute episode of pancreatitis is dependent on the severity of damage to the pancreas and the magnitude of the inflammatory response. Fluid may accumulate around the pancreas or extend beyond its immediate vicinity to involve the rest of the retroperitoneal space as well as small- and large-bowel mesentery. Fluid may also accumulate in the peritoneal cavity, initially in the lesser sac and posterior to the stomach, but, in more severe cases, ascites may develop. The degree of autodigestion may be of an extent that produces necrosis of a part or whole of the pancreas. The inflammatory process may affect adjacent organs, such as the colon, to reduce their mucosal barrier and allow migration (translocation) of bacteria to infect the necrotic tissue, thus forming an abscess. Oedema of the pancreas may also compress the bile duct and result in obstructive jaundice. Similarly, the oedema may obstruct the duodenum and result in an upper small-bowel obstruction, which will manifest as vomiting.

Necrosis of the pancreas and surrounding fatty tissue also results in deposition of calcium, which may result in a precipitous fall in serum calcium levels. In addition, with the massive shift of fluid that may occur with severe pancreatitis, there is a relative loss of fluid from the circulating volume, resulting in hypovolaemic shock.

Surgical pathology and complications

The pathological appearance of the pancreas in a patient with acute pancreatitis is that of an acute inflammatory condition characterised by oedema, increased vascularity and haemorrhage. In addition, and depending on the severity of an episode, an area of necrosis as well as scattered calcium deposits may be present. The pathological changes in acute pancreatitis represent a continuum, with interstitial oedema and minimal histological evidence of necrosis at the minor end of the scale, and confluent macroscopic necrosis at the other extreme. The complications of acute pancreatitis are subdivided into local and systemic (Box 17.1).

Box 17.1 Complications of acute pancreatitis

Local (these complications occur with increasing severity of the disease)

- *Acute fluid collections.* These occur early in the disease and are located near the pancreas. The fluid collects in anatomical spaces such as the lesser sac. They usually resolve with regression of the disease.
- *Pancreatic necrosis.* This may be diffuse or focal and is typically associated with peripancreatic fat necrosis. In its most severe form it may result in no viable pancreatic tissue being present and thus lead to exocrine and endocrine pancreatic secretion insufficiency. It may become infected and is then known as infected pancreatic necrosis. This condition has a high mortality.
- *Acute pseudocyst.* This is a collection of pancreatic fluid enclosed by a wall of fibrous or granulation tissue that arises as a consequence of acute pancreatitis. The fluid usually accumulates in the lesser sac of the abdomen and is called a 'pseudo' as opposed to a 'true' cyst because it is not lined by epithelial cells. The pseudocyst clinically presents with pain and a palpable abdominal mass. If large enough, it may produce gastric outlet obstruction by compressing the duodenum, or jaundice by compressing the bile duct.
- Pancreatic abscess. This is a circumscribed intra-abdominal collection of pus, usually in proximity to the pancreas. It is distinct from infected pancreatic necrosis and usually has a better outcome following treatment. Patients present with features of abdominal infection (i.e. fever, abdominal tenderness, an abdominal mass).

Systemic

- The generalised complications of acute pancreatitis are those of shock and organ failure. Severe pancreatitis may be associated with adult respiratory distress syndrome and lead to either cardiac or pulmonary failure. Furthermore, acute tubular necrosis may occur in the kidneys and result in renal failure. These systemic complications may lead to multisystem organ failure (see Chapter 6).

Clinical presentation

Acute pancreatitis is characterised by an acute episode of epigastric to central abdominal pain, usually of rapid onset. The pain often radiates into the middle of the back. In some instances the patient may complain of vomiting; however, this is not a constant feature. There may be a history of significant alcohol consumption (>40 g/day) or the presence of gallstones.

Examination reveals a person in distress from the pain and varying signs of shock, dependent on the severity of the attack. Vital signs may range from totally normal to severe hypotension, tachycardia and tachypnoea. Abdominal examination will reveal tenderness in the epigastrium, and, depending on severity, there may be signs of peritonism. A tender mass may be palpable and abdominal distension evident due to a developing ileus. In severe cases, flank ecchymosis (Grey–Turner sign) or periumbilical ecchymosis (Cullen's sign) may be seen.

Investigation

The diagnosis of acute pancreatitis is made on the clinical features and demonstration of an abnormally elevated serum amylase. Amylase is one of the major enzymes of the pancreas. It is also present in salivary glands but has a different molecular size. Damage to the pancreas is associated with a release of amylase into the bloodstream, demonstrating a rapid rise in the serum level. The amylase is then rapidly cleared from the serum; therefore, the peak is only short-lived (i.e. 24 hours). For this reason, the rise in the amylase level does not correlate with the severity of pancreatitis because there is no way of predicting the timing of the sample to coincide with the peak amylase level.

Other enzymes have also been used for the diagnosis of pancreatitis, including serum lipase and serum trypsinogen levels. These investigations are more difficult to perform and, therefore, in most institutions, reliance is placed on serum amylase estimation. As all of these enzymes are cleared from the serum by the kidneys and excreted in urine, estimation of urinary enzyme levels (i.e. urinary amylase or lipase) can be used to assist in the diagnosis in patients where there may be some doubt. The peak rise for the urinary levels occurs 24–48 hours later than the serum peaks and hence allows for subsequent estimation.

The severity of pancreatitis is estimated by determining systemic criteria, which have been shown by carefully conducted studies to relate to outcome. The more of these positive systemic criteria, the greater is the severity of illness. These objective criteria are named after their originators and are known as Ranson or Imrie (Glasgow) scores. In addition, a more general

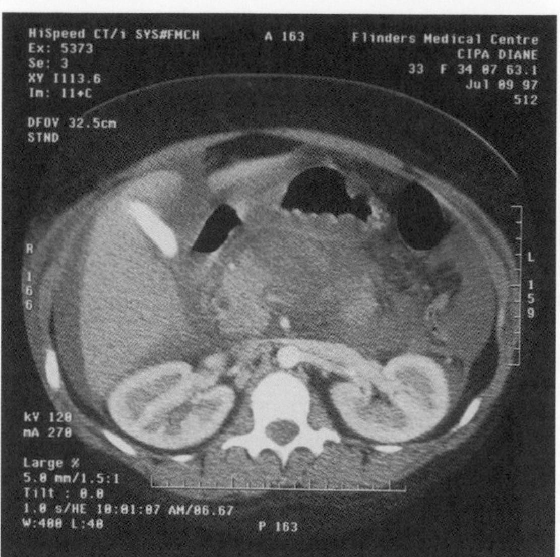

Fig. 17.2 A contrast-enhanced CT scan in a patient with severe acute pancreatitis. It demonstrates an area of hypoperfusion that reflects necrosis of the pancreas.

score, which is also used for other severely debilitating conditions, is the APACHE II score, which may be used. If three or more of the Ranson/Imrie criteria or eight or more of the APACHE II criteria are abnormal, then pancreatitis is defined as severe. Criteria that are measured include systolic blood pressure, $Pa\text{O}_2$, creatinine, blood sugar level, urea, albumin, calcium, white cell count and level of liver transaminases. A positive score for each is registered when an abnormal value is detected within the initial 48 hours of the disease.

Structural changes of the pancreas may be demonstrated using computed tomography (CT), and when this is combined with contrast to perform a contrast-enhanced CT scan, areas of necrosis can be visualised, thus determining the degree of local complications.The optimal time for the CT is approximately 5 days after the onset of the disease (Fig. 17.2.). CT scan is also used to determine the presence or absence of fluid collections and pseudocysts. Ultrasound is used to determine any evidence of gallstones in the gall bladder.

Treatment

The treatment of a patient with acute pancreatitis is directed four ways: general, local, complications and cause.

General

Depending on the severity of the fluid loss, patients with acute pancreatitis are treated for their fluid loss and given appropriate cardiovascular support. In the most common situation of mild pancreatitis, this consists of intravenous fluid replacement via a peripheral intravenous line. However, in severe pancreatitis, careful fluid replacement with central venous pressure measurements may be necessary. Oxygen is given via nasal mask or speculum as hypoxia is a common association of acute pancreatitis. In addition effective pain control needs to be ensured, and usually this means administration of parenteral opiate analgesics such as morphine.

Local

There is no specific treatment for the pancreatic inflammation. Therefore, treatment is directed at minimising the progression of the disease and preventing complications. Initially, the patient is fasted; however, enteral feeding has been shown to minimise the fasting-associated breakdown of the gut mucosal barrier and hence prevent bacterial translocation. Furthermore, enteral nutrients have been shown to decrease the incidence of pancreatic abscess formation in patients with severe pancreatitis. Consequently once it has been determined that the pancreatitis is severe nasoenteric feeding is commenced. In some instances it may not be possible to deliver the total nutritional needs of the patient via the enteral route, because the ileus, which accompanies the inflation, limits the volume of the feed. In such circumstances parenteral nutrition is added to supplement the patient's needs.

Early studies in the management of acute pancreatitis have not shown a role for antibiotics. However, recent studies that have used antibiotics whose effects are concentrated in the pancreatic parenchyma (imipenen) have shown a decrease in complications. Consequently, prophylactic antibiotics that are taken up by the pancreatic parenchyma are used in patients demonstrating evidence of pancreatic necrosis on CT scan. Antibiotics are also used if there is clear evidence of infection.

Complications

Complications are treated as they arise and often require surgery via an endoscopic, percutaneous or open approach. Surgical intervention in pancreatitis is reserved for the treatment of complications and in gallstone pancreatitis for the treatment of the cause.

In severe pancreatitis with infected necrosis, there is a need for operation to debride the pancreas of infected necrosed tissue. Infection may be diagnosed from either the presence of gas in the necrosed tissue as demonstrated by CT or the presence of organisms in tissue that has been aspirated from the pancreas following a percutaneous radiologically guided needle approach. Pancreatic abscesses may be drained via percutaneous techniques but usually require open surgical drainage. Pseudocysts are treated either by a combination of percutaneous and endoscopic techniques, or by open surgery.

In severe acute pancreatitis of a biliary cause (i.e. gallstones), acute intervention by endoscopic retrograde cholangiopancreatography (ERCP) often demonstrates the cause (i.e. a stone), and treatment by endoscopic sphincterotomy results in a greatly improved outcome for these patients when compared to either a more conservative approach or intervention by open surgery.

Cause

In one third of patients with acute pancreatitis, the cause is gallstones that pass from the gall bladder into the duodenum. Following recovery from an acute attack of pancreatitis, the patients are treated by cholecystectomy, which in the majority is done via a laparoscopic approach. No further episodes of pancreatitis occur after cholecystectomy.

In patients with the rare cause of sphincter of Oddi dysfunction, division of the sphincter of Oddi is also associated with cure. In patients where the cause is alcohol consumption, abstinence is accompanied with a decreased frequency and ultimately cure of pancreatitis. However, in many instances alcohol addiction is a major problem and patients require much community and social support before abstention is achieved.

Thus acute pancreatitis is a debilitating acute abdominal disorder that, in the majority of patients, has a benign outcome when appropriately diagnosed and treated. In a small number of patients the disease may be severe and may be associated with complications that ultimately may lead to the patient's death. The progression of the disease is unpredictable, hence all patients given the diagnosis of acute pancreatitis should be observed carefully in the initial period and a severity score determined. Once the severity of the disease is defined, appropriate treatment can be given.

Chronic pancreatitis

Chronic pancreatitis is a fibrotic disease of the pancreas that is characterised by recurrent episodes of abdominal pain, and gastrointestinal symptoms and signs of malabsorption. In some patients, involvement of the islet cells also results in diabetes.

Aetiology and pathogenesis

The most common cause of chronic pancreatitis in Australia and other developed countries is chronic alcohol abuse. Less commonly, three other forms of chronic pancreatitis may be seen: hereditary, nutritional and distal pancreatitis.

Hereditary pancreatitis is a disease of recurrent inflammation of the pancreas that leads to chronic pancreatitis. The disease occurs in blood relatives across at least two generations. It is an autosomal dominant condition with variable expression and the first attack of pancreatitis usually occurs in childhood. Nutritional pancreatitis is also known as tropical pancreatitis and fibrocalcific pancreatic diabetes. It is a non-alcoholic form of calcific pancreatitis and occurs in young adults in low-income populations of developing nations. Recurrent attacks begin in early childhood. Distal pancreatitis occurs following trauma to the pancreas (e.g. after a motor vehicle accident).

The pathogenesis of chronic pancreatitis is probably different for each form of the disease, and an underlying theory does not exist. A number of mechanisms have been proposed in the pathogenesis. Hypersecretion of pancreatic enzymes is thought to be one cause. These enzymes precipitate in the ducts, forming plugs that may calcify and cause obstruction. An alternative suggestion is that the plugs form as a result of high concentrations of intraductal mucoproteins, or clusters of desquamated epithelial cells associated with a high viscosity of pancreatic juice. A direct toxic effect of alcohol on pancreatic lipids has also been proposed as a pathogenic mechanism. Following destruction of lipid-containing membranes of the cells there is cell necrosis, which over the years leads to chronic pancreatitis.

Surgical pathology and complications

The pancreas of a patient with chronic pancreatitis is typically fibrosed and reduced in size (atrophied). There is extensive calcification throughout the parenchyma. Initially, the pancreatic islet cells are preserved; however, with progressive atrophy, these may also become involved in the process and atrophy. The pancreatic ducts develop multiple strictures and demonstrate post-stenotic dilatation. Calcified calculi may be found within the ducts.

Complications of chronic pancreatitis include the formation of a pseudocyst when an acute episode is superimposed on the chronic disease. In view of the atrophy, malabsorption and diabetes may result.

Clinical presentation

Patients with chronic pancreatitis present with recurrent episodes of epigastric abdominal pain that radiates into the back. These episodes of pain occur over a prolonged period and, in alcohol-related pancreatitis, initially occur after bouts of heavy drinking. However, as the disease progresses, episodes of pain also occur independently of alcohol consumption. In due course, the pain may be constant, with more severe attacks occurring intermittently. The pain at its worst is very debilitating because the patient often cannot find a position of comfort and needs high doses of parenteral analgesia for relief. The disease may be associated with varying degrees of malabsorption characterised by steatorrhoea and weight loss. In addition, symptoms and signs of diabetes may develop.

Investigation

The diagnosis is made on the characteristic presentation plus confirmatory radiological investigations. Serological tests, in particular serum amylase, may be entirely normal in chronic pancreatitis. A plain abdominal X-ray may reveal calcification in the region of the pancreas. This may be confirmed by CT scanning, which may also show direct dilatation and atrophy of the pancreas. The most specific investigation is an ERCP. In patients with moderate to severe pancreatitis, changes will be demonstrated in the pancreatic duct. These changes include stricture formation and duct dilatation. Pancreatic calculi may also be demonstrated.

The only useful test of pancreatic function is the measurement of faecal fat content to determine whether the patient has significant steatorrhoea. This is usually done by collecting faeces for 3 days and measuring the fat content of the faeces in the laboratory. An abnormal amount of faecal fat supports the diagnosis of malabsorption. A number of other tests of pancreatic enzyme function have been developed, but all are invasive and require prolonged study, thus making their indication of low value.

Treatment

Chronic pancreatitis is one of the most difficult abdominal conditions to treat as there is no specific treatment for the ongoing chronic inflammatory disease and treatment is largely aimed at the symptoms and complications.

For alcoholic patients, it is crucial that they abstain from alcohol consumption; otherwise no other form of treatment will be effective. It is important to realise that in alcoholic patients, the epigastric pain experienced after heavy drinking may not be solely due to pancreatitis and may be caused by alcoholic gastritis. Therefore, antacid therapy and treatment with gastric acid suppressing medication is important.

The role of surgery in the treatment of chronic pancreatitis is limited and confined to those patients in whom it can be demonstrated that the cause is non-alcoholic or who have abstained from alcohol.

Because pain is the major symptom of chronic pancreatitis, measures that aim to alleviate this are usually taken. Administration of oral pancreatic enzyme replacement medication reduces the hormone drive on the pancreas and may assist in the control of pain, in addition to appropriate oral analgesics. The pancreatic enzyme replacement therapy will also treat the steatorrhoea and assist with the treatment of malabsorption.

Operative management

Surgery in chronic pancreatitis is usually aimed at relieving an obstruction to pancreatic secretion, by either removing stones and debris from the duct or bypassing a stricture. In patients with a dominant pancreatic duct stricture and a dilated duct, a bypass operation between the duct and small bowel (Puestow procedure) is often effective in relieving symptoms and improving malabsorption. Unfortunately, in many patients single strictures are uncommon and what is more likely are multiple strictures throughout the gland, making bypass surgery inappropriate.

Placement of a plastic stent in a pancreatic duct with multiple strictures has been associated with relief in some patients and this technique may be appropriate for a group of patients with chronic pancreatitis.

For some patients the extent of the disease is such that only removal of a large part of the pancreas can alleviate the symptoms. This may require either a Whipple, pancreatoduodenectomy resection or a newer operation that removes the head of the pancreas whilst preserving the duodenum (Beger operation).

Chronic pancreatitis in Western countries is mainly a self-inflicted disease with disastrous results for the patient because it is difficult to treat specifically. In patients who abstain from alcohol the symptoms of pain may be relieved by surgical bypass or stenting of the duct or by resection of the part of the pancreas in which the disease predominates.

Pancreatic cancer

Introduction

Among all of the cancers, pancreatic cancer has one of the worst reputations and, despite improvements in both diagnostic and surgical techniques, survival has not significantly improved during the past 50 years. Furthermore, unlike most other cancers, its incidence appears to be increasing and, in certain parts of the world, including Australia, it has an incidence approaching 100 per million of population per year.

The incidence of pancreatic cancer is greater in males compared with that in females, and in general is a disease of people in their seventh decade and older. The poor outcomes may relate to the fact that it often presents late and after there has been spread of the disease beyond the pancreas.

Aetiology and pathogenesis

The cause of cancer of the pancreas is unknown. The only environmental factor associated with cancer of the pancreas has been cigarette smoking. There have not been any dietary factors conclusively associated with the development of pancreatic malignancy. A recent multicentre study has demonstrated that patients with chronic pancreatitis, which primarily has an alcohol aetiology, have an increased risk of developing cancer (the rate being 4%).

As in many other malignancies, alterations in cell genes are thought to be the basis of cancer development in the pancreas. Alterations have been demonstrated in the *ras* oncogene family and the *p53* tumour suppressor gene. However, their significance in either the aetiology or development of pancreatic cancer is not known.

Growth factors and their receptors have been demonstrated to be important in the biological behaviour of pancreatic cancer. A number of tissue growth factors have been associated with the growth of the cancers, including epidermal growth factor (EGF) and tumour growth factor-alpha (TGF-α). In addition, a number of gastrointestinal and other hormones have been associated with tumour growth. These include cholecystokinin, secretin, oestradiol, progesterone and testosterone. The significance of these growth factors and hormones in the development of pancreatic cancer is also not known. However, an understanding of the molecular basis of these tumours may provide new markers for diagnosis, for prognosis and ultimately for therapy.

Surgical pathology and complications

Cancers of the pancreas are subdivided into different types, depending on their site and histological type. While the majority of pancreatic cancers are adenocarcinomas of the main pancreatic gland, it is important to identify the rarer cancers because these have a much better prognosis after successful excision.

Adenocarcinoma

Adenocarcinoma cancers originate from the ductular lining and usually occur in the head of the pancreas. Less commonly they may arise in the body or tail of the gland. Owing to the extensive vascularity of the pancreas, metastatic spread occurs early in the evolution of the disease. Metastases initially spread to the draining lymph nodes in the region of the coeliac axis and may involve the sensory nerves in this area. Cancer metastases also preferentially involve the liver and, in more advanced cases, there may be spread throughout the peritoneal cavity.

Ampullary cancers

Ampullary cancers are adenocarcinomas that originate in the region of the ampulla of Vater, which is made up of the intraduodenal components of the bile duct and pancreatic duct as well as their common channel. These tumours have a lower malignant propensity when compared to cancers of the head and body of the pancreas and thus have a much better prognosis following surgical excision. However, this may reflect the fact that due to their position diagnosis is made early in the evolution of the disease. Ampullary cancers are not a common malignancy; however, when they do occur it is important that diagnosis be made early because surgical resection can be curative.

Cystic tumours

Cystic tumours are quite rare lesions of the pancreas, representing 1% of malignant neoplasms of the pancreas. Histologically, they range from benign tumours of adenomatous appearance to cystadenocarcinomas. The tumours may have either mucous or serous fluid-containing cysts; the former having a greater malignant propensity. Recognition and differentiation from benign cysts is important because surgical excision is associated with cure.

Clinical presentation

The typical presentation of a patient with adenocarcinoma of either the ampulla or the pancreas is a person with 'painless jaundice'. There may also have been a period of anorexia with associated weight loss. The patient may report pale-coloured stools, occasionally said to have silver streaks on their surface. In addition, the urine is dark and the skin yellow. On examination, an abdominal mass may be detected; however, more commonly the tumour will not be palpable. A distended gall bladder may be palpated under the right costal margin and this sign in a patient with painless obstructive jaundice is strongly suggestive of a malignant pancreatic cause (Courvoisier's Law).

In patients in whom the bile duct is not involved early in the disease, presentation may be due to early spread of the tumour and resulting pain in the epigastrium or mid-back. Pain is a poor prognostic factor in a patient with pancreatic cancer because it invariably signals spread of the disease.

Investigation

Patients with pancreatic malignancy usually present with symptoms and signs of obstructive jaundice.

Therefore, investigations are directed at the differential diagnosis of this condition. Ultrasound examination will demonstrate a dilated extrahepatic biliary system, often with dilated intrahepatic ducts and a distended gall bladder. Depending on its size, a mass may be seen in the head of the pancreas. With ampullary tumours a mass will not be detected but the pancreatic duct may be seen to be dilated.

The most precise investigation, providing the most information, is endoscopic retrograde cholangiopancreatography (ERCP). This endoscopic procedure allows for direct visualisation of the ampulla, and after cannulation of the bile and pancreatic ducts, contrast may be injected into the ducts and X-rays taken to visualise any signs of obstruction. Cancer of the head of the pancreas shows a characteristic narrowing of both ducts on ERCP (the double duct sign).

Biopsy of any visualised abnormality, or cytology from the strictured areas, can provide histological confirmation of the diagnosis. Computed tomography (CT) scanning may demonstrate a mass in the pancreas, but often small masses may not readily be seen. For larger masses and when histological confirmation is needed prior to treatment, a percutaneous biopsy may be done under either CT scan or ultrasound guidance.

Serum tumour markers have been used for the diagnosis of various abdominal neoplasms. The tumour-associated antigen CA19-9 has been extensively investigated to assess its role in the diagnosis of pancreatic cancer. This antigen is certainly detected in the serum of patients with pancreatic cancer, and there appears to be a direct correlation between tumour size and level of CA19-9. However, its specificity is low as is its sensitivity for small tumours. Its main value currently is in the follow-up of patients with high values to assess response to treatment.

Treatment

The only form of therapy that potentially may cure patients with cancer of the pancreas is surgical resection. For surgery to be effective early diagnosis is essential in order to detect lesions of relatively small size. Put another way, the best surgical results are achieved in patients with small tumours. In general, a diameter of 3 cm or less will be resectable and potentially give the best outcome. Due to their position, ampullary cancers tend to present earlier than cancers of the rest of the pancreas and, consequently, have the best outcome following surgery. In addition, surgical removal of cystic tumours is associated with an excellent outcome. Cancers of the body of the pancreas tend to present late and, in general, are not resectable. Similarly, most cancers of the head of the pancreas are not resectable for cure. Occasionally, however, they may become symptomatic early and can be resected with good results.

Thus, despite the generally gloomy picture regarding the curative treatment of these cancers, it should be remembered that for certain tumours curative resection is possible and all attempts should be made to identify these patients and not place all patients in the incurable category.

For the majority of patients with cancer of the pancreas, treatment is directed at palliation. The most common presentation is that of obstructive jaundice, which is associated with anorexia and pruritus. Treatment that aims to relieve the obstruction relieves the pruritus and also improves the patient's well-being. The life expectancy of a patient with an inoperable cancer of the pancreas is approximately 10 months. Therefore, the aim of palliation is to do the least invasive procedure that will achieve drainage of the bile duct and relieve the obstructive jaundice.

In the majority of patients excellent palliation is achieved by inserting an endoprosthesis (stent) through the obstruction using an endoscopic approach. The stent drains bile from the proximal bile duct into the duodenum and the jaundice is relieved. If the endoscopic approach is not successful a percutaneous route through the liver may be used to place the stent. However, in general, the morbidity and results of this approach are not as good as the endoscopic route. The advantage of the endoscopic and percutaneous treatment is the fact that it avoids the need for laparotomy, and the patient's recovery is therefore rapid. It should be emphasised that this procedure should only be used in patients in whom pre-operative investigations have determined that the tumour is inoperable.

Surgical bypass of the tumour to drain the biliary tract and relieve the jaundice is done in patients who have undergone laparotomy to assess resectability but in whom curative resection was not possible. Patients with inoperable cancers often inquire about the use of chemotherapy and radiotherapy, but these treatments have not been shown to be effective in the treatment of pancreatic cancer. It should be remembered that unless it can be shown that these forms of treatment can prolong survival they should not be used because there are significant side effects.

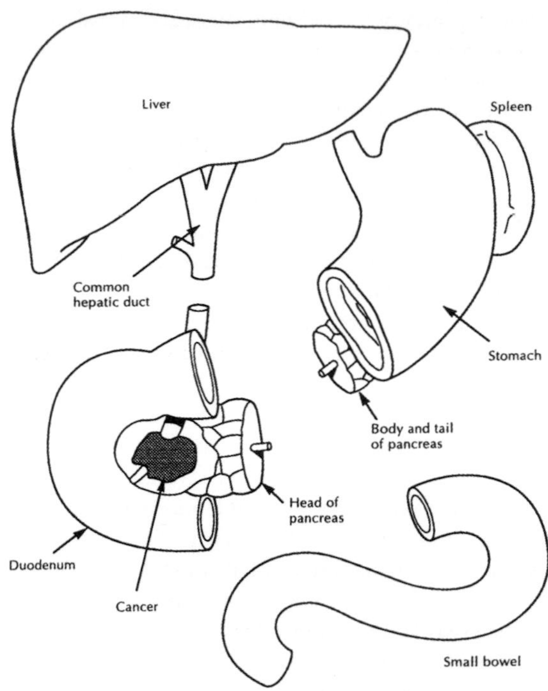

Fig. 17.3 Pancreaticoduodenectomy, which consists of partial gastrectomy, partial pancreatectomy, and excision of the distal bile duct and all of the duodenum.

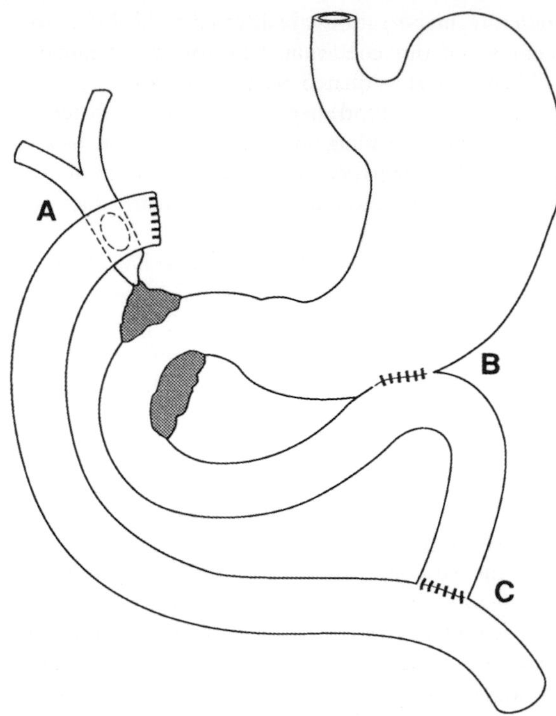

Fig. 17.4 Palliative bypass of the bile duct and stomach in a patient with a non-resectable pancreatic cancer.
(A) Choledochojejunostomy, (B) gastroenterostomy, (C) entero-enterosotomy.

Most patients with pancreatic cancer will develop pain, especially in the terminal stages of the disease. Modern analgesics and techniques that aim to inhibit sensory transmission are effective in controlling this debilitating symptom, and patients should be informed of their availability in order to avoid unnecessary suffering.

Operative management

The operation done for cure of ampullary or head of pancreas cancers is a pancreaticoduodenectomy (Whipple procedure; Fig. 17.3). In this operation the head of the pancreas and adjacent duodenum plus lower bile duct and half the stomach are removed. This extensive surgical resection ensures that not only is the tumour removed but also the adjacent lymph nodes. The pancreas, bile duct and stomach are re-anastomosed and thus continuity is re-established. This operation had a bad reputation in the past; however, with modern surgical techniques the operative mortality and morbidity is low and is now advised for patients with operable tumours.

Palliative bypass operation (Fig. 17.4) consists of an anastomosis between the dilated bile duct and a segment of the small intestine. Occasionally, the gallbladder may be used for the bypass instead of the bile duct. In addition, a prophylactic bypass of the duodenum may be done via a gastroenterostomy in order to prevent the vomiting that may occur in approximately 30% of patients due to duodenal obstruction in the terminal stage of the disease.

Prognosis

The overall survival of patients with pancreatic cancer is poor, with less than 5% survival at 5 years from diagnosis. However, in patients having successful curative resection, survival is greater than 30% at 5 years, and for patients with ampullary tumours it is greater than 50%. Patients with cystadenomas have the best results, with cure reported in the majority of patients.

Pancreatic cancer is one of the worst malignancies in terms of outcome following diagnosis and treatment. Undoubtedly, early diagnosis when the tumour is differentiated and of a smaller size is associated with a better outcome. Surgical excision remains the best available therapy and only chance for cure.

MCQs

Select the single correct answer to each question.

1 The following are causes of pancreatitis:
a gallstones
b alcohol
c mumps
d ampulla of Vater tumours
e all of the above

2 The pancreas is protected from autodigestion by:
a only secreting enzymes following stimulation by a meal
b secreting enzymes in an inactivated form
c secreting activated enzymes into the pancreatic duct
d packaging the activated enzymes in zymogen granules
e all of the above

3 Severity of acute pancreatitis is determined by:
a concentration of serum amylase
b amount of urinary amylase secreted over 24 hours
c clinical scoring systems (Ranson/Imrie)
d amount of peripancreatic fluid collection as determined by CT scan
e all of the above

4 The only feature regarding antibiotic use in acute pancreatitis which is not of importance is:
a antibiotic uptake by pancreatic necrotic tissue
b therapeutic level in serum
c effective against *Staphylococcus aureus*
d broad-spectrum cover, including anaerobes
e none of the above

5 Patients who suffer from chronic pancreatitis are totally cured of their disease by:
a surgical removal of the pancreas
b endoscopic drainage of the pancreatic duct via a stent
c total abstinence from alcohol
d all of the above
e none of the above

6 Which of the following is an incorrect statement about pancreatic carcinoma:
a most pancreatic cancers are incurable
b palliation can be achieved with a biliary stent
c palliation can be achieved by surgical bypass of the tumour
d ampullary cancer has a worse prognosis than carcinoma of the body of the pancreas
e survival rate of 5% at 5 years from diagnosis can be expected

7 Which of the following investigations has little value in determining the curability of pancreatic carcinoma:
a Ultrasound
b ERCP
c CT scanning
d Serum markers
e Pancreatic biopsy

18 Portal hypertension

C. Christophi and V. Muralidharan

Introduction

The term *portal hypertension* was first mentioned in 1906 by Gilbert and Vilaret, when the association between cirrhosis, ascites and gastrointestinal haemorrhage was described. The normal pressure of the portal venous system is 5–10 mm Hg and maintains the liver blood flow at approximately 1 L/min. Portal hypertension is defined as portal venous pressures greater than 10 mm Hg.

Anatomy

The portal venous circulation is one of three venous systems in the human which is formed and terminates in a capillary system. It provides approximately 60% to 80% of total hepatic blood flow. The portal vein is formed by the confluence of the splenic and superior mesenteric vein behind the neck of the pancreas. The superior mesenteric vein is formed by venous tributaries from the jejunum, ileum and colon, the predominant being middle, right and iliocolic veins. The left gastric vein (coronary vein) and the right gastric vein drain into the main portal vein close to its origin while the right gastroepiploic vein drains into the superior mesenteric vein near its termination. The left gastroepiploic and inferior mesenteric veins enter the portal system in the vicinity of the splenic and portal vein junction. There are no valves in the portal venous system. This allows an increase in portal venous pressure to be equally distributed across the entire system, including potential collateral sites.

Aetiology

Portal hypertension may be caused by increased blood flow into the portal venous system or by portal venous outflow obstruction.

Increased portal blood flow is an uncommon cause of portal hypertension. This is usually caused by arteriovenous fistulas, which may occur secondary to trauma, arteriovenous malformations or tumours. Massive splenomegaly secondary to myeloproliferative disorders is a rare cause of portal hypertension where the hyperdynamic splenic blood flow results in increased portal venous pressure.

Obstruction to the portal circulation is by far the most common cause of portal hypertension. It is further classified on the basis of the anatomical site of obstruction as pre-sinusoidal, sinusoidal or post-sinusoidal portal hypertension

Pre-sinusoidal obstruction accounts for 10–15% of cases of portal hypertension and may occur in the intra- or extra-hepatic parts of the portal system. These include splenic and portal vein thrombosis. Rarely, congenital absence or abnormality of the portal vein may also be a cause. Portal vein thrombosis in the child is predominantly related to umbilical sepsis. In the adult, hypercoagulable states such as polcythaemia rubra vera or myeloproliferative disorders are the major causes of portal vein thrombosis. Isolated splenic vein thrombosis may occur secondary to tumours of the pancreas or pancreatitis. Intrahepatic causes of pre-sinusoidal portal hypertension include schistosomiasis, congenital hepatic fibrosis and other rarer causes such as primary portal hypertension and infiltration by sarcoidosis and reticulosis.

Post-sinusoidal obstruction accounts for approximately 2–5% of patients with portal hypertension and is mainly caused by veno-occlusive disease or Budd–Chiari Syndrome. Veno-occlusive disease occurs in the sublobular branches of the hepatic veins. Factors causing this condition include antineoplastic drugs and irradiation. Other causes of post-sinusoidal obstruction are Budd–Chiari Syndrome and constrictive pericarditis. The Budd–Chiari syndrome may be caused by hepatic vein stenosis and membranous webs of the hepatic veins. The most common cause of this syndrome is thrombosis caused by hypercoagulable states or myeloproliferative conditions

Sinusoidal obstruction is predominantly caused by cirrhosis and accounts for the majority of cases of portal hypertension. Alcohol ingestion and viral infection (Hepatitis B and C) are the major causes of cirrhosis. Other causes include primary biliary cirrhosis, schlerosing cholangitis, autoimmune disorders, Wilson's disease and other enzyme deficiencies. The major implication in this group of patients with portal hypertension is the underlying presence of hepatocellular damage. This has both prognostic and management implications.

Pathophysiology

The main consequence of raised portal venous pressure (>10 mm Hg and usually >20 mm Hg) is the development of collaterals with the systemic circulation at multiple sites. The most common sites include the oesophagogastric junction (oesophageal varices), peri-umbilical area (caput medusae), superior haemorrhoidal veins (haemorrhoids) and retroperitoneal collaterals. These anastomotic channels progressively become engorged, leading to increased blood flow and gradual dilatation. The major sequelae of portal hypertension are gastrointestinal haemorrhage, the development of ascites, chronic porta-systemic encephalopathy and hypersplenism secondary to splenomegaly.

Oesophageal varices

Fine anastomoses develop between the systemic and portal circulation in the submucous plexus of the oesophagus and stomach. Eventually the submucosa disappears and the wall of the veins becomes the lining of the oesophagus. Rupture of these vessels cause significant bleeding. The two most important factors contributing to bleeding varices are the underlying increase in portal venous pressure and ulceration secondary to oesophagitis. Patients with cirrhosis have a higher incidence of variceal bleeding in contrast to other noncirrhotic causes of portal hypertension. The incidence of varices is also related to the severity of the underlying liver disease. Bleeding from ruptured oesophagogastric varices is the most severe complication of cirrhosis and is the cause of death in about one third of these patients.

Ascites

A reduction in the colloidal osmotic pressure related to hypoalbuminaemia, sodium and water retention caused by abnormal hormonal and circulating vasoactive agents and vasodilation of the splanchnic circulation ultimately lead to the formation of ascites. The development and severity is often aggravated by surgery, systemic infection, gastrointestinal bleeding and hepatic decompensation. Spontaneous bacterial peritonitis may complicate pre-existing ascites.

Hypersplenism

This frequently accompanies portal hypertension. It is characterised by anaemia, thrombocytopenia and leukopenia.

Encephalopathy

Neuropsychiatric symptoms commonly develop in patients with portal hypertension and underlying hepatocellular dysfunction. Encephalopathy is related to impaired ammonia metabolism caused by extensive collaterals which bypass the liver and by the underlying hepatocellular dysfunction. The early stages are characterised by mental confusion and delirium, followed by stupor and coma. It is a prominent feature in patients with bleeding varices, as this leads to increased production of nitrogen compounds within the gastrointestinal tract.

Classification of the severity of the underlying liver disease in a patient with portal hypertension is important from a prognostic and management point of view. The Child–Pugh classification (see Table 18.1) is the most commonly used grading to assess the severity of underlying liver disease.

Table 18.1 Child–Pugh classification of severity of liver disease

Points	1	2	3
Encephalopathy grade	None	1–2	3–4
Ascites	Absent	Slight	Moderate
Albumin (g/L)	>3.5	2.8–3.5	<2.8
Prothrombin time (sec)	<4	4–6	>6
Bilirubin level (mg/dL) (In cholestatic disease)	<2(<4)	2–3(4–10)	>3(>10)

Clinical features

The major clinical differentiation in patients with portal hypertension is the presence of underlying chronic hepatocellular liver disease and the detection of complications.

History

A history of liver disease, cirrhosis and gastrointestinal bleeding should be specifically requested. Detailed information relating to the aetiology of the liver disease should be sought. This should include the duration and extent of alcohol intake, previous episodes of jaundice and hepatitis, previous blood transfusions and any risky behaviour for the transmission of blood-borne diseases. A family history of liver disease may provide clues to genetic causes of liver disease. Routine medications which the patient may be on, especially oral contraceptives, and particularly of recent onset, should be listed.

Previous upper or lower gastrointestinal bleeding should be documented, including frequency and severity of episodes. Any associated symptoms of ascites or encephalopathy should be noted as well as a history of umbilical sepsis, pancreatitis or coexistent malignancy.

Examination

This should aim to elucidate features of the underlying chronic liver disease, signs specific to the aetiology of the disease and the presence of portal hypertension. Apart from the common signs of chronic liver disease such as gynaecomastia, testicular atrophy spider naevi, the presence of bilateral parotid enlargement, Dupytren's contractures and Keiser–Fleischer rings may provide a clue to the aetiology of the disease. Splenomegaly, ascites, caput medusae and abdominal wall collaterals are specifically indicative of portal hypertension. A venous hum may be present in the peri-umbilical area.

Investigations

The presence of chronic liver disease and clinical evidence of portal hypertension should lead to investigations tailored to the identification of the underlying disease, the severity of the disease and identification of potential complications.

Blood tests

Full blood examination

A low haemoglobin or decreased hematocrit may indicate either continued bleeding or anaemia of chronic liver disease. Thrombocytopenia or low white cell count may indicate hypersplenism. A coagulation profile is essential for the management and for prognostic contribution to the Child–Pugh system. An elevated prothrombin time or International Normalised Ratio (INR) is a strong indicator of synthetic dysfunction and indicates severe hepatocellular disease. Plasma fibrinogen may also be a useful indicator to the risk of bleeding.

Renal function tests

Electrolyte imbalance, especially low sodium levels, may occur in patients with chronic liver disease. The urea and creatinine levels may not only be an indicator of renal dysfunction but may also be a useful indirect guide to liver function.

Liver biochemistry

Serum bilirubin is important in assessing liver function as well as contributing to the Child-Pugh score. Albumin levels may indicate underlying synthetic function, the degree of malnutrition and also contribute to prognostic evaluation. Alkaline phosphatase and gamma gluteryl transferase reflect underlying cholestasis. Increased aspartate aminotransferase (AST) and alanine aminotransferase (ALT) are an indication of acute hepatocellular damage.

Serology

The main role of serology is in the diagnosis and assessment of viral hepatitis as the underlying cause. Viral antigen and antibody levels should be investigated as appropriate for Hepatitis A, B and C as well as cytomegalovirus (CMV) and human immunodeficiency virus. Quantitation of viral DNA and RNA levels by more sophisticated techniques allow assessment of viral load and replication. Antimitochondrial antibodies, antinuclear antibodies, alpha-1-antitrypsin levels and genetic testing for Wilson's disease may provide clues to the underlying aetiology of the liver disease.

Radiology

Abdominal ultrasound should always be performed as an initial screening test to assess liver parenchyma in terms of the degree of cirrhosis, possible space occupying lesions, enlarged lymph nodes or incidental gallstones. A Doppler ultrasound of the portal vein, splenic and superior mesenteric vein, hepatic artery and hepatic veins assesses patency, and the direction and volume of blood flow. Multiphasic CT l scans and MRI scans of the abdomen may also be required to delineate specific aspects of liver anatomy. MR angiography and CT angiography have evolved in sophistication to the point where percutaneous invasive angiography has been made redundant. Angiography and venography are used on specific occasions to define certain aspects of the portal circulation and hepatic venous anatomy especially prior to surgery or other interventional techniques.

Occluded hepatic vein wedge pressure is the most accurate indirect objective measurement of the portal venous pressure and is performed via percutaneous internal jugular vein catheterisation.

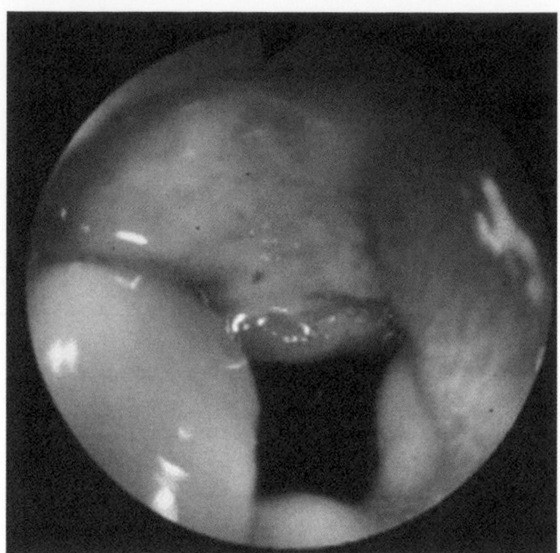

Fig. 18.1 Oesophageal varices with ulceration of the mucosa.

Endoscopy

An upper gastrointestinal endoscopy should always be performed in any patient with suspected portal hypertension, in order to define the extent, size and characteristics of oesophageal varices (see Fig. 18.1), as well as any evidence of gastric varices and portal hypertensive gastropathy. It also allows the prophylactic treatment of oesophageal varices, as well as excluding other causes of gastrointestinal haemorrhage such as malignancy and peptic ulcer disease.

Liver biopsy

This is performed if the nature and severity of the underlying liver disease is unknown. It may be performed percutaneously under ultrasound guidance or by the internal jugular vein to minimise complications of haemorrhage.

Management

The management of the patient with portal hypertension involves the assessment and treatment of any underlying liver disease as well as specific attention to the complications of bleeding, ascites and encephalopathy.

Bleeding varices

Acute variceal bleeding requires a multidisciplinary approach, including surgeons, gastroenterologists, radiologists and intensive care personnel. The management of variceal bleeding involves initial aggressive resuscitation, early diagnosis, measures to control the acute bleeding and strategies to prevent re-bleeding.

Resuscitation

The first priority in the management of patient with acute variceal bleeding is active resuscitation. Intravenous access, including multiple wide-bore peripheral venous cannulae and central venous access, should be established immediately. A Swan–Ganz catheter may be required in the severely comprised patient. A urinary catheter should be inserted to monitor urine output. Blood is withdrawn for grouping and cross-matching. Tests including full blood examination, liver and renal biochemistry and a coagulation profile are performed. Resuscitation usually requires the infusion of large volumes of blood and crystalloid. Most patients will require correction of coagulation defects using platelets, coagulation factors and vitamin K. The gastrointestinal tract should be cleared using cathartics such as lactulose. Non-absorbable antibiotics may be used to achieve selective gut sterilisation. Systemic antibiotics are administered as these patients are susceptible to infection. The aim of resuscitation is to achieve cardiovascular stability with a view to urgent endoscopy.

Diagnosis

An urgent endoscopy within 6 hours should be done to confirm the cause and site of bleeding. Repeat endoscopy may be required to achieve this.

Control of bleeding

The initial control of acute variceal bleeding can be achieved in 90–95% of patients by endoscopic sclerotherapy or banding. Endoscopic sclerotherapy involves the injection of one of several agents directly into the varix, leading to thrombosis and fibrosis. Banding of varices is achieved by applying a rubber band to strangulate the varix under endoscopy. It is superior to sclerotherapy in achieving haemostasis and has fewer side effects.

Balloon tamponade of the varices using a Sengstaken–Blakemore tube may be indicated on rare occasions when sclerotherapy and banding fail. This is required in less than 5% of patients and is usually used as a temporising measure to stabilise the patient prior to further attempts at banding or sclerotherapy. The tube is inserted endoscopically and has both gastric and oesophageal balloons, inflated to specific pressures for a limited period, since potentially lethal complications of asphyxia and oesophageal perforation may occur.

Apart from locally applied techniques, variceal bleeding may be decreased temporarily by lowering the underlying portal venous pressure using pharmacological agents, such as continuous infusions of octreotide (a synthetic analogue of somatostatin) or terlipressin, which lower portal pressure and are beneficial in preventing early recurrence of variceal bleeding.

Placing of transjugular intrahepatic portal systemic shunts (TIPS) may be performed under local anaesthetic via percutaneous access of the right internal jugular vein. An internal stent is placed through the liver parenchyma between the right or middle hepatic vein and a branch of the portal vein, creating in essence a side-to-side porta-systemic shunt. Major complications are rare but may include haemorrhage or the development of encephalopathy.

Surgical procedures

Surgical Procedures are now seldom required for variceal bleeding and are used only when other measures fail. These procedures include local devascularisation procedures and porta-systemic shunts. The local devascularisation procedures include components of splenectomy or splenic artery ligation, oesophageal transection and devascularisation of the oesophagus and stomach by ligation of appropriate vessels. There is a high incidence of re-bleeding with these procedures.

Porta-systemic shunts create an artificial or surgical communication between the portal and systemic venous systems and lower portal pressures. These procedures include portacaval and mesocaval shunts and more selective techniques such as the lieno-renal shunts. These shunts have a significant mortality and morbidity and may be complicated by ascites and encephalopathy.

Prevention of recurrent bleeding

Once the initial bleeding has ceased, measures are instigated to prevent recurrence. These include prophylactic banding or sclerotherapy and the use of pharmacological agents such as oral β-blockers. If patients re-bleed during the primary therapy TIPS may be also be used in the acute setting. Liver transplantation is the procedure of choice to prevent recurrent variceal bleeding in selected patients with cirrhosis, once control of the acute haemorrhage has been achieved. It not only lowers portal venous pressures, but also corrects the underlying liver disease.

Prophylactic therapy

Prophylactic therapy may be employed to reduce the incidence of bleeding in patients with oesophageal varices before the first episode of variceal haemorrhage. Measures used include routine surveillance gastroscopy, sclerotherapy, banding and the use of β-blockers. Even though the incidence of bleeding is reduced, the effect on overall mortality is not affected.

Ascites

The presence of ascites is a bad prognostic sign and usually indicates severe underlying liver disease. It results from a combination of portal hypertension, altered fluid and electrolyte imbalance and hypoalbuminaemia. Major complications of ascites include primary peritonitis and renal failure (hepatorenal syndrome).

Evaluation

Evaluation should include a detailed history and examination for the presence of ascites, portal hypertension and the severity of the underlying liver disease. Liver and renal biochemistry should be performed. An ascitic tap is undertaken and the ascitic fluid tested for bacteriology and albumin content.

Management

The management of ascites should initially include sodium and fluid restrictions and specific diuretics which block tubular reabsorption of sodium (spironolactone). If these measures are unsuccessful, large volume paracentesis and intravenous infusion of albumin should be considered. For a small percentage of patients with refractory ascites despite these measures, consideration should be given to performing TIPS.

Liver transplantation should be considered in patients with chronic liver disease and intractable ascites. Liver transplantation is also indicated in patients with encephalopathy and progressive liver disease.

Hepatic encephalopathy

This is a complex neuro-psychiatric syndrome with a wide spectrum of clinical manifestations. It may occur due to the loss of hepatocellular function or the formation of porta-systemic shunts which bypass the liver parenchyma. The underlying cause for the encephalopathy dictates the clinical outcomes.

Aetiology

The aetiology of porta-systemic encephalopathy is thought to be multifactorial. The most widely implicated substance is ammonia in the portal circulation. Other nitrogenous substances as well as amino acid imbalances and false neurotransmission have also been implicated. An increase in urea-splitting gut bacteria, gastrointestinal haemorrhage and protein-rich diet may all increase the ammonia content of the portal venous blood. Reduction in intestinal bacteria by oral antibiotics, prevention of gastrointestinal haemorrhage and strict dietary measures contribute to minimising their effects. In addition changes in cerebral neurotransmitters have also been identified, making the brain of the encephalopathic patient more sensitive to insults that would not affect normal individuals.

Assessment

Assessment should include detailed history and examination. Patients may often be unable to provide coherent history depending on the severity of encephalopathy. Clinical features include alterations in conscious state along with slurring of speech. More subtle changes may be seen in chronic porta-systemic encephalopathy. These include personality changes and intellectual deterioration. The most characteristic neurological abnormality is the 'flapping tremor' hat occurs with attempted dorsi-flexion of the wrist. The Reitan trail-making test, where the patient is required to connect numbers on a test page is a routinely used objective test of higher function.

Diagnosis

Definitive diagnosis of hepatic encephalopathy may be achieved by electroencephalogram supported by CT evidence of chronic cerebral atrophy. The latter also serves to exclude other causes of impaired consciousness, including intra-cranial haemorrhage and tumours.

Summary

The effective management of portal hypertension requires early diagnosis, surveillance, prevention and early diagnosis and, when necessary, rapid treatment of its complications. Concurrent identification of the underlying disease and early aggressive management are paramount to a successful outcome.

MCQs

Select the single correct answer to each question.

1 Regarding the portal circulation in the normal healthy adult, which one of the following is true?
- **a** normal portal venous pressure is between 20 and 30 mm Hg
- **b** the portal vein is formed by the confluence of the superior mesenteric vein and the splenic vein behind the neck of the pancreas
- **c** splenic vein thrombosis does not cause localised portal hypertension
- **d** portal venous flow provides approximately 30–40% of total liver blood flow
- **e** the portal venous system contains unidirectional valves at specific points

2 Which one of following physical signs is not usually found in a patient with portal hypertension?
- **a** caput medusae
- **b** hepatomegaly
- **c** ascites
- **d** splenomegaly
- **e** lower limb varicose veins

3 Regarding patients suffering from portal hypertension, which one of the following is true?
- **a** hepatocyte destruction caused by cirrhosis account for the majority of the causes of portal hypertension
- **b** the main diseases leading to cirrhosis in the Australian population are alcoholic liver disease and chronic viral hepatitis
- **c** encephalopathy is the most common cause of death in patients with portal hypertension
- **d** peritonitis complicating ascites in these patients is usually due to perforated duodenal ulcer
- **e** the commonest source of bleeding varices are the haemorrhoidal veins

4 Considering the management of patients with portal hypertension, which one of the following statements is true?
- **a** upper gastrointestinal endoscopy should not be performed unless there is evidence of variceal bleeding
- **b** liver biopsy is rarely required as a part of the diagnostic process in determining the underlying disease
- **c** intravenous infusion of drugs such as octreotide and terlipressin which reduce splanchnic blood flow play an important role in the prevention of early re-bleed of oesophageal varices
- **d** the mainstay of management of bleeding oesophageal varices is the insertion of a Sengstaken–Blakemore tube
- **e** surgical porto-caval shunts remain the definitive management of bleeding varices

5 Which of the following does not play an important role in the prevention of the first variceal bleed in patients with portal hypertension?
- **a** surveillance upper gastrointestinal endoscopy
- **b** prophylactic banding of visible varices
- **c** the use of β-blockers
- **d** prophylactic sclerotherapy
- **e** surgical porta-systemic shunt

Lower Gastrointestinal Surgery

19 Small bowel obstruction

Joe J. Tjandra

Introduction

Mechanical small bowel obstruction is one of the most common surgical emergencies. A traditional adage, 'let the sun never set or rise' on a bowel obstruction, indicating the need for immediate operative intervention, does not apply to all patients. However, it does highlight the importance of careful evaluation of patients with small bowel obstruction. Aggressive non-operative and operative management has reduced mortality from 50% to 5% over the past 50 years.

Aetiology

The causes of small bowel obstruction vary widely with geographic region and patient's age group. The most common cause in Western society is post-surgical adhesions, followed by external hernias (Box 19.1). The pathogenesis of adhesions is not well understood and, until recently, there was no clinically useful medication or manoeuvre that prevents formation of adhesions. Recently there has been interest in various bioresorbable membranes or gel (Seprafilm™ or Spraygel™) placed between the viscera and abdominal wall at the end of surgery which may help prevent adhesions.

Box 19.1 Causes of small bowel obstruction

- Adhesions
- Hernias: ventral, inguinal, femoral, internal
- Neoplasms: malignant (primary/metastatic), benign
- Strictures: Crohn's disease, ischaemia
- Radiation enteritis
- Intussusception
- Volvulus
- Gallstone ileus
- Bezoar
- Superior mesenteric artery syndrome

Pathophysiology

Small bowel obstruction leads to rapid accumulation of fluid and gas in the bowel proximal to the site of obstruction. In typical cases, there is initial active peristalsis proximal to the obstruction. Within a few hours, the peristaltic activity declines. Oedema and increasing distension supervene. Stasis and bacterial overgrowth make the fluid faeculent. Appearance of faeculent fluid with a foul odour in the vomitus or from a nasogastric tube confirms the diagnosis of obstruction.

Clinical features

Classic presentations of small bowel obstruction include:

- crampy abdominal pain
- nausea and vomiting
- abdominal distension
- constipation.

Patients with a proximal small bowel obstruction are likely to present early (within a day) with pain and vomiting; abdominal distension and constipation are less likely. Patients with a distal obstruction frequently have a more prolonged symptom complex with a 2–3-day history of crampy abdominal pain prior to vomiting; distension and constipation are predominant features. The bowel sounds are initially hyperactive and high-pitched. In delayed presentation, the bowel sounds may be reduced, indicating onset of secondary ileus.

The symptom complex also varies with the underlying aetiology. Small bowel obstruction due to hernia tends to present early and more acutely with a tense and irreducible external hernia, that associated with a neoplasm is more indolent and that due to adhesions intermediate in presentation.

Recognition of strangulated obstruction with bowel ischaemia and impending perforation is important. Clinical features of bowel ischaemia include constant and severe abdominal pain associated with tenderness and guarding, tachycardia, fever and leucocytosis.

Radiology

Supine and erect abdominal radiographs

Specific radiographic findings suggestive of small bowel obstruction include a dilated small bowel with air-fluid levels, often in a stepladder distribution on the erect film (Fig. 19.1). Presence of colonic gas may indicate an incomplete obstruction or the presence of an adynamic ileus rather than a complete mechanical obstruction.

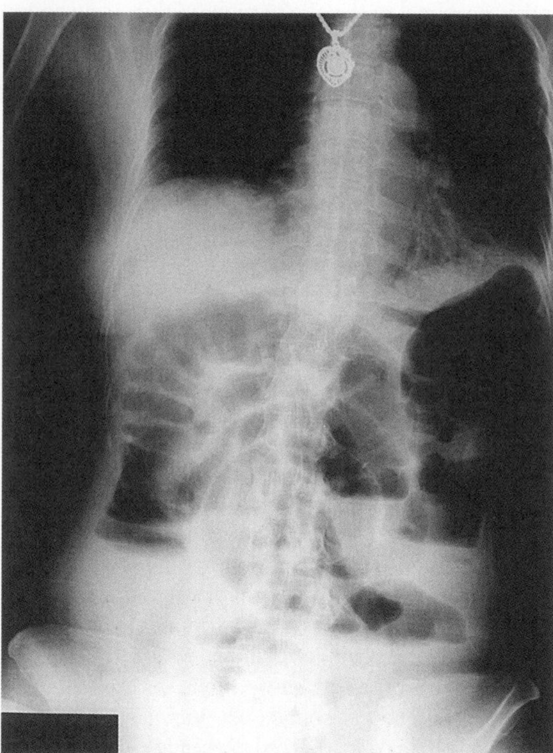

Fig. 19.1 Plain X-ray of the abdomen showing a mechanical small bowel obstruction with multiple loops of distended small bowel with 'step-ladder' air-fluid pattern in the erect film.

Presence of foreign bodies causing obstruction, such as gallstones, should be noted. Plain radiographs are not always diagnostic. In a proximal obstruction, there may be few radiographic abnormalities.

Contrast radiography

The use of barium is unpopular because of the risk of inspissation of barium proximal to the point of obstruction and the potential for peritioneal contamination if bowel perforation is present.

A gastrografin small bowel follow-through study will establish the extent (complete vs. incomplete) and degree of small bowel obstruction (Fig. 19.2). Gastrografin is hyperosmolar and may stimulate peristaltic activity of the small bowel. Caution is exercised in the dehydrated patient because gastrografin may exacerbate dehydration by sequestration of third-space fluid in the intestinal lumen. The intestinal mucosa is not well defined by the water-soluble gastrografin study. A good alternative, providing better anatomic detail, is a mixture of half barium and half water-soluble contrast.

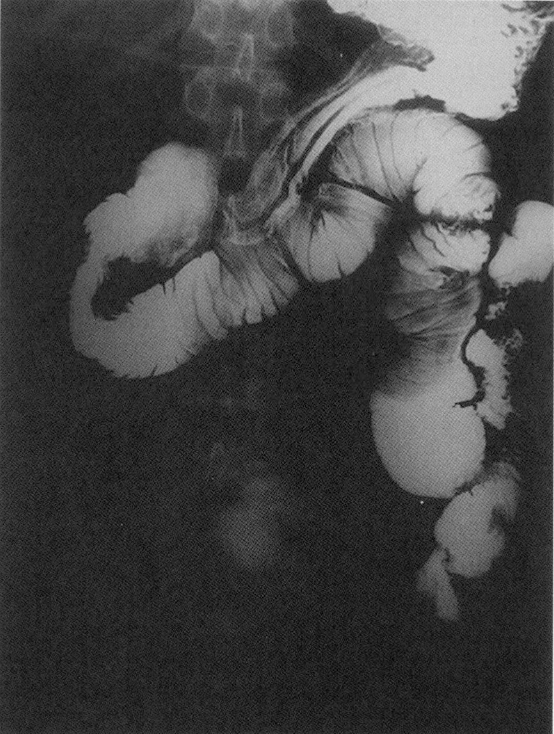

Fig. 19.2 Gastrografin small bowel follow-through showing an obstruction in the mid-small bowel.

Laboratory studies

There is no specific laboratory test that is diagnostic of intestinal obstruction. However, with a more protracted history, a hypokalaemic, hypochloraemic metabolic alkalosis may develop. Full blood examination may show leucocytosis if there is impending bowel ischaemia, and anaemia may indicate a malignant cause. Deranged liver function tests with hypoalbuminaemia may be associated with poor nutrition or sepsis.

Therapy

General support

Fluid and electrolyte replacement

Careful assessment of fluid and electrolyte status is important. A patient whose obstruction has been present for many hours, when there has been vomiting and sequestration of large amounts of fluid in the intestinal third-space, may require intravenous administration of several litres of isotonic saline to replace the deficit.

Monitoring

Pulse, blood pressure and tissue turgor are monitored as indices of fluid status. Urine output is also monitored. A urine output of at least 0.5 mL/kg per hour is a useful index of adequate fluid replacement. In critical cases, insertion of a urinary Foley catheter is useful. Central venous or pulmonary artery pressure monitoring is considered in older patients with a history of cardiac disease.

Nasogastric tube

Decompression of the upper gastrointestinal tract is initiated early in the management to avoid vomiting, and to reduce gastric and small bowel distension.

Analgesia

Analgesia is prescribed with caution so as not to mask signs of peritoneal irritation, which may indicate impending bowel ischaemia.

Non-operative management

Most patients with small bowel obstruction undergo an initial phase of resuscitation and decompression. Any signs of intestinal strangulation with vascular compromise should prompt immediate surgical intervention. Non-operative management is continued in patients with a partial small bowel obstruction and without signs of intestinal strangulation. Repeated evaluation of the abdomen and the general status of the patient is important. If there has been no significant improvement after 48 hours, operative intervention is generally indicated.

Operative treatment

In adhesive obstruction, surgery is indicated where there are concerns of intestinal ischaemia or the patient fails to improve after a short period of non-operative management. Constant, rather than intermittent, pain suggests bowel ischaemia. Bowel obstruction due to hernia in the inguinal or femoral area requires prompt surgery, as the bowel entrapped within the hernia can develop irreversible ischaemia and gangrene.

Pre-operative preparations include adequate fluid and electrolyte replacement, prophylaxis with broad-spectrum antibiotics covering aerobes and anaerobes, anti-thrombotic prophylaxis with compressive stockings and subcutaneous heparin.

Avoidance of aspiration pneumonitis is ensured with adequate nasogastric decompression and a rapid-sequence induction of anaesthesia with cricoid pressure until the endotracheal tube has been inserted.

Surgery is sometimes easy when a single adhesive band or an external hernia is the cause of obstruction, and surgery may be complex where there are dense adhesions. Closed-loop obstruction, with occlusion at both ends of the loop of bowel, may arise from torsion or complex adhesions of the small bowel, and obstructed external hernia. The intraluminal pressure rapidly rises and the risk of perforation is accelerated. The object at surgery is to find the junction of the dilated and collapsed bowel. The viability of a segment of intestine is determined by observation. In doubtful cases, a warm pack is placed over the bowel in question and the bowel re-examined several minutes later. If the bowel is not viable, a simple resection and primary anastomosis is performed. Sometimes, as with carcinomatosis or extensive pelvic adhesions, a side-to-side bypass is the better choice.

Obstruction due to external hernia is usually dealt with through the herniorrhaphy incision. The entrapped bowel is examined prior to returning it to the general peritoneal cavity. The hernia is then repaired. Local signs of inflammation at the hernia site may indicate strangulation of the entrapped bowel or omentum.

Special problems

Recurrent small bowel obstruction

After the initial operation of adhesiolysis for obstruction, the recurrence rate of further adhesive obstruction is about 20%. Repeated bouts of adhesive small bowel obstruction can be incapacitating: moreover, repeated operative intervention can be met with increasing technical difficulties and further episodes of adhesive obstruction. The first episode of adhesive small bowel obstruction is usually managed by prompt surgical intervention because of the risk of strangulation. When obstruction recurs, a non-operative management with nasogastric decompression and maintenance of fluid and electrolyte balance is generally preferred, provided that there is no evidence of bowel compromise. Increasing pain, fever, leucocytosis, high nasogastric output, lack of bowel function, abdominal distension and increasing bowel dilatation on plain abdominal X-ray are indicators for swift surgical intervention.

At surgery, gentle handling of the bowel and precision in dissection is important. A long intestinal tube introduced through a gastrostomy may help to splint the small bowel. Such a tube is left in place for at least 3 weeks but its efficacy has not been fully established.

Early post-operative small bowel obstruction

Mechanical small bowel obstruction presenting early in the post-operative period following abdominal surgery presents a diagnostic and therapeutic dilemma. The diagnosis may be obscured by paralytic ileus and the clinical features may be confused with the 'normal' convalescence following a laparotomy. With any prolongation of ileus beyond 5 days, mechanical obstruction should be suspected. Post-operative adhesions are most extensive about 10–21 days after a laparotomy. A gradual process of resolution then occurs. Apart from adhesions, other causes of mechanical small bowel obstruction include internal hernias, peritoneal defects and intra-abdominal abscesses.

Strangulation of the bowel in post-operative obstruction is uncommon. Careful repeated observation is important. Nasogastric decompression and replacement of fluid and electrolytes are essential. Parenteral nutritional support is often indicated if the obstructive episode lasts longer than 7 days. Plain radiograph of the abdomen is helpful in diagnosis. The presence of gas throughout the small and large bowel suggests a paralytic ileus. In cases where the diagnosis is uncertain, the use of dilute barium or gastrografin follow-through study will determine the severity of the obstruction and may lead to relief of the obstruction.

Timing of surgical intervention is difficult. Most patients will settle with non-operative management. The presence of complete obstruction, intra-abdominal sepsis or an excessively prolonged obstructive course are common indications for exploratory operation. In many situations, localised sepsis may be drained percutaneously under computed tomographic or ultrasonic guidance.

Metastatic malignant tumours

A history of neoplasm should not necessarily imply that carcinomatosis is the cause of small bowel obstruction. Some of these patients can have a benign cause of obstruction, such as an adhesive band. Management of patients with documented recurrent malignancy must be individualised. Peritoneal seedlings may lead to multiple narrowed segments. Strangulation is rare as the bowel loops are relatively fixed. Retroperitoneal and mesenteric deposits may contribute to the impaired motility.

A minimal-residue diet may reduce obstructive symptoms and acute episodes usually settle with nasogastric decompression. In patients with a relatively good prognosis, operative intervention with resection or bypass may achieve effective palliation.

Crohn's disease

Treatment of small bowel obstruction secondary to Crohn's disease is usually non-operative initially. Treatment with steroids and metronidazole reduces oedema and inflammation. If obstruction persists, surgery is necessary. A phlegmonous segment is resected and a fibrotic stricture is treated with strictureplasty.

Gallstone ileus

Gallstones may ulcerate through the gall bladder into the duodenum and pass down the small bowel. For a gallstone to cause mechanical small bowel obstruction, it is usually larger than 2.5 cm. The common site of impaction is about 60 cm from the ileocaecal valve because this is the narrowest part of the small bowel. Patients are often elderly, presenting with a subacute small bowel obstruction. Plain radiograph of the abdomen reveals a small bowel obstruction with a gallstone in the right lower quadrant and gas in the biliary tree. At surgery, the obstructing gallstone is crushed and emptied into the large bowel. Alternatively, an enterotomy is made and the gallstone removed from the small bowel. The gall bladder is left alone so as not to disturb the cholecyst–duodenal fistula.

Further reading

Chen SC, Lin FY, Lee PH, et al. Water-soluble contrast study predicts the need for early surgery in adhesive small bowel obstruction. *Br J Surg*. 1998;85:1692–1695.

Ellis H, Moran BJ, Thompson JN, et al. Adhesion-related hospital readmission after abdominal and pelvic surgery: a retrospective cohort study. *Lancet*. 1999;353:1476–1478.

Fevang BT, Fevang J, Lie SA, Soreide O, Svanes K, Viste A. Long-term prognosis after operation for adhesive small bowel obstruction. *Ann Surg*. 2004 Aug;240(2):193–201.

Tjandra JJ, Ng K. A sprayable hydrogel adhesion barrier facilitates closure of defunctioning loop ileostomy: a randomized trial. *Dis Colon Rectum*. 2004;47.

MCQs

Select the single correct answer to each question.

1 A 52-year-old man develops symptoms of small bowel obstruction over a 24-h period. Which of the following MOST SUGGESTS development of bowel strangulation?
- **a** profuse vomiting
- **b** constant abdominal pain associated with abdominal guarding
- **c** tachycardia
- **d** high nasogastric aspirate
- **e** hypokalaemic alkalosis

2 In acute proximal small bowel obstruction:
- **a** the symptoms are prolonged with abdominal distension prior to vomiting
- **b** there is a tendency towards dehydration, with hyponatraemia and hypokalaemic, hypochloraemic metabolic alkalosis
- **c** the vomitus is usually faeculent
- **d** a common cause is gallstone ileus
- **e** decompression with nasogastric tube is not often required

3 Spontaneous cholecystoenteric fistula:
- **a** occurs more frequently in young patients
- **b** can be diagnosed by plain abdominal X-rays
- **c** most frequently occurs between the gall bladder and ileum
- **d** frequently causes obstructive jaundice
- **e** is the most common cause of small bowel obstruction in females

4 Common causes of small bowel obstruction do NOT include:
- **a** post-surgical adhesions
- **b** inguinal hernia
- **c** incisional hernia
- **d** small bowel tumour
- **e** faecal impaction

5 Investigations in a patient with acute small bowel obstruction would NOT include:
- **a** supine and erect abdominal radiographs
- **b** blood urea and electrolyte estimation
- **c** gastrografin small bowel follow-through
- **d** technetium-labelled iminodiacetic acid (HIDA) scan
- **e** computed tomography of the abdomen

20 Large bowel obstruction

Adrian L. Polglase

Introduction

Large bowel obstruction is usually an acute blockage of the colon or rectum occurring in the elderly age group and requiring expeditious medical and surgical treatment. The urgency of management relates to the possibility of rupture of distended or compromised colon with the risk of faecal peritonitis. The three most common causes of mechanical obstruction are carcinoma of the colon, sigmoid volvulus and diverticular disease. Pseudo-obstruction (Ogilvie's syndrome), where there is acute dilatation of the colon without mechanical obstruction, presents with similar clinical features to an organic obstruction with the same potential complications, but is usually associated with some other illness.

Clinical features of large bowel obstruction

The typical clinical features are:

- Abdominal pain due to distension and colic.
- Abdominal distension due to retention of faeces and flatus.
- Constipation, and in a complete obstruction this will be absolute, ie. without the passage of faeces or flatus.
- Peritonism if perforation has occurred.
- Vomiting can be a late symptom.

Aetiology of large bowel obstruction

Carcinoma of the colon or rectum

At least 50% of large bowel obstructions are due to carcinoma. The most common site is the sigmoid colon, accounting for 30% of all cases. This is not only because the sigmoid colon is a common site for colonic carcinoma, but also because the lumen is relatively narrow and the faeces are firm rather than liquid. The second most common site is the splenic flexure, where the combination of a sharp kink in the colon together with luminal narrowing by the tumour and relatively firm stools leads to blockage. Right-sided obstructions are less frequent because the caecum and ascending colon are relatively capacious and the faecal material is liquid. The features of a right-sided large bowel obstruction may be less obvious than those of left-sided colonic lesions because only a small proportion of the colon is distended. An obstruction at the ileocaecal valve will produce features of a low small bowel obstruction.

Sigmoid volvulus

In Western countries sigmoid volvulus is essentially a condition of the elderly and frail, often with a long history of constipation and laxatives. In Africa, however, younger age groups can be afflicted and this is probably associated with the very high fibre dietary intake. Caecal volvulus is relatively uncommon and tends to occur in the younger age group. Volvulus of the colon involves twisting of the bowel on its mesentery, leading to ischemia and subsequent risk of perforation of the volved portion of the bowel and the caecum if it becomes overdistended because of unrelieved obstruction.

Diverticular disease

Diverticular disease can involve any part of the colon but in the vast majority of instances the sigmoid colon is most severely affected. Diverticulosis with subsequent scarring as well as muscular wall hypertrophy can cause stricturing of the colon, which can lead to large bowel obstruction and can be confused with carcinoma.

Less common causes

Less common causes of mechanical large bowel obstruction include stricturing as a result of inflammatory bowel disease (both ulcerative colitis and Crohn's disease) as well as ischaemic and radiation strictures, intussusceptions, adhesions (much more likely to cause a small bowel obstruction) and faecal impaction. Faecal impaction occurs when a faecal mass cannot be evacuated and it can affect any age group, but most commonly occurs in the elderly. The symptoms may be those of inability to evacuate, but not infrequently and paradoxically patients will present with faecal incontinence. This is because the impacted faecal bolus relaxes the rectosphincteric reflex and more proximal liquid stool escapes around the faecal bolus.

Pseudo-obstruction (Ogilvie's syndrome)

Pseudo-obstruction is a form of ileus of the large intestine, and in most patients is associated with some other ongoing medical condition. It tends to affect the older generation, and the symptoms and potential complications are essentially the same as those due to mechanical large bowel obstruction, including perforation. It is believed that the associated medical condition or metabolic abnormality may cause an imbalance of the autonomic nervous system, with a predominance of sympathetic activity.

Examination and investigations

Examination of a patient with a typical large bowel obstruction will reveal a distended and tender abdomen, often worst in the right iliac fossa because of caecal distension. Guarding or peritonism will be present if there has been vascular compromise or perforation of the colonic wall. The abdomen is highly tympanitic to percussion, with high-pitched bowel sounds. An abdominal mass might be present but the distension may prevent it being palpable. Digital rectal examination and/or sigmoidoscopy may reveal a rectal or sigmoid carcinoma or tell-tale blood within the lumen of the bowel indicative of a higher lesion. Sometimes a 'corkscrew sign' may be detected at sigmoidoscopy, suggesting volvulus or torsion of the sigmoid colon. The differential diagnosis should include tense ascites and gross bladder distension secondary to urinary retention. A patient with a late large bowel obstruction may be dehydrated and toxic because of vomiting or peritonitis. Peritonitis with a large bowel obstruction is a serious complication with a high mortality rate due to faecal peritonitis, most likely as a result of perforation of the

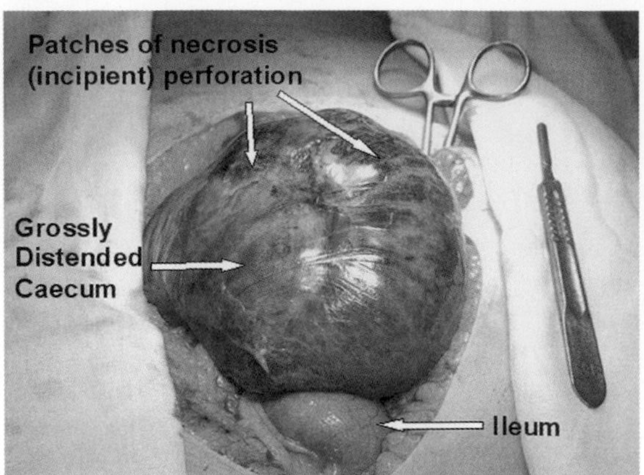

Fig. 20.1 Grossly distended caecum with incipient perforation.

caecum (as a result of Laplace's Law) (Fig. 20.1) or at the site of the obstruction, particularly at the point of torsion in a sigmoid volvulus.

The key investigation to be performed urgently is a plain X-ray of the abdomen, which will confirm

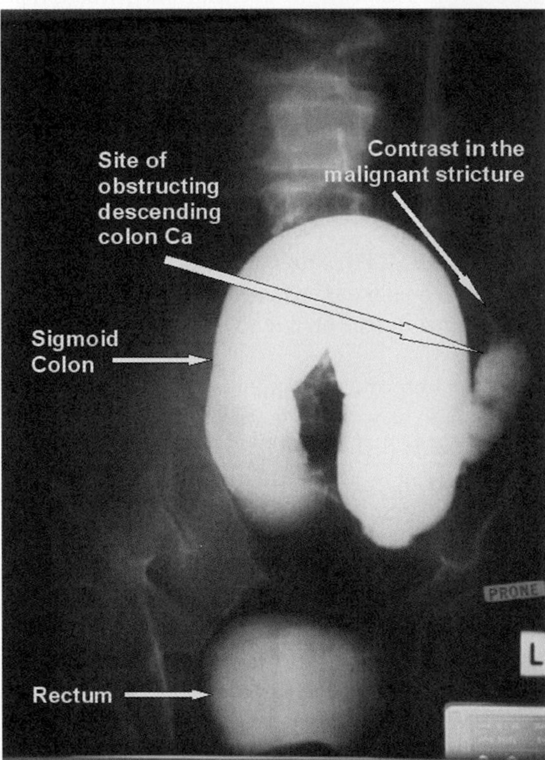

Fig. 20.2 Gastrografin enema showing obstructed descending colon.

marked colonic distension. A gastrografin enema should differentiate between a mechanical obstruction and colonic pseudo-obstruction. (Fig. 20.2) This differentiation is important as it will determine management. A plain X-ray may reveal the typical features of a sigmoid volvulus, with a distended sigmoid colon in the right upper quadrant. Free intraperitoneal gas indicates colonic perforation. A water-soluble contrast enema should define the level of the obstruction and in most instances the nature of the obstructing lesion. Sometimes the use of such water-soluble contrast enemas can be therapeutic by dislodging faeces from a narrowed large bowel lumen. Ultrasound examination of the liver and CT scanning of the abdomen and pelvis may also be useful in determining the presence of occult malignancy and aiding in management planning. Routine haematology and medical assessment is indicated, as in most instances surgical intervention is required.

Management of large bowel obstruction (Fig. 20.3)

Surgery

Immediate surgery will be required if the patient has overt peritonitis. Such immediate management, however, will usually depend on the result of a water-soluble contrast enema. If a mechanical obstruction is present then it is most likely due to a colonic carcinoma. For a distal obstruction (most commonly a sigmoid carcinoma) where obstruction is complete, relatively urgent surgery is necessary. Conventionally the most common approach would be a three-staged surgical management. The first stage is establishment of a proximal colostomy followed within weeks by a second stage involving resection and anastomosis, and finally some weeks or months later the closure of the colostomy.

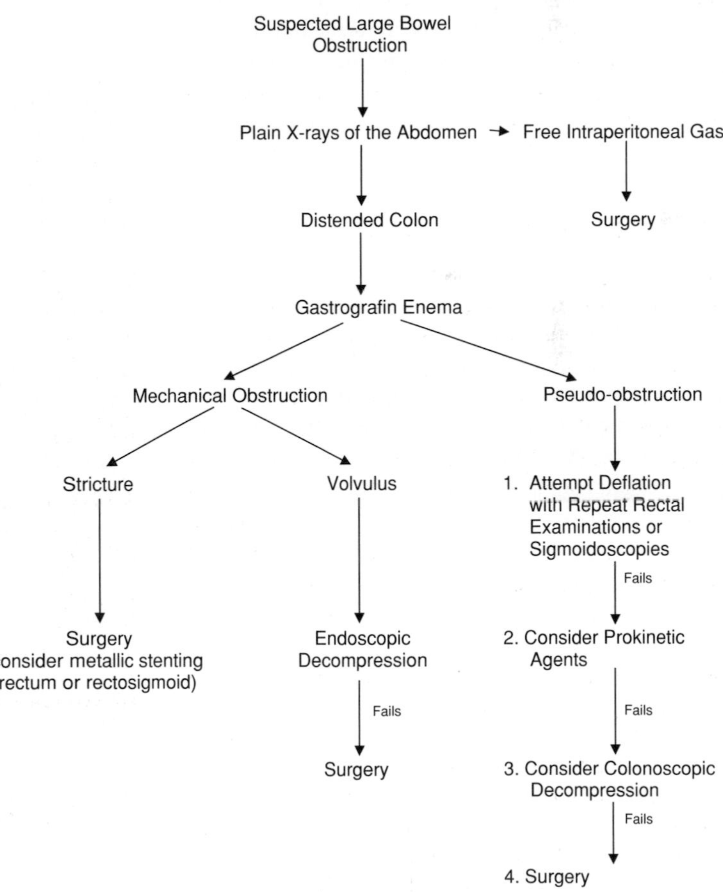

Fig. 20.3 Management of suspected large bowel obstruction.

A one-stage resection and anastomosis has been considered hazardous because, in general, the patients are elderly and often with co-morbidities. There is usually luminal disparity making anastomosis difficult and the proximal colon is loaded with faeces, which may increase the risk of anastomotic disruption. Recently, however, with improvement in resuscitation and anaesthesia the introduction of a one-stage resection and anastomosis, most often with on-table total colonic lavage to remove faecal material, has been demonstrated as safe and is a technique being used more frequently. Any perforation or sepsis at the site of the carcinoma mandates resection of the lesion, establishment of a sigmoid colostomy and oversewing of the rectal stump (Hartman's procedure). A second stage is done at a later time to re-establish bowel continuity.

Obstructing carcinoma of the splenic flexure and more proximal colon, including the transverse and ascending colons as well as the caecum, will usually be dealt with by a resection and end-to-end ileocolonic anastomosis. In this operation the tumour and all of the proximal distended colon is resected, and the well vascularised and relatively healthy ileum is suitable for anastomosis to the collapsed distal large intestine. Some patients may not be well enough for this one-stage procedure and still require a proximal stoma.

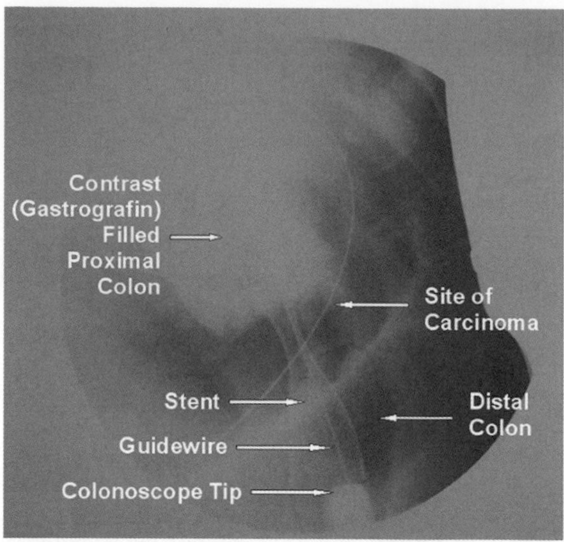

Fig. 20.4 Metallic stenting of an obstructing carcinoma of the sigmoid colon.

Colorectal stenting

Self-expandable metal stents are now being used more widely in the management of malignant low left-sided large bowel obstruction. These stents are placed endoscopically under fluoroscopic control through the obstructing lesion (Fig. 20.4) and can remain in place for a prolonged period where the stent is definitive palliative treatment or alternatively can decompress the colon so that within some weeks a one-stage resection and anastomosis may be possible. The stents are expensive but they appear to be cost-effective. Complications of perforation and bleeding are possible but uncommon, and it is likely this technique will be used more widely in the future.

Sigmoid volvulus

In the first instance after diagnosis of the sigmoid volvulus endoscopic decompression should be attempted. This can be performed with a rigid sigmoidoscope or a colonoscope. Such decompression can be achieved in most instances. If it is performed with a colonoscope it has the advantage of potentially being able to decompress the proximal colon. Endoscopic decompression is not without risk as the instrument then being passed through the spiral lumen at the level of the volvulus may perforate the colon, particularly if there is an area of ischaemia. If decompression is successfully achieved it may be useful to pass a long flatus tube through the lumen of a rigid sigmoidoscope to 'splint' the sigmoid colon in the hope of preventing early recurrence. Unfortunately, recurrence tends to occur in about half of the patients. Under these circumstances surgical resection with either end-to-end anastomosis or a Hartman's procedure is required. In general, if the acute situation is successfully dealt with by decompression, then an elective sigmoid colostomy should be performed when the patient's physical condition has improved and the bowel is deflated.

Diverticular stricture

In general, the principles of surgical management applicable to obstructing carcinoma of the sigmoid colon apply to obstruction due to a diverticular stricture. A definitive resection, whether it is performed at the time of the initial resection of the stricture (i.e. a Hartman's procedure) or if there is an end-to-end anastomosis, will usually require complete resection of the sigmoid colon to effectively eradicate the diverticulosis. Any sepsis in association with the diverticular stricture, such as a perforation or contained abscess, will usually mandate resection and a Hartman's procedure, although in some instances drainage of sepsis and a temporary proximal defunctioning stoma may be appropriate.

Pseudo-obstruction (Ogilvie's syndrome)

If a gastrografin enema confirms the diagnosis of pseudo-obstruction, provided there is no evidence of colonic perforation, which would mandate urgent surgical intervention, then conservative measures which address the patient's general medical condition including fluid and electrolyte balance are required. If rectal examination or sigmoidoscopy achieve the passage of flatus then this should be carried out three or four times each day to continue to decompress the colon. About half the patients with pseudo-obstruction may respond to this management, but if not then neostigmine, which is a potent parasympathomimetic, should be administered intravenously. Such treatment has the potential for complications, including cardiac arrhythmias and perforation if there happens to be mechanical obstruction. If sigmoidoscopy and neostigmine or other prokinetic agents such as erythromycin or cisapride are unsuccessful, then colonoscopic decompression should be attempted. This is likely to be successful, but without bowel preparation may be dangerous. Satisfactory decompression may be achieved in most patients, but there is a significant recurrence rate. If these measures fail then the establishment of a colostomy or caecostomy may be required.

Further reading

De U, Ghosh S. Single stage primary anastomosis without colonic lavage for left-sided colonic obstruction due to acute sigmoid volvulus: a prospective study of one hundred and ninety-seven cases. *ANZ J Surg.* 2003;73:390–392.

Goyal A, Schein M. Current practices in left-sided colonic emergencies. *Dig Surg.* 2001;18:399–402.

Kahi CJ, Rex DK. Bowel obstruction and pseudo-obstruction. *Gastroenterol Clin North Am.* 2003;32:1229–1247.

Keymling M. Colorectal stenting. *Endoscopy.* 2003;35:234–238.

Moons V, Coremans J, Tack J. An update on acute colonic pseudo-obstruction (Ogilvie's syndrome). *Acta Gastro-Enterologica Belgic.* 2003;April–June:150–153.

MCQs

Select the single correct answer to each question.

1 The following are common causes of large bowel obstruction except:
- **a** intra-abdominal adhesions
- **b** sigmoid volvulus
- **c** carcinoma of the colon
- **d** diverticular disease
- **e** carcinoma of the rectum

2 Large bowel obstruction requires urgent treatment because:
- **a** fluid and electrolyte imbalance is often life threatening
- **b** intracolonic bacterial overgrowth leads to septicaemia
- **c** there is a significant risk of colonic perforation
- **d** small bowel obstruction with ischaemia will eventually occur

3 Sigmoid volvulus:
- **a** is common in the under 50 years age group
- **b** is uncommon in Africans
- **c** may lead to ischaemia and perforation of the colon
- **d** is rarely treated successfully by sigmoidoscopic decompression
- **e** is best treated surgically by subtotal colectomy

4 Colonic pseudo-obstruction:
- **a** is common in the elderly and debilitated
- **b** should initially be treated by colonoscopic decompression
- **c** should be treated with sympathetomimetic agents
- **d** is not associated with a risk of caecal perforation
- **e** is liable to require surgical treatment

5 Complete left-sided large bowel obstruction:
- **a** should be treated by self-expandable metallic stents
- **b** will mostly require treatment by a three-staged surgical procedure
- **c** is commonly caused by a Crohn's disease stricture
- **d** should be treated by Hartman's procedure

21 Mesenteric vascular disease

Joe J. Tjandra

Introduction

Mesenteric vascular disease encompasses a family of diseases in which the end result is ischaemic injury to the small or large bowel. Early recognition and appropriate management offers the best outcome, but this is not easily achieved because in the early stages the presentations are vague and non-specific.

The intestinal tract has a generous overlapping blood supply. The three main vessels supplying circulation to the bowel include the coeliac axis (CA), the superior mesenteric artery (SMA) and the inferior mesenteric artery (IMA). Important collateral vessels emanate from the hypogastric vessels at the level of the sigmoid colon. The CA communicates with the SMA system via the pancreaticoduodenal loop and, to a lesser extent, from the dorsal pancreatic artery. The SMA communicates with the IMA system via the marginal artery (and sometimes a separate collateral, the arc of Riolan, at the base of the mesentery) between the left branch of the middle colic artery and the left colic artery.

In general, acute occlusion of any of the three main mesenteric vessels may lead to acute bowel infarction. Gradual occlusion of any one, two or even three of these vessels can occur without injury, depending on the efficacy of the collateral circulation.

Acute mesenteric ischaemia

Aetiology and pathology

The main blood supply to the intestine is via the SMA. Inadequate intestinal perfusion is due to either a low-flow state or to focal vascular occlusion. Non-occlusive intestinal ischaemia results from inadequate perfusion secondary to hypotension, spasm or intestinal distension. In patients with underlying atherosclerosis and in whom other organ systems are already impaired, a vicious cycle may be initiated. Occlusive vascular diseases include SMA embolism, thrombosis and venous thrombosis. Mesenteric embolus is uncommon. Acute thrombosis certainly occurs, but the relationship between the vascular and the intestinal lesion is not clear-cut. However, stenoses and even complete occlusion of the mesenteric vessels can be found in asymptomatic individuals.

The early phase of acute intestinal ischaemia leads to intense loss of circulating blood volume and metabolic acidosis. At this early stage the acute process is still reversible. Vasoactive substances released in response to intestinal ischaemia further diminish perfusion. Partial reduction of molecular oxygen results in the production of oxygen free radicals. These superoxide radicals lead to increased vascular permeability and mucosal injury, and are central to the reperfusion injury. The intestinal mucosa is uniquely rich in the enzyme xanthine oxidase, which contributes to superoxide production. This particularly applies to the phase of reperfusion when the intestinal mucosa is flooded with oxygen. Thus tissue damage tends to occur during reperfusion rather than during the period of ischaemia. Later in the course, mucosal disruption and bacterial invasion develop with endotoxin release, septicaemia and shock, indicating an irreversible injury.

Clinical features

Patients are usually elderly with associated cardiac or peripheral vascular disease. They present with severe central abdominal pain that is often out of proportion to the objective abdominal signs. A history of chronic intestinal ischaemia may be present. Superior mesenteric artery thrombosis is distinguishable from embolism by the more insidious onset of symptoms. Vomiting and diarrhoea may be present. Bloody diarrhoea is evident only late, when mucosal infarction has occurred. Peritoneal irritation indicates full-thickness bowel infarction and the process becomes irreversible.

Non-occlusive mesenteric ischaemia is diagnosed with increasing frequency in intensive care unit settings among critically ill patients with a low blood flow state. This entity should be suspected in anyone with abdominal pain following a prolonged episode of hypotension.

The white blood cell count usually is elevated. It may be used as an indicator to monitor the progress of the disease. Serum phosphate levels, while not specific for bowel ischaemia, may be elevated and these may precede irreversible ischaemic injury. Metabolic acidosis is a late finding and suggests bowel necrosis. In the early stages, the patient appears sicker and in more pain than is suggested by the physical examination. Within a very short period (hours to 1–2 days), the damage progresses and the patient becomes desperately ill with ileus, peritonism and dehydration. Hypovolaemic and septic shock develops and multi-organ failure ensues.

Radiographic changes

In the early stages, plain radiograph of the abdomen may appear normal. Later, features of ileus develop and air may appear in the portal vein and the liver. In patients with doubtful clinical features who are haemodynamically stable, visceral angiography of the CA, SMA and IMA via the femoral artery is helpful. With thromboembolism, a sharp cut-off is present at the site of obstruction. A normal mesenteric angiogram, however, does not exclude ischaemia, because approximately one-third of cases are 'non-occlusive' in nature and are due to a low-flow state.

General management

Intravenous rehydration

Vigorous replacement of water and electrolytes is initiated with balanced saline or colloid solution. Adequacy of replacement is monitored by serial measurements of the urine output, vital signs and central venous or wedged pulmonary arterial pressure.

Intravenous antibiotics

Blood culture is taken and broad-spectrum antibiotics covering Gram-negative organisms and anaerobes are commenced. This will usually be a second- or third-generation cephalosporin together with metronidazole.

Correction of metabolic acidosis

Metabolic acidosis is due to a combination of low tissue perfusion, absorption of products of tissue necrosis, and impaired respiratory exchange. Restoration of circulating blood volume will help to correct acid–base equilibrium. Occasionally, bicarbonate therapy may be necessary.

Heparin

Continuous infusion with heparin is given for thromboembolic disease to prevent clot extension and to counteract disseminated intravascular coagulation. This therapy is interrupted during surgery.

Specific management

Thrombolytic therapy

If clot is demonstrated within the mesenteric system and signs of irreversible ischaemia (i.e. peritonism) are absent, lysis may be performed with fibrinolytic agents infused via a catheter placed in the SMA immediately proximal to the occlusion. Streptokinase is commonly used but there are problems with anaphylaxis, febrile reactions and bleeding. Newer agents such as recombinant tissue plasminogen activator (rTPA) or anisoylated plasminogen streptokinase activator complex (APSAC) may be more efficacious. Clinical reports on these agents are awaited.

Vasodilatation

Angiographic catheter infusion of papaverine is best for non-occlusive mesenteric ischaemia and, less often, for embolic disease. Epidural block may also help relieve the reflex component of the vasospasm.

Laparotomy

This remains the standard surgical treatment when the diagnosis of acute mesenteric ischaemia is suspected or made. Once the metabolic defects are brought under control, swift surgical action is taken, unless the clinical condition has progressed beyond salvage and is preterminal.

Laparotomy

The diagnosis is usually obvious, with the characteristic 'musty' smell of ischaemic bowel. Thrombosis of the SMA occurs at the origin and produces ischaemia throughout the midgut from the ligament of Treitz to the splenic flexure of the colon. Emboli usually lodge at or distal to the origin of the middle colic artery from the SMA, thus sparing the proximal jejunum and sometimes the right transverse colon. Small emboli may migrate peripherally to cause segmental damage.

A number of surgical options are available.

First, the abdomen can be closed without further action. This procedure is adopted if a large length of intestinal tract is dead such that the patient will be committed to long-term parenteral nutrition and there are severe co-morbid factors.

Second, the infarcted bowel can be resected and both bowel ends exteriorised. This is the safest option and allows inspection of both bowel ends for their viability. Anastomosis and restoration of continuity of bowel is deferred for 4–6 months to allow restoration of health and maturation of intra-abdominal adhesions. Occasionally, a primary anastomosis is performed if viability is assured. In these latter cases, or in cases in which viability is uncertain, the use of a second-look laparotomy may maximise intestinal salvage. The re-exploration is planned and done 24–48 hours later, regardless of apparent clinical improvement. Support with parenteral nutrition is invaluable.

Third, revascularisation of the bowel may be undertaken. Embolectomy for embolic disease or aortomesenteric bypass grafting for arterial thrombosis may be performed. The need for small bowel resection often may be avoided by re-evaluating the viability of the bowel 15–30 minutes after restoration of blood flow. Such operations are technically difficult and the results are variable. Reperfusion of ischaemic bowel also imposes a heavy physiological burden on the patient.

Post-operatively, intensive care with cardiovascular and respiratory monitoring is important. Fluid replacement, antibiotics and inotropic agents are continued. Central intravenous lines, urethral catheter and nasogastric tube are in place. Often a period of assisted ventilation is continued.

Outcome

Mesenteric infarction is associated with mortality of between 90% and 100%. Embolic disease has a better outcome than thrombotic disease as it tends to present more acutely and earlier. Non-occlusive mesenteric ischaemia tends to have a poor prognosis because of the severity of the underlying illness that precipitates the ischaemic event.

Mesenteric venous thrombosis

Aetiology

Mesenteric venous thrombosis accounts for less than 10% of cases of mesenteric infarction. Approximately 20% are idiopathic but the underlying causes include portal hypertension, haematological diseases, malignancy, inflammatory bowel disease, sepsis, reactions to oral contraceptives and trauma.

Clinical presentation

Mesenteric venous thrombosis is insidious in onset with vague abdominal discomfort, distension, altered bowel habits and nausea. Later, features of an acute abdomen with tenderness and guarding, and leucocytosis may appear. This is differentiated from arterial occlusion by one of the associated diseases that is commonly present.

Diagnosis

A plain radiograph of the abdomen usually shows features of an ileus with dilated loops of small bowel and air-fluid levels. Gas is usually present in the large bowel as well. Mesenteric angiography is less useful; the features include prolongation of the arterial phase, non-opacification of the superior mesenteric vein and visible contrast within the bowel lumen. Diagnostic peritoneal lavage may reveal serosanguineous fluid. In practice, the diagnosis is made at surgery. Operative findings include the presence of a congested, cyanotic, oedematous bowel with pulsatile mesenteric arteries.

Treatment

Treatment includes fluid resuscitation, antibiotics and prompt surgical intervention. With venous infarction, the damage is often limited and a segmental resection with primary end-to-end anastomosis is performed. A short bowel syndrome is less likely to occur than with arterial occlusion. Anticoagulation therapy is initiated during or immediately after surgery, initially with heparin and subsequently converted to Warfarin. Recurrences occur in 20% of patients and, therefore, anticoagulation therapy is continued for 6 months post-operatively.

Short bowel syndrome

Introduction

Intestinal failure results from reduction in the amount of functioning gut to below the minimal amount necessary for adequate digestion and absorption of nutrients. A major cause is short bowel syndrome secondary to major resections of the small bowel. The outlook for these patients has improved dramatically with the advent of total parenteral nutrition (TPN) and home parenteral nutrition (HPN).

The length of normal small bowel measured at surgery is variable but is about 350 cm. In general, loss of more than 50–70% or a remaining length of less than 100 cm of small bowel results in significant malabsorption and malnutrition.

Pathophysiology

Loss of intestinal length leads to a loss of mucosal absorptive surface and an associated shortened transit time. There is a reduced interaction between the nutrients, the biliary and pancreatic secretions, and the intestinal mucosa. Carbohydrate absorption is usually less affected than protein or fat absorption. Fat absorption is most severely affected.

Bile salts are resorbed only by the ileum, and approximately 100 cm of distal ileum is necessary for complete bile salt resorption. With less than 100 cm of ileum, enterohepatic circulation of bile salts is impaired, leading to fat malabsorption and steatorrhoea, which in turn leads to malabsorption of the fat-soluble vitamins A, D, E and K.

Loss of ileum is more disabling than an equal loss of jejunum. The ileum is the selective site for resorption of bile salts as well as the intrinsic factor-bound vitamin B_{12}. The jejunum has a lesser potential for adaptation than the ileum. Motility in the ileum is also slower than in the jejunum, allowing more time for absorption. Loss of jejunum leads to a reduction in several enterohormones. Lactose intolerance may also be noted. Absorption of minerals and electrolytes is disturbed.

Adaptation

The residual small bowel undergoes adaptation, which is most pronounced within the first 6 months. However, adaptive change is a slow process and may continue for up to 3 years after resection. The adaptive changes include cellular hyperplasia, increases in villous height and crypt depth, intestinal lengthening and dilatation, increased absorptive ability and activity of brush border enzymes, and increased transit time. Enteral feeding stimulates intestinal adaptation and should be introduced as soon as the clinical situation allows. Patients maintained on TPN alone do not undergo adaptation as readily.

Outcome

The following factors may influence the outcome.

- Extent of resection of small bowel.
- Site of resection. Jejunal resections are better tolerated than ileal resections.
- Age of the patient. Younger patients adapt better both physically and mentally than older patients.
- Presence of stomach or colon. Diarrhoea is lessened if the stomach and colon are intact; however, unabsorbed bile salts following massive ileal resection may have a choleretic effect on the colon, causing diarrhoea and fluid–electrolyte loss.
- Presence of ileocaecal valve. The ileocaecal valve reduces bacterial colonisation of the ileum from the colon and slows intestinal transit.
- Health of the residual bowel. Absorption and adaptive potential of the remaining bowel is impaired by the presence of any residual disease.

Management

After massive bowel loss, the immediate problems are dehydration and electrolyte imbalance. These problems may last for several weeks and intravenous fluid replacement is needed to keep apace with ongoing losses (diarrhoea, fistula or stoma effluent), as well as daily maintenance needs. Assessment of fluid and electrolyte balance is made by clinical examination, fluid-balance charts, and biochemical analysis of urine and serum electrolytes, as well as electrolyte analysis of other losses (fistula or stoma effluent). In the short term, TPN is usually necessary while intestinal recovery and adaptation occur.

Enteric feeding is commenced as soon as the clinical condition allows. If massive bowel resection has been performed, enteric feeding through a thin silastic naso-enteric tube may be preferred. Initially, a solution of 5% dextrose with half normal saline is used. When the patient's fluid status stabilises, one of the defined formula diets may be initiated. These contain glucose or other simple sugars, amino acids and peptides, electrolytes, small amounts of fats, vitamins and trace elements. These formulae are hyperosmolar and should be diluted initially to avoid bloating or worsening diarrhoea. Monthly injections of vitamin B_{12} may be necessary. Glutamine infusions or enteral supplements produce mucosal growth. Additional nutritional needs are supplemented with TPN, and additional fluids and electrolytes are replaced as necessary. Nutritional support is instituted early in the treatment of short bowel syndrome. It prevents malnutrition and improves survival. As adaptation occurs, the enteral intake is increased and the TPN tapered. This phase may take several weeks to a year. In others, a more prolonged HPN may be necessary.

Antidiarrhoeal agents, such as loperamide or codeine are added in increasing dosages tailored to the response. Liquid preparations generally are more readily absorbed and work better. Bulking agents such as Metamucil® may also be used. If bile salt malabsorption is a problem, cholestyramine can be added. Gastric secretion is decreased with H_2 antagonists (cimetidine or ranitidine) or proton pump inhibitors (omeprazole). Somatostatin and its analogues (e.g. octreotide) help to reduce diarrhoea or fistula output. Somatostatin acts by slowing intestinal transit, thus improving absorption and by suppressing gastric acid and pancreatic fluid secretion.

Chronic mesenteric vascular disease

Aetiology and pathology

Chronic mesenteric vascular disease or 'intestinal angina' is poorly defined and poorly understood. The clinical studies on this disease are limited but there is underlying atheromatous occlusion of the visceral arteries. There is poor correlation between angiographic findings and clinical symptoms. Because of the rich collateral network, high-grade arterial stenosis may be present without any symptoms of ischaemia.

Clinical presentation

The presenting symptoms are variable but include postprandial pain, weight loss and malabsorption. The patient often refuses to eat because of fear of subsequent pain, which occurs soon after a meal and lasts for several hours.

Treatment

Surgery should be considered only when the clinical presentation is typical of intestinal ischaemia and there is angiographic evidence of critical stenosis in two of the three vessels. The favoured surgical option is bypass grafting with prosthetic grafts or with autogenous vein grafts. Some early success has been reported following percutaneous transluminal angioplasty. If symptoms recur following a previously successful angioplasty, a favourable outcome may be expected from surgical reconstruction. However, technical failure in the mesenteric circulation could be catastrophic. For this reason, angioplasty should be used only where facilities for immediate operation are available.

Ischaemic colitis

Aetiology and pathology

The colon has a generous overlapping blood supply with contributions from the SMA, IMA and hypogastric arteries. All parts of the colon are susceptible to ischaemia. However, two regions are anatomically vulnerable: 'Griffith's point', at the splenic flexure corresponding to the junction of the SMA and the IMA; and 'Sudeck's critical point', in the midportion of the sigmoid colon corresponding to the junction of the IMA and hypogastric arteries.

Occlusive events and low-flow states both have been associated with ischaemic colitis.

- Surgery: aortic surgery with ligation of a patent IMA or colonic surgery.
- Hypotension or low-flow states from any cause.
- Underlying diseases such as atherosclerosis, vasculitis and polycythaemia.
- Medications such as oral contraceptives, antihypertensive agents, vasopressors and digoxin.

The severity of ischaemic colitis will depend on the duration of reduction in blood flow, the adequacy of collateral circulation and, if the mucosal barrier is disrupted, the concentration of colonic bacteria in the colon. Distension of the involved colon will further impair the transmural blood flow.

Pathophysiology

Three phases of ischaemic colitis have been described (Box 21.1).

Box 21.1 Phases of ischaemic colitis

- Transient ischaemia. This phase is reversible. Histological changes of inflammation are predominantly confined to the mucosa and submucosa. Characteristic radiological 'thumb-printing' of the bowel lumen is seen on plain radiograph of the abdomen. This is caused by submucosal haemorrhage or oedema.
- Ischaemic stricture. Partial thickness injury to the mucosa and muscular layers of the bowel leads to delayed presentation with fibrosis and stricture.
- Gangrene. This is due to full-thickness necrosis and infarction. Perforation, sepsis and death ensue unless surgical intervention is undertaken promptly. Contrast studies should be avoided if this is suspected.

Clinical presentation

The clinical features depend on the phase of the disease. Common symptoms include left iliac fossa pain if the left colon is the site affected. There may be bloody diarrhoea and often fever and abdominal distension. The patient usually is not grossly ill or shocked.

Investigations

Laboratory tests and angiography usually are not helpful. Barium enema has been a useful tool in diagnosis, by demonstrating 'thumbprinting' in the early stages (Fig. 21.1) and later with mucosal ulceration and strictures. CT scan may also be helpful by showing mucosal oedema, thickening and associated inflammatory changes. A limited colonoscopy performed in the unprepared large bowel during the acute phase is particularly useful with the more severe disease where barium enema is contraindicated. Biopsy may be helpful in differentiating the disease from inflammatory bowel disease.

Management

In the acute phase, clinical and early endoscopic evaluation will distinguish ischaemic colitis from inflammatory bowel disease or diverticulitis. The treatment for the most part is expectant and will include bowel rest, intravenous fluid replacement and combination antibiotics that cover for Gram-negative organisms and anaerobes. When a protracted course is suspected, TPN may be helpful. Most patients will recover

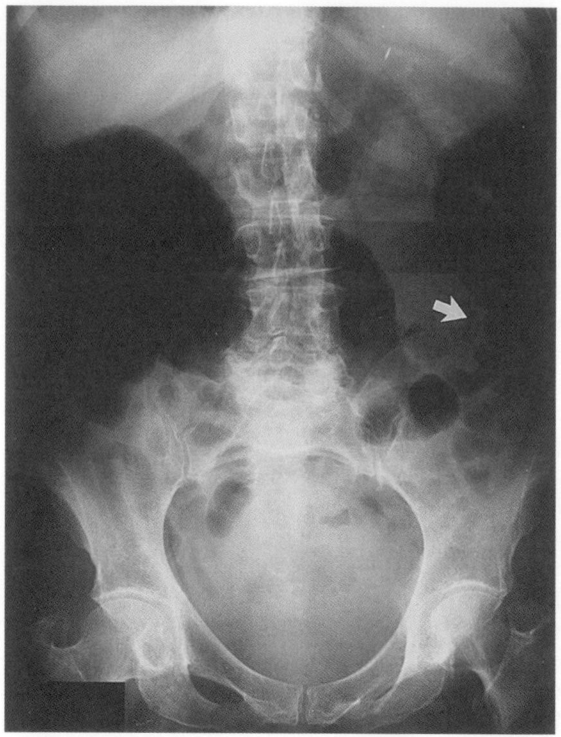

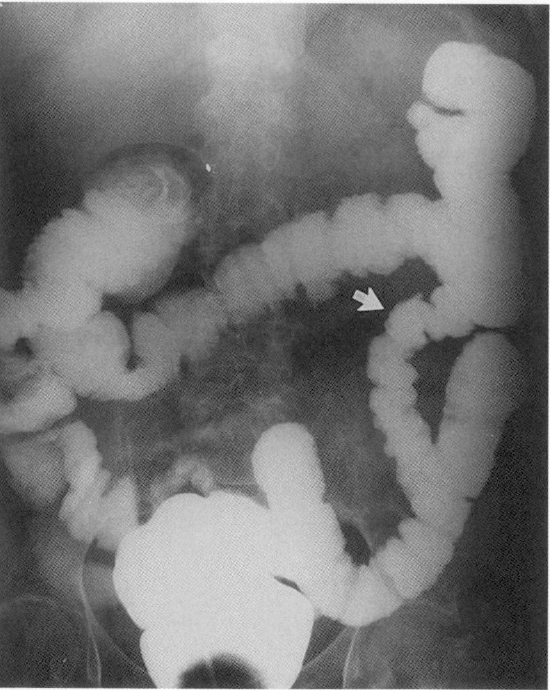

Fig. 21.1 Early ischaemic colitis with 'thumbprinting' in the splenic flexure.

spontaneously. Progression to gangrene or perforation is rare. Fibrous stricture is a late and unpredictable event.

Surgery is rarely necessary in ischaemic colitis. Specific indications for surgery include peritonitis, perforation and sepsis. A wide resection of non-viable colon is performed with exteriorisation of the proximal colon as a stoma. The distal part of the large bowel is either stapled or oversewn, or exteriorised as a mucous fistula. Primary anastomosis is unsafe in this acute setting with unprepared bowel. Post-operative progression of the ischaemia may compromise the anastomosis as well.

Surgery is generally not indicated for strictures without clinical symptoms of obstruction. Obstructing strictures may require resection. Occasionally, resection for strictures is indicated because malignancy cannot be ruled out.

Ischaemic colitis following aortic surgery

Ischaemic colitis following aortic surgery is unique because the most likely aetiology is a sudden loss of blood flow from ligation of a patent IMA. The incidence of ischaemic colitis is higher following emergency than elective repair of abdominal aortic aneurysm (see Chapter 52). Other factors include duration of cross-clamping of the aorta, hypotension, presence of hypogastric blood flow, collateral circulation and cholesterol emboli. The mortality of clinical ischaemia following elective aortic aneurysm surgery is around 20% and is much higher after emergency operation.

Further reading

Oldenburg WA, Lau LL, Rodenberg TJ, Edmonds HJ, Burger CD. Acute mesenteric ischemia: a clinical review. *Arch Intern Med.* 2004 May 24;164(10):1054–62.

Horgan PG, Gorey TF. Operative assessment of intestinal viability. *Surg Clin North Am.* 1992;72:143–155.

Chou CK, Mak CW, Tzeng WS, Chang JM. CT of small bowel ischemia. *Abdom Imaging.* 2004 Jan–Feb;29(1):18–22.

MCQs

Select the single correct answer to each question.

1 Three days after elective repair of an abdominal aortic aneurysm, a 70-year-old man developed left iliac fossa pain, abdominal distension, bloody diarrhoea and a fever of 38°C. The most helpful investigation would be:
a mesenteric angiography
b limited flexible sigmoidoscopy and biopsy
c gastroscopy
d barium small bowel follow-through
e abdominal ultrasound

2 Three days after a myocardial infarction with cardiogenic shock, a 75-year-old man develops abdominal pain and distension. The abdomen is slightly tender with reduced bowel sounds. A plain abdominal X-ray shows distended small bowel without fluid levels. Blood tests reveal a metabolic acidosis. The most likely diagnosis is:
a perforated peptic ulcer
b mesenteric ischaemia
c pseudo-obstruction of the colon
d acute pancreatitis
e diverticulitis

3 Following massive small bowel resection for mesenteric venous thrombosis, the following may develop EXCEPT:
a dehydration
b malnutrition
c lactose intolerance
d fat malabsorption
e adaptation of the colon to absorb vitamin B_{12}

22 The appendix and Meckel's diverticulum

Joe J. Tjandra

Acute appendicitis

Acute appendicitis is common and affects one in seven persons. The diagnosis of appendicitis can be difficult. Delays in diagnosis complicate the illness.

Surgical pathology

With acute appendicitis, organisms invade the wall of the appendix and are lodged in the submucosa. Eventually, the full thickness of the wall is involved by acute inflammation and becomes swollen and reddened. With delay in diagnosis, the appendix becomes distended, especially if there is obstruction of the lumen. Venous stasis and then arterial occlusion result in gangrene at the tip of the appendix, where the blood supply is precarious, or at the site of obstruction in the appendix because of pressure necrosis.

Perforation may follow and can be localised by the greater omentum and loops of small bowel or may become generalised with diffuse contamination of the peritoneal cavity.

Clinical features

Symptoms

Abdominal pain

The nature of the pain may be highly variable. The most common initial presentation is a periumbilical, gnawing pain that migrates within a few hours to the right iliac fossa. There may be a preceding period of anorexia, nausea and vomiting that lasts 12–24 hours. Severe vomiting is uncommon. The usual sequence is anorexia, followed by central abdominal pain, then vomiting and finally pain in the right iliac fossa.

The initial periumbilical pain is due to obstruction and inflammation of the appendix and is mediated through the visceral pain fibres as a mid-gut pain. When appendicitis becomes transmural, the serosa of the appendix and the parietal peritoneum are involved, causing a localised pain mediated through the somatic pain fibres in the right iliac fossa.

Atypical presentations include a right upper quadrant pain from a long appendix or a right loin pain from a retrocaecal appendix. Patients presenting with peritonitis from perforated appendicitis have generalised abdominal pain.

Diarrhoea

Early in the course of the illness, patients may have one or two loose bowel movements as a response to visceral pain. Diarrhoea and tenesmus are most likely in the presence of an inflamed pelvic appendix irritating the rectal wall or a retroileal appendix irritating the terminal ileum. Severe and persistent diarrhoea is more likely to be due to gastroenteritis or inflammatory bowel disease.

Signs

General

With more advanced inflammation, the patient may look unwell. Moderate fever and tachycardia may be present and reflect the underlying infective process.

Local

Tenderness over the site of the appendix is the most important sign of appendicitis. The tenderness is localised and persistent and is classically at McBurney's

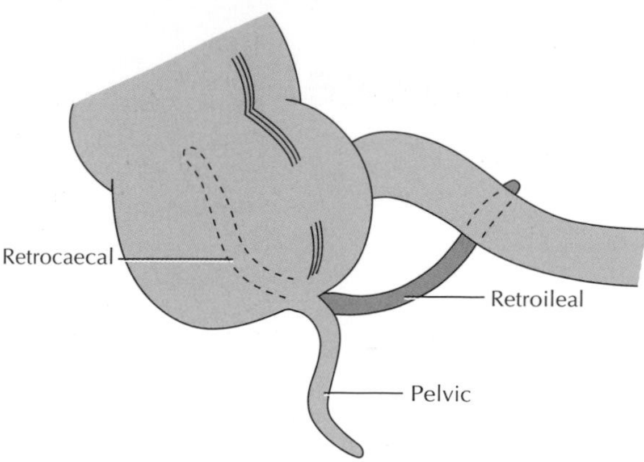

Fig. 22.1 The various positions of the appendix.

point (one-third of the way from the anterior superior iliac spine to the umbilicus), although it may vary depending on the location of the appendix (Fig. 22.1). Tenderness may be minimal early in the course of the illness and hard to elicit in the obese or if the appendix is retrocaecal.

Local muscular rigidity in the right iliac fossa is produced by inflammation of the parietal peritoneum overlying the appendix. Subtle rigidity can be detected by gently moving the palpating hand toward the area of maximal pain in the right iliac fossa while talking with the patient. This helps to differentiate true rigidity or guarding from voluntary spasm associated with nervousness. It is also helpful to ask the patient to cough or to sit up while watching the patient's facial expression; a grimace further suggests the presence of local peritonitis.

With local peritonitis, palpation in the left lower quadrant may cause pain in the right lower quadrant (Rovsing's sign). Signs of local peritonitis may be minimal in patients with a retrocaecal or pelvic appendicitis. The Psoas sign – pain caused by the extension of the right hip to stretch the psoas muscle – is generally present in retrocaecal appendicitis. Pelvic appendicitis is often difficult to differentiate from pelvic inflammatory disease but is usually associated with a right-sided tenderness on rectal examination.

Patients who present late with appendicitis may have generalised tenderness and rigidity, indicating perforation and peritonitis. Rebound tenderness indicates peritoneal inflammation and is best elicited by percussion. The delayed presentation of a tender, inflammatory appendiceal mass may occur in the right iliac fossa after 3 or more days.

Box 22.1 Investigations in appendicitis

- Leucocytosis is usual in the range of 11 000 to 17 000/mL with a neutrophilia.
- Urinalysis by ward test and microscopy is useful in doubtful cases, as it may diagnose urinary tract infection. However, pyuria may occur due to irritation of the bladder or ureter by an inflamed appendix.
- Plain abdominal X-rays are rarely helpful. They may detect non-specific changes that suggest intra-abdominal mischief, such as localised ileus in the right lower quadrant, free intra-peritoneal air or a faecalith in the appendix area.
- Ultrasound may show a thick-walled appendix with a dilated lumen. The sensitivity and specificity for appendicitis using ultrasound are 75% and 95%, respectively. However its greatest value is to rule out gynaecological pathology.
- Computed tomography scan has a sensitivity and specificity of about 80% and is insufficiently accurate for early diagnosis of acute appendicitis. It allows percutaneous drainage of a localised peri-appendiceal abscess and is useful in the evaluation of patients with atypical pain. Ingestion of oral contrast media is necessary for the examination.

Investigations

Investigations that are useful in the diagnosis of appendicitis are given in Box 22.1.

Differential diagnosis

Diagnosis of appendicitis is particularly difficult with a retrocaecal appendicitis. The pain is not as severe as that associated with abdominal or pelvic appendicitis and the pain rarely localises well to the right iliac fossa. The pain vaguely localises to the right side of the abdomen and rarely to the right flank or right upper quadrant. In neglected cases, a retrocaecal abscess develops as a result of perforation of the appendix.

Diagnosis in the elderly is often delayed because of late and less typical presentation. The incidence of perforation is therefore higher. Most elderly patients have fever and right-sided abdominal tenderness at presentation.

During pregnancy the appendix may be displaced, cephaled by the gravid uterus. In the second trimester of pregnancy, the appendix is displaced upwards to the right upper flank. Appendicitis may be confused with pyelonephritis, as pyuria is common during pregnancy. Owing to abdominal laxity, the abdominal findings are also less acute. Mild leucocytosis is also a normal physiological response in pregnancy.

Mesenteric adenitis

About 5% of patients undergoing an appendicectomy for 'acute appendicitis' are found to have mesenteric adenitis. The patient has clinical features similar to those of appendicitis; however, the appendix is normal and there are several enlarged lymph nodes in the mesentery of the terminal ileum.

The condition is most common in children. Some have a history of a recent sore throat together with a high fever. There is no muscle rigidity on presentation. The cause of the illness is obscure but is self-limiting, with spontaneous improvement over 24–36 hours.

At surgery, the appendix should be removed to avoid future confusion because a right iliac fossa incision is present.

Gynaecological conditions

Mittelschmerz pain occurs at mid-menstrual cycle from the rupture of a follicle at ovulation. Fever is uncommon and most patients have had previous painful ovulation.

In pelvic inflammatory disease, including salpingitis and tubo-ovarian abscess, there is a longer duration of symptoms, higher fever, greater leucocytosis and more pelvic pain. Gonococcal and chlamydial infection are the most common causes. Careful gynaecological history and examination are helpful.

Torsion of a fallopian tube and torsion or haemorrhage of an ovarian cyst tend to present with pain of sudden onset. Pelvic examination and ultrasound will help with the diagnosis.

Urological conditions

Urinary tract infection presents with urinary symptoms and rigors. Lack of abdominal rigidity and presence of pus and organisms in the urine indicate the diagnosis.

Right ureteric colic may cause confusion but the radiation of pain and haematuria should give the diagnosis.

Other conditions

Bacterial or viral gastroenteritis causes vomiting, profuse diarrhoea and diffuse abdominal pain without localised tenderness. Diarrhoea associated with appendicitis is rarely prolonged or severe. Non-specific ileitis may be secondary to *Yersinia* or *Campylobacter* infection.

Perforated caecal carcinoma with a pericolic abscess may mimic appendicitis, but the patients are usually elderly.

Acute cholecystitis may be confused with a high retrocaecal appendicitis.

Diverticulitis of a long redundant sigmoid colon lying on the right of midline may cause confusion. Rarely, a solitary caecal diverticulum becomes inflamed; this is usually seen in Asian patients.

Meckel's diverticulitis is rare and the diagnosis is usually made at surgery.

Management

If the diagnosis is clear, an appendicectomy is performed. If the diagnosis is suspected but not definite, a period of observation (usually in the hospital) is appropriate. Over the following 12–24 hours, the nature of the illness should clarify itself. The risk of perforation is low in the first 24 hours of symptomatic appendicitis.

Conventionally, open surgery is performed. A skin crease incision is made over the point of maximal tenderness in the right iliac fossa. Under anaesthesia, a mass may be palpable. The external and internal oblique muscles are split. The caecum is identified and the appendix is traced at its base on the posteromedial aspect. The mesoappendix is ligated and divided. The base of the appendix is ligated and transected. The appendix stump may be inverted using a purse-string in the caecum, although there is no firm evidence to suggest that this is necessary. All patients should receive prophylactic antibiotics administered preoperatively, usually in the form of a second- or third-generation cephalosporin and metronidazole. When there is severe sepsis, a full course of 5 days of therapy is recommended.

Alternatively, an appendicectomy can be performed laparoscopically. This approach has a lesser role if the diagnosis of appendicitis is firm because the conventional open approach involves only a small incision, is associated with a rapid recovery phase, and particularly incurs much less expense. Laparoscopy is helpful if the diagnosis is uncertain even after a period of observation and helps to diagnose pelvic inflammatory disease.

Patients presenting late may have a right iliac fossa mass. A computed tomography (CT) scan is performed to determine whether it is an abscess or a phlegmon. If an abscess is present, it is drained percutaneously under CT guidance. This obviates the need for surgery in most cases in patients with active sepsis. An appendiceal phlegmon is treated with bowel rest and intravenous antibiotics. Non-operative therapy is successful in 85% of cases and most patients are sent home after 7–10 days.

Because the risk of recurrent sepsis is about 25%, interval appendicectomy is generally performed 6–8 weeks after resolution of the acute illness. In patients older than 35 years, this is preceded by a barium enema examination or colonoscopy.

Meckel's diverticulum

Meckel's diverticulum is a congenital condition that arises from failure of embryonic obliteration of the omphalomesenteric duct connecting the foetal gut to the yolk sac. As distinct from other small bowel diverticula, Meckel's diverticulum is antimesenteric, contains all coats of the bowel and has its own blood supply (Fig. 22.2). It is present in 2% of the population and is commonly within 1 m of the ileocaecal valve. In 20% of cases, the mucosa contains heterotopic epithelium of gastric, colonic or pancreatic origin. Symptomatic cases are usually males.

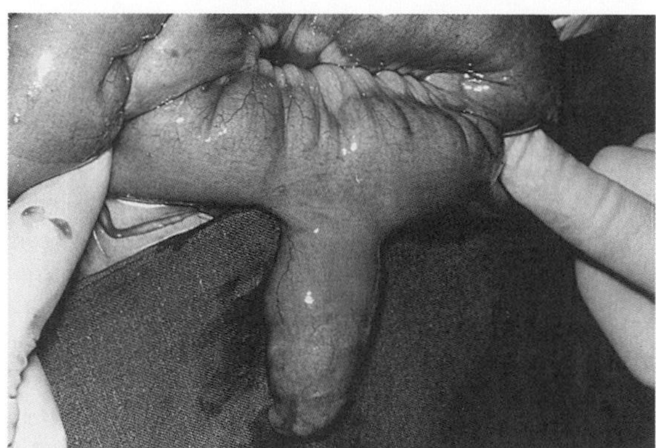

Fig. 22.2 Meckel's diverticulum.

Clinical syndromes

Bleeding peptic ulceration adjacent to ectopic gastric epithelium is found. This usually occurs in young patients.

Small bowel obstruction due to intussusception may occur. The apex of intussusception is usually the inflamed heterotopic tissue at the mouth of the diverticulum. Obstruction of the small bowel may also be caused by the presence of a band between the apex of the diverticulum and the umbilicus, causing kinking or volvulus.

Meckel's diverticulitis is usually due to lodgement of enteroliths or a sharp foreign body in the diverticulum, or narrowing of the mouth of the diverticulum. The clinical features are similar to appendicitis. Perforation may occur, causing generalised peritonitis.

Gastric heterotopia may cause peptic ulcer–like symptoms, with meal-related pain around the umbilicus because of its mid-gut location.

Diagnosis

Barium small bowel follow-through does not always demonstrate Meckel's diverticulum because the mouth of the diverticulum is often narrowed with oedema. A sodium technetium-99 m scan will localise heterotopic gastric mucosa in Meckel's diverticulum in 90% of cases.

Treatment

Complicated or symptomatic Meckel's diverticulum should be treated with resection of the diverticulum or of the involved small bowel. If diverticulectomy is performed, care is taken to remove any peptic ulcer in the adjacent ileum.

Incidental Meckel's diverticulum found at laparotomy is usually left alone because most remain asymptomatic. Any band to the umbilicus or other viscus is divided. Resection is considered in children younger than 2 years; with the presence of palpable heterotopia (especially in men); and with evidence of prior Meckel's diverticulitis, such as adhesions.

Further reading

Birnbaum BA, Wilson SR. Appendicitis at the millennium. *Radiology* 2000;215:337–348.

Schumpelick V, Dreuw B, Ophoff K, Prescher A. Appendix and caecum. Embryology, anatomy and surgical applications. *Surg Clin North Am.* 2000;80:295–318.

Sajja S, Schein M Laparoscopic appendectomy: an advance or a gimmick? *Curr Surg.* 2004 Mar–Apr;61(2):136–41.

McKinlay R, Mastrangelo MJ, Jr. Current status of laparoscopic appendectomy. *Curr Surg.* 2003 Sep–Oct;60(5):506–12.

Martin JP, Connor PD, Charles K. Meckel's diverticulum. *Am Fam Physician.* 2000;61:1037–1042.

MCQs

Select the single correct answer to each question.

1 Right iliac fossa pain and nausea in a 62-year-old woman may be due to the following EXCEPT:

a acute appendicitis
b caecal cancer
c urinary tract infection
d mittelschmerz pain
e sigmoid diverticulitis

2 The INCORRECT statement on sepsis associated with appendicectomy for acute appendicitis is:

a may present with a pelvic abscess
b may present as a wound infection
c is reduced by prophylactic peri-operative antibiotics
d is increased by laparoscopic rather than open appendicectomy
e is most often associated with anaerobic bacteria

3 The incorrect statement on Meckel's diverticulum:

a may cause small bowel obstruction due to intussusception
b may simulate acute cholecystitis
c may present with meal-related central abdominal pain
d may present with melaena and a normal upper gastrointestinal endoscopy
e may be diagnosed with a sodium technetium-99 m scan in some cases

23 Tumours of the small bowel

Joe J. Tjandra

Introduction

Neoplasms of the small bowel are unusual. Although the small bowel comprises 75% of the length of the gastrointestinal tract, less than 2% of all malignant neoplasms arise there. Small bowel tumours generally manifest with non-specific symptoms and frequently can be missed in the usual screening tests of the gastrointestinal tract.

Epidemiology

Small bowel cancers are more common in developed Western countries. The incidence of small bowel malignancy is about 1.5 cases per 100 000 population. There is no racial predilection for adenocarcinoma, although lymphoma is more common in Caucasians.

Clinical presentation

The peak incidence occurs in the 60–70 years age group. Small bowel neoplasms occur with equal frequency in men and women. They usually present insidiously with non-specific and intermittent symptoms (Table 23.1). Malignant neoplasms are less common than benign tumours, but are more likely to produce symptoms. Symptoms vary with site of origin and nature of the tumour. Diagnosis is often delayed until the disease is advanced.

Abdominal pain is the most common complaint and is related to underlying subacute bowel obstruction. The pain may be a dull ache or crampy in nature. More than 50% of patients present as emergencies with complications of the tumour. Small bowel obstruction and bleeding are the most common complications. Obstruction may be secondary to luminal narrowing, volvulus or occasionally intussusception, with the tumour acting as the lead point. When all causes are considered, small bowel tumour is an uncommon (<5%) cause of small bowel obstruction. Bleeding from small bowel tumours may be occult with symptoms due to anaemia, or occasionally overt with maroon-coloured stools. Massive haemorrhage is rare and is more likely with small bowel angioma and leiomyosarcoma. Abdominal masses are more likely with leiomyosarcoma and lymphoma than with adenocarcinoma.

Table 23.1 Clinical presentation of small bowel tumours

	Maligant	Benign
Weight loss	Yes	No
Abdominal pain	Yes	Yes
Small bowel obstruction	Yes	Yes
Gastrointestinal bleeding	Yes	Yes
Abdominal mass	Yes	Rare
Acute abdomen (perforation)	Yes	No
Miscellaneous		
Obstructive jaundice	Periampullary tumour	No
Malabsorption	Extensive lymphomas	No
Carcinoid syndrome	Carcinoid tumours	No
Asymptomatic	Rare	Yes

Diagnosis

When more common causes for small bowel obstruction, such as adhesion or external hernia, are absent a small bowel tumour should be considered. Plain abdominal radiograph will confirm a small bowel obstruction. In patients with partial or subacute small bowel obstruction, barium studies may be diagnostic. Enteroclysis or a barium small bowel enema is more sensitive than a standard barium small bowel series. An enteroclysis study is performed by first passing an intestinal tube through the stomach into the duodenum or jejunum. Dilute barium is then slowly and steadily infused. This technique provides excellent visualisation of the small bowel mucosa. Computed tomography (CT) with oral contrast may show the extraluminal extent and nodal or liver metastases, thereby aiding the pre-operative staging. Upper gastrointestinal endoscopy is diagnostic of duodenal neoplasms. Capsule enteroscopy provides excellent images of the stomach, duodenum and small bowel. It involves swallowing a small camera which relays digitised images to a computer recorder over an 8-hour duration. Push enteroscopy can visualise the proximal small bowel but is no more sensitive than a capsule endoscopy.

In patients with anaemia secondary to occult gastrointestinal bleeding, small bowel barium studies are the best way to diagnose a small bowel tumour. If bleeding is massive, mesenteric angiography will localise the bleeding site if the rate of bleeding is faster than 0.5 mL/min. Radiolabelled red blood cell scans are useful if the bleeding is less severe or is intermittent. Upper gastrointestinal endoscopy and colonoscopy are helpful to exclude gastroduodenal and colonic sources of haemorrhage. Despite these investigations, the diagnosis of small bowel tumour is made at operation in most patients.

Management

The management of small bowel tumours is surgical. Details of management depend on the pathology of the tumour.

Benign tumours

Most benign tumours are relatively asymptomatic and are undiagnosed until autopsy. Benign tumours arise from any of the endothelial or mesenchymal cells within the bowel wall (Table 23.2). Leiomyomas, adenomas and lipomas are most common.

Table 23.2 Tumours of the small bowel, in order of frequency

Benign	Maligant
Leiomyoma	Adenocarcinoma
Adenoma	Carcinoid tumour
Lipoma	Lymphoma
Hamartoma (Peutz–Jeghers syndrome)	Leiomyosarcoma
Haemangioma	
Neurogenic	
Fibroma	
Lymphangioma	

Leiomyoma

Leiomyoma occurs most frequently in the jejunum as a firm, grey–white lesion. Histologically, it contains well-differentiated smooth muscle cells without mitoses. Radiographically, it appears as a smooth filling defect with intact mucosa. It enlarges extraluminally and may cause obstruction or intussusception. Treatment requires simple segmental resection.

Adenoma

Villous adenoma of the small bowel occurs most frequently in the duodenum, especially in the periampullary region. It has the same malignant potential as villous adenoma of the colon. There is an association with familial adenomatous polyposis (see Chapter 24). A large periampullary villous adenoma may bleed or cause duodenal or biliary obstruction. The diagnosis is confirmed by gastroduodenoscopy and biopsy. If the pre-operative evaluation suggests that the lesion is benign, a duodenotomy is made and a local submucosal excision is performed. With more extensive tumours, a formal pancreaticoduodenectomy (Whipple's operation) may be required. Lesions in the third or fourth part of the duodenum are treated with segmental resection.

Tubular adenoma is also most common in the duodenum. It is usually asymptomatic and is amenable to endoscopic polypectomy. It has a very low malignant potential. Brunner's gland adenoma is hyperplasia of the exocrine glands of the first portion of the duodenum. Most are asymptomatic and are found incidentally.

Lipoma

Lipoma arises from submucosal fat and usually occurs in the distal ileum. Computed tomography can confirm the diagnosis by defining the density of the lesion. Lipoma has no predisposition to malignancy. Excision is performed only if the lesion is symptomatic.

Peutz–Jeghers syndrome

This condition is discussed in Chapter 24.

Malignant tumours

There are four major types of malignant small bowel tumour: adenocarcinoma, carcinoid tumour, lymphoma and leiomyosarcoma (Table 23.3). Tumours metastatic to small bowel may also mimic primary small bowel tumours.

Adenocarcinoma

Pathology

This neoplasm occurs with decreasing frequency from duodenum to ileum. Within the duodenum, two-thirds occur in the periampullary region. By contrast, adenocarcinoma associated with Crohn's disease is most common in distal ileum.

Clinical features

Adenocarcinoma of the small bowel may be associated with Crohn's disease, familial adenomatous polyposis and adult coeliac disease. It occurs in patients in the sixth or seventh decade. On gastrointestinal contrast study, the lesion may appear as an apple-core defect with mucosal ulceration. Sometimes, the diagnosis is made only at laparotomy for small bowel obstruction of unknown cause.

Adenocarcinoma of the duodenum is diagnosed by endoscopic examination with biopsy. As surgical treatment for duodenal lesions may be extensive, pre-operative staging with CT is performed. In periampullary lesions, endoscopic retrograde cholangiopancreatography to delineate biliary and pancreatic involvement is helpful.

Management

Surgical management is determined by the location of the tumour. Unless the disease is extensive and disseminated, surgical exploration is indicated in most patients. The extent of the disease is evaluated intraoperatively. Wide segmental small bowel resection including the draining of the mesenteric lymph nodes is performed. However, resection of involved mesenteric lymph nodes should not be unduly extensive as it may jeopardise the viability of the remaining normal small bowel. Extensive lymph node metastases are associated with a poor outcome. Distal ileal lesions are managed by a right hemicolectomy and ileotransverse anastomosis. Even in advanced disease with hepatic metastases, palliative small bowel resection is performed to prevent bleeding or obstruction. If the disease is locally advanced and unresectable, a side-to-side enteroenteric bypass is performed.

For most duodenal lesions, pancreaticoduodenectomy (Whipple's operation) is the treatment of choice. Presence of lymph node metastases in the field of surgery is not a contraindication for resection. For small lesions affecting the first or fourth portions of the duodenum, segmental resection may be performed. In patients with unresectable duodenal adenocarcinoma, gastrojejunostomy and biliary stenting or bypass will provide palliation.

There is no proven value for radiotherapy or chemotherapy in the adjuvant or palliative setting.

Outcome

Overall prognosis is poor because of the advanced state of presentation. Overall 5-year survival averages 20%. Without nodal metastases, survival improves to 60%.

Table 23.3 Malignant tumours of the small bowel

Tumour type	Overall (%)	Duodenum (%)	Jejunum (%)	Ileum (%)
Adenocarcinoma	40	40	40	20
Carcinoid tumour	30	10	40	50
Lymphoma	20	10	10	80
Leiomyosarcoma	10	Rare	40	60

Carcinoid tumour

Pathology

Carcinoid tumours arise from enterochromaffin cells of the gastrointestinal tract. These pleuripotential, neuroendocrine cells are part of the amine precursor uptake and decarboxylation (APUD) system and can synthesise vasoactive amines and regulatory peptides. The majority (85%) of all carcinoids occur in the appendix. The small bowel (usually distal ileum) is the next most common site and, overall, 30% are multicentric.

The tumours have a characteristic yellow–orange colour and are usually small (<2 cm) and submucosal. These tumours have a variable malignant potential. They may cause an intense desmoplastic reaction in the mesentery, probably from local release of serotonin, with secondary mesenteric ischaemia and infarction or kinking of small bowel with subsequent obstruction.

Clinical features

Most appendiceal and many small bowel carcinoids remain asymptomatic. Appendiceal carcinoid tumours follow a very benign clinical course and are usually diagnosed following appendicectomy. Appendiceal carcinoids less than 2 cm in size require no therapy other than appendicectomy. Tumours larger than 2 cm require a right hemicolectomy to resect the draining lymph nodes.

Some small bowel carcinoids are more aggressive. Symptoms arise from the primary tumour itself or from the metastatic disease (anorexia, weight loss, lethargy or carcinoid syndrome). Diagnosis of carcinoid tumours necessitates a high index of suspicion. Barium small bowel series may show tethering of distal ileal loops without visualising the tumour itself. Computed tomography may show mesenteric nodal metastases or hepatic metastases. The operative management includes a segmental resection of the small bowel, *en bloc* mesenteric resection and primary anastomosis. Careful inspection for synchronous lesions should be performed because 30% are multicentric. Even with extensive disease, palliative resection will help to debulk the disease and often delay the occurrence of carcinoid syndrome. Lymphadenectomy will also prevent the desmoplastic reaction in the mesentery. Solitary or isolated liver metastases are resected if, technically, it is simple to perform and there are no contraindicating co-morbid factors.

Carcinoid syndrome

Carcinoid syndrome is thought to be caused by the release of vasoactive substances into the systemic circulation. The pharmacology of the mediators remains uncertain. Bradykinin, serotonin, tachykinins (substance P, neuromedin A), histamine, dopamine and prostaglandins may act in concert. For carcinoid syndrome to occur from gastrointestinal primary tumours, hepatic metastases must be present. The carcinoid syndrome may also be seen in carcinoid tumours of the lung, testis and ovary, where venous drainage allows systemic circulation of the vasoactive substances directly.

Classic clinical features include diarrhoea, flushing of the face and upper trunk, which lasts seconds or a few minutes, and bronchospasm. Symptoms may be precipitated by foods, alcohol or emotional stress. Venous telangiectasias, pellagra (dementia, dermatitis, diarrhoea) and right-sided endocardial valvular fibrosis may develop in reaction to circulating vasoactive amines. Progress to tricuspid insufficiency, pulmonary stenosis and, ultimately, right-sided heart failure may occur. The carcinoid crisis is a rare life-threatening event involving intense flushing, severe diarrhoea, cardiovascular abnormalities (tachycardia, arrhythmias, hypertension or hypotension) and central nervous system problems that range from dizziness to coma.

Treatment of carcinoid syndrome is aimed at symptomatic relief. The synthetic somatostatin analogue, sandostatin, is the most effective therapy. It improves cutaneous flushing and diarrhoea. Improvement is sustained in 30% of patients for up to 2.5 years. Chemotherapy may also be used. Modest responses to doxorubicin, 5-fluorouracil or streptozotocin are obtained in 20% of patients. Chemotherapy is more effective if combined with hepatic artery ligation. Debulking of hepatic metastases has a short-lived response. Liver transplantation is still experimental.

Outcome

Carcinoid tumours are slow growing. Many patients live for prolonged periods despite distant metastases. After curative resection of localised intestinal carcinoid tumour, survival is equivalent to that for the the general population. Following resectable nodal metastases, median survival is 15 years. With non-resectable intestinal disease or liver metastases, survivals are 5 and 3 years, respectively.

Lymphoma

Pathology

Lymphoma of the small bowel arises either as a primary gastrointestinal tumour or as a manifestation of generalised lymphomatous disease. With primary gastrointestinal lymphoma, mesenteric lymph node involvement is limited to the area of involved bowel, white blood cell count is normal and there is no peripheral or mediastinal lymphadenopathy or splenomegaly. In Western countries, gastric lymphomas are most common, followed by small bowel lymphomas.

Clinical features

Small bowel lymphoma usually presents in the fifth decade and is multifocal in 15% of cases. Patients with Crohn's disease, coeliac disease or immunosuppressive diseases such as AIDS are susceptible to gastrointestinal lymphomas. Small bowel lymphomas predominate in the ileum. Most are intermediate or high-grade non-Hodgkin's B-cell lymphomas. T-cell varieties occur sporadically or with coeliac disease.

An abdominal mass is common. Obstruction, perforation, intussusception or haemorrhage occurs in 25% of patients. Malabsorption from diffuse mucosal involvement occurs occasionally. Small bowel contrast studies may suggest the presence of a tumour mass and CT may reveal bulky mesenteric nodes associated with thickened bowel or a large mass. Percutaneous cytology is not adequate for characterising the lymphoma, although core biopsies are more helpful.

Management

Management includes diagnosis, staging, resection or debulking, and treatment of complications. Liver biopsy and sampling of nodes outside the field of resection are important, although splenectomy is not indicated. In patients with localised disease, resection of the involved bowel with a wide margin of adjacent mesentery is performed. Resection of primary duodenal lymphomas is controversial; Whipple resections have a high morbidity and mortality rate. Without surgery, perforation and bleeding occur in 20% of patients during combined radiation and chemotherapy. Adjuvant multi-drug chemotherapy regimens containing adriamycin are often offered after curative resection, on the premise that lymphomas are systemic diseases. With advanced disease, debulking or palliative resection is performed to prevent complications of bleeding or perforation, provided excessive removal of normal small bowel is avoided. If resection is not possible, tissue is obtained for histological diagnosis and classification, the extent of tumour is staged and an enteric bypass is performed to prevent obstruction. Responses to chemotherapy and radiotherapy are variable and short-lived but are dramatic in some patients.

Outcome

Outcome depends on the stage of disease. With 'curative' resection for localised disease, 5-year survival is 80%. With more advanced disease, the prognosis is much less favourable and depends on response to chemotherapy.

Leiomyosarcoma

Pathology

Leiomyosarcoma arise from the smooth muscle cells of the small bowel. They are often encapsulated and subserosal in location. They often grow to a large size before causing symptoms.

Clinical features

An abdominal mass is evident in 50% of patients. As these highly vascular tumours reach a large size, necrosis within the tumour may cause haemorrhage or, less commonly, perforation. Small bowel obstruction may result from intussusception or from extramural and mural compression. Barium small bowel studies often show extrinsic compression of the small bowel and CT shows a large, extraluminal mass with central necrosis.

Management

Surgical resection is the key treatment. Frozen section is unreliable in determining the malignancy of these tumours. Thus, all tumours of smooth muscle origin, whether they are thought to be benign or malignant, should be treated similarly with adequate surgical resection. In tumours of the distal duodenum and the remainder of the small bowel, segmental resection with primary anastomosis is the treatment of choice. As leiomyosarcoma tends to spread haematogenously, an extended lymphadenectomy is not necessary. Fifteen per cent of patients do have metastatic involvement of mesenteric lymph nodes. Resection of duodenal lesions requires pancreaticoduodenectomy because of the bulky tumour size. Both radiotherapy and chemotherapy are of little benefit.

Outcome

Prognosis depends on the stage of the disease and histological grade. Histological grade is determined by cellularity, nuclear atypia and number of mitoses. Survival at 5 years after curative resection for low-grade tumour approaches 60%, but with high-grade lesions survival is less than 20%. Distant metastases (lung, liver, bone) are present in 30% of patients at presentation. Palliative resection of small bowel leiomyosarcoma in this situation is worthwhile and may be associated with 5 years' survival in as many as 20%.

Further reading

Burkard PG. Mucosa-associated lymphoid tissue and other gastrointestinal lymphomas. *Curr Opin Gastroenterol.* 2000;16:107–112.

Martini C, Sturniolo GC, De Carlo E, et al. Neuroendocrine tumor of small bowel. *Gastrointest Endosc.* 2004 Sep;60(3):431.

Joensuu H, Kindblom LG. Gastrointestinal stromal tumors–a review. *Acta Orthop Scand Suppl.* 2004 Apr;75(311):62–71.

Rosch T. DDW Report 2004 New Orleans: Capsule Endoscopy. *Endoscopy.* 2004 Sep;36(9):763–9.

MCQs

Select the single correct answer to each question.

1 Adenocarcinoma of the small bowel is most commonly associated with:

a familial adenomatous polyposis
b tuberculosis of the small bowel
c lymphoma
d prolonged use of cytotoxic chemotherapy for breast cancer
e ulcerative colitis

2 Carcinoid tumour of the appendix is associated with the following features EXCEPT:

a most are asymptomatic
b tumours less than 2 cm in size require no further therapy other than appendicectomy
c it is always malignant
d carcinoid syndrome arises when hepatic metastases have occurred
e synchronous carcinoid tumour in the distal ileum may be present

24 Colorectal cancer and adenoma

Joe J. Tjandra

Introduction

Cancer of the colon and rectum is the most common internal cancer in the Western world. It is the second most common cause of death from cancer after lung cancer. The prognosis for colorectal cancer is relatively good compared with that for other solid tumours such as lung cancer and stomach cancer. Improvement in outcome has come from meticulous surgical techniques and more sophisticated medical management. Endorectal ultrasound has enabled a more precise staging of low rectal cancer and has allowed stratification of surgical treatment. Excision of the rectum and anus and a permanent colostomy is now rarely performed. Early trials of adjuvant therapy offer possibilities for further reduction in deaths from cancer recurrence. Strategies for mass screening for polyps and cancers are yet to be finalised but may further reduce mortality from colorectal cancers.

Epidemiology

Rectal cancers are twice as common in men, and right-sided cancers are more common in women. For the rest of the large bowel, the incidence is almost equal between the sexes. Colorectal cancers are common in the urban Western world but rare in Asia, Africa and most of South America. The lifetime risk for colorectal cancer is 1 in 18 for men and 1 in 28 for women, but its occurrence under 50 years of age is very low. After that age, the incidence increases rapidly. The peak incidence is in the seventh decade, some 5–10 years later than the peak for adenoma.

Aetiology

Epidemiological studies suggest that environmental factors predominate in the causation of most large bowel cancers. A diet rich in fat and meat, and low in fibre, is commonly associated with colorectal cancers. Dietary fibre increases the bulk of stool by retaining water and decreases the colonic transit time in most people. Fibre alters the colonic bacterial flora and absorbs luminal toxins. The net result is to reduce the carcinogenic capacity of the luminal contents. A number of minor dietary constituents may also inhibit carcinogenesis. These include beta-carotene, selenium and vitamins C and E.

Other risk factors for colorectal cancer are listed in Box 24.1.

Pathology

The outcome of colorectal cancer depends on its biological behaviour. More aggressive cancers may present with a shorter history and are advanced at the time of presentation. The clinicopathological stage (thus the amount of spread) of the disease is a 'snapshot' in the life of a cancer; together with the histopathological features, it provides the most accurate prognostic index at the moment. Other phenotypic features, as yet unidentified, may provide further prognostic information.

Staging

The most common staging methods are Dukes' classification (Table 24.1) and its various derivatives, including the Australian clinicopathological staging (ACPS),

Box 24.1 Risk factors for colorectal cancer

- Adenomatous polyps. Most if not all cancers originate within an adenoma. However, most adenomas do not become malignant.
- Genetic factors. Familial adenomatous polyposis syndromes (FAP); hereditary non-polyposis colon cancer (HNPCC); other polyposis syndromes such as Peutz–Jegher's syndrome and juvenile polyposis.
- Family history. Individuals with a family history of colorectal cancer or large (>1cm) adenoma have an increased risk of developing colorectal cancer. The risk is increased twofold if one first-degree relative is diagnosed with colorectal cancer at age 55 or older, rising to sixfold if the age at which diagnosis of cancer is made is less than 55 years or if two first-degree relatives are diagnosed with colorectal cancer at any age.
- Inflammatory bowel disease. Ulcerative colitis, Crohn's colitis when the disease is longstanding and extensive.
- Irradiation. The risk of rectal cancer is increased following radiation therapy for cancer of the cervix. These cancers may appear 10–20 years later.
- Surgical procedures. Ureterosigmoidostomy was used at one time for urinary diversion. This is associated with colon cancer at the site of ureterocolic anastomosis and may be related to the effect of toxic compounds excreted in the urine, upon the colonic mucosa.
- Cholecystectomy. This is associated with an increased risk of right colon cancer, probably from increased delivery of bile acids to the colon.

or the Union Internationale Centre Cancer (UICC) TNM classification.

Dukes' staging has the attraction of its simplicity but it is relatively imprecise because several important prognostic factors are not included. These include the depth of cancer penetration, the extent of spread outside the bowel, the number of lymph nodes involved and the presence of distant metastases. Patients with Dukes' C cancers are more likely to have occult liver metastases than B or A cancers.

Histopathology

Poorly differentiated cancers have a worse outlook than those that are well to moderately differentiated. Other adverse features include lymphovascular or perineural invasion and a histology of signet ring, mucinous and small cell cancers.

Table 24.1 Staging methods for colorectal cancer

Modified Dukes' Staging	
A	Tumour confined to bowel wall
B	Tumour invading through serosa
B_1	Through muscularis propria
B_2	Through serosa or perirectal fat
C	Lymph node involvement
C_1	Apical node clear
C_2	Apical node involved
UICC TNM Staging	
Tumour depth (T)	
T_1	Submucosa
T_2	Muscularis propria
T_3	Subserosa or pericolic tissues
T_4	Invade adjacent organs or visceral peritoneum
Nodes (N)	
N_0	Nodes not involved
N_1	1–3 pericolic nodes involved
N_2	$\geq$4 pericolic nodes involved
Metastasis (M)	
M_0	No distant metastases
M_1	Distant metastases
Stage I	$T_{1,2}$ N_0
Stage II	$T_{3,4}$ N_0
Stage III	$T_{1–4}$ $N_{1,2}$
Stage IV	M_1

Other characteristics

The anatomic site of the cancer has an influence on the outcome. Rectal cancers tend to have a better outcome than colonic cancers because of earlier detection. However, there is a higher incidence of local recurrence in rectal cancer from technical failure in radical removal of the tissues at risk. Stage for stage, right-sided colonic cancers tend to have a better prognosis than left-sided cancers.

Prognosis

Tumour stage is the main determinant (Table 24.2) of prognosis. The survival of patients with Dukes' A

Table 24.2 Prognosis in colorectal cancer

Stage	5-Year survival (%) Colon cancer	Rectal cancer
Dukes' A	99	90
Dukes' B	80	60
Dukes' C	50	40
Distant metastases	10	10

cancers after adequate resection is similar to that of the general population of similar age. Patients with superficial cancers confined to the submucosa will be cured by adequate surgery. The adverse prognostic effects of lymph node metastases are dependent on their number and extent. While metastatic disease may develop somewhat later than for other solid tumours, such as breast or lung cancer, few develop metastases beyond 5–10 years after surgical resection of the primary disease. The majority (85%) of patients with liver metastases die within 1 year of diagnosis.

Clinical presentation

The clinical presentations vary with the primary site and extent of disease. About 50% of cancers occur at the rectosigmoid junction or in the rectum.

Caecal and right-sided carcinoma

Caecal and right-sided carcinoma account for 20% of all large bowel cancers. Clinical presentations include:
- Insidious onset of iron deficiency anaemia from occult faecal blood loss. This is the most common finding.
- Distal ileal obstruction. As the faecal content entering the caecum is liquid, this is a relatively late presentation.
- Palpable right iliac fossa mass.
- Lethargy or fever of unknown origin. These symptoms are due to a small occult, localised perforation or from tumour burden. Metastases tend to be more aggressive and grow more rapidly than the primary tumour. Ischaemic infarction and necrosis may occur in the metastases, producing pain, fever and malaise.
- Acute appendicitis. This occasionally develops following occlusion of the appendiceal orifice by caecal cancer.

Left-sided and sigmoid carcinoma

By the time the stool reaches the left colon, it becomes harder because most of the fluid is absorbed. The diagnosis is sometimes confused with irritable bowel syndrome or diverticular disease. Common clinical presentations include:
- Alteration of bowel habit: constipation alternating with diarrhoea.
- Lower abdominal colic, distension and a desire to defecate.
- Passage of altered blood and sometimes mucus. Rectal bleeding is usually intermittent, with a small amount of dark blood mixed with the stool.
- A palpable mass in the left side of the abdomen.

Complications of colon cancer

Large bowel obstruction with abdominal distension is more common with right-sided cancers. The caecum becomes very distended and tender. If the ileocaecal valve is incompetent, the obstructed large bowel decompresses into the small bowel, producing a mixed clinical picture of large and small bowel obstruction.

Local invasion into the lateral abdominal wall or a loop of small bowel may occur, producing either a small bowel obstruction or an ileocolic fistula with severe diarrhoea. Sigmoid cancers may invade the bladder to form a colovesical fistula. Patients present with recurrent urinary tract infection, haematuria and later with pneumaturia and faecaluria. Other organs that may be invaded include the uterus and ovaries.

Rectal cancer

Rectal cancers generally cause symptoms early in their course and the tumours are accessible to digital examination or rigid sigmoidoscopy. However, the diagnosis is often delayed because the symptoms are attributed to haemorrhoids or anal fissure. There is a general reluctance of both the patients and primary care physicians to undertake anorectal examination. Clinical presentations include:
- Rectal bleeding. The blood may be dark and mixed with stool or bright and quite separate from the faeces.
- Changes in bowel habit, such as frequent bowel movement or mucous diarrhoea. Passage of potassium-rich mucus and resultant hypokalaemia is particularly associated with a large villous adenoma, often with malignant foci.

- Tenesmus or a continuous urge to defecate is indicative of a large rectal neoplasm, causing a fullness in the rectum.
- Anal and perineal pain, initially on defecation and later continuous, occurs with low rectal cancer invading the anal sphincters. Sacral pain, sometimes radiating down the legs, results from tumour invasion of the sacrum and sacral nerve plexus.

Metastatic disease

Local transcoelomic spread within the peritoneal cavity may produce an ascites rich in protein. Sometimes a chylous ascites results from obstruction of the lymphatics by widespread peritoneal seeding. A Sister Marie Joseph nodule may develop at the umbilicus from tumour infiltration.

Liver metastases are quite asymptomatic in the early stages. Initially, hepatomegaly, vague hepatic pain and later jaundice may ensue. Lung metastases may produce a persistent cough. Bone marrow infiltration may produce leucoerythroblastic anaemia.

Clinical assessment

A careful history and physical examination remain the most important assessment with regard to the diagnosis, the extent of spread and the patient's fitness for surgery. An estimation of the nutritional state preoperatively is also important. Digital rectal examination is important in order to feel for a rectal mass, its location and relationship to the anal sphincters, its fixity to adjacent structures and to feel for any enlarged extrarectal nodule.

A proctosigmoidoscopic examination of the rectum and anus should follow. Rigid sigmoidoscopy allows examination of the rectum without any bowel preparation. The mucosa, faeces, blood and mucus are examined in their natural state. A flexible sigmoidoscopy allows examination of the rectum, the sigmoid colon and a variable portion of the left colon with comfort.

Investigations

Faecal occult blood

Two main types of tests are available.

- Guaiac tests (Hemoccult, Hemoccult SENSA), based on the pseudoperoxidase activity of haematin, a degradation product of haemoglobin, to produce a blue colour on the test strip.
- Immunochemical tests (HemeSelect, Hemolex) use antibodies to human haemoglobin.

The traditional guaiac tests will detect 40–80% of asymptomatic colorectal cancer, especially left-sided cancer. Dietary restrictions are necessary (not with immunochemical tests) to prevent a false positive result. Red meat, melons, horse-radish, vitamin C and non-steroidal inflammatory drugs must be avoided for 3 days before testing. Ninety-eight per cent of healthy subjects (specificity) will test negative for faecal occult blood. In general, the greater the sensitivity, the lower the specificity of the test.

The newer guaiac tests and immunochemical tests are more sensitive. They may detect 80% of cancers at an earlier stage than those diagnosed at the time when symptoms occur. They will be positive in 70% of patients with adenomas larger than 1 cm. The specificity is lower than that of guaiac tests.

In general, faecal occult blood testing is used for screening asymptomatic individuals and not for investigating symptoms. A positive faecal occult blood test must be followed by further investigation of the entire colon and rectum.

Colonoscopy or barium enema

Colonoscopy enables a detailed study of the entire colon, visualising lesions of less than 0.5 cm. Any lesion visualised may be biopsied and small polyps may be removed by cautery. Colonoscopy is more involved than a barium enema as sedation is needed and there is a small risk of perforation.

Double-contrast barium enema provides good anatomical information of the colon and any lesion seen (Fig. 24.1). However, detection of small lesions and mucosal abnormalities such as inflammation is much more limited than colonoscopy. Any abnormality identified by barium enema often needs confirmation by colonoscopy and biopsy. A sigmoidoscopy is a mandatory adjunct to barium enema as the rectum is not well visualised in barium enema.

In most specialist colorectal centres, the first-line test is a colonoscopy. Barium enema is performed if the colonoscopy is incomplete owing to anatomical or pathological factors.

Endorectal ultrasound

A rigid endorectal ultrasound probe is a new but established method of assessing the depth of penetration

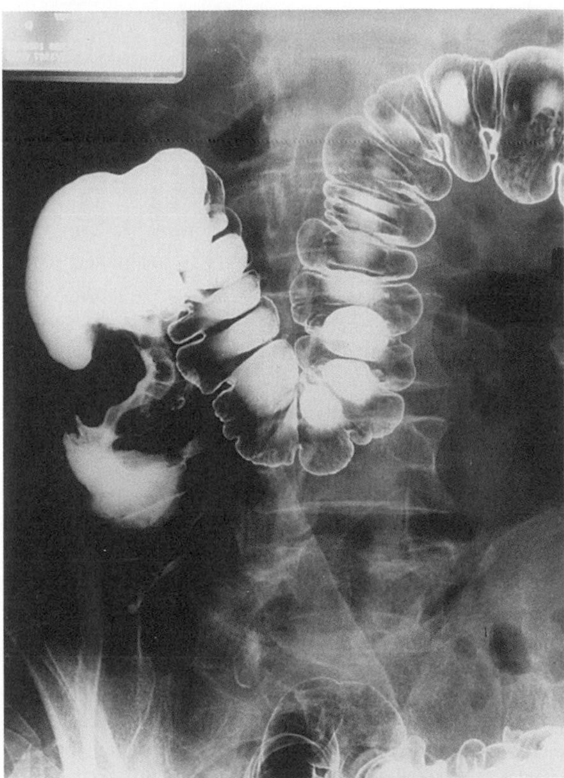

Fig. 24.1 Double contrast barium enema showing a cancer in the ascending colon.

of a rectal tumour through the bowel wall (Fig. 24.2). Enlarged mesorectal lymph nodes can be identified, although confirmation of nodal metastases is less reliable. The test is performed as an outpatient procedure without any sedation or bowel preparation. While the test is simple, it is best performed by a colorectal specialist with a detailed knowledge of the rectum and anal canal.

This improved diagnostic information is helpful in planning a transanal local excision of an early-stage rectal tumour and sometimes when choosing between an abdominoperineal excision of the rectum and an ultra-low anterior resection. A locally advanced rectal cancer may benefit from pre-operative adjuvant chemoradiotherapy.

Computed tomography, ultrasound or magnetic resonance imaging

Either computed tomography (CT) or ultrasound may be used to screen for intra-abdominal metastases, although CT scan (Fig. 24.3) tends to provide more

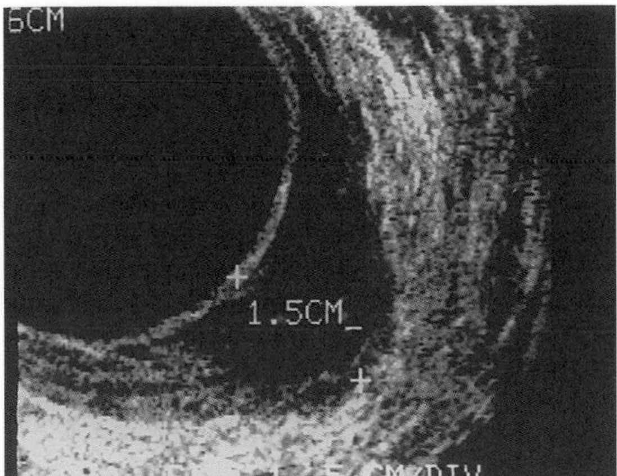

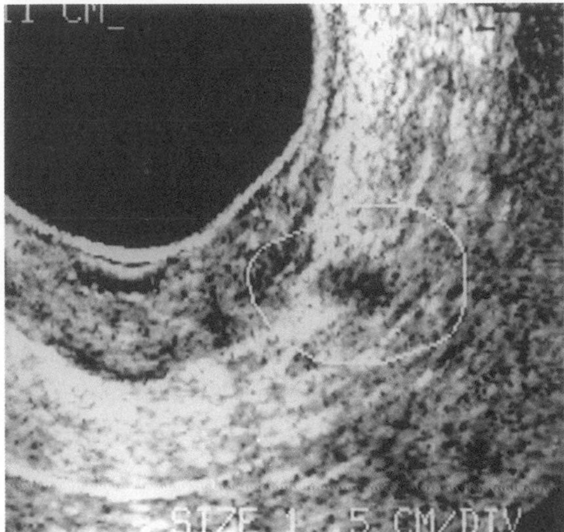

Fig. 24.2 Endorectal ultrasound showing (A) tumour invasion through the muscular wall to the perirectal fat, T3 and (B) an enlarged lymph node in the mesorectum.

information than an ultrasound. Routine screening for distant metastases by CT scan or ultrasound incurs significant costs and has not been shown to alter the outcome significantly. Pre-operative CT scan or ultrasound should be reserved for patients in whom distant metastases are suspected, or in the elderly and frail when a less radical surgical treatment may be justified. Magnetic resonance imaging (MRI) is helpful in defining the extent of loco-regional invasion of rectal cancer.

Intra-operative hepatic ultrasound

This is useful in detecting secondary liver deposits and locating their site in the anatomic segments of the liver. It helps in assessment of the resectability of

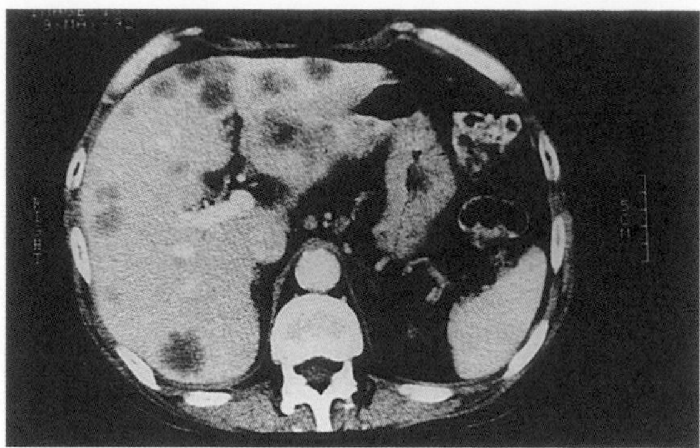

Fig. 24.3 Computed tomography scan of the abdomen showing multiple metastases in both the right and left lobes of the liver.

liver metastases and in planning the extent of liver resection. Intra-operative hepatic ultrasound is more sensitive than transabdominal ultrasonography and complements pre-operative CT scan.

Carcinoembryonic antigen

Carcinoembryonic antigen (CEA) is a non-specific, circulating, tumour-associated antigen in colorectal cancer. It has little diagnostic value but has a limited use in the follow-up after resection for cancer. While a rise in CEA may antedate clinical recurrence, the practice of routine CEA monitoring has not affected the cancer-related mortality significantly, because of limitations by its sensitivity and specificity.

Treatment

The principle of potential surgical cure demands that the cancer be excised with an adequate margin of surrounding tissue and lymphovascular clearance. It is rare for a cancer to spread up or down the bowel as much as 2 cm from the primary unless it is a mucinous or undifferentiated tumour. Distal spread exceeds 2 cm in less than 3% of patients. Most of these patients are Dukes' C cases with high-grade malignancy. A large segment of the colon (up to 10–15 cm) is usually resected because of the extent of lymphovascular clearance.

For rectal tumours, less of the bowel is removed to allow restoration of bowel continuity. A 5 cm margin of clearance is usually preferred, although as little as 2 cm may be taken for a small mid-rectal tumour. Spread is equally likely into surrounding tissues such as the mesorectum. Thus, a wide lateral resection including all of the mesorectum is important for a rectal cancer.

Meticulous handling of tissues and the techniques used are more important than the material with which the anastomosis is made. The anastomosis may be stapled or hand-sewn using an inverting, interrupted technique.

A laparoscopically assisted technique is being developed. Most of the large bowel is mobilised using laparoscopic techniques. The large bowel is delivered through a small abdominal incision where the mobilisation, resection and anastomosis or stoma are completed extracorporeally by hand. Alternatively, the entire operation may be performed laparoscopically. Certain tumours, such as those in the transverse colon or distal rectum or locally advanced tumours are less amenable to laparoscopic resection. Laparoscopic colorectal surgery is technically more difficult to perform, and there is a steep learning curve. When performed expertly, patients undergoing laparoscopic resection have significant benefits with smaller and more cosmetic scars, a shorter hospital stay and much earlier return to normal activity. The oncologic outcome is similar to conventional open surgery. However the success of laparoscopic colorectal surgery is very dependent on surgical experience; otherwise protracted long operations or conversion to open surgery after prolonged attempts at laparoscopic surgery are detrimental to patient outcome.

Peri-operative preparation

Bowel preparation

Mechanical preparation with Golytely, Fleet phosphosoda or picolax on the pre-operative day are currently the most widely used methods. Reduction of faecal load reduces both the wound and anastomotic sepsis (see Chapter 33).

In patients with partial bowel obstruction, a more gentle and prolonged bowel preparation over 2–3 days is necessary. In the more acute situation with a complete obstruction, intra-operative antegrade lavage of the colon using a small Foley catheter through the appendix stump or the distal ileum may be performed if a primary anastomosis is intended.

Antibiotic prophylaxis

Prophylactic broad-spectrum antibiotics against aerobic and anaerobic bowel pathogens have greatly reduced incidence of wound infection and intra-abdominal sepsis (see Chapter 33). While one good dose may be adequate, most clinicians would continue the prophylactic antibiotics for 24 hours post-operatively. An unnecessarily prolonged course of antibiotics is expensive, predisposes to pseudomembranous colitis and may encourage growth of antibiotic-resistant organisms.

Thromboembolism prophylaxis

Patients undergoing surgery for colorectal carcinoma have many risk factors for deep vein thrombosis. Increasing age, malignancy, immobilisation and operations of the abdomen and pelvis are all well recognised risk factors (see Chapter 1).

Colon cancer

Carcinoma of caecum or ascending colon

Right hemicolectomy is the standard operation (Fig. 24.4). The ileocolic vessels are divided at their origins while maintaining the blood supply to the residual terminal ileum. The right colic vessels and the right branch of the middle colic vessels are also removed. The amount of bowel removed is influenced by the extent of lymphovascular clearance, which, in turn, is dependent on the site of the primary colon cancer. More terminal ileum and less transverse colon may need to be removed for tumours in the caecum. Less terminal ileum and more transverse colon may be removed for cancers near the hepatic flexure.

Carcinoma of transverse colon

The blood supply to this area is derived from the middle colic vessels as well as from the right and the left colic vessels. If the cancer is at the hepatic flexure end of the transverse colon, a right hemicolectomy is performed. Lesions of the mid-transverse colon are treated by extended right hemicolectomy, which entails an anastomosis between the terminal ileum and the descending colon. The omentum is removed *en bloc* with the tumour.

A carcinoma at the splenic flexure can spread to regional lymphatics along the middle colic and left colic arteries. Thus, a more radical operation of subtotal colectomy, which allows an easy anastomosis between the terminal ileum and the sigmoid colon, is undertaken.

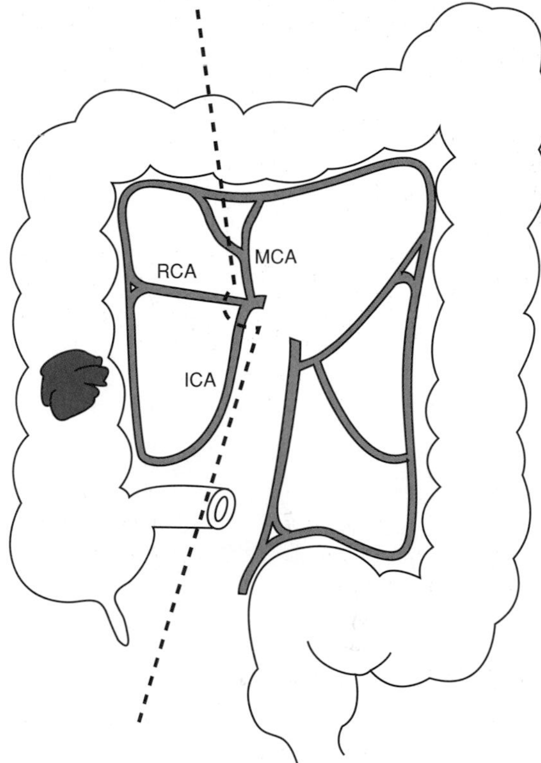

Fig. 24.4 Right hemicolectomy for ascending colon cancer. (---) Resected material; RCA, right colic artery; MCA, middle colic artery; LCA, left colic artery.

Carcinoma of descending colon

Left hemicolectomy is the operation of choice (Fig. 24.5). The inferior mesenteric artery is divided at its origin and the left colic vessels, and the sigmoid vessels are included in the resection. The anastomosis is performed between the mid-transverse colon and the upper rectum.

Carcinoma of sigmoid colon

A high anterior resection is favoured, anastomosing the mid-descending colon to the upper rectum. The inferior mesenteric artery and the left colic vessels together with the sigmoid branches are resected. If the sigmoid colon is redundant, or in a frail patient, a more limited sigmoid colectomy is performed.

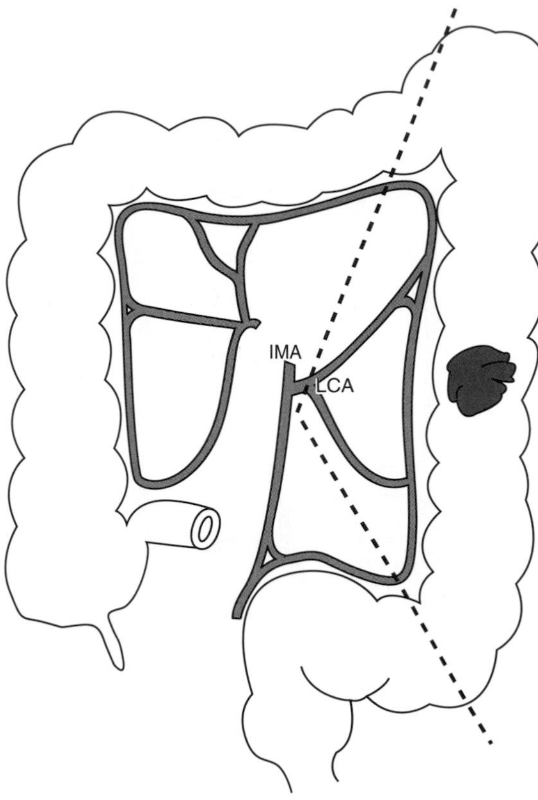

Fig. 24.5 Left hemicolectomy for descending colon cancer. (---) Resected material; IMA, inferior mesenteric artery; LCA, left colic artery.

Obstructing colon carcinoma

Obstructing carcinoma of the right and transverse colon usually can be treated by resection and primary anastomosis. The treatment of a left-sided obstruction is more controversial. A resection with or without a primary anastomosis is favoured. The surgical options include:

- Hartmann's operation: The obstructing lesion is resected. The proximal colon is brought out as a left iliac fossa colostomy and the distal bowel is oversewn or stapled closed. Re-anastomosis is established 4–6 months later.
- Subtotal colectomy and ileosigmoid or ileorectal anastomosis: This removes all the obstructed and often ischaemic colon and allows a primary anastomosis without bowel preparation. However, increased stool frequency is likely because of the more extensive resection.
- Single-stage resection with intra-operative on-table colonic lavage and a primary colorectal anastomosis: This has good results with a clinical anastomotic leak rate of 5% but is not always possible because of oedematous bowel wall.
- Proximal diverting stoma alone without resection. This is considered if the proximal colon is very dilated, if resection is hazardous and the patient is very unwell. Elective resection can be undertaken 2 weeks later.
- Colonic stent can be placed endoscopically under guidance with fluoroscopy to relieve obstruction. There is a risk of colonic perforation and stent migration. A colonic stent is generally deployed in a palliative setting.

Perforated carcinoma of the colon

Perforation is less common than obstruction and is usually via the tumour as a result of tumour necrosis. The prognosis is poor and the risk of local recurrence is high. Hartmann's operation is generally performed with *en bloc* excision of the contained perforation. The proximal end is brought out as an end colostomy and the distal end either oversewn or brought out as a mucous fistula. A primary anastomosis is generally not performed because it is more likely to leak in the presence of sepsis. The peritoneal cavity should be lavaged with saline to reduce faecal contamination.

Rectal cancer

Management of rectal cancer is challenging because of the technical expertise and clinical judgement required. About 25% of large bowel cancers develop in the rectum. Skill and judgement comes in selecting patients for restorative anterior resection, transanal local excision, abdominoperineal resection (APR) or a palliative procedure. About 30 years ago, nearly all patients with a rectal cancer were treated by an APR of the rectum and anus with a permanent left iliac fossa end colostomy. In more recent times, APR is used in less than 10% of rectal cancers.

Factors influencing choice of operation

Level of lesion

The distance of the lower edge of the tumour from the dentate line is the most important factor in the choice of operation. As a rule, a tumour that is less than 5 cm from the dentate line requires APR. A 2 cm distal margin is acceptable and may permit restorative resection in most cases without damaging the anal sphincter complex.

Nature of carcinoma

A high-grade, poorly differentiated tumour tends to be more widely infiltrative. This is best treated by rectal resection with a greater margin. Evidence of tumour invasion into the anal sphincters or fixation in the pelvis will contraindicate sphincter preservation procedures.

Patient factors

The age and medical fitness of the patient and the presence of metastases are important factors in deciding the magnitude of the operation. Pre-operative sphincter impairment usually precludes a restorative procedure.

Mesorectal lymph node status

Endorectal ultrasound examination will give some guidance as to the presence of lymph node metastases. Resection should be performed in the presence of lymph node metastases.

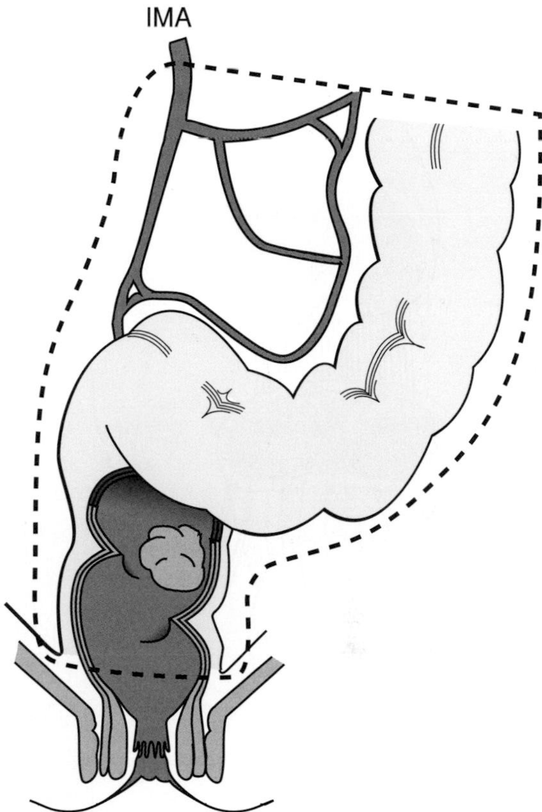

Fig. 24.6 Anterior resection for rectal cancer. (---) Resected material; IMA, inferior mesenteric artery.

Anterior resection

Anterior resection (Fig. 24.6) is the standard radical operation for cancers of the upper and mid-rectum. It is also used for the smaller tumours of the distal rectum when a 2 cm distal margin of resection is possible without damaging the anal sphincters. The level of colorectal anastomosis may be as low as the dentate line (coloanal anastomosis).

The sigmoid colon and the rectum are resected. The inferior mesenteric artery and left colic artery are divided at the highest possible level to enable a tension-free anastomosis between a well-vascularised left colon and the rectum, while ensuring an adequate resection of the lymphovascular pedicle. The mesorectum is removed as completely as possible beyond the distal line of rectal transection.

Anterior resection has a similar incidence of pelvic recurrence to APR provided a wide lateral margin and adequate distal margins are achieved. Both operative approaches deal with the proximal lymphovascular pedicle in an equivalent manner.

Anterior resection is high or low depending on whether the colorectal anastomosis is intraperitoneal or extraperitoneal. Colorectal anastomosis may be constructed by hand-sewn or stapled anastomosis (Fig. 24.7).

The functional results after anterior resection are usually good but vary with the level of anastomosis. Bowel function continues to improve spontaneously for 12 to 18 months post-operatively. With a very distal anastomosis, there is a loss of rectal reservoir and impairment of the internal anal sphincter function. There may be stool frequency of 3–6 times in 24 hours, urgency and impaired continence.

With improved techniques, anastomotic leakage has become less common. Clinically significant anastomotic leaks for high anterior resection and low anterior resection are 1% and 4%, respectively. Although neither a protective defunctioning colostomy nor a pelvic drain prevents anastomotic leaks, it may abrogate generalised sepsis should anastomotic leakage occur.

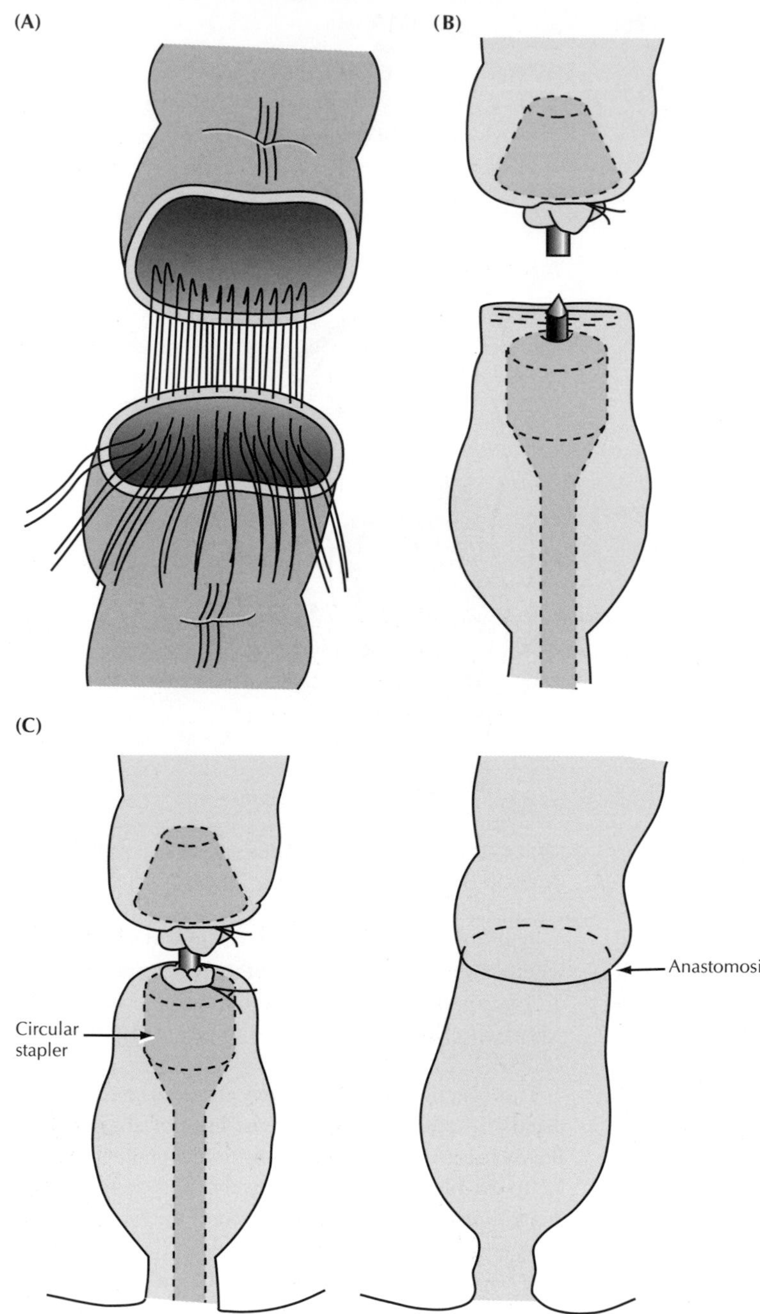

Fig. 24.7 (A) Hand-sewn anastomosis. (B) Double-stapled anastomosis where the rectal stump has been occluded with a linear stapler followed by construction of a colorectal anastomosis with a circular stapler. (C) Single-stapled anastomosis using a circular stapler.

Abdominoperineal resection of the rectum

Abdominoperineal resection of the rectum is now largely reserved for larger T_2, T_3 or poorly differentiated tumours of the distal rectum (Fig. 24.8). The rectum is mobilised down to the pelvic floor through an abdominal incision. The large bowel is divided and the sigmoid colon brought out as a left iliac fossa end colostomy. A separate perianal elliptical incision is made to mobilise and deliver the anus and distal rectum. The surgery may be expedited by having the abdominal and perineal surgeons operating simultaneously.

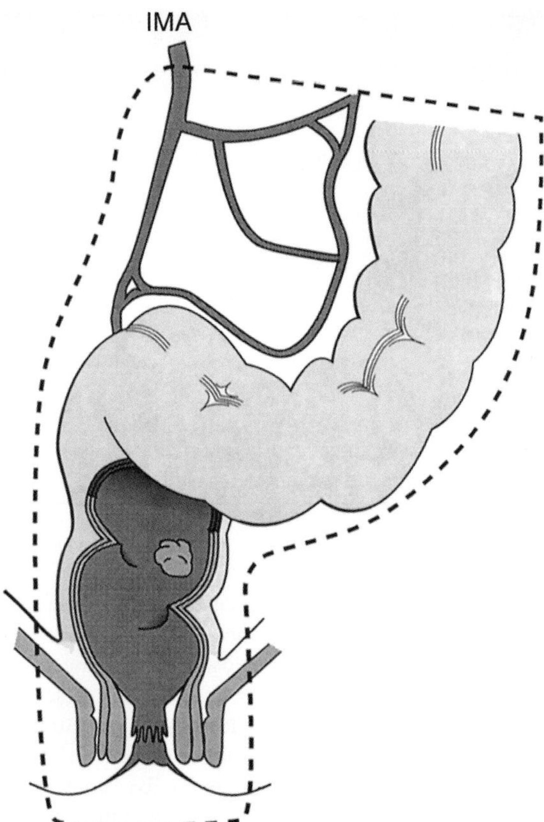

Fig. 24.8 Abdominoperineal resection of the rectum. (---) Resected material; IMA, inferior mesenteric artery.

Hartmann's operation

Hartmann's operation is an anterior resection of the rectum without an anastomosis (Fig. 24.9). The operation is usually reserved for palliation or as a preliminary procedure for acute malignant obstruction or perforation.

Transanal local excision

Transanal local excision is considered in early-stage rectal cancers that are too distal to allow restorative resection, or when age or infirmity of the patient or presence of metastases precludes major resection. Appropriate guidelines for a curative local excision are:

- mobile tumour located in the lower third of the rectum
- tumour size <3 cm
- T_1 (submucosal invasion) or T_2 (muscularis propria) tumour on endorectal ultrasound
- well or moderately differentiated histology on biopsy
- no detectable mesorectal lymph nodes clinically or by endorectal ultrasound.

Long-term surveillance is essential.

Palliative procedures

Palliative procedures include a diverting stoma, radiotherapy and chemotherapy. Local therapy includes laser therapy, electrocoagulation and cryosurgery. Severe pelvic and perineal pain may be improved by a variety of nerve block procedures.

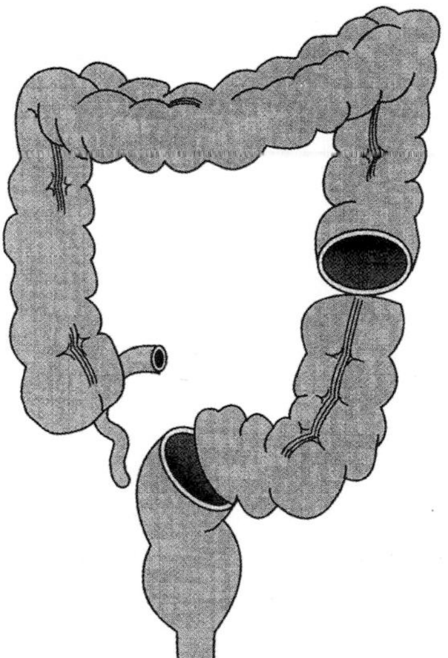

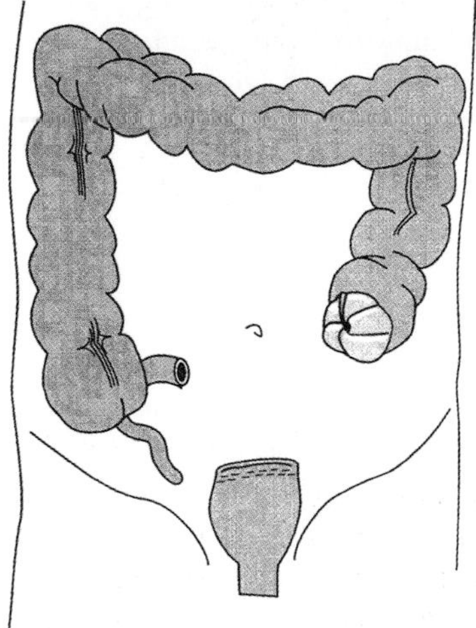

Fig. 24.9 Hartmann's procedure for cancer of the sigmoid colon or upper rectum and sigmoid end colostomy.

Locally advanced colorectal carcinoma

En bloc resection of the cancer with adherent viscera and portions of the abdominal wall is performed. This reduces the risk of seeding viable tumour cells. Sometimes the adherence is inflammatory rather than neoplastic. The increased morbidity of such radical *en bloc* resection should be weighed against the likelihood of cure and the effect on the patient.

If vital structures such as the inferior vena cava or pancreas are involved, a palliative operation (e.g. bypass with ileocolic anastomosis) is preferred. A diverting stoma is considered if an internal bypass is not possible.

Adjuvant therapy

Patients with more bulky disease (T_3, N_1, N_2) are at greatest risk of having microscopic residual disease. Chemotherapy, radiotherapy and immunotherapy have all been tried alone and in various combinations as adjuvant treatments after and, less often, before surgery with variable success. However, the regimens of adjuvant therapy in various trials are not uniform, further compounding the confusion. Various new protocols are in trial, but currently most centres would recommend post-operative adjuvant therapy for Dukes' C colon cancer with 6 months of 5-fluorouracil and folinic acid, and 6 months of 5-fluorouracil and pelvic radiotherapy for Dukes' C and some B_2 rectal cancer. Pelvic radiotherapy may, however, adversely affect fertility, sexual and bowel function.

Combined chemotherapy and radiotherapy may be administered pre-operatively to 'downstage' or shrink a large T_3 or T_4 rectal cancer fixed to the pelvis. This is followed by a resection 6 to 8 weeks later.

Treatment of metastases

The magnitude of treatment should be weighed against any potential gain, in the relief of symptoms and the quality of remaining life. The prospect of cure to some extent justifies radical therapy of isolated metastases. The treatment options include surgery, radiotherapy, chemotherapy and drug management of symptoms (Box 24.2).

Box 24.2 Treatment of metastases

Liver
- Resection
- Hepatic artery embolisation or ligation
- Chemotherapy
- Cryosurgery or radiofrequency ablation

Small bowel
- Resection
- Bypass

Pelvis
- Radiotherapy: 35–55 cGy
- Systemic chemotherapy: 5-fluorouracil and folinic acid, immunotherapy (e.g. monoclonal antibody)

Liver metastases

The presence of liver metastases usually indicates incurability. Occasionally, a liver metastasis is isolated and allows liver resection, to be followed by prolonged survival. Hepatic lobectomy may be necessary if several metastases are confined to one lobe. Intra-operative ultrasonography is a useful adjunct to exclude other occult liver metastases and to define the liver anatomy.

Generally, hepatic resection is delayed until after resection of the primary colorectal cancer. Patients are carefully monitored with CT scan after 2–3 months to assess the growth of the metastasis and the development of other metastases by a positron emission tomography (PET). In a fit patient with a truly isolated liver metastasis, hepatic resection remains the mainstay of therapy. Other treatments such as radiofrequency ablation, cryosurgery and chemotherapy given systemically or via hepatic artery infusion are useful in a palliative role but are unlikely to lead to any long-term survival.

Follow-up

The need for and the intensity of follow-up is controversial. Most would agree that routine follow-up should cease after the patient reaches 75 years of age. Follow-up review provides reassurance for patients and allows a surgical audit of outcome. Occasionally, a structured and directed review protocol (CT scan, chest X-ray, CEA, liver function test) may detect minimal recurrent disease, which enables earlier treatment. This may

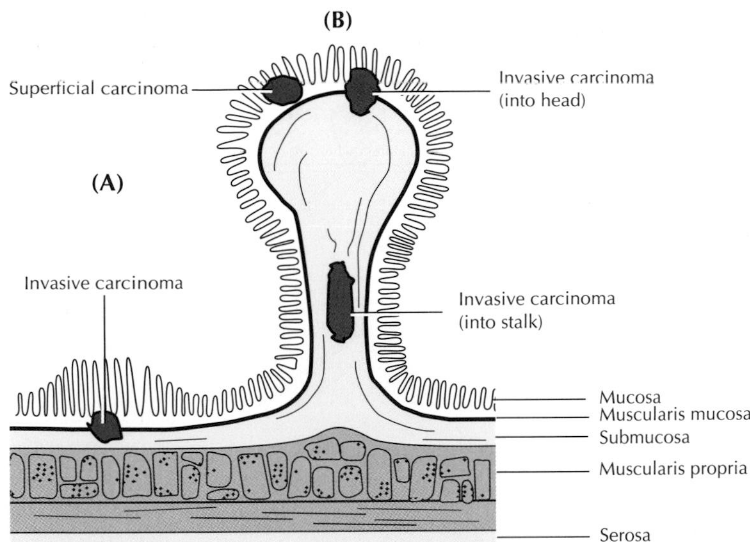

Fig. 24.10 Sessile (A) and pedunculated (B) polyp.

improve survival and give better palliation. However, detection of minimal disease requires more than clinical examination and a proctosigmoidoscopy. As there is an increased risk of metachronous colorectal neoplasm, routine colonoscopy surveillance every 3 to 5 years is recommended.

Adenoma

Adenoma is a benign neoplasm of the large bowel that is associated with colorectal cancers. The most common variety is a tubular adenoma that is usually well differentiated and more often pedunculated (Fig. 24.10). By contrast, a villous adenoma is less differentiated and is sessile, often extending as a carpeting lesion over several centimetres. Tubulovillous adenoma lies between the two both in frequency and morphology and is polypoid with a fairly broad base or a short stalk.

Adenoma–carcinoma sequence

Most colorectal carcinomas arise from, or within, pre-existing benign adenomas. The risk of carcinoma is significant in adenomas greater than 1 cm and polypectomy should be performed. The risk of malignancy increases with the size and the histology of the adenoma. Large villous adenomas have the greatest risk (Table 24.3). Carcinoma in polyps smaller than 1 cm in diameter is uncommon.

Clinical features

Most adenomas are silent and only diagnosed during the investigation of bowel symptoms. They may cause episodic bleeding. The bleeding is usually occult and is detected by faecal occult blood testing. Less commonly, the bleeding is copious and mixed in the faeces, especially when a large polyp partially sloughs from its pedicle. Large villous adenomas may cause urgency at stool, mucous diarrhoea and hypokalaemia from excessive loss of potassium-rich mucus.

Management

Double-contrast barium enema may reliably detect polyps 0.5 cm or more in diameter. Colonoscopy can detect smaller lesions and has the added benefit of being therapeutic as well as diagnostic. Very small adenomas

Table 24.3 Relationship of adenoma to invasive carcinoma

Size	Incidence of malignancy (%) Tubular	Tubulovillous	Villous
<1 cm	0.3	1.5	2.5
1–2 cm	4	6	6
2–3 cm	7	12	17
>3 cm	11	15	20

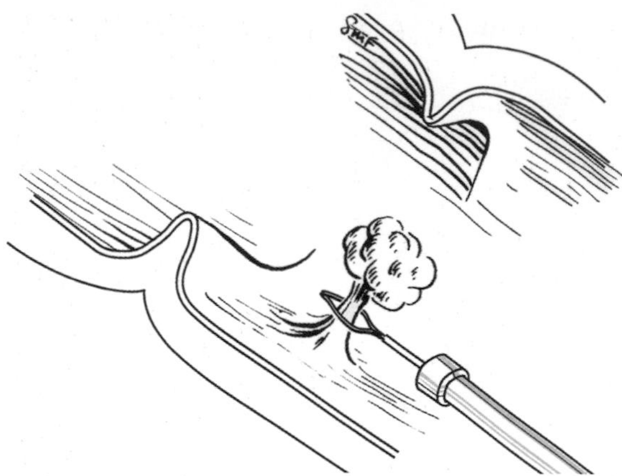

Fig. 24.11 Endoscopic snare polypectomy during colonoscopy.

are treated with biopsy cautery. Bigger polyps are snared (Fig. 24.11). Very large, flatter polyps are snared in a piecemeal fashion.

Low rectal villous adenomas are treated by transanal disc excision. Larger and more proximal rectal villous adenomas may be treated with anterior resection of the rectum, especially if the patient is young.

Follow-up

The incidence of further polyps is 25% when one polyp is found initially and 50% when more than one polyp is detected. Most of these probably represent polyps that were overlooked at the initial colonoscopy. Most centres would recommend, after colonoscopic clearance of two or more polyps and of any polyp greater than 1 cm, repeat colonoscopy annually until the colon is clear of polyps, after which the intervals are increased to 3–5 years. For smaller single polyps, the first follow-up colonoscopy may be performed after 3 years.

Screening

Population screening for cancer or adenoma requires the use of a simple, non-invasive, cheap and accurate method of testing. The protocol for screening for colorectal cancer or adenoma is controversial. The following is modified from the guidelines published by the National Health and Medical Research Council.

Average risk

Average risk refers to people aged between 50 and 75 years, who have no bowel symptoms and no special risk factors. The need for screening is not clear. Options are either faecal occult blood testing and sigmoidoscopy or a full colonoscopy. The interval between screenings is uncertain but current evidence suggests that, in a well-structured screening program, 2-yearly faecal occult blood testing will reduce mortality due to colorectal cancer.

Colonoscopy is clearly the best method of diagnosing and treating the cancer precursors, adenomas. There is considerable interest in once-in-a-lifetime colonoscopy surveillance between 50 and 55 years. However, it is too invasive and expensive to be an acceptable means of screening the entire population. Its use is still limited to screening subjects at higher risk of developing colorectal cancer.

Above-average risk

Previous colorectal cancer or adenoma

A colonoscopy surveillance program that entails colonoscopy every 3 years is recommended. More frequent examinations should be made if there are large or multiple adenomas.

Chronic inflammatory bowel disease

For total or extensive ulcerative colitis, surveillance colonoscopy is started 8 years after onset of symptoms, and is carried out at 2–3-year intervals. Multiple biopsies are taken randomly throughout the colon to detect dysplasia, and from plaque-like or mass lesions. Cancer risk is not increased with distal proctosigmoiditis, and surveillance colonoscopy is not necessary.

The need for surveillance colonoscopy in Crohn's colitis is unclear but is generally similar to ulcerative colitis.

Family history of colorectal cancer: uncertain genetic basis

Colonoscopy surveillance is offered every 5 years from the age of 50 or at an age 5 years younger than the age of the earliest diagnosis of cancer in the family (whichever comes first). Faecal occult blood testing is offered annually in the intervening years.

Familial adenomatous polyposis and hereditary non-polyposis colorectal cancer (HNPCC–Lynch syndrome)

These are discussed below.

Hereditary colorectal cancer syndromes

Introduction

Polyp is a descriptive term that refers to a lump arising from an epithelial or endothelial surface. Histological types of intestinal polyps are neoplastic, hyperplastic, inflammatory, hamartomatous or lymphoid. The neoplastic polyp or adenoma is the type most commonly associated with colorectal cancer. Multiple polyps of the colon and rectum (polyposis) are usually related to an inherited predisposition of the colorectal mucosa towards abnormal growth; however, hereditary polyposis is uncommon. Of all forms of colonic polyposis, familial adenomatous polyposis (FAP) is the most common. Its association with colorectal cancer is strongest and much is known about its molecular and genetic background. Other conditions to be considered are hereditary non-polyposis colorectal cancer syndrome, juvenile polyposis and Peutz–Jeghers syndrome.

Familial adenomatous polyposis

Familial adenomatous polyposis is an autosomal dominant disorder characterised by the formation of multiple colorectal adenomas. However, spontaneous new mutations account for about 25% of new cases, so patients may present without a family history. It is a generalised growth disorder affecting 1:10 000 individuals per year. Offspring of FAP patients have a 50% chance of developing the disease. If left untreated, all FAP patients will develop colorectal carcinomas with time; FAP is responsible for 0.5% of all colorectal cancers.

Familial adenomatous polyposis registries have been instrumental in developing a knowledge of FAP and in tracing affected family members. With the help of the registries, the risk of FAP patients dying of colorectal cancer (previously the main cause of death) has been halved by appropriate prophylactic colorectal surgery.

Progressive development of hundreds of colorectal adenomas begins during the teenage years. A number of extra-colonic manifestations of FAP have been recognised: intra-abdominal desmoid tumours, osteomas, sebaceous cysts (Gardner's syndrome), pigmented ocular lesions and brain tumours (Turcot syndrome).

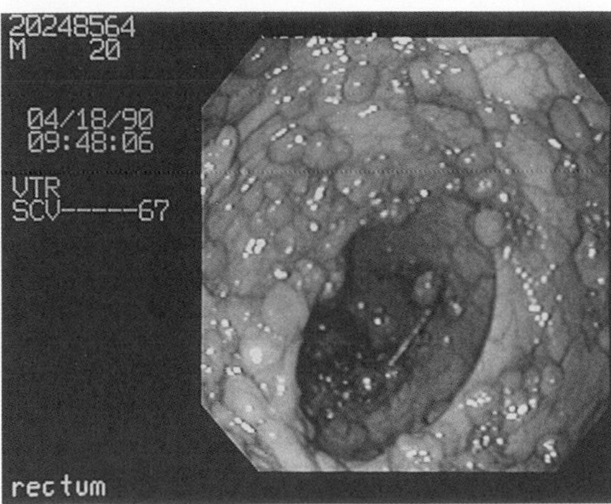

Fig. 24.12 Colonoscopic views of familial adenomatous polyposis.

Diagnosis

Most affected individuals develop polyps by the age of 10 years, although there is wide variation in age of expression. Rarely, patients may present at as late as 70 years of age. There is also variation in the numbers and location of polyps. Most individuals have more than 100 colorectal adenomas with rectal involvement (Fig. 24.12). An attenuated form of FAP with a few polyps and a frequently spared rectum has been recognised. This has a specific genotypic correlation to mutations in exons 3 and 4 and at the distal (3′) end of the gene.

Molecular genetics

The adenomatous polyposis coli (*APC*) gene is associated with FAP. The *APC* gene is one of the tumour suppressor genes responsible for regulation of cell growth in normal cells. Inactivation of tumour suppressor genes can result in a loss of control over cell proliferation, thus promoting neoplasia.

The *APC* gene is a large gene located on the long arm of chromosome 5 (5q21). Individuals affected with FAP have a germline mutation in one of the two alleles of the *APC* gene. It is likely that both *APC* alleles have to be inactivated for the development of colorectal tumorigenesis. Because FAP patients already have one inactivated allele in their cells, loss of both alleles can occur much more frequently in the colonocytes. Hence, these patients are predisposed to the development of hundreds to thousands of colonic neoplasms.

Polyposis registry

A careful genetic history and construction of family pedigrees are vital. The aim is to screen parents and children at the same time. This facilitates education and helps to allay anxieties. A FAP registry is available to facilitate this.

Surveillance strategies

Patient education relating to FAP is very important. Symptoms associated with FAP usually indicate the development of cancer. Therefore, it is crucial to diagnose the condition at a presymptomatic stage. The conventional strategy of endoscopic surveillance is giving way to the rapidly developing molecular genetic tests.

Molecular diagnosis

Presymptomatic carrier risk assessment of the offspring of FAP patients can be performed by either linkage analysis or direct mutational analysis of the *APC* gene.

Linkage analysis used to be the mainstay of most early diagnosis programs that assign individuals into high-risk and low-risk groups. The method depends on the presence of the microsatellite sequences that are closely associated with the *APC* gene and does not involve the direct characterisation of the *APC* mutations. The performance of linkage analysis is dependent on the availability of DNA (from blood or formalin-embedded tissues) from parents and other members of the family. Linkage analysis is now rarely required because of progress in direct mutational analysis of the *APC* gene.

Direct mutational analysis of the *APC* gene is now performed as a diagnostic test for families with clinical FAP. About 85% of such families will have a mutation identified, either by the detection of a truncated *APC* protein *in vitro* (PTT) or tests seeking deletions of the *APC* gene that are not dependent on DNA amplification. Inactivation of *APC* function results in a premature signal for the end point of translation, resulting in the generation of a truncated protein product. Functional assays for *APC* mutation detection have been developed based on detection of the truncated protein on electrophoresis. This protein truncation test is a rapid and efficient means of obtaining *de facto* evidence of the presence of a causative mutation.

If a mutation is characterised in a family, other clinically unaffected members in the family can be offered predictive DNA testing for FAP. If a mutation is identified, the risk of the individual developing FAP is 100%. Those family members who tested negative on molecular genetic testing are not at risk for FAP but are still at risk for common colorectal cancers as they get older. Application of molecular technology has revolutionised the management of FAP. Presymptomatic diagnosis using molecular technology will reduce anxiety in low-risk individuals and increase compliance with regards to surveillance in high-risk patients. Considerable savings are made by avoiding multiple screening endoscopies if an individual is recognised as not carrying a mutated allele. An important application is the correlation between different mutations and the clinical severity and spectrum of disease.

Flexible sigmoidoscopy

The rectum is invariably involved with polyps in FAP, although the number of polyps in various sites in the colon and rectum varies between individuals. Flexible sigmoidoscopic examination of family members is commenced around puberty and continues to the age of 40 years at 1–2-year intervals. The presence of a rectal adenoma dictates the need for a colonoscopy to assess the numbers of polyps in the large bowel and to exclude cancer. With development of molecular genetics, a more selective endoscopic screening policy is evolving. Family members at no risk on the basis of negative molecular genetic testing for the family-specific mutation do not need special surveillance other than that appropriate for average-risk individuals from 50 years of age onwards.

Extracolonic manifestations

Osteomas

Gardner's syndrome is characterised by the presence of sebaceous cysts and osteomas, particularly of the skull and mandible. These extracolonic manifestations may precede the expression of colorectal polyps. Almost all individuals with FAP will have these manifestations if

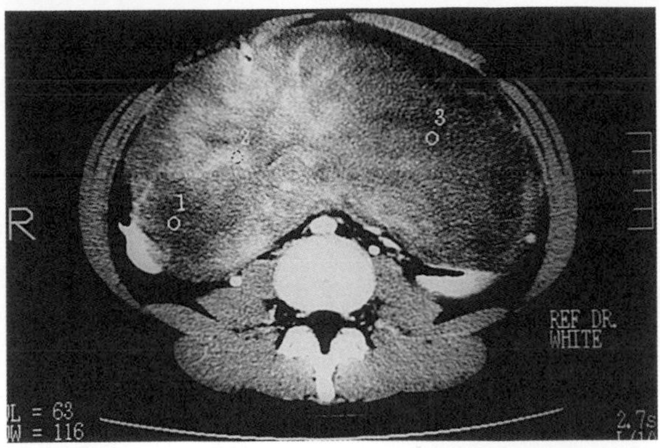

Fig. 24.13 Computed tomography scan of an abdomen showing a large desmoid tumour occupying almost the entire peritoneal cavity.

sufficiently sensitive clinical and radiological examinations are undertaken.

Desmoid tumours

Desmoid tumours can be found in about 10% of FAP patients (Fig. 24.13). These are fibroblastic tumours commonly affecting the abdominal wall or small bowel mesentery. They are benign because they do not metastasise but can be lethal because of aggressive local growth with pressure on the neighbouring viscera.

Desmoid tumours may present as a discrete lump or more commonly as an area of thickening. Trauma of any abdominal surgery precipitates the rapid growth of desmoid tumour, which may preclude subsequent ileo–anal pouch procedures. These patients tend to have unusually dense post-operative adhesions. With reduction in mortality from colorectal cancer, desmoid tumours are now a common cause of death, usually from mesenteric strangulation.

No treatment has proven consistently efficacious for intra-abdominal desmoid tumours. Response to medical management with sulindac, a non-steroidal anti-inflammatory drug, or tamoxifen is variable. Surgery is performed to deal with the complications. The recurrence rate is very high but aggressive desmoid tumours are fortunately uncommon. As a last resort, chemotherapy may be attempted (see Chapter 42).

Gastroduodenal polyps

Almost all FAP patients have gastroduodenal polyps, although only 5% will develop fatal duodenal cancer. Gastric polyps are usually hamartomas (fundic gland polyps) and cause no symptoms. Duodenal polyps are usually adenomatous. Patients with FAP do not generally suffer an excess risk of gastric cancer. The risk of duodenal cancer in FAP is, however, increased to more than 100 times that of the normal population. Adenomas around the ampulla of Vater are particularly prone to development of cancer. Duodenal cancer now accounts for most cancer deaths after successful colorectal surgery for FAP.

The screening strategy for gastroduodenal polyps is not well defined. Diagnosis of periampullary adenoma requires side-viewing upper gastrointestinal endoscopy. Asymptomatic patients should have their first upper gastrointestinal endoscopy between the ages of 20 and 25 years or at the time of colorectal surgery. The presence of a large number of duodenal polyps more than 5–10 mm in size is an indication for annual surveillance. Otherwise, surveillance can be every 5 years, and more frequent after 45 years of age.

As there is no genetic marker that predicts the likelihood of progression of adenoma to cancer, the degree of dysplasia is currently the best index for potential surgical intervention. Large polyps may be treated endoscopically using laser or argon plasma coagulation, although the consequences of complications such as perforation are severe at this site. Surgery is indicated if polyps show villous change, severe dysplasia, rapid growth or induration at endoscopic probing. Radical surgery with pancreaticoduodenectomy is done in younger patients with severe duodenal polyposis. Local excision is associated with a higher recurrence rate. Sulindac is not effective for gastroduodenal polyps.

Retinal pigmentation

The overall incidence of congenital hypertrophy of the retinal pigment epithelium (CHRPE) in patients with FAP is 80%. There appears to be an inverse relationship between the presence of CHRPE lesions and desmoid tumours. The presence of CHRPE is associated with mutations at specific locations in the *APC* gene. While CHRPE lesions are themselves harmless, their presence or absence will guide the search for the causative mutations in FAP families.

Surgical management

In affected individuals, the principal treatment is surgery. There are essentially two groups presenting for prophylactic colorectal surgery: screen-detected members of a known FAP family (usually in teenage years) and symptomatic individuals (mostly in their 30s). Colectomy before the age of 20 years is desirable to prevent cancer (the risk of cancer by the age of 20 years is 5%).

Total abdominal colectomy and ileorectal anastomosis

Total abdominal colectomy and ileorectal anastomosis eliminates the colonic polyps, and rectal polyps may regress after surgery. Careful surveillance of the rectal remnant by flexible sigmoidoscopy is performed every 6 months. Small polyps can safely be left but larger ones need to be removed.

Colectomy with ileorectal anastomosis has a low complication rate, good post-operative bowel function and is ideally suited to young patients. In most cases, the surgery can be performed laparoscopically. The risk of cancer in the rectum is about 15% at 15 years. Advanced-stage rectal cancer may develop insidiously despite careful surveillance by sigmoidoscopy. The risk of cancer in the retained rectum increases with age and with the number and size of polyps in the rectum. Removal of the retained rectum and conversion to ileal pouch–anal anastomosis is generally recommended in patients older than 40.

Restorative proctocolectomy and ileal pouch–anal anastomosis

Restorative proctocolectomy and ileal pouch–anal anastomosis removes the entire colon and rectum and thus eliminates the risk of colorectal cancer. Faecal continence is preserved by construction of an ileal reservoir anastomosed to the upper anal canal. The morbidity is higher than for an ileorectal anastomosis and the function is marginally worse. With improvement in surgical techniques and surgical results, pouch surgery is becoming increasingly popular as the primary prophylactic surgery for FAP, especially for individuals with mutations associated with dense rectal and colonic polyposis.

Total proctocolectomy and permanent end ileostomy

Total proctocolectomy and permanent end ileostomy is now rarely performed except in FAP patients presenting with a very low-risk rectal cancer.

Hereditary non-polyposis colorectal cancer syndrome

Hereditary non-polyposis colorectal cancer (HNPCC) is inherited in an autosomal dominant pattern. Gene carriers have a very high risk of colon cancer, with an estimated lifetime penetrance of 85%. The cardinal features are early age of colorectal cancer onset (approximately 44 years), proximal colonic cancer predilection (approximately 70%), an excess of synchronous and metachronous colorectal cancers (approximately 45% at 10 years after primary resection), and often an excess of certain extracolonic cancers (endometrial carcinoma, transitional cell carcinoma of the ureter and kidney, adenocarcinomas of the stomach, small bowel, ovary, pancreas and biliary tract). Polyposis is not a feature of HNPCC and the incidence of adenomas in HNPCC approximates that observed in the general population. The colon cancers of HNPCC have histological features highly suggestive of the syndrome; they are more likely to be poorly differentiated and mucinous.

The clinical diagnosis of HNPCC once depended entirely on family history and was imprecise because it lacks definitive clinical features. The genes linked to HNPCC have now been defined by the genes *MSH2* at chromosome 2p, *MLH1* at chromosome 3p, and *PMS2* at chromosome 7q, *hMSH6* and *TGFBRII*. The critical genes on 2p, 3p and 7q are concerned with DNA mismatch repair, a proofreading function that helps ensure replication fidelity. Defective DNA mismatch repair results in a steady accumulation of mutations. The mutation load can be detected as errors in long tandem repeat sequences; that is, errors that produce microsatellite instability (MSI). Microsatellite instability is much more frequent in colorectal cancers in young HNPCC patients than in sporadic cases but the reverse is true for older patients. Microsatellite instability testing in tissue sections is frequently used as an adjunct to select families for mutational analysis, where there is doubt about HNPCC on pedigree studies. However, MSI is not specific for colon cancer and may be present in other cancers associated with HNPCC.

Management

Genetic counselling, with discussions about surveillance and management, should be extended to all available first-degree relatives of HNPCC-affected patients, starting in the late teenage years. Because of the proximal predominance of colon cancer, a colonoscopy should be given at the age of 25 years and repeated at 2-year intervals through to the age of 35 years, then annually thereafter.

In subjects who have undergone DNA testing and were found to have one of the HNPCC germline mutations, a more intensive surveillance program is initiated. Colonoscopy is started at age 20 and is repeated annually. If a patient develops colorectal cancer, abdominal colectomy and ileorectal anastomosis is recommended because of the risk for synchronous and metachronous colonic cancers. Prophylactic colectomy may be offered in patients with proven evidence of the HNPCC germline mutations.

The role of screening for endometrial and ovarian cancers in female kindreds of an HNPCC family is less certain. It entails endometrial aspiration biopsy and transvaginal ovarian ultrasound, respectively, and CA125 blood testing. Screening for ovarian cancer is particularly limited. Women presenting with colonic cancer in HNPCC (Lynch syndrome II) families and who have completed their families, should be considered for prophylactic total abdominal hysterectomy and bilateral salpingo-oophorectomy at the same time as their abdominal colectomy.

Hamartomatous polyposis

A hamartoma is the result of disordered differentiation during embryonic development and is a disorganised caricature of normal tissue components. Common variants include juvenile polyposis and Peutz–Jeghers syndrome.

Juvenile polyposis

The juvenile polyp is the most common large bowel polyp observed in children. It is usually pedunculated and has a smooth surface with a distinctive cherry-red appearance. The long-term risk of developing colorectal cancer is probably similar to that in the general population, although adenomatous and carcinomatous change may develop.

In juvenile polyposis, multiple (more than five) juvenile polyps occur in the colon, rectum and even in the small bowel and stomach. The disease is inherited in an autosomal dominant pattern, although in some individuals the pattern of inheritance is not obvious. Juvenile polyps, particularly those located in the rectum, are prone to prolapse and trauma and often present with rectal bleeding. Auto-amputation of the pedunculated juvenile polyps may occur.

Endoscopic polypectomy will remove isolated and smaller juvenile polyps. Continued colonoscopic surveillance at 3-year intervals is performed. When the polyps are too many or too large for endoscopic therapy, abdominal colectomy with ileorectal anastomosis is performed. The rectal polyps can be treated through an operating sigmoidoscope. First-degree relatives of patients with juvenile polyposis are screened with colonoscopy, starting in the early teenage years.

Peutz–Jeghers syndrome

This is an autosomal dominant, inherited condition in which dozens of polyps (usually less than 100) occur throughout the stomach, small bowel, colon and rectum. They arise from glandular epithelium on a branching muscular framework. These polyps may be quite large, up to 4 cm in diameter, and may be sessile or pedunculated. Symptoms usually occur in the third decade of life. Clinical presentations include:

- small bowel intussusception from small bowel polyp, causing colicky abdominal pain and bowel obstruction
- rectal bleeding from colorectal polyps
- prolapsing rectal polyps
- melanin deposition in the mouth, around the lips, on the eyelids and fingers.

There are associations with gastric, small bowel and colorectal cancer. The estimated frequency of gastrointestinal cancer is 2%. Neoplastic transformation may occur in the hamartomatous polyps or from adenomas occurring synchronously. There are also lesser associations with cancers of the cervix, endometrium, ovary, breast and pancreas.

Management of Peutz–Jehgers syndrome is symptomatic. If endoscopic polypectomy is not possible, removal via laparotomy is required. Small bowel polyps need to be removed at laparotomy. Intra-operative endoscopy is an important part of the surgery. Because the hamartomatous polyps are present diffusely throughout the gastrointestinal tract, prophylactic colectomy is not recommended.

Surveillance colonoscopy and gastroduodenoscopy should be performed at intervals determined by the rate of formation of polyps. Regular abdominal and pelvic examination, breast examination and Papanicolaou (PAP) smear should also be performed.

Further reading

Ooi BS, Tjandra JJ, Green M. Morbidity of adjuvant chemotherapy and radiotherapy for resectable rectal cancer. *Dis Colon Rectum.* 1999;42:403–418.

Gibbs P, Chao MW, Tjandra JJ. Optimizing the outcome for patients with rectal cancer. *Dis Colon Rectum.* 2003;46:389–402.

Sengupta S, Tjandra JJ. Transanal excision of rectal cancer: what is the evidence ? *Dis Colon Rectum.* 2001;44:1345–1361.

Prichard PJ, Tjandra JJ. Colorectal cancer. *Med J Aust.* 1998;169:493–498.

Tjandra JJ. Surgical management of the locally advanced pelvic malignancy – the colorectal surgeon's view. *Ann Acad Med Singapore* 1995;24:271–276.

NHMRC. *NHMRC Guidelines for the Prevention, Early Detection and Management of Colorectal Cancer (CRC).* Commonwealth of Australia; 1999.

Tjandra JJ, Fazio VW, Church JM, et al. Functional results after restorative proctocolectomy are similar in patients with familial adenomatous polyposis and mucosal ulcerative colitis. *Am J Surg.* 1993;165:322–325.

Morpurgo E, Vitale GC, Galandiuk S, Kimberling J, Ziegler C, Polk HC Jr.Clinical characteristics of familial adenomatous polyposis and management of duodenal adenomas. *J Gastrointest Surg.* 2004 Jul–Aug;8(5):559–564.

Jass JR. Diagnosis of hereditary non-polyposis colorectal cancer (HNPCC). *Gut.* 2004 Jul;53(7):1055.

Church J, Kiringoda R, LaGuardia L. Inherited colorectal cancer registries in the United States. *DisColon Rectum.* 2004 May;47(5):674–678. E-pub 2004 Mar 25.

MCQs

Select the single correct answer to each question.

1 The following are appropriate managements for familial adenomatous polyposis EXCEPT:

- **a** restorative proctocolectomy and ileoanal pouch anastomosis
- **b** regular surveillance with flexible sigmoidoscopy
- **c** enrolment in a familial adenomatous polyposis registry
- **d** identification of presymptomatic carrier by molecular genetic testing
- **e** prophylactic histamine H2 receptor antagonist, as duodenal cancer is a common cause of death

2 The INCORRECT statement on FAP:

- **a** inheritance is in autosomal dominant fashion
- **b** the condition accounts for 10% of all colorectal cancers
- **c** most affected individuals develop polyps by the age of 10 years
- **d** desmoid tumour is an association
- **e** all affected patients will develop colorectal carcinomas with time

3 The HNPCC syndrome:

- **a** is inherited in an autosomal dominant pattern
- **b** tends to affect younger patients
- **c** has a predilection for cancer in the proximal colon
- **d** is often associated with metachronous colorectal cancers
- **e** is linked to hereditary adenomatous polyposis

4 Hamartomatous polyposis includes:

- **a** Peutz–Jeghers syndrome
- **b** familial adenomatous polyposis
- **c** HNPCC syndrome
- **d** tubulovillous adenoma
- **e** haemangioma

5 The oncologic outcome of rectal cancer is:

- **a** improved by precise pre-operative staging, including endorectal ultrasound
- **b** better if the surgery is performed by a surgeon who has large case volume of rectal cancer
- **c** improved by multimodality therapy for high-risk cancer
- **d** improved by pre-operative chemotherapy alone, if pre-operative endorectal ultrasound indicates that it is a T_3 cancer
- **e** equivalent whether laparoscopic or conventional open resection is performed.

25 Diverticular disease of the colon

Joe J. Tjandra

Introduction

The term *diverticulum* indicates an abnormal pouch opening from a hollow organ such as the colon. Literally, *diverticulum* means a wayside house of ill-repute. Diverticular disease is a problem associated with a Western lifestyle. The incidence increases with age and is more common in females. It is infrequent before the age of 40 years but increases thereafter so that at least half the population aged 80 years has diverticula present in the colon.

Pathology

Diverticular disease of the colon comprises acquired mucosal herniations protruding through the circular muscle at sites weakened by entry blood vessels. The incidence appears to be related to the amount of intake of fibre in the diet. The over-refined and fibre-deficient diet of Western countries produces small, hard stools. As the faecal stream is more viscous by the time it reaches the sigmoid colon, hypersegmentation of the colon occurs to generate higher pressures to propel these stools. Diverticular disease is thus the result of increased intraluminal pressure within the colon.

Diverticula break through the circular muscle in four main sites, each relating to penetrating vasa recta (Fig. 25.1). Characteristically, the diverticula are of the pulsion type and occur in two rows between the mesenteric and antimesenteric taeniae. Diverticula project into the appendices epiploicae and may not be apparent on external examination of the colon. In about 40% of cases, diverticula occur between the antimesenteric taeniae.

The sigmoid colon affected by diverticular disease appears shortened and thickened. The muscular abnormality is the most important and consistent feature. There is gross thickening of both the longitudinal and circular muscles of the colon, and progressive elastosis of the taeniae coli. This muscular abnormality often precedes the development of diverticulosis and occurs predominantly in the sigmoid colon. The muscle of the sigmoid colon and rectosigmoid is different from that of the more proximal colon, in that it is thicker and more prone to spasm. The colonic mucosa is pleated, with a saccular appearance. Narrowing of the lumen is due to muscular hypertrophy, redundant mucosal folds and pericolic fibrosis.

In classic situations, diverticula with associated muscular hypertrophy occur predominantly on the left side of the colon and are characterised by inflammation and perforative complications. There appears to be another kind of diverticular disease that is present throughout the entire colon without associated muscle abnormality. This latter group tends to occur in younger patients and may be due to a connective tissue abnormality that allows development of diverticula. Bleeding as a complication is more common in this atypical group. Right-sided diverticulitis with right-sided abdominal pain occurs almost exclusively in the Asian population but whether this is due to genetic or dietary factors remains undetermined.

Microscopically, diverticula have two coats, an inner mucosal and an outer serosal layer. An artery, vein or attenuated muscle may be present close to the neck of the diverticulum. Antimesenteric diverticula do not herniate fully through the circular muscle coat and have a thinned layer of circular muscle in their wall.

Complications

Most patients remain asymptomatic. The presence of diverticula is often referred to as diverticulosis. Of those with symptomatic diverticular disease, about 30% will develop troublesome complications that

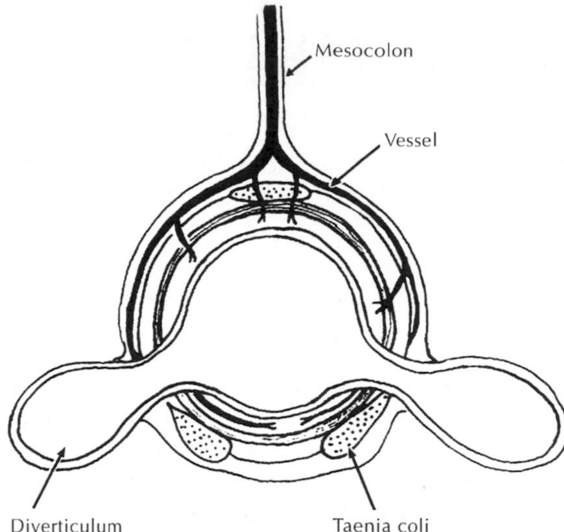

Fig. 25.1 Diverticular disease. Diverticula protrude through the circular muscle at the points where the blood vessels penetrate the colonic wall.

require an operation in their management. The disease tends to pursue a more aggressive course in the young. The likelihood of complications is unrelated to the number of diverticula present. Common complications are listed in Box 25.1.

Symptomatic diverticular disease

Common symptoms of symptomatic diverticular disease include left iliac fossa pain, which may be an ache or colicky in nature. Associated symptoms of flatulence, altered bowel habit (usually constipation) and nausea may occur. On examination, the sigmoid colon is often palpable, and on rectal examination the thickened sigmoid colon may be palpated in the pelvis.

Box 25.1 Common complications of diverticular disease

- Symptomatic diverticular disease
- Acute diverticulitis
- Inflammatory phlegmon
- Pericolic or mesenteric abscess
- Perforation with local or generalised peritonitis
- Fistula
- Diverticular stricture
- Colonic bleeding

Box 25.2 Differential diagnosis of symptomatic diverticular disease

- Colonic carcinoma
- Irritable bowel syndrome
- Crohn's colitis
- Pelvic inflammatory disease/endometriosis
- Pyelonephritis/ureteric colic

Rigid sigmoidoscopy will often be limited to the rectosigmoid junction, as the thickened muscular changes in the bowel wall will make advancement beyond that level difficult. Saint's triad, which refers to the association of diverticular disease, cholelithiasis and hiatus hernia (Saint's triad), has also been stressed. Differential diagnoses are listed in Box 25.2.

Investigations

AIR-CONTRAST BARIUM ENEMA

Typical changes include colonic spasm, segmental 'zigzag' deformity of the sigmoid colon and multiple diverticula that rarely extend distal to the upper rectum. In chronic cases, the bowel lumen may become stenotic. In severe cases, radiological examination is often unsatisfactory. Cleansing of the bowel in preparation for air-contrast barium enema is often incomplete. Residual faecal debris may produce filling defects in the colon that cause concern about possible tumours. The presence of diverticula in an area of colonic narrowing favours the diagnosis of diverticular disease but in no way rules out the presence of a concomitant carcinoma (Fig. 25.2).

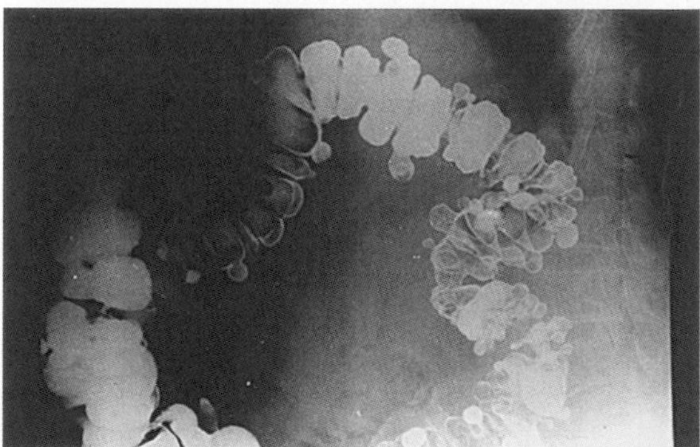

Fig. 25.2 Double-contrast barium enema showing extensive diverticular disease, which is most severe in the sigmoid colon.

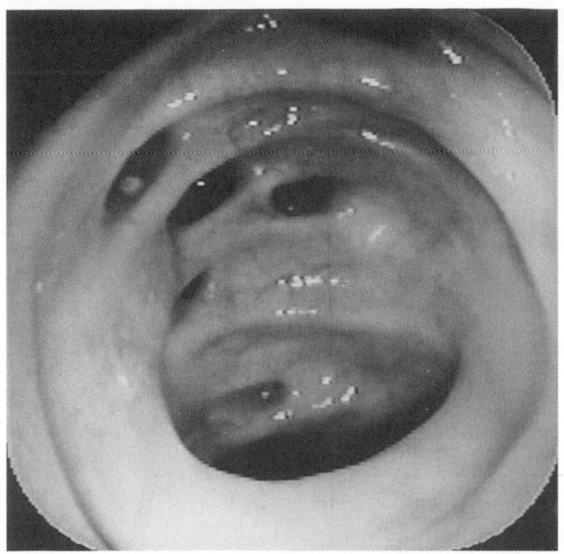

Fig. 25.3 Colonoscopic views of sigmoid diverticular disease.

COLONOSCOPY OR FLEXIBLE SIGMOIDOSCOPY
Colonoscopy or flexible sigmoidoscopy is most useful in differentiating diverticular disease from carcinoma (Fig. 25.3). However, the area of colonic narrowing must be traversed and fully evaluated. The presence of colonic bleeding strongly suggests the presence of other concomitant lesions such as a carcinoma or polyp. Diverticula are often better appreciated on contrast enema than on flexible endoscopy.

Medical treatment

DIET AND BULK-FORMING AGENTS
A high-fibre diet and ingestion of bran (20 to 30 g/day) are effective in producing a significant increase in stool weight, a decrease in transit time and a lower intraluminal pressure in the colon. Coarse bran is more effective than fine bran. Because a high-fibre diet is often unpalatable, the addition of bulk-forming agents such as psyllium derivatives is helpful. While the use of bran and bulking agents are helpful in controlling the symptoms of pain, there is no evidence that once the diverticula are formed dietary management will prevent the complications of diverticular disease.

ANALGESICS
Non-constipating analgesics should be used. Morphine should be avoided because it increases intracolonic pressure.

ANTIBIOTICS
Antibiotics are not indicated in the absence of septic complications.

ANTICHOLINERGICS
Anticholinergics are often prescribed because some symptomatic patients have hypermotility of the sigmoid colon. Their value, however, has never been proven.

Indications for operative treatment

Determining factors include the patient's age, general health, and the severity and frequency of the symptoms. Indications for surgery include:

- chronic symptoms despite the use of a high-fibre diet and bulk-forming agents
- recurrent acute diverticulitis
- persistent tender mass
- inability to distinguish colonic lesion from carcinoma (Table 25.1).

Elective operations for symptomatic diverticular disease are more commonly recommended in younger patients (<55 years), in those who are immunosuppressed (e.g. after renal transplantation) because of the morbidity of complications, and in patients with significant radiological abnormalities such as extravasation of contrast or a sigmoid stricture.

Table 25.1 Features differentiating diverticular disease from carcinoma

Features	Diverticular disease	Carcinoma
Previous attacks	Frequent	Rare
Onset	Intermittent, acute	Gradual
Pain	Colic or dull	Colic
Rectal bleeding	Uncommon	Common
Anaemia	Uncommon	Common
Fever and leucocytosis	Common	Uncommon
Affected bowel	Longer segment, gradual transition, mucosa preserved	Shorter, abrupt, mucosa destroyed

Resection

The timing of elective operation should ideally be about 8 weeks after the most recent attack of diverticulitis. Only the segment of colon affected by the inflammatory reaction to the diverticula needs to be removed. In general, this includes the entire sigmoid colon and the rectosigmoid junction. The distal margin of resection must extend below the level of muscular thickening and is usually in the upper rectum. The proximal extent of transection should include all induration palpable at the junction of the mesocolon with the colon itself and is usually in the descending colon. It is not usually necessary to resect the entire diverticula-bearing proximal colon. A primary colorectal anastomosis is generally utilised. In most cases, a laparoscopic approach is possible, rather than the conventional big incision.

Acute diverticulitis

Pathology

Approximately 20% of patients with known diverticulosis will develop one or more bouts of diverticulitis. Among patients who require hospitalisation, 20% require an emergency operation. The primary pathogenesis is presumably related to obstruction at the neck of the diverticulum, giving rise to an inflammatory reaction in the pericolic tissues. In severe cases, an inflammatory phlegmon will form. Resolution may result in fibrosis. Progression of sepsis can result in perforation, which is often contained locally in the form of an abscess. Pericolic abscesses are usually walled off and, with repeated episodes, the colon may become ensheathed in fibrous tissue and adherent to surrounding structures. Less commonly, free perforation from the diverticulum or the pericolic abscess may ensue, resulting in pelvic or generalised peritonitis. Fistulisation to adjacent organs such as bladder, small bowel or vagina may occur.

Clinical features

Acute diverticulitis is associated with a constant and protracted pain in the left iliac fossa, with systemic symptoms and fever, leucocytosis and sometimes an abdominal mass. Alteration of bowel habit, with constipation or diarrhoea, may occur. If the inflammatory process involves the bladder, urinary symptoms may be present. In more severe cases, abdominal distension is also present, either secondary to ileus or to partial colonic obstruction. Rectal examination may reveal tenderness in the pelvis and a mass or pelvic collection may be felt. Use of rigid sigmoidoscopy is usually limited because of pain. Differential diagnoses are listed in Box 25.3.

Box 25.3 Differential diagnosis of acute diverticulitis

- Pelvic inflammatory disease
- Appendicitis. When the diverticulitis occurs in the mid-sigmoid area of a redundant colon that lies on the right side of the abdomen
- Crohn's colitis
- Ischaemic colitis
- Perforated colonic carcinoma
- Pyelonephritis

Investigations

Plain abdominal X-ray is rarely helpful because there are no specific features.

Computed tomography (CT) scanning provides good definition of the extraluminal extent of the disease and is particularly helpful in diagnosing complications such as abscesses and colovesical fistula. Percutaneous drainage of localised collection of pus can also be performed under CT guidance.

Ultrasound can provide information similar to a CT scan and can facilitate percutaneous drainage of a localised abscess. However, with the extent of gaseous dilatation of the bowel during acute diverticulitis, images from sonography may be limited.

Flexible sigmoidoscopy adds little useful information and risks perforating an acutely inflamed bowel. It may have a role if ischaemic colitis, Crohn's colitis or carcinoma is strongly suspected.

Air-contrast barium enema is generally contraindicated during the acute episode because instillation of the contrast may disrupt a well-contained sepsis. Contrast examination and flexible endoscopy are best deferred for 3 weeks after an acute episode has settled.

Medical management

MILD DIVERTICULITIS

Patients can be managed with broad-spectrum antibiotics (ciprofloxacin and metronidazole; augmentin) for

7 days, as outpatients. Clear liquids by mouth should be taken for 2–3 days, followed by bland solid food as symptoms subside.

SEVERE DIVERTICULITIS

Patients need to be hospitalised for bowel rest with nil by mouth. Intravenous fluid replacement is provided. A nasogastric tube is used if there is evidence of significant ileus or bowel obstruction. In severe cases, intravenous antibiotics (e.g. cefotaxime and metronidazole) that cover Gram-negative organisms and anaerobes are prescribed. Pethidine is usually effective in providing analgesia. Morphine should be avoided because it increases intraluminal pressure.

The patient's symptoms should begin to subside within 48 hours. If resolution continues, further investigation with colonoscopy or contrast enema is performed 3 weeks later. If medical therapy should fail, further investigation with a CT scan may be necessary. Approximately one-fifth of patients with severe diverticulitis will require operation during the first hospital admission.

For patients with an initial uncomplicated attack of diverticulitis who have responded to medical therapy, 70% will have no recurrence. It is not clear whether the complication rate increases with subsequent attacks.

Operative management

Indications for operative management include generalised peritonitis and failure of non-operative therapy after 3–5 days. The decision to intervene depends on the severity and extent of peritonism and systemic disturbance.

Operative options

PERCUTANEOUS DRAINAGE OF DIVERTICULAR ABSCESSES

With a confined pericolic or pelvic abscess, CT- or ultrasound-guided percutaneous drainage is helpful (Fig. 25.4). The optimal timing for subsequent elective resection is probably after a period of 6 weeks.

The drainage catheter is kept patent by regular irrigation with normal saline and kept in place until drainage ceases and the abscess cavity is completely collapsed. Sinography is performed once or twice a week to assess shrinkage of the abscess cavity and closure of the fistula.

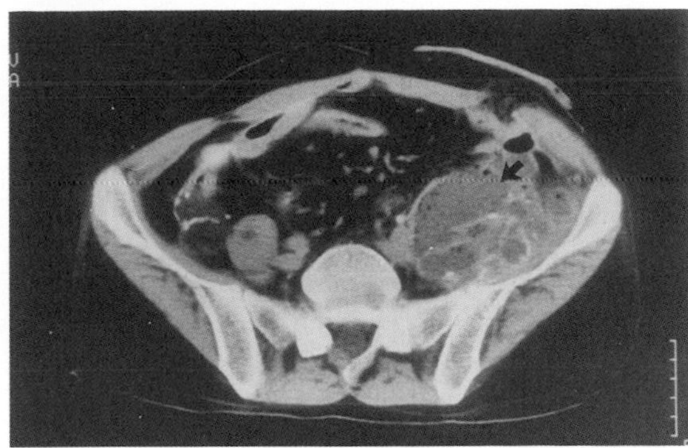

Fig. 25.4 Computed tomography scan showing a localised abscess in the left pelvic region due to complicated diverticulitis.

HARTMANN'S PROCEDURE

Hartmann's procedure (Fig. 25.5) has the advantage of removing the septic focus (i.e. phlegmonous or perforated sigmoid colon) and avoids an anastomosis in the presence of gross sepsis and faecal contamination. However, a second-stage operation is necessary after 4–6 months to re-establish intestinal continuity and entails a further laparotomy, bowel mobilisation and further resection, and colorectal anastomosis with all its attendant risks.

Hartmann's procedure has evolved as the treatment of choice for patients with purulent or faecal peritonitis. It is no longer the treatment of first choice in patients

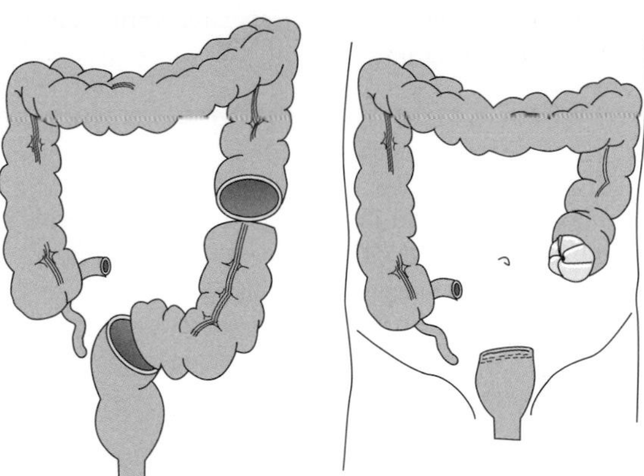

Fig. 25.5 Hartmann's procedure.

with an abscess, which should be treated primarily by percutaneous drainage.

RESECTION AND PRIMARY COLORECTAL ANASTOMOSIS

Resection and primary colorectal anastomosis has the advantage that the diseased segment is resected and the anastomosis is established. In most cases of severe acute diverticulitis a proximal diverting colostomy or ileostomy is used. Subsequent closure of the diverting stoma is easier than the second-stage reversal of Hartmann's procedure. However, it involves extensive dissection in the presence of intraperitoneal sepsis with the attendant risk of spreading the infective process. The diverting stoma is generally closed after 2–3 months. A limited gastrografin enema is performed prior to closure of the stoma to ensure healing and patency of the colorectal anastomosis.

With on-table large bowel irrigation, resection and primary colorectal anastomosis may be performed without a protecting proximal stoma. On-table colonic washout is performed to wash out the faecal residue in the otherwise unprepared colon. This manoeuvre is cumbersome and may contaminate the operative field. This surgical option should be considered only in highly selected situations where the sepsis is confined with minimal bowel distension and oedema.

TRANSVERSE COLOSTOMY AND DRAINAGE

This outdated three-stage procedure involves an initial diverting transverse loop colostomy and tube drainage of the septic area, a subsequent sigmoid resection and, finally, closure of the colostomy. The combined morbidity and mortality of the three stages of operations are high and the procedure is associated with long periods of hospitalisation.

Fistula

Fistulas develop from localised perforations to which an adjacent viscus becomes adherent. Eventually the abscess or faeces drains through that viscus.

Colovesical fistula

Most patients are male; presumably the uterus acts as a protective shield between the bladder and colon in females. Common symptoms are those of cystitis. There is usually a history of recurrent urinary tract infections that fail to respond to appropriate antibiotic therapy. Faecaluria is diagnostic. Pneumaturia that occurs at the end of voiding is strongly suggestive but gas-forming organisms in the bladder can simulate the condition. Bowel symptoms may be absent.

Flexible sigmoidoscopy will rule out inflammatory bowel disease and may identify the fistula and the presence of diverticula. Barium enema will show the diverticular disease but demonstrates the fistulous communication in only about 50% of cases. Cystoscopy may reveal cystitis and the fistulous opening. Cystograms may demonstrate the fistula in 30% of cases. A CT scan may be most useful because it defines the extent and degree of pericolic inflammation and may detect air in the bladder that is associated with a colovesical fistula.

Treatment involves separation of the sigmoid colon from the bladder, and sigmoid resection followed by a primary colorectal anastomosis. The opening in the bladder is often not obvious. If an opening in the bladder is seen, it is repaired. The omentum is interposed between the colorectal anastomosis and the bladder.

Other fistulas

Other rarer forms of fistulas present with discharge of purulent fluid, flatus or faeces on the abdominal wall (colocutaneous fistula), via the vagina (colovaginal fistula) or with diarrhoea (coloenteric fistula).

Bleeding diverticular disease

Massive diverticular bleeding probably arises from injury to the vasa recta. The characteristic presentation is that of an otherwise well individual who suddenly passes a large amount of maroon-coloured stool. Bleeding stops spontaneously in about 70% of cases. Physical examination is usually unrevealing. Proctoscopy and rigid sigmoidoscopy are performed to exclude bleeding haemorrhoids. In addition, a neoplasm and inflammatory bowel disease of the rectum can be excluded.

Management of massive rectal bleeding is discussed in Chapter 61. Considerable difficulty exists in identifying the source and cause of the colonic bleeding. In patients with a minor degree of persistent rectal bleeding, the bleeding should not be attributed too readily to the diverticular disease. In many patients, there is a coexistent carcinoma or polyp of the colon. If diverticular disease is identified confidently as the source of recurrent colonic bleeding, segmental resection is recommended.

Special problems

Crohn's colitis

There is an association between Crohn's colitis and diverticulitis in elderly patients. Involvement of the diverticula by Crohn's disease may result in an increased incidence of diverticulitis. The clinical, radiological and endoscopic differentiation between the two entities is often difficult. The diagnosis is often made only after microscopic examination of the resected specimen. Presence of Crohn's disease should be suspected when there is anorectal disease or perirectal fistulas.

Immunosuppressed patients

Immunosuppressed patients may not give a classic picture of diverticulitis but may present with complications in an unexpected fashion and with few signs. Sepsis is the major cause of the high morbidity and mortality in this group in whom the diagnosis is often delayed.

Further reading

Lawrimore T, Rhea JT. Computed tomography evaluation of diverticulitis. *J Intensive Care Med.* 2004 Jul-Aug;19(4):194–204.

Aydin HN, Remzi FH. Diverticulitis: when and how to operate? *Dig Liver Dis.* 2004 Jul;36(7):435–445.

Killingback M, Barron PE, Dent OF. Elective surgery for dIverticular disease: an audit of surgical pathology and treatment. *ANZ J Surg.* 2004 Jul;74(7):530–536.

So J, Kok K, Ngoi S. Right-sided colonic diverticular disease as a source of lower gastrointestinal bleeding. *Am Surg.* 1999;65:299–301.

MCQs

Choose the single correct answer to each question.

1 A 72-year-old woman presents with left iliac fossa pain, fever and abdominal distension. Abdominal X-ray reveals two dilated loops of small bowel. The most likely diagnosis is:
a left ureteric calculus
b tubo-ovarian abscess
c irritable bowel syndrome
d acute diverticulitis
e sigmoid volvulus

2 Diverticular disease of the colon is associated with:
a thickening of the longitudinal but not circular muscle of the colon
b narrowing of the lumen from mucosal hyperplasia
c increased intraluminal pressure within the colon
d high-fibre and high-fat diet
e a high incidence of anastomotic breakdown in elective surgery

3 Surgical management of perforated diverticular disease with faecal peritonitis includes:
a pre-operative mechanical bowel preparation
b Hartmann's procedure and sigmoid end colostomy
c pre-operative barium enema to define the anatomy
d anterior resection and primary colorectal anastomosis whenever possible
e use of peri-operative antibiotics optimally with penicillin and gentamycin

4 The complications of sigmoid diverticular disease include the following EXCEPT:
a sigmoid inflammatory phlegmon
b colonic bleeding
c purulent peritonitis
d colovaginal fistula
e colon cancer

26 Inflammatory bowel disease

Joe J. Tjandra

Ulcerative colitis

Introduction

Ulcerative colitis occurs most commonly in temperate climates and in Caucasians. It is rare in Africa and the East. Ulcerative colitis is about two to three times more common than Crohn's disease, although the incidence of Crohn's disease is increasing. The disease is usually diagnosed between 15 and 45 years of age. The aetiology of ulcerative colitis is uncertain although familial clusters occur and some as yet unknown environmental factors may be relevant.

Pathology

Ulcerative colitis is a mucosal disease that almost invariably affects the rectum and spreads proximally in a continuous manner. Inflammation is limited to the mucosa, except in fulminant cases, where transmural changes occur. The mucosa is congested and friable, with varying degrees of ulceration. Microscopy shows diffuse infiltration of acute and chronic inflammatory cells limited to the mucosa. The glandular structure is distorted, with goblet cell depletion and crypt abscesses. In chronic quiescent phases, the glands may be shortened and atrophic, although the endoscopic appearances may be relatively normal.

Differentiation between ulcerative colitis and Crohn's disease is most difficult when the disease is severe. In fulminant cases, the colitis is transmural, with deep ulceration and fissures. The histopathology can be confusingly similar to that of Crohn's disease. In some cases, diagnosis is made only after the rectum is removed or when Crohn's disease appears in the small bowel or the perianal region. Sometimes, the diagnosis remains uncertain and is labelled as 'indeterminate colitis'.

Ulcerative colitis and dysplasia

Long-standing colitis may be associated with dysplasia of the epithelium. The absence of any dysplasia or the presence of high-grade dysplasia are generally well recognised by pathologists. The other categories of indefinite or low-grade dysplasia are much more variable and are subject to considerable inter-observer variation. Severe dysplasia is frequently associated with cancer elsewhere in the large bowel and represents a general field change. The incidence of dysplasia in long-standing total colitis is probably around 5–10%.

Risk for cancer rises significantly with the presence of a dysplasia-associated mass lesion (a plaque or large polyp) or stricture. The risk for cancer in colitis increases with the extent and duration of the disease. When carcinoma does occur, patients almost always have had the disease for at least 7 years. Carcinoma rarely occurs before 7 years. This time frame applies only to pancolitis (total colitis) and extensive colitis (from rectum to transverse colon and beyond). For total colitis, the risk for cancer is 3% at 10 years, rising by 1–2% per year thereafter. Patients with colitis cancers tend to be 10–20 years younger at presentation than those without inflammatory bowel disease. The tumours are more likely to be multiple and are more likely to occur in the right or transverse colon. Carcinoma in ulcerative colitis may occur in flat mucosa and may be missed on colonoscopy or barium enema. This fact provides a strong argument for routine colonoscopy surveillance with biopsy.

Surveillance for cancer in ulcerative colitis is controversial and there is no clear evidence that biopsy surveillance saves lives. In addition, cancer does arise in the non-dysplastic bowel. Surveillance with colonoscopy and biopsy is generally commenced after 7 years of disease in patients with extensive or total colitis at 2-year intervals. Biopsy specimens are taken either of specific lesions or from random sites of the colon, as dysplasia in one area may indicate the presence of an unsuspected cancer elsewhere in the colon. The risk of cancer in patients with left-sided colitis is much lower but rises sharply after 25–30 years of disease. Patients with a rectal stump after subtotal colectomy should be screened for dysplasia and carcinoma.

Clinical features

The clinical features depend on the severity and extent of colitis (Box 26.1). Extra-intestinal manifestations are listed in Box 26.2.

The most common presentation is bloody diarrhoea in an otherwise fit patient. Patients with proctosigmoiditis may complain of tenesmus as well. More severe disease with extensive colonic involvement may cause severe diarrhoea with abdominal cramps and urgency at stool. Sigmoidoscopy shows a confluent proctitis with mucosal friability, contact bleeding, ulceration and granularity.

Box 26.1 Spectrum of ulcerative colitis

- Proctitis
- Proctosigmoiditis
- Acute ulcerative colitis
- Chronic ulcerative colitis
- Relapsing chronic ulcerative colitis
- Complicated ulcerative colitis
  - Toxic colitis/toxic megacolon
  - Perforation
  - Haemorrhage
  - Dysplasia/carcinoma
- Extra-intestinal manifestations

Box 26.2 Extra-intestinal manifestations of ulcerative colitis

Present with active disease
- Skin: erythema nodosum, pyoderma gangrenosum
- Mucous membranes: aphthous ulcers of mouth and vagina
- Eyes: iritis
- Joints: flitting arthralgia/arthritis of large joints

Present independent of disease activity
- Joints: sacroilitis, ankylosing spondylitis
- Hepatobiliary: chronic active hepatitis, cirrhosis, sclerosing cholangitis

Acute toxic colitis

Toxic colitis and toxic megacolon are part of the spectrum of ulcerative colitis with severe attacks, and are more common in patients with pancolitis. While acute fulminating colitis usually occurs as an acute exacerbation of ulcerative colitis, it presents as an initial manifestation of inflammatory bowel disease in more than 60% of patients.

Acute toxic colitis is characterised by the abrupt onset of bloody diarrhoea, urgency, anorexia and abdominal cramps. Patients often are ill with severe anaemia and dehydration. A patient is toxic when, in addition to severe colitis, there is evidence of at least two of the following:
- tachycardia >100/min
- temperature >38.6°C
- leucocytosis $>10.5 \times 10^9$/L
- hypoalbuminaemia <3.0g/100 mL.

Other features commonly present include stool frequency of more than nine per day, abdominal distension, tenderness, mental changes, electrolyte disturbances (hyponatraemia, hypokalaemia) and alkalosis.

Abdominal distension often indicates colonic dilatation, and tenderness suggests impending perforation. Toxic dilatation or megacolon is usually defined as a diameter exceeding 6 cm in the transverse colon on plain abdominal X-ray. Signs of septicaemia may be masked by the use of steroids.

Investigations

Colonoscopy

Characteristic appearances include an erythematous mucosa with contact bleeding. The normal vascular pattern is lost and there may be blood and pus in the lumen. Biopsies are taken to establish the extent of the disease and the presence of dysplasia. A full colonoscopy is generally not performed in acute colitis because of the risk of perforation.

Double-contrast barium enema

Double-contrast barium enema will demonstrate the full extent of macroscopic disease, showing a tubular colon and mucosal ulceration.

General investigations

General investigations include full blood examination, erythrocyte sedimentation rate and liver function test.

Therapy for chronic ulcerative colitis

Ulcerative colitis is a disease of remissions and exacerbations. Most management decisions are made on clinical grounds. Endoscopic evaluation is not essential but it may facilitate decisions on therapy. Colonoscopy and biopsy are more accurate than barium enema to define the extent of disease.

Corticosteroids

Steroids may be used orally, intravenously or topically as an enema. Although steroids are effective in inducing remission, they are not effective for maintaining remission. Side effects of corticosteroids are dose- and duration-related. Moon facies, acne, weight gain, mood swings, sleep disturbances and diabetes are common problems. Infections and perforations may be masked. Osteoporosis, aseptic necrosis and cataracts are problems that arise from long-term use. When steroids have been administered continuously for more than 1 month, adrenal suppression may ensue.

Sulphasalazine and aminosalicylates

Sulphasalazine is composed of sulphapyridine and 5-aminosalicylate (5-ASA) joined by an azo-bond. 5-ASA is the active therapeutic moiety, and sulphapyridine alone has no therapeutic effect and is responsible for most of the side effects. A small amount (approximately 20%) is absorbed by the small bowel and most of the sulphasalazine enters the colon, where the azo-bond is cleaved by colonic bacteria. 5-ASA is poorly absorbed from the colon and remains intraluminal, where it exerts the therapeutic effect. Sulphapyridine is absorbed and metabolised by the liver.

Sulphasalazine (4 g daily) benefits about 80% of patients with active mild or moderate colitis regardless of the extent of involvement. It is never used alone in severe colitis. Most patients respond within 2–3 weeks. Sulphasalazine is effective for maintenance therapy (2 g daily) in preventing relapses. It can be continued during pregnancy.

Side effects may occur in 20% of patients. Common dose-related problems of dyspepsia, nausea, anorexia and headache can be prevented by starting slowly with 500 mg qid daily for 3 or 4 days and then increasing the dose incrementally to 4 g daily. Enteric-coated tablets may be helpful. Allergic reactions with rash or fever, haematological side effects of haemolysis or neutropenia and sperm abnormalities are indications for cessation of sulphasalazine. Sulphasalazine interferes with dietary folate absorption. Folic acid supplementation is helpful in patients on long-term treatment with sulphasalazine.

When 5-ASA is taken alone by mouth, rapid absorption occurs in the upper small bowel. Various slow-release preparations of 5-ASA have been developed and are effective in treating mildly or moderately active ulcerative colitis. They are the drug of choice in patients intolerant of sulphasalazine; however, they are more expensive. Common side effects of 5-ASA are diarrhoea, nausea and headache. Occasionally, there is a cross-allergic reaction between sulphasalazine and 5-ASA.

Immunosuppressive agents

Azathioprine or its metabolite, 6-mercaptopurine (6-MP), is not effective as a single agent to treat acute colitis or to maintain remission. However, a steroid-sparing effect is noted. Use is limited by a slow onset of action.

Although these agents have potentially serious side effects, adverse effects associated with the lower doses used in treating inflammatory bowel disease are infrequent. Pancreatitis and leucopenia are the most common side effects. Whenever possible, these drugs should be ceased 3 months before a patient becomes pregnant.

Cyclosporine may have a limited role in stabilising a patient with severe, steroid-resistant colitis to avoid emergency surgery. It has a rapid onset of action but has significant renal toxicity.

Antidiarrhoeal agents

Antidiarrhoeal agents should be avoided in severe ulcerative colitis because of the risk of precipitating toxic megacolon. When the patient is not acutely ill, judicious use of loperamide, diphenoxylate or codeine and bulking agents is helpful to control symptoms and to retain medicated enemas.

Diet and nutrition

A balanced, nutritious diet is important. Some alteration in diet may help to minimise symptoms.

Therapy of proctitis and proctosigmoiditis

With proctitis alone, topical therapy with 5-ASA suppositories is effective. Other alternatives include steroid foam or 5-ASA enemas. This is usually prescribed for 4 weeks. If the symptoms have resolved, alternate-night therapy is continued for another 2 weeks. If remission has been achieved clinically and endoscopically, therapy can be stopped. Maintenance therapy is not routinely used unless the symptoms are difficult to control or there are frequent flares. If maintenance therapy is necessary, oral sulphasalazine 2 g daily may be preferred.

With proctosigmoiditis, steroid foam or 5-ASA enemas are more appropriate than suppositories. These preparations distribute medicine up to the splenic flexure. If there is no clinical response in 2–3 weeks, a trial of twice-daily enemas or oral sulphasalazine can be added. In refractory cases, oral prednisolone is prescribed to induce remission.

Therapy of extensive colitis

When colitis involves the colon proximal to the splenic flexure, systemic agents are usually necessary. The activity of the disease dictates which agents are used.

Mild/moderate disease

Patients with mild/moderate disease have diarrhoea, bleeding, flatus and abdominal cramps but they do not feel or look ill. About 80% of these patients respond to sulphasalazine alone. With repeated flares, long-term maintenance therapy with sulphasalazine is indicated. When patients have shown no clinical improvement after 4 weeks of sulphasalazine or 5-ASA alone, prednisolone may be added and then tapered. A check sigmoidoscopy or colonoscopy may be helpful to note the extent and severity of mucosal inflammation. Some patients have troublesome tenesmus and will respond to topical steroids or 5-ASA enemas.

While most patients can be withdrawn from steroids and maintained on sulphasalazine or 5-ASA until the next flare of disease, some patients require continuous steroid therapy. Immunosuppressive agents may be added for their steroid-sparing effect.

Severe colitis

Patients with severe colitis are systemically ill and should be hospitalised. Initial investigations include a complete full blood examination and a serum biochemical profile. With severe toxic attacks, blood cultures and coagulation studies are also performed. A plain abdominal and erect chest radiograph is obtained to note whether there is any colonic dilatation and/or free intraperitoneal gas from perforation.

A limited unprepared sigmoidoscopy (preferably flexible) with minimal air insufflation is helpful, particularly in patients where a firm diagnosis has not been made. This will help to exclude pseudomembranous colitis and ischaemic colitis. Barium enema and colonoscopy are contraindicated in the presence of acute fulminating colitis. Stool cultures for enteric pathogens, *Clostridium difficile*, *Campylobacter jejuni*, *Salmonella* spp., *Shigella* spp., *Escherichia coli* and *Amoeba* are carried out.

Resuscitation

Intravenous fluids are initiated to correct dehydration, hyponatraemia and hypokalaemia. Blood transfusion is sometimes necessary for anaemia. Total parenteral nutrition may be beneficial in severely ill patients.

Antibiotics

Antibiotics are reserved for fulminant cases and are used to reduce the consequences of sepsis associated with microperforations from the friable bowel. Antibiotics effective against aerobes and anaerobes are used.

Steroids

Therapy is initiated with 100 mg intravenous hydrocortisone given every 6 hours, or an equivalent dose of 60 mg prednisolone daily. In patients in whom a satisfactory response is obtained, the intravenous steroid dose is reduced after 5 days and changed to oral prednisolone. Immunosuppressive agents have little place in the treatment of toxic colitis, particularly if it appears that surgery may be indicated.

Other measures

Narcotics are used with caution because of the potential of exacerbating toxic megacolon. Antidiarrhoeal agents are contraindicated.

Monitoring

Careful and regular clinical review with monitoring of heart rate, temperature, stool frequency, abdominal girth, leucocyte count and albumin level indicate clinical response to treatment. Serial plain radiographs of the abdomen will detect progressive colonic dilatation.

Therapy during pregnancy and nursing

Sulphasalazine and prednisolone do not have teratogenic effects. The neonate does not suffer adrenal suppression from the mother's steroid use. Immunosuppressives are not used in pregnancy, although there is a suggestion that azathioprine and 6-MP are safe in pregnancy.

Surgical management

Indications for surgery

Acute illness

Evidence of free perforation, generalised peritonitis and massive colonic haemorrhage indicates the need for emergency surgery. Surgery is indicated with deterioration of acute colitis (increasing toxicity or colonic dilatation) at any time after initiation of adequate medical management or if there has not been a clear improvement within 24–72 hours of admission. Development of toxic megacolon is usually an indication for early surgery. If the improvement has been minor after 5–7 days of adequate medical management, it is unlikely to sustain a long-term remission. In these cases, surgery is also indicated.

With adoption of more aggressive resuscitation, a coordinated plan of management and early operative intervention, mortality is less than 3%. In contrast, colonic dilatation complicated by perforation has a mortality of 33%. About half the patients with acute fulminating colitis respond to medical therapy, thereby avoiding emergency surgery. The majority of these patients develop repeated episodes of toxic dilatation or incapacitating chronic symptoms, ultimately requiring surgery.

Chronic illness

The main indication for elective surgery is chronic illness that responds poorly to medical treatment or that is troubled by recurrent acute colitis. The threshold for surgery by gastroenterologists and patients is variable. With the advent of sphincter-preserving restorative proctocolectomy, surgery is now better accepted. Severe extra-intestinal manifestations are rare indications for surgery.

Cancer risk

Dysplasia is currently the most sensitive marker of premalignancy. Its limitations have been discussed earlier. Presence of dysplasia from a villous or polypoidal lesion or from a stricture is an indication for prophylactic proctocolectomy. The presence of severe dysplasia from an area of flat mucosa at two separate sites in the colon is also an indication for surgery. The presence of low-grade dysplasia in flat mucosa is an indication for increased vigilance, and may ultimately require surgery.

Pre-operative preparation

The patient and the family are counselled jointly by the gastroenterologist and colorectal surgeon. The need for a stoma is discussed and the stoma site is marked pre-operatively. Steroids are continued and broad-spectrum antibiotic prophylaxis is used. Mechanical bowel preparations are used for elective surgery but are contraindicated in emergency surgery. Prophylaxis for deep vein thrombosis is prescribed.

Surgical options

Restorative proctocolectomy

Restorative proctocolectomy entails removal of the entire colon and rectum. A close rectal dissection allows

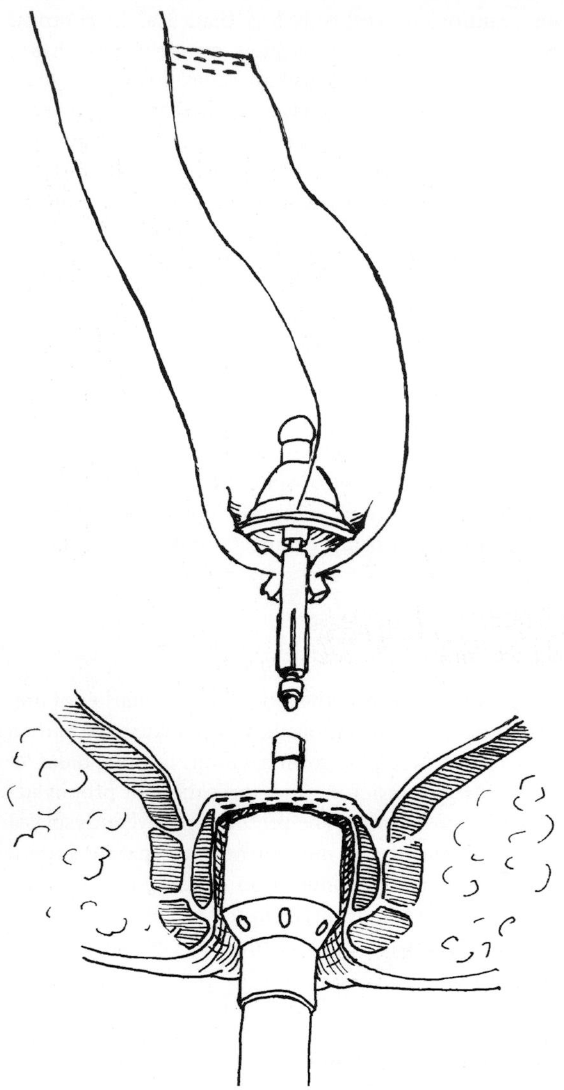

Fig. 26.1 A stapled ileal pouch–anal anastomosis.

preservation of the pelvic autonomic nerves, especially the nervi erigentes. The technique is associated with sexual dysfunction in less than 1% of patients. A pouch is constructed using loops of the terminal 40–50 cm of ileum to replace the rectum and is anastomosed to the upper anal canal (Fig. 26.1). Various designs of the ileal pouch have been described: two-loop J pouch, three-loop S pouch and four-loop W pouch (Fig. 26.2). The functions of various pouch designs are comparable. The two-loop J pouch is most popular because of its simplicity.

Controversies remain as to the distal level of anorectal transection: flush transection at the anorectal ring and a stapled ileal pouch–anal anastomosis, preserving a 2 cm strip of the anal transitional zone, or a hand-sewn anastomosis and stripping of the entire anorectal mucosa to the level of the dentate line. A stapled ileal pouch–anal anastomosis without mucosectomy is generally favoured because of technical expediency. The functional outcome with a stapled anastomosis is probably also superior.

Because of the large number of suture and staple lines involved and because many patients are on steroids, a temporary diverting loop ileostomy is generally performed. The diverting ileostomy is then reversed through a small parastomal incision about 3 months later. In selected 'healthier' patients, a diverting stoma may safely be omitted if the surgery proceeds smoothly.

Despite the technical complexity of restorative proctocolectomy, the procedure is safe. Specific postoperative complications include pelvic sepsis, with or without anastomotic breakdown, adhesive small bowel obstruction and ileostomy-related problems. Overall, 80% recover uneventfully and 20% experience some morbidity.

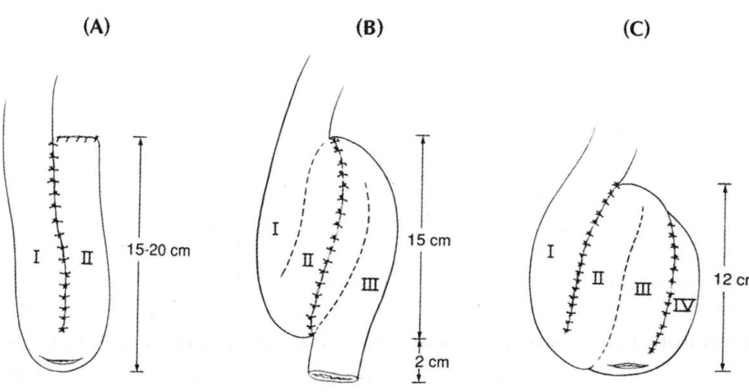

Fig. 26.2 Different designs of an ileal pouch: (A) 2-loop J pouch, (B) 3-loop S pouch, (C) 4-loop W pouch. (With permission from Fazio VW, Tjandra JJ, Lavery IC. Techniques of pouch construction. In: Nicholls J, Bartolo D, Mortensen N, eds. *Restorative Proctocolectomy*. Oxford: Blackwell Science; 1993:18–33.)

Functional results following restorative proctocolectomy continue to improve within the first 18 months after surgery. Most patients defecate five to six times daily and will be able to defer defecation without urgency. Few patients suffer severe faecal incontinence, although minor faecal spotting occurs in up to 25% during the day and 40% at night. Some 50% of patients use antidiarrhoeal or bulking agents at least intermittently.

Major failure requiring excision of the pouch occurs in only 2% of patients. The usual causes are persistent pelvic sepsis, unsuspected Crohn's disease or poor faecal continence.

Long-term sequelae of the ileal pouch are uncertain. 'Pouchitis' is a vague syndrome associated with diarrhoea, abdominal cramps, low-grade fever, tenesmus and general ill health. It may be associated with endoscopic and histologic evidence of inflammation of the ileal pouch. Its pathogenesis is not known. Treatment of pouchitis is empirical. Most cases respond to metronidazole. Some require long-term low-dose metronidazole. In refractory cases, enemas containing steroid or 5-ASA can be used. In very severe cases, Crohn's disease must be excluded.

Complete proctocolectomy and permanent end ileostomy

With the advent of restorative surgery, complete proctocolectomy and permanent end ileostomy is currently indicated only in elderly patients with weak anal sphincters, in patients with advanced-stage rectal cancer and in those unwilling to undergo the more complicated restorative proctocolectomy.

Colectomy with ileorectal anastomosis

Colectomy with ileorectal anastomosis is rarely performed because it leaves the rectum with a continuing risk for inflammation and cancer. It might be considered in patients with coexisting severe portal hypertension where rectal dissection is hazardous or in children to allow them to pass through adolescence without a stoma or until conversion to a pouch.

Emergency surgery for severe acute colitis

The optimal operation is subtotal colectomy and end ileostomy (Fig. 26.3) because of its simplicity and because it allows the later possibility of restorative surgery. Restorative proctocolectomy in the emergency situation is associated with a higher operative morbidity, especially in patients on high-dose steroids, and should be avoided. The diagnosis of ulcerative colitis and Crohn's disease is also often not clear in the acute situation.

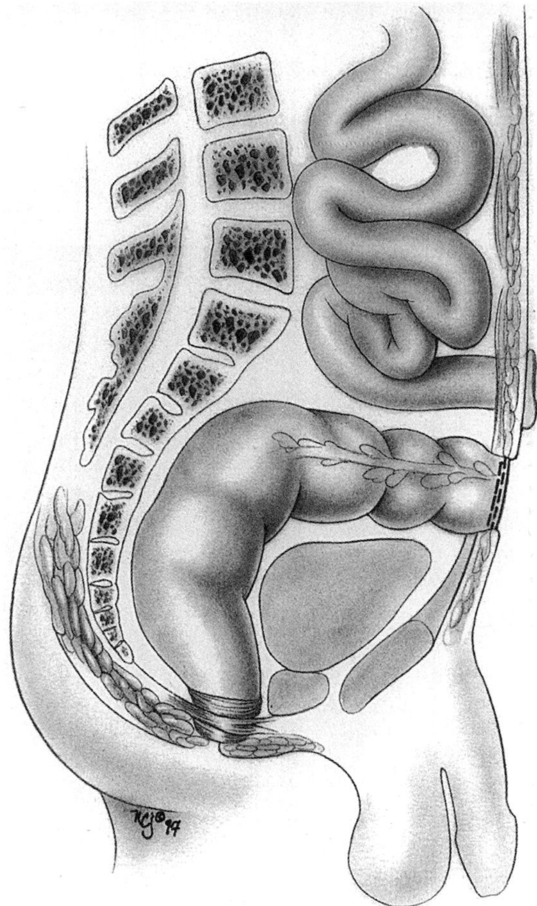

Fig. 26.3 Abdominal colectomy for toxic megacolon. Lateral view showing the end ileostomy and the implanted rectosigmoid stump. (With permission from Tjandra JJ. Toxic colitis and perforation. In: Michelassi F, Milsom JW, eds. *Operative Strategies in Inflammatory Bowel Disease*. New York: Springer-Verlag; 1999:239.)

The splenic flexure is usually the most dangerous area in an emergency colectomy because of inadvertent perforation. If the omentum is adherent to the colon, it should be resected together with the colon to minimise iatrogenic perforation.

The best way to manage the distal rectosigmoid stump remains undecided. Our preferred technique, in most cases, is to staple-transect the distal sigmoid colon at a level where it will lie without tension in the subcutaneous plane at the lower end of the midline incision. This technique avoids a troublesome discharging mucous fistula but allows for discharge of blood and pus through the wound should the distal stump break down. It also allows the rectum to be easily identified at a future laparotomy.

Crohn's disease

Introduction

In 1932, Crohn and his colleagues described an inflammatory disease of the terminal ileum characterised by ulceration and fibrosis with frequent stenosis and fistula formation. They called it 'regional ileitis'. It was later recognised that a similar inflammatory process could also affect the colon and perianal region. The cause of Crohn's disease remains unknown although immunological mechanisms play a role in the pathogenesis of mucosal inflammation.

Crohn's disease is a disease of young adults. The age at which Crohn's disease is first diagnosed peaks between 20 and 29 years, with a second smaller peak between the ages of 60 and 80 years.

Pathology

Crohn's disease can affect any part of the gastrointestinal tract. Multiple areas may be involved with intervening areas of normal bowel, referred to as skip areas (Fig. 26.4). The mesentery is thickened and the mesenteric fat creeps along the sides of the bowel wall toward the antimesenteric border. This is termed 'fat wrapping'. The disease involves all layers of the bowel wall. Ulcerations range from small, shallow aphthous ulcers to deep fissuring ulcers. The fissuring of the mucosa and submucosal oedema can give the bowel a cobblestone appearance with the formation of pseudopolyps. Fistulas and abscesses result from full-thickness penetration of the ulcers. The bowel wall may become thickened with fibrosis, leading to stricture formation.

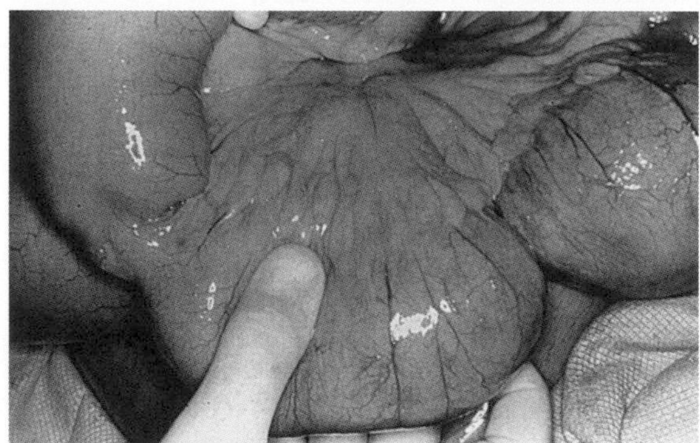

Fig. 26.4 Short strictures of the small bowel separated by normal skip areas.

Perianal Crohn's disease includes large oedematous skin tags, deep fissures, perianal fistulas or abscesses.

The histological appearance varies depending on the severity of the disease but a lymphocytic infiltrate is usually seen in all layers of the bowel. Non-caseating granulomas are noted in about 50% of surgical specimens.

Crohn's disease and cancer

The risk of gastrointestinal malignancy in Crohn's disease is increased. The small bowel cancers are predominantly adenocarcinomas in the distal small bowel and the tumours have a poor prognosis. Colorectal cancers associated with Crohn's disease have a similar distribution when compared with colon cancer occurring *de novo*. The value of surveillance programmes for Crohn's disease are even more uncertain than that for ulcerative colitis because the small bowel is relatively inaccessible to examination.

Extra-intestinal manifestations

Extra-intestinal manifestations are similar to those described for ulcerative colitis (see Box 26.2).

Clinical manifestations

Patterns of intestinal involvement in Crohn's disease are often separated into three main categories: colonic (25%), ileocolic (40%) and small intestine alone (30%). Duodenal involvement occurs in only about 2%. The symptoms depend on the location of disease.

Small intestinal Crohn's disease

Clinical features

The most common symptoms of small intestinal Crohn's disease are diarrhoea (90%), abdominal pain

Box 26.3 Complications of Crohn's disease

- Obstruction from fibrous stricture or inflammatory oedema.
- Fistulas to neighbouring loops of small or large bowel, or to bladder or vagina.
- Perforation and intra-abdominal abscesses.
- Massive haemorrhage.
- Gallstones, especially if the terminal ileum has been resected for the disease. This is due to interruption of the enterohepatic circulation, and eventual depletion, of bile salts.
- Right ureteric involvement from ileocolic phlegmon may lead to a recurrent pyelone-phritis or a right hydronephrosis. Renal stones, especially oxalate stones, are common, especially in the presence of steatorrhoea.
- Amyloidosis is rare.
- Adenocarcinoma of the small bowel, usually in the terminal ileum. The prognosis is poor.

(55%), anorexia, nausea and weight loss. Malaise, lassitude and anaemia are frequently present. Borborygmus denotes obstruction.

Most patients present with long-standing symptoms. Some patients present acutely with a complicated episode such as obstruction, inflammatory phlegmon, abscesses or fistulas. Occasionally, the initial presentation is with a more acute history of right iliac fossa pain and fever, and a misdiagnosis of acute appendicitis is made. The true diagnosis is revealed only at operation. Careful questioning often reveals a more chronic history that suggests Crohn's disease.

Complications of small intestinal Crohn's disease are given in Box 26.3.

Investigations

Barium small bowel follow-through will demonstrate the presence of strictures (Fig. 26.5), gross mucosal changes and internal fistulas. The length of the small bowel is also noted.

Small bowel enema (enteroclysis) allows better definition of the mucosal pattern than a conventional barium small bowel follow-through and demonstrates aphthous ulcers, fissures and mucosal oedema well.

Colonoscopy enables a full assessment of the colon. Focal inflammation and granulomas can be seen histologically even when the mucosa is macroscopically normal. Colonoscopy may also allow biopsy of the terminal ileal orifice when the radiological appearances of the terminal ileum are not conclusive.

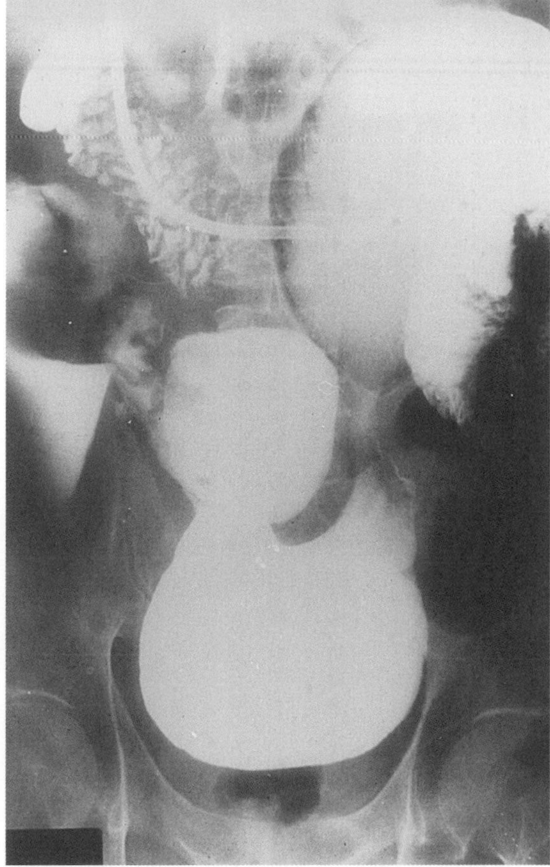

Fig. 26.5 Barium small bowel series showing small bowel strictures with proximal small bowel dilatations.

Computed tomography (CT) scan may demonstrate internal fistulas, intra-abdominal abscesses and thickening of the bowel wall (Fig. 26.6).

Symptoms in Crohn's disease may be due to active inflammation or obstruction or result from previous surgery or bacterial overgrowth. Laboratory tests including full blood examination, albumin and erythrocyte sedimentation rate frequently help to determine the disease activity.

Labelled white cell scan (indium- or technetium-labelled granulocytes) helps to differentiate whether the symptoms are primarily inflammatory or obstructive. It complements barium radiographs in detecting microperforation with abscess formation. This test is not widely used.

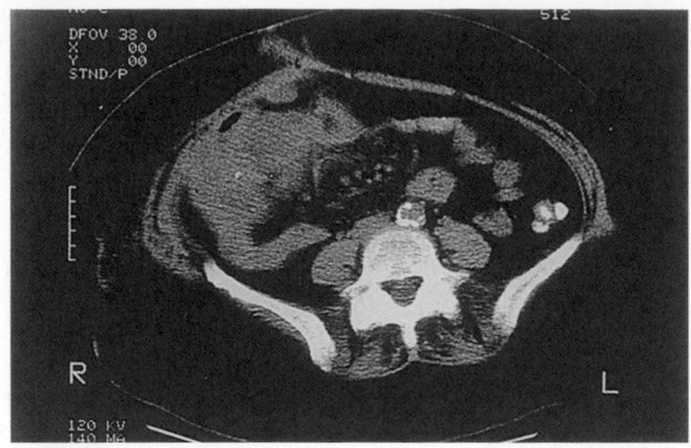

Fig. 26.6 Computed tomography scan showing thick-walled bowel loops in a patient with recurrent Crohn's disease after a prior ileocolic resection.

Medical management

Crohn's disease cannot be cured. The principles of management include palliation of symptoms, control of inflammation and correction of nutritional deficiencies. About 80% of patients will require at least one operation during their lifetime.

For patients with mild to moderate disease, a 5-aminosalicylate, such as mesalazine, together with metronidazole can be used either alone or in combination. For patients with greater disease activity, oral prednisolone can be given. A short sharp course of corticosteroids is given. If the disease is going to respond to corticosteroids, this is usually complete after 4 weeks of therapy.

In severe Crohn's disease, the patient has symptoms of active disease such as diarrhoea, abdominal pain and weight loss, as well as being systemically unwell with fever and tachycardia. An abdominal mass may be present. These patients are hospitalised and are treated with intravenous hydrocortisone or high-dose prednisolone. Fluids and electrolytes are replaced. Blood transfusion may be necessary for anaemia. Intravenous broad-spectrum antibiotics such as second- or third-generation cephalosporins and metronidazole are often given empirically. Most patients settle with this regimen of treatment. Parenteral nutrition is considered if serious complications such as fistulas are present or if surgery is likely.

In patients with chronic active disease, flare-ups of symptoms occur whenever the prednisolone dosage falls below 15 mg daily. They may benefit from immunosuppressive therapy. Either azathioprine or 6-mercaptopurine is used. These drugs take several weeks before a benefit is evident and may allow withdrawal of the prednisolone. Their mode of action and duration of treatment are not clear. In general, if a benefit has been demonstrated, the immunosuppressant is maintained for 1–2 years. Side effects include nausea and diarrhoea. Full blood examination at 2-month intervals is performed because bone marrow suppression occasionally occurs. The role of cyclosporine A is still being evaluated in clinical trials.

Maintenance of remission

In contrast to ulcerative colitis, there is no convincing evidence that any drug is useful in maintaining remission of small bowel Crohn's disease.

In a few studies, mesalazine in high doses has been shown to have some effectiveness in maintaining remission and might reduce relapse following surgical resection or strictureplasty. Low-dose prednisolone may also have a small benefit.

Symptomatic treatment

Treatment of diarrhoea depends on its causation; treatment of active disease has been discussed and bacterial overgrowth is treated with metronidazole. A bile salt–induced diarrhoea following ileal resection is treated with cholestyramine. Finally, antidiarrhoeal agents such as codeine phosphate, loperamide and diphenoxylate hydrochloride may have a small role.

Surgery for small bowel Crohn's disease

Crohn's disease is a diffuse intestinal problem and there is a high incidence of recrudescence of Crohn's disease at various sites. The rate of recurrence increases with the length of follow-up. The cumulative operation rate for patients with distal ileal disease is 80% at 5 years from the time of diagnosis. Crohn's disease cannot be cured by surgical excision and a group of patients will require repeated resections with time. Thus, there is a tendency towards more conservative or minimal surgery to minimise the risk of short-bowel syndrome from excessive resections of the small bowel. Surgery is mainly indicated for:

- stricture-causing obstructive symptoms
- phlegmonous disease not responding to medical therapy
- enterocutaneous or enterovesical fistulas

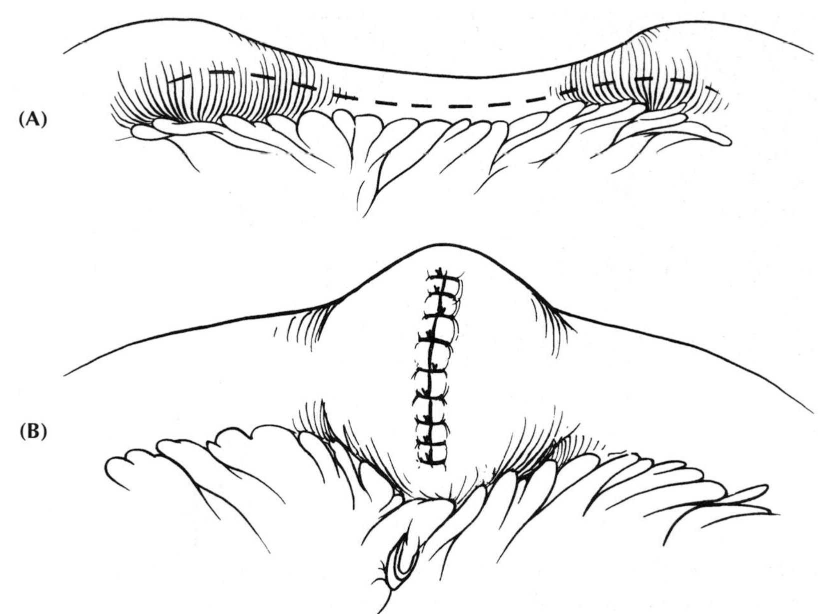

Fig. 26.7 Heineke–Mikulicz strictureplasty. The stricture is (**A**) incised longitudinally along the antimesenteric border and (**B**) then sutured transversely.

- intra-abdominal abscesses (most of these are now drained by percutaneous radiological techniques)
- acute or chronic blood loss (this is a rare indication).

Surgical options

CONSERVATIVE RESECTION

The severely diseased segment is resected with a 2-cm margin of macroscopically normal bowel on either side. With extensive disease, minor evidence of Crohn's disease at the anastomotic site does not matter. The emphasis should be on preserving bowel length.

The cumulative re-operation rate after the first resection for distal ileal disease is 25% at 5 years after the first operation. Aphthous ulceration on the ileal side of the ileocolic anastomosis is present in almost all patients within 12 months of ileocolic resection. Although recurrent disease after surgery is common, surgery rapidly restores patients with incapacitating obstructing symptoms to good health.

STRICTUREPLASTY

In selective cases, strictures of the small bowel may be overcome by strictureplasty without resection. The stricture is incised longitudinally along the antimesenteric border and then sutured transversely as in Heineke–Mikulicz strictureplasty (Fig. 26.7) or in a side-to-side bypass as in Finney strictureplasty (Fig. 26.8). Strictureplasty can be accomplished with a surgical morbidity similar to resection. It relieves obstruction, modifies the progression of the disease and allows preservation of functional small bowel.

Fistula and abscess

Fistula and abscess often coexist. Small bowel enema or contrast follow-through is used to evaluate the extent of Crohn's disease in the small bowel and the presence of fistulas. Colonoscopy is performed to rule out severe disease in the colon, and especially the rectum. A CT scan will demonstrate any abscesses that may be appropriately treated by CT-guided percutaneous drainage. Fistulography sometimes provides useful information about the complexity of the fistulous tracks.

Internal fistulas are often asymptomatic and are identified incidentally at surgery. Ileosigmoid fistulas are usually due to ileal disease. Enterovesical fistulas will cause recurrent urinary tract infections and pneumaturia. The small bowel disease is resected and the viscera that is secondarily involved is closed locally. Following repair of an enterovesical fistula, a Foley catheter is left in the bladder for at least a week.

Enterocutaneous fistula in the early post-operative period is a challenging problem. It arises from anastomotic breakdown or from inadvertent damage to

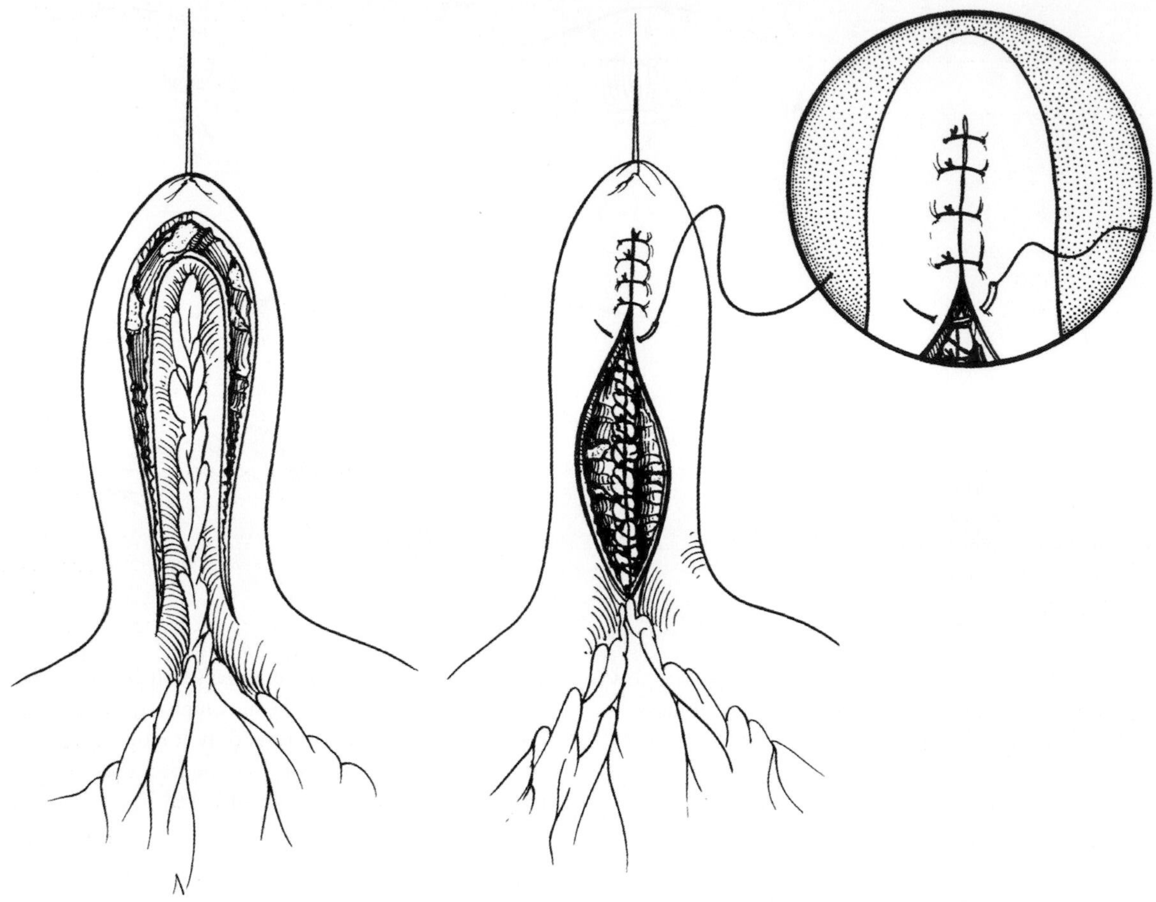

Fig. 26.8 Finney strictureplasty for a longer stricture using a side-to-side bypass. (With permission from Tjandra JJ, Fazio VW. Strictureplasty in Crohn's disease. In: Cameron JL, ed. *Current Surgical Therapy*, 4th ed. Philadelphia: Mosby Year Book; 1992;108–113.)

the small bowel unrecognised at the time of surgery. Principles of management are discussed in Chapter 28.

Crohn's colitis

Clinical features

Colonic disease presents with bloody diarrhoea, urgency and frequency. Fibrosis and stricture may lead to subacute large bowel obstruction. Fistulation to adjacent viscera include colovesical or rectovaginal fistula. Perianal disease commonly accompanies Crohn's colitis: fleshy anal skin tags, anorectal strictures, relatively painless chronic anal fissures and painful anal canal ulcers with complex perirectal fistulas. The differences between ulcerative colitis and Crohn's colitis are given in Table 26.1.

Medical management

Steroids and mesalazine are the mainstay therapy for Crohn's colitis. Occasionally azathioprine is used for severe disease. Nutritional support is important.

Surgical management

EMERGENCY SURGERY

Acute fulminant colitis with toxic dilatation and perforation may occur as in ulcerative colitis. Perforation can occur without toxic dilatation. The procedure of

Table 26.1 Differentiation between ulcerative colitis and Crohn's colitis

	Ulcerative colitis	Crohn's colitis
Distribution	Continuous	Segmental
Inflammation	Mucosal and submucosal	Transmural
Mucosa	Granular, ulcerated	Cobblestone, patchy inflammation
Small bowel involvement	No	Common
Complex anal lesions	No	Common
Internal fistula	No	May be
Granulomas	No	Common
Fibrosis	No	Common
Carcinoma	Common in extensive and long-standing cases	Common in extensive and long-standing cases

choice is a subtotal colectomy with formation of an end ileostomy.

Severe colonic bleeding may also necessitate urgent surgery. Subtotal colectomy and ileorectal anastomosis is appropriate if the rectum is relatively free of disease and the patient is fit.

ELECTIVE SURGERY

Subtotal colectomy and ileorectal anastomosis is indicated in patients with severe diffuse colonic disease and rectal sparing, especially in younger patients. This operation is unwise if there is severe perianal or rectal disease or if the anal sphincters are functionally inadequate. Recurrent disease tends to occur in the pre-anastomotic segment of ileum or in the retained rectum. Many of these recurrences may be treated medically.

Total proctocolectomy and end ileostomy is indicated for extensive Crohn's colitis involving the rectum, with or without perianal disease. Sometimes this is performed for severe perianal Crohn's disease. There is a high incidence of delayed perianal wound healing, especially if there is severe perianal Crohn's disease. Preliminary faecal diversion prior to proctocolectomy may expedite healing of the perineal wound.

Perianal Crohn's disease

More than half the patients with Crohn's disease have anal lesions, especially those with rectal disease. The most common anal lesions are fleshy anal skin tags or anal fissure. These anal fissures are often at atypical sites and cause little pain, unless there is a cavitating ulcer or an associated abscess. Perianal fistulas and abscesses are often multiple and complex. Stricture at the anorectal ring is common as well.

Conservative medical and surgical treatment is the key. The underlying anal sphincter is preserved as much as possible. Many anal lesions are relatively asymptomatic and do not require specific treatment. Metronidazole, ciprofloxacin, steroids and azathioprine can have good therapeutic effects. Anti-tumour necrosis factor-α antibody is the latest development in the medical treatment of severe perianal Crohn's disease.

Proper assessment may demand an examination under anaesthesia, especially in the presence of anorectal stricture and undrained pus. Endorectal ultrasound facilitates assessment of complex fistulous tracts and abscesses.

Haemorrhoids are common problems but most have few symptoms. Dietary and topical management alone are adequate. In troublesome cases, elastic-band ligation may be performed. A haemorrhoidectomy should be avoided because of the risk of secondary sepsis and fistula formation. Anal surgery for fissure should be avoided whenever possible. Associated abscesses are drained but the anal sphincters must be preserved as much as possible. With more complex fistulous abscesses, a long-term seton through the fistula functions as an effective drain. A tube drain is also effective. If the disease is progressive or fails to respond to adequate local drainage procedures, consideration should be given to faecal diversion, followed by a proctectomy in severe cases.

Rectovaginal fistula poses a special problem in Crohn's disease. Asymptomatic patients need no treatment. A low anovaginal tract may be laid open with division of a minimal amount of the anal sphincters. In a more proximal fistula where there is no severe rectal disease, a mucosal–submucosal flap of the rectum may be advanced to repair the fistula, constituting the advancement rectal flap.

Further reading

Bernstein CN. A balancing view: dysplasia surveillance in ulcerative colitis—sorting the pro from the con. *Am J Gastroenterol.* 2004 Sep;99(9):1636–1637.

Tjandra JJ. Surgical treatment of specific complications of ulcerative colitis: toxic colitis and perforation. In: Michelassi F, Milsom JW, eds. *Operative Strategies in Inflammatory Bowel Disease.* New York: Springer-Verlag; 1999:234–245.

Tjandra JJ, Fazio VW. Indication for and results of ileal pouch. *Curr Pract Surg.* 1993;4:22–28.

Kurtovic J, Segal I. Recent advances in biological therapy for inflammatory bowel disease.*Trop Gastroenterol.* 2004 Jan–Mar;25(1):9–14.

Tjandra JJ. Small bowel Crohn's disease. In: Wexner SD, Vernava AM III, eds. *Clinical Decision Making in Colorectal Surgery.* New York: Igaku-Shoin; 1995;413–417.

Tjandra JJ, Fazio VW. Crohn's disease – the benefits of minimal surgery. *Can J Gastroenterol.* 1992;7:254–257.

Wild GE. The role of antibiotics in the management of Crohn's disease. *Inflamm Bowel Dis.* 2004 May;10(3):321–323.

Singh B, McC Mortensen NJ, Jewell DP, George B. Perianal Crohn's disease. *Br J Surg.* 2004 Jul;91(7):801–814. Review.

Tjandra JJ, Fazio VW. Strictureplasty without concomitant resection for Crohn's strictures of the small bowel. *Br J Surg.* 1994;81:561–563.

Tjandra JJ, Fazio VW. Crohn's disease: surgical management. In: Bayless TM, ed. *Current Therapy in Gastroenterology and Liver Disease.* 4th ed. Philadelphia: Mosby-Year Book Inc; 1994:336–341.

MCQs

Select the single correct answer to each question.

1 Extra-intestinal manifestations of ulcerative colitis include the following EXCEPT:
- **a** pyoderma gangrenosum
- **b** iritis
- **c** sacroileitis
- **d** sclerosing cholangitis
- **e** eczema

2 The following features may occur in both ulcerative colitis and Crohn's disease EXCEPT:
- **a** proctitis
- **b** erythema nodosum
- **c** toxic megacolon
- **d** non-caseating granuloma
- **e** response to mesalazine

3 Which of the following statements about Crohn's disease is correct?
- **a** adenocarcinoma of the small bowel is a recognised complication of Crohn's disease
- **b** when operative resection is required, the sites of anastomosis should be completely normal
- **c** strictureplasty is associated with a much higher surgical morbidity than resection
- **d** perianal Crohn's disease is more commonly associated with Crohn's jejunitis than colitis
- **e** haemorrhoidectomy should be performed as early as necessary because severe symptoms are likely

4 Ulcerative colitis:
- **a** is a mucosal disease that affects both the large and small bowel
- **b** in contrast to Crohn's disease, does not have an increased risk of colorectal cancer
- **c** surveillance for colon cancer is mandatory, starting at diagnosis
- **d** toxic megacolon may be the initial manifestation
- **e** salphasalazine is most effective for acute colitis

5 Indications for restorative proctocolectomy in ulcerative colitis include:
- **a** toxic megacolon
- **b** a 2-cm villous adenoma in the hepatic flexure of the colon
- **c** ulcerative proctitis
- **d** severe sacroileitis
- **e** low-grade dysplasia on rectal biopsy

6 Pathological findings in Crohn's disease of the small bowel include:
- **a** enlarged blood vessels, creeping along the sides of bowel wall towards the mesenteric border
- **b** caseating granulomas occurring in the bowel wall and mesenteric lymph nodes
- **c** continuous rather than segmental involvement of the small bowel
- **d** inflammation confined to the mucosa and submucosa of the bowel
- **e** a cobblestone appearance of the bowel arising from fissuring of the mucosa and submucosal oedema

27 Radiation injuries to the small and large bowel

Michael J. Solomon and Joe J. Tjandra

Introduction

Radiation therapy is an important treatment modality for malignancies of the cervix, uterus, prostate, bladder, testes and rectum. Although radiation therapy is generally well tolerated, a small percentage of patients will suffer significant radiation-induced damage. The complication rates following radiation therapy range from 0.5 to 36%, depending on the bias of the reports. The incidence of clinically significant radiation-related complications is about 5–20%. Many of the more serious injuries occur in the gastrointestinal tract, with damage to the small bowel, colon and rectum. Tolerance of normal tissues to radiation is dependent on the organ involved and the total radiation doses delivered.

Pathophysiology

Ionising radiation generates free radicals from intracellular water, which in turn affect DNA synthesis. Cells with a high proliferation rate tend to be more susceptible to radiation injury. The gastrointestinal tract is second only to the kidneys in radiosensitivity. While the small bowel is more radiosensitive than the large bowel, it is injured less frequently because of its mobility within the peritoneal cavity. Because of its relative fixity, the terminal ileum is the most commonly injured segment of the small bowel. Acute changes are inflammatory and chronic changes are sclerotic and fibrotic.

Acute radiation damage may occur within hours to days after radiation. Early radiation injuries result in oedematous, thickened and hyperaemic mucosa. Superficial ulceration or necrosis may be present. In the small bowel the villi become blunted, and in both the small and large bowel the crypts become shortened. The submucosa may show bizarre and enlarged fibroblasts with cytological atypia and is replaced with a hyalin-type substance. Infiltration by leucocytes is seen throughout the full thickness of the bowel wall. Spasm and thrombosis may affect arterioles. Hyalin thickening of the artery wall occurs (Fig. 27.1).

Chronic radiation damage is frequently progressive. Late injuries are characterised by fibrosis. Unlike acute damage, which mainly involves the mucosa, chronic damage represents involvement of the entire bowel wall. The bowel appears pale and shortened. The mesentery is thickened and shortened. Loops of small bowel may be fused with obliterative fibrous adhesions, often called a 'frozen pelvis' or 'frozen abdomen'. Long strictures affecting the bowel are present. Ulcers within the bowel wall develop and may progress to a fistula or perforation. Incidence of severe delayed toxicity among women treated for cervical cancer is 10% at 20 years. Up to 10% of chronic persistent radiation enteropathy will die from the disease. Microscopic features include thrombosis, obliterative endarteritis, submucosal fibrosis and hyalinisation, and lymphatic and venous ectasia. The ganglion cells in the rectum may degenerate, affecting sphincter function, rectal compliance, contractability and continence.

Predisposing factors

The incidence and severity of intestional radiation toxicity depends on dose, volume of bowel irradiated, fractionisation schedule, use of concomitant chemotherapy, co-morbidity and duration of follow-up.

Cumulative total dosage of radiation delivered to the tissues

Cumulative total dosage of radiation delivered to the tissues is an important determinant of subsequent radiation damage. Toxicity has been quantified as the

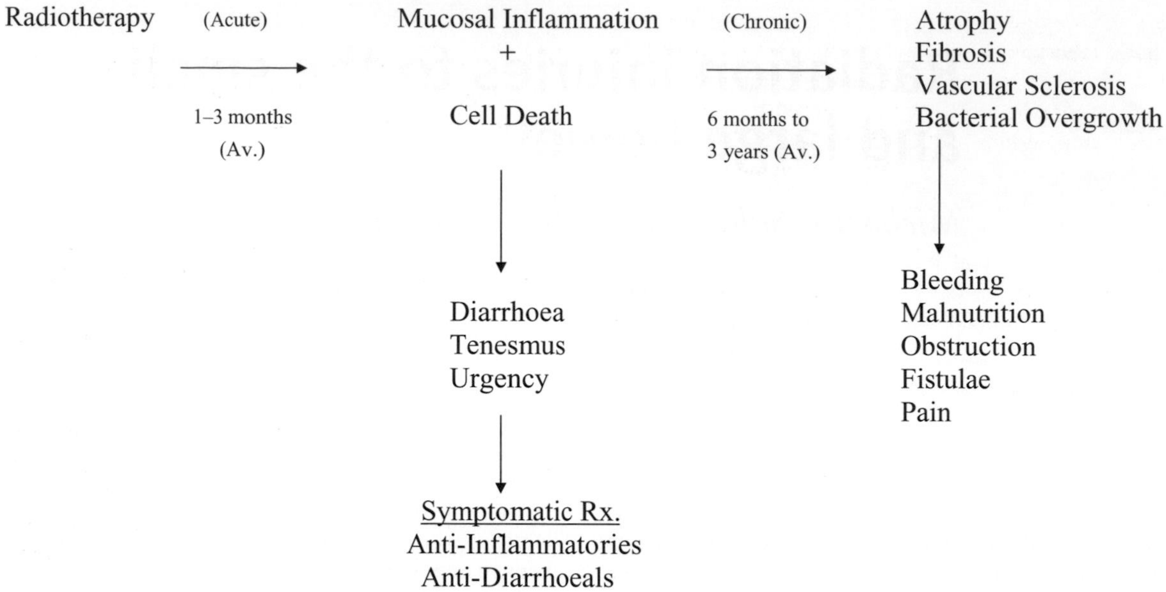

Fig. 27.1 Flow chart of radiation injury to bowel.

minimum tolerance dose (TD 5/5) and maximum tolerance dose (TD 50/5). TD 5/5 is defined as that dosage that leads to the development of clinical damage in up to 5% of patients within 5 years, and TD 50/5 indicates the dosage that produces radiation-related complications in up to 50% of patients within 5 years. When the total radiation dose is less than 3000 cGy intestinal injury is rare; the injury rate increases to 36% among patients receiving 7000 cGy.

Rate of delivery of radiation

Normal cells are more tolerant of frequent dosing of radiation than malignant cells because the latter do not self-repair as well as normal cells. External beam radiation uses doses less than 200 cGy per day. With intracavitary radiation the dosing is particularly crucial; dosage rates greater than 60 cGy per hour are associated with a higher incidence of visceral injuries.

Techniques of radiation delivery

Exposure of the small bowel to radiation can be decreased by careful positioning of the patient during radiotherapy, by distending the bladder and by using multiple fixed or rotational fields. Whenever possible, intracavitary irradiation is used because it also limits the extent of radiation exposure of normal tumours. Surgical manoeuvres during laparotomy may also minimise adhesion of the small bowel in the pelvis (see under 'Prevention').

Co-morbid factors

Cardiovascular diseases and diabetes potentiate radiation-induced vascular injury (obliterative endarteritis). Concurrent chemotherapy, such as adriamycin and 5-fluorouracil, enhances radiation-induced cell injury.

Previous laparotomy with adhesion formation and pelvic inflammatory disease predispose to radiation injury because of the relative fixation of the bowel in the pelvis.

Clinical presentation

Early injuries or reactions usually occur within the first 3 months of therapy. These injuries usually result in mucositis. About 50% of patients develop early reactive symptoms after radiation therapy to the abdomen or pelvis, usually within 6 weeks of the first treatment. The symptoms are usually transient and readily amenable to conservative therapy. In some patients, the symptoms are severe enough to warrant temporary cessation of radiation therapy. Rarely, an early injury is severe enough to cause necrosis and perforation of the bowel.

Late complications typically develop 6–36 months after completion of therapy, although some cases develop many years later. The underlying pathophysiology of chronic radiation injury is obliterative endarteritis and ischaemic fibrosis. Late effects may be the continuation of early reactions but more commonly they arise *de novo*. The incidence of late complications following abdominal and pelvic radiation range from 1 to 17%; overall, about 1–5% of patients will require surgery for these delayed effects and 10% may die from chronic persistent complications.

The clinical presentation of chronic radiation injury varies with the segment of bowel affected.The symptoms may be hard to distinguish from those of recurrent cancer.

Radiation enteritis

The most common symptoms include colicky abdominal pain, bloody diarrhoea, steatorrhoea or weight loss. More acute presentations include obstruction, perforation, fistula or bleeding. Extensive disease may lead to malnutrition from malabsorption and bowel obstruction.

Diagnosis

Enteroclysis is more reliable than barium small bowel series in defining changes and extent of radiation enteritis. Suggestive radiological findings include mural thickening, thickened valvulae conniventes, strictures, separation of bowel loops secondary to oedema and/or fibrosis and fixation of small bowel loops within the pelvis. Fistulae, internal or enterocutaneous, may also be present. Small bowel ischaemia, when present, manifests as 'thumbprinting' nodular-filling defects. Radiological changes may be difficult to distinguish from neoplastic invasion. Most radiation injuries appear in the terminal ileum, while recurrent malignancy may affect the duodenum and jejunum.

Medical management

Acute toxicity is best treated with anti-diarrhoeal, antiemetic, and spasmolytic agents.

Diet

A low-residue diet and a diet low in fats and lactose are helpful. In more severe cases, an elemental diet may improve diarrhoea while maintaining nutrition.

Drugs

Antispasmodics, anticholinergics and opiates can improve symptoms of pain and diarrhoea by reducing motility. Oral antibiotics may improve diarrhoea in patients with bacterial colonisation of the small bowel. Enteric-coated acetylsalicylic acid (ASA) may improve symptoms, possibly because of its anti-inflammatory effects. If the bile salt absorption is abnormal, cholestyramine can decrease diarrhoea. However, cholestyramine should not be given concurrently with other drugs because it binds other oral medications. Occasionally synthetic somastatin analogues can be tried for resistant diarrhoea.

Total parenteral nutrition

Bowel rest and total parenteral nutrition (TPN) may be used for severe symptomatic disease and malnutrition and for enterocutaneous fistulas, although spontaneous closure is uncommon. Total parenteral nutrition is also invaluable in preparing the malnourished patient for surgery.

Surgical management

Indications for surgery include bowel obstruction, perforation, abscess, fistula unresponsive to TPN, intractable bleeding or diarrhoea, and occasionally malabsorption. Surgery is associated with a high operative morbidity (65%) and mortality (40%), with poor nutritional status, delayed wound healing and high risk for wound dehiscence and fistula. Clinical judgement on timing and type of operation is critical. Surgical decision-making is sometimes influenced by uncertainty about recurrent malignancy (Fig. 27.2).

Pre-operative preparation

Patients should be carefully evaluated pre-operatively for the extent of radiation damage, unless emergency surgery is required. This includes a careful review of the patient's general medical condition and

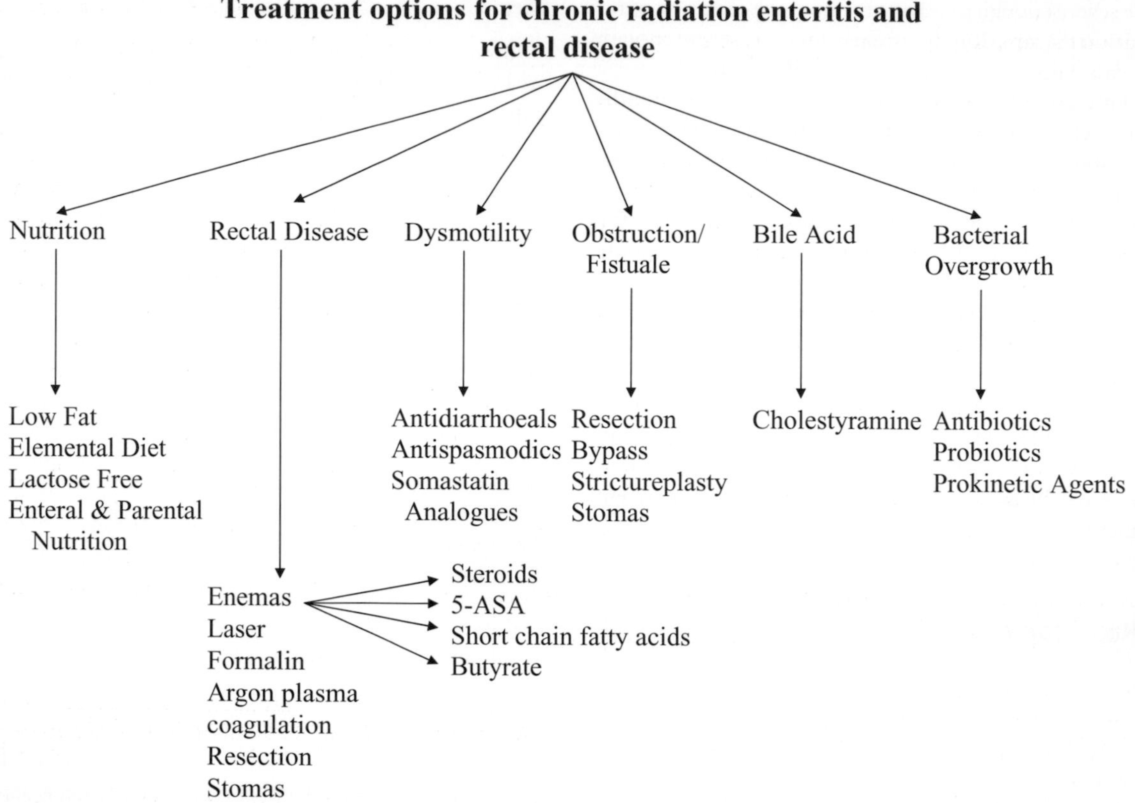

Fig. 27.2 Treatment options for chronic radiation enteritis and rectal disease.

correction of any fluid and electrolyte abnormalities. A decompressive nasogastric tube is inserted if the patient is obstructed. Broad-spectrum antibiotics that cover Gram-negative organisms and anaerobes are prescribed if there is active sepsis. Preliminary treatment with TPN should be considered in patients who are malnourished. Appropriate bowel cleansing programs are initiated.

Surgical treatment: Resection versus bypass

Major controversy surrounds surgical treatment, by resection or bypass, of the abnormal bowel. The argument against resection with primary anastomosis is the concern about the viability of bowel ends and that dissection around adhesions increases the risk of later fistula formation. However, bypassing an irradiated segment leaves behind a diseased portion of bowel that is prone to perforation, sepsis, fistula formation and development of a blind-loop syndrome.

An individualised approach with regard to the choice of treatment is desirable. Resection is preferable if only a short segment of small bowel is diseased or if ileocolic anastomosis to normal colon can be performed. The caecum and right colon are frequently in the radiation field and are not ideal sites for anastomosis. The transverse colon is generally preferred for the ileocolic anastomosis. In patients with extensive disease and considerable adhesions in the pelvis, a bypass procedure without resection is prudent. Anastomosis or stoma formation should be constructed in non-irradiated bowel whenever possible. Lysis of adhesions should be undertaken with great caution. Careless adhesion lysis is associated with ischaemia or inadvertent enterotomies. These may lead to fistula formation or perforation.

Management of fistulas in the presence of radiation enteritis poses special problems. The radiation damage is generally severe and the fistula is unlikely to close with bowel rest and TPN. Surgery is complicated and often difficult.

Colonic and rectal injuries

Patients with radiation damage to the colon and rectum usually present with bleeding, urgency, diarrhoea, tenesmus, constipation from stricture, anal and pelvic floor pain and faecal incontinence. A digital examination may reveal an anorectal stenosis, and a bimanual examination can detect a frozen pelvis. Proctosigmoidoscopy may reveal oedematous and pale rectal mucosa with petechial haemorrhages. Colonoscopy defines the extent and distribution of radiation damage. With radiation damage to the rectosigmoid region, barium enema studies reveal shortening and narrowing of the rectosigmoid region, with loss of the normal curvature. With chronic cases, the rectum may appear rigid and narrowed. Multiple strictures may be present.

Ulcerations may appear, especially on the anterior rectal wall following irradiation for cervical or prostatic cancer. The ulcers probably result from ischaemia and thrombosis of small mucosal vessels. Biopsies may be required to rule out malignancy, but these must be performed with care or a rectal perforation can result. Frequently, the rectal ulcers are extremely painful. With progression of disease, perforation and fistulisation may develop. Erosions may lead to massive haemorrhage. Fibrosis leads to strictures with obstructive symptoms.

Medical management

Low-residue diet and stool softeners minimise damage to the rectal mucosa. Salazopyrine and prednisolone can help some patients. For radiation proctitis, 5-ASA or steroid enemas are helpful and short chain fatty acids and butyrate enemas have been tried more recently. Belladonna and opiate suppositories may improve rectal pain. Gentle dilatation may be useful for treating low rectal strictures. Troublesome haemorrhage sometimes occurs. For acute bleeding from proctitis, an adrenaline enema with 50 mL 1 : 100 000 solution is effective. For recurrent bleeding, endoscopic argon plasma coagulation or laser ablation of the petechiae or telangiectasias is useful, although repeated applications are necessary. In refractory cases, gentle topical application of formalin solution has shown some promise.

Surgical management

Most colorectal radiation injuries do not require surgery. If obstruction, perforation, fistula, persistent bleeding, intractable pain or severe faecal incontinence develops, surgery should be considered, especially if there are no other co-morbid factors.

Surgical options include a diverting stoma (colostomy or ileostomy), and resection and, rarely, anastomosis. Diversion alone may ameliorate pain or ulceration in the distal large bowel. Its efficacy for bleeding is less predictable. A healthy loop of bowel should be adequately exteriorised to form the stoma.

With severe rectal disease, especially in younger patients, formal resection may be preferred. Conventional anterior resection with a low colorectal anastomosis is associated with high operative risks and significant anastomotic leaks. This should be attempted only if the colon and rectum have received less than 4000–4500 cGy, and a protective ileostomy or colostomy is generally performed. Mucosal proctectomy and coloanal sleeve anastomosis between a well-vascularised, non-irradiated proximal colon and the anal canal has met with some success, although this is a major surgery.

Prevention

Technological advances in radiation oncology have allowed a more focused delivery of radiation to the areas of interest while sparing normal adjacent tissues unnecessary radiation. Fractionating radiation doses, altering the size of the radiated field and use of various positioning techniques, such as the prone position and bladder distension, have helped to minimise small bowel exposure. Several surgical techniques have been developed following proctectomy to exclude the small bowel from the pelvis before irradiation.

Further reading

Hauer- Jensen M, Wang J, Denham JW. Bowel injury: current and evlolving management strategies. *Semin Radiat Oncol.* 2003;13(3).

Schofield PF. Iatrogenic disease. In: Nicholls RJ, Dozois RR, eds. *Surgery of the Colon and Rectum.* New York: Churchill Livingstone; 1997:847–852.

Wheeler JMD, Warren BF, Jones AC, Mortensen NJMcC. Preoperative radiotherapy for rectal cancer: Implications for surgeons, pathologists and radiologists. *Br J Surg.* 1999;86:1108–1120.

MCQs

Select the single correct answer to the following question.

1 Radiation enteritis:
  - **a** is related to techniques of delivery of radiation therapy
  - **b** may present acutely with perforation and peritonitis
  - **c** may present late with recurrent small bowel obstruction
  - **d** is associated with a high operative morbidity
  - **e** may benefit from a high-fibre diet

28 Enterocutaneous fistula

Joe J. Tjandra

Introduction

Enterocutaneous fistula is an abnormal communication between the bowel and skin (Fig. 28.1). It is often accompanied by intra-abdominal abscesses. Despite improvement in its management with the use of parenteral nutrition, newer antibiotics, somatostatin analogues, improved intensive care and better imaging techniques and surgical treatments, the mortality rate is still around 10%.

Aetiology

Most cases develop following surgery for inflammatory bowel disease, cancer or lysis of adhesions. These complications usually occur in patients who are poorly prepared or who have had radiation therapy, with emergency surgery or because of poor surgical judgement. Anastomotic breakdown, sepsis and traumatic enterotomy are common predisposing factors. Malnutrition is also an important contributing factor. Less commonly, enterocutaneous fistulas develop spontaneously as part of the disease process in Crohn's disease or diverticulitis.

Some of the complications of enterocutaneous fistulas are listed in Box 28.1.

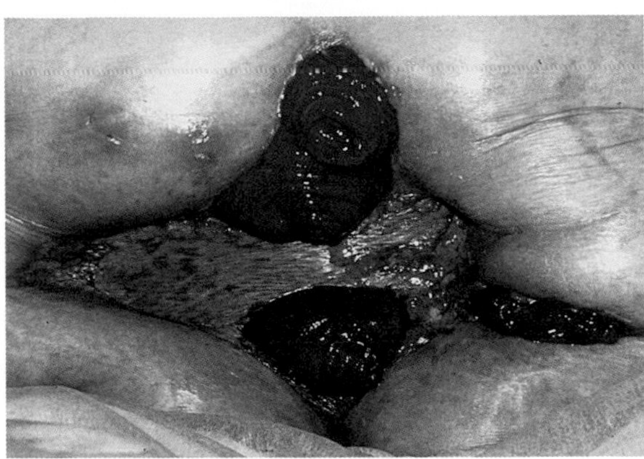

Fig. 28.1 Enterocutaneous fistula.

Box 28.1 Complications of enterocutaneous fistulas

- Electrolyte disturbances. These usually involve potassium, sodium, magnesium and, especially when parenteral nutrition is used, phosphate.
- Malnutrition. This is most common with high-output fistulas and when there is severe sepsis.
- Sepsis. This is commonly associated with anastomotic leaks, and intra-abdominal and pelvic abscesses from enteric contamination. Cutaneous sepsis from irritation of the abdominal wall by the enteric effluent is also common.

Classification

Enterocutaneous fistulas are classified in the following manner:

- high output: output greater than 500 mL per 24 hours
- moderate output: output between 200 and 500 mL per 24 hours
- low output: output less than 200 mL per 24 hours.

Moderate- or high-output fistulas are usually related to the small bowel. Higher-output fistulas are more prone to electrolyte imbalance and malnutrition. The site of origin in the gastrointestinal tract is also helpful in the prediction of its outcome.

Diagnosis and medical management

In the usual setting in which fistulas develop postoperatively, the patient will have done poorly for 5 or 6 days. There is often fever and persistent ileus. A wound abscess appears and is drained. Within the next 24 hours, intestinal contents appear from the wound. By that stage, the patient is often dehydrated, anaemic and malnourished. Optimisation of the patient follows the following schema.

Nutritional support

Adequate nutritional repletion and bowel rest may allow spontaneous closure of a fistula. Unless there is prominent paralytic ileus or the fistula arises from a proximal part of the gastrointestinal tract, enteric nutritional support is encouraged because it provides some of the immunological and other hormonal functions of the gut. However, adequate caloric and nitrogen support with enteral nutrition is usually not possible for 4 or 5 days after its implementation. Supplementation with parenteral nutrition through a central venous line is helpful.

Enteric support requires the presence of approximately 120 cm of small bowel. If enteric nutrition is provided through the stomach, the osmolarity is increased first until hyperosmolarity is tolerated, followed by an increase in volume. If enteric support is provided directly into the small bowel, the volume should be increased first and then osmolarity. The small bowel does not tolerate hyperosmolar solutions well. Enteric nutritional support tends to increase fistula drainage, at least initially.

Provision of parenteral nutrition may be established as an elective procedure to provide bowel rest and maintain nutrition. Whenever possible, parenteral nutrition should be deferred until major sepsis is contained because haematogenous seeding of the central venous catheter may occur with repeated bacteraemia or septicaemia.

Management of fluid and electrolytes

The amount of fistula drainage is carefully quantified so that fluid balance is achieved. In most cases electrolytes may be adequately replaced in the parenteral nutrition solution. Occasionally, additional replacement for fluid and electrolytes may be necessary in patients with very high (>3 L per 24 hours) fistula outputs. A large amount of sodium is lost in proximal enteric fistulas. Acid-base balance must be carefully monitored in these difficult cases.

Control of fistula drainage

Bowel rest

Complete bowel rest is useful in the initial management until stabilisation and evaluation is complete, especially if there is underlying sepsis and the fistula output is high. Gradually, enteric nutrition can be initiated. The placement of a decompressive tube, either nasogastric or long gastrointestinal, should be avoided unless severe paralytic ileus or mechanical obstruction is present. The presence of an indwelling nasogastric tube for a prolonged period is not only uncomfortable for the patient but may result in pneumonia, reflux oesophagitis and serous otitis media. If long-term decompression is thought to be necessary, a gastrostomy tube is preferred.

Somatostatin

Somatostatin analogues such as sandostatin reduce fistula output, facilitate skin care and may contribute to the closure of fistulas, especially those of biliary or pancreatic origin.

H_2 antagonists

These decrease gastric secretion and may prevent bleeding from gastric stress ulceration. On their own, they have little impact on fistula output.

Skin care

With higher fistula output, care of the skin surrounding the fistula is best accomplished by sump drainage of the fistula and application of various skin-protective preparations. Care is taken to avoid skin maceration, cellulitis and cutaneous necrosis. When this occurs, subsequent surgical therapy is more difficult. An enterostomal therapist should be involved with the care of these patients.

Control of sepsis

If there is clinical evidence of sepsis with swinging fever and leucocytosis, broad-spectrum antibiotics covering Gram-negative organisms and anaerobes are prescribed after preliminary work-up for sepsis (i.e. urine culture, blood culture and examination of the wound). Use of antibiotics should be judicious and guided by the cultures and sensitivity studies.

Computed tomography (CT) scans are useful in detecting closed-space infection and abscesses that are amenable to percutaneous drainage, guided by CT or ultrasonography. Uncontrolled sepsis remains the major cause of mortality in these patients. Sometimes an exploratory laparotomy may be performed to drain abscesses that are not accessible to percutaneous drainage.

General management

The process of recovery from enterocutaneous fistula may be protracted and the patient may need several operations. Because most fistulas will heal spontaneously it is important to maintain good morale from the outset. Ambulation is maintained to avoid thromboembolic complications. In less ambulant patients, compressive stockings and subcutaneous heparin prophylaxis are prescribed.

Investigation

After the initial 48 hours most patients will have stabilised enough to allow investigation and definition of the fistula. Radiological investigations are usually the most important step in defining the anatomy of the fistula. Collaboration between the surgeon and radiologist is important for optimal management.

Computed tomography scan

Computed tomography scan determines whether there are any drainable septic collections. Because the presence of contrast in the bowel or in the peritoneal cavity will distort CT images, whenever possible the CT scan should be done prior to other contrast examinations.

Sinography

The fistula orifice is cannulated with a small feeding tube or catheter, and the water-soluble contrast such as gastrografin is injected through the tube. The following information is sought:

- nature of the fistulous tract
- site of entry into the bowel
- nature of adjacent bowel (whether strictured, damaged or inflamed)
- intestinal continuity (whether it is a side or an end fistula).

Contrast small bowel follow-through or contrast enema

Contrast small bowel follow-through or contrast enema provides information on the underlying bowel and demonstrates the presence of intestinal obstruction distal to the fistula. The fistulas may not be visualised as clearly as in a sinogram.

Treatment

The aim of therapy is to restore intestinal continuity enabling the patient to take nutrition orally. This is best achieved by spontaneous closure. However, in complicated fistulas, this occurs only in approximately one-third of patients. The following factors are important for clinical decision making.

Fistula drainage

Usually fistula output decreases with bowel rest and total parenteral nutrition. If it does not decrease, surgery will probably be required. If the fistula output has not reduced markedly after a 4–5-week period without sepsis and with adequate nutritional support, it is unlikely that the fistula will close spontaneously.

Nature of fistula

The site of the fistula is important. Ileal and gastric fistulas are less likely to undergo spontaneous closure than lateral oesophageal, lateral duodenal and jejunal fistulas, or pancreatic and biliary fistulas (Box 28.2).

Abnormal underlying bowel

With inflammatory bowel disease such as Crohn's disease, radiation or malignancy, the fistulas may close

Box 28.2 Adverse factors to spontaneous closure of fistulas

- Loss of intestinal continuity (e.g. complete disruption of an anastomosis or a large (>1 cm) defect in the bowel).
- Persistent intestinal obstruction distal to the fistula.
- Large adjacent abscess cavity.
- Presence of a foreign body (e.g. sutures, gauze or prosthesis).
- Epithelialisation of the fistula.

readily but then re-open. In these circumstances, the fistula is allowed to heal and surgery is then performed with a formal resection and end-to-end anastomosis. Fistulas occurring in association with a carcinoma should be resected whenever feasible.

General condition of the patient

In patients who are severely malnourished with significant co-morbid factors, a period of non-operative management is preferred. If severe sepsis is present, salvage procedures that include drainage of abscesses and proximal diversion, with or without resection of the phlegmon, are indicated. A macerated abdominal wall further affects the surgical outcome adversely.

In most cases, a period of bowel rest and total parenteral nutrition is indicated to restore nutritional balance and to allow for healing of the skin surrounding the fistula. With control of sepsis and restoration of nutrition, about 50% of enterocutaneous fistulas close spontaneously over a 3–6-week period. Following recent surgery and the fistulising process, dense peritoneal reaction in the form of obliterative peritonitis is commonly encountered. Thus, definitive surgery is best deferred for at least 4 months to allow resolution of this peritoneal reaction.

Operative therapy

Prevention

Because most fistulas follow surgical mishaps, the foremost principle in management is prevention. This may be accomplished by adherence to strict surgical principles in performing intestinal anastomosis and sepsis prevention.

Salvage procedures

Sometimes early surgical intervention is necessary because of uncontrolled sepsis or a high fistula output, despite the poor general condition of the patient. The surgical procedures include:

- drainage of abscesses
- proximal diversion of bowel
- exteriorisation of the fistulising segment of bowel
- resection of the phlegmonous segment of bowel without anastomosis.

Definitive surgery

Major indications for surgery are persistent drainage following 2–3 months of maximal non-operative management, significant sepsis or presence of underlying diseased bowel (Crohn's disease, malignancy, radiation). Operations for fistulas are not to be taken lightly and require meticulous planning. If a recent surgery has been performed, an interval of at least 3–4 months should elapse before the definitive surgery.

Pre-operative preparations include appropriate bowel preparation, prophylaxis for deep vein thrombosis and adequate nutritional repletion. Samples from the fistula site and wound should be cultured and sensitivities obtained to guide the antibiotic prophylaxis. Blood should be cross-matched. The stoma site should be marked pre-operatively and its possibility discussed with the patient.

The operation should be performed through an adequately healed abdominal wall in which a secure abdominal closure can be obtained. Meticulous dissection and lysis of adhesions are performed to ensure that more distal obstruction of bowel is not present. Care is taken not to cause an unnecessary enterotomy, which, if it occurs, must be repaired with care. If technically possible, the entire gastrointestinal tract is carefully examined. Pre-operative imaging studies will have indicated the site of the fistula.

There are a number of surgical options: resection and anastomosis, which is the preferred option whenever feasible (the anastomosis is performed using healthy bowel in a clean field distant from the site of sepsis); resection with exteriorisation of bowel ends if there are factors adverse to optimal anastomotic healing; and wedge excision of the fistulising segment of bowel and primary repair if the fistula is small.

Post-operative management

Post-operative paralytic ileus is often prolonged and a period of decompression with a nasogastric tube is helpful. Antibiotics are continued for 72 hours after surgery, unless otherwise indicated. Parenteral nutritional support is continued post-operatively. Reintroduction of enteric intake may be slower in patients who have not eaten for several months. A minimal caloric intake of 1500 calories is necessary before parenteral nutrition can be discontinued.

Further reading

Chamberlain RS, Kaufman HL, Danforth DN. Enterocutaneous fistula in cancer patients: etiology, management, outcome, and impact on further treatment. *Am. Surg.* 1998; 64: 1204–1207.

Memon AS, Siddiqui FG. Causes and management of postoperative enterocutaneous fistulas. *J Coll Physicians Surg Pak.* 2004 Jan;14(1):25–8.

MCQs

Select the single correct answer to each question.

1 The following treatments are appropriate for a high-output enterocutaneous fistula EXCEPT:

a a high-fibre diet
b total parenteral nutrition
c intravenous fluid and electrolyte replacement
d sandostatin
e skin care by an enterostomal therapist

2 An enterocutaneous fistula that occurs 5 days after a small bowel resection for Crohn's disease may be associated with the following EXCEPT:

a anastomotic breakdown
b persistent intestinal obstruction distal to the fistula
c the presence of an inadequately drained abscess adjacent to the anastomosis
d traumatic enterotomy during adhesion lysis, which has been overlooked
e recurrent Crohn's disease

29 Rectal prolapse

Joe J. Tjandra

Introduction

Rectal prolapse has been described at all ages. Peaks of incidence are observed in the fourth and seventh decades of life. In the Western adult population, females are much more commonly afflicted. About 20% of patients with prolapse have an associated history of psychiatric illness. The key to rectal prolapse and its treatment is to first understand the terminology (Box 29.1, Fig. 29.1).

Pathogenesis

The cause of rectal prolapse is unknown but abnormal motor activity of the pelvic floor muscles may play a central role. A number of anatomical and physiological abnormalities are noted but it is unclear whether these abnormalities are primary and causative or secondary to the prolapse.

The primary support of the rectum is the levator ani. The puborectalis pulls the rectum anteriorly and its muscle fibres intermingle with the external anal sphincter to provide further support. Anatomic features associated with prolapse include:

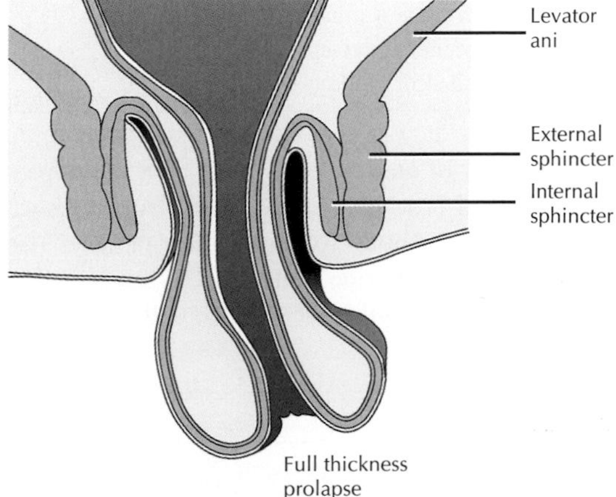

Fig. 29.1 Anatomic features of rectal prolapse.

- a deep peritoneal cul-de-sac
- a long mesorectum and poor posterior fixation of the rectum
- a redundant rectosigmoid
- a lax and atonic levator ani.

In some cases, functional disturbances result from intense straining against a pelvic floor that does not relax concomitantly. This may lead to rectal wall intussusception, causing a sensation of incomplete evacuation leading to further straining. In response to chronic and prolonged straining when passing stools, the pelvic floor muscles become stretched. In turn, the perineum descends, stretching the pudendal nerve. Pudendal neuropathy further leads to denervation of the anal sphincters and puborectalis. Over time, and with continued straining, the rectum protrudes beyond the anal orifice (Fig. 29.1). Faecal incontinence occurs in about 50% of patients and is caused both by progressive denervation of the external anal sphincter and by the presence of the intussuscepted rectum dilating the anal canal. Despite sphincter dysfunction, faecal incontinence is not invariably present.

Box 29.1 Definitions of rectal prolapse

- **Occult rectal prolapse** is caused by intussusception of the full thickness of the rectum, which does not protrude through the anal canal and may represent an early stage of complete prolapse.
- **Mucosal rectal prolapse** is protrusion of rectal mucosa through the anal canal and may be circumferential.
- **Complete rectal prolapse** (procidentia) is defined as full-thickness rectal protrusion through the anal orifice.

Box 29.2 Clinical presentation of complete rectal prolapse

- Prolapsing anorectal lump, which may occur only at defecation or may occur with coughing or walking or even spontaneously
- Rectal bleeding
- Mucous discharge
- Tenesmus

Associated features

- Faecal incontinence in about 50% of patients
- Constipation causing straining
- Concomitant uterine prolapse or cystocoele
- Solitary rectal ulcer syndrome

About 40% of women presenting with rectal prolapse have had previous gynaecological surgery, such as hysterectomy. About 20% of female patients also have an associated uterine prolapse. This suggests that an anatomic abnormality of the pelvic floor may be contributory.

Clinical presentation

The clinical presentations and associated features of complete rectal prolapse are given in Box 29.2.

Differential diagnosis

Rectal prolapse can be difficult to distinguish from extensive prolapsing internal haemorrhoids. With rectal prolapse, concentric rings of mucosa line the prolapsed tissue and a sulcus is present between the anal canal and the rectum. Two layers of the rectal wall are palpated. Haemorrhoids are separated by radial grooves and the sulcus is absent.

Evaluation

History

Careful history is directed at establishing the duration of the prolapse, the presence of coexistent symptoms of faecal incontinence or constipation and the patient's general medical status.

Physical examination

Physical examination includes a full anorectal and sigmoidoscopic examination to evaluate the anal sphincters and to document any concomitant abnormalities in the rectum. If the rectal prolapse is not obvious, the patient is asked to strain on the toilet until the prolapse is reproduced and viewed by the examiner.

Colonoscopy

If there is rectal bleeding or any change in bowel habits, a full colonic evaluation with colonoscopy should be performed.

Defecating proctogram

If the diagnosis is not obvious and an occult rectal prolapse is suspected, a defecating proctogram is diagnostic.

Anorectal physiological assessment

Anorectal physiological assessment is not generally helpful in rectal prolapse but may be valuable in the assessment of patients with faecal incontinence, because it may sometimes influence the operative approach.

Colonic transit studies

Colonic transit studies may be useful in constipated patients.

Treatment

Surgery is generally indicated for the treatment of complete prolapse, except in the very elderly. Conservative management is generally prescribed initially for occult or mucosal rectal prolapse. Elastic-band ligation of the prolapsing anterior rectal mucosa is sometimes helpful. Patients with persistent and unacceptable symptoms are considered for surgery; the types of procedures are similar to those performed for complete prolapse.

A large number of operations have been described for complete prolapse. Evaluation of their respective effectiveness is often limited by short or incomplete post-operative follow-up, as the patients are often elderly. Recurrence of prolapse has been observed up to 10 years post-operatively. The choice of surgical operation for rectal prolapse depends on the patient's general medical condition and the presence of associated features, such as constipation, diverticular disease and faecal incontinence. In general, a transabdominal repair is used for younger patients and a perineal repair for the elderly and frail patients. A full mechanical bowel preparation and parenteral antibiotic prophylaxis are essential for minimising septic complications.

Abdominal approach

Sacral fixation/rectopexy

The rectum is mobilised postero-laterally down to the level of the coccyx. The lateral ligaments are preserved during lateral dissection. Anterior dissection is usually not necessary. Fixation of the rectum to the sacrum may be performed by non-absorbable sutures (suture rectopexy) or a synthetic mesh. A partial wrap using the synthetic mesh, leaving the anterior surface of the rectum free, is sometimes described as the modified Ripstein operation (Fig. 29.2). Complete recurrence is around 3%, although mucosal prolapse is more common. Post-operative constipation is a common complaint after a Ripstein operation, as a tight sling may obstruct defecation. Rectal mobilisation with division of lateral ligaments per se may result in constipation from disruption of rectal innervation.

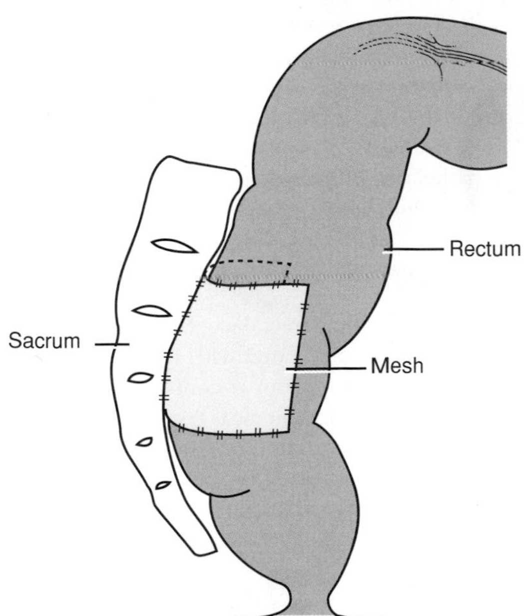

Fig. 29.2 Mesh rectopexy (modified Ripstein operation).

Abdominal sutured rectopexy with sigmoid resection (Frykman–Goldberg operation)

A sigmoid colectomy is performed. The rectum is mobilised as described earlier and sacral fixation with non-absorbable sutures is performed. Resection of redundant rectosigmoid may reduce post-operative constipation, either by eliminating the potential for kinking above the sling, as in the Ripstein operation, or by shortening the colon. The recurrence rate is probably slightly lower than rectopexy alone. The complication rate, especially sepsis, is higher because of the associated sigmoid resection. This surgical option is best reserved for good-risk patients with severe constipation and rectal prolapse.

Faecal continence

Faecal continence improves post-operatively in about 50% of patients following either abdominal repair of rectal prolapse. Improvement in continence post-operatively is mainly due to improvement in resting anal pressure. Pre-operative resting pressure does not seem to be predictive of post-operative continence.

Perineal approach

Perineal proctosigmoidectomy (Altemeier operation)

The procedure may be performed under general or regional anaesthesia. Patients are placed in a prone 'jack-knife' position. A circumferential incision is made about 1 cm above the dentate line. The prolapsed rectum is unfolded and the redundant rectum transected. The mesorectum is serially ligated and divided to deliver redundant rectum through the anal opening. A coloanal anastomosis is then performed either by sutures or a circular stapler. The levator muscles may be approximated, constituting a 'levatorplasty', which may improve faecal continence. Some surgeons also plicate the anal sphincters. Post-operative care is the same as for any bowel anastomosis. Pain is minimal, which is a major benefit of the procedure. The most common early post-operative complications are anastomotic dehiscence or bleeding. The recurrence rate is commonly quoted as less than 10%, although longer follow-up suggests that the cumulative rate may be much higher. Constipation is rarely a problem.

Mucosal sleeve resection (Délorme's procedure)

The procedure is performed with the patient in a prone jack-knife or lithotomy position under local, regional or general anaesthesia. The submucosa is infiltrated with a 1:200 000 adrenaline solution. A circumferential incision is made at the level of the dentate line. Dissection is performed in the submucosal plane to the proximal extent of the prolapse. The redundant mucosa is then excised. The underlying rectal muscle wall is plicated and the mucosal defect is then closed by sutures. Supplemental plication of anal sphincters may be performed. The most common complication is postoperative bleeding from the denuded muscle surface. The operation is generally well tolerated by frail patients, although the recurrence rate is probably higher than in other procedures and faecal incontinence is not improved. This perineal approach is probably best for the smaller complete prolapse or mucosal prolapse because a perineal proctosigmoidectomy is technically difficult in these cases.

Occult prolapse

This starts as an infolding of the anterior rectal wall 6–8 cm from the anal verge. The prolapse may descend into the anal canal but not through the anus. About 40% of asymptomatic subjects have occult rectal prolapse and it is not clear whether these will invariably progress to a complete rectal prolapse. Common symptoms include sensation of obstructed or incomplete defecation, pelvic pain, rectal bleeding and faecal incontinence. Solitary rectal ulcer may be present. Some patients have underlying psychological abnormalities on formal testing.

The initial management is conservative with careful explanation of the condition to the patient. Medical management includes the use of bulk-forming agents and judicious use of suppositories or enemas. Biofeedback is effective if paradoxical contraction of the puborectalis muscle is identified by anorectal physiological studies. Elastic-band ligation of the redundant anterior rectal mucosa may provide short-term relief for constant urge to strain.

In refractory cases with severe symptoms, surgery may be considered. Surgical options are essentially the same as for overt prolapse. Symptomatic outcome is often unpredictable. Pre-operative symptoms may not have been due to the internal prolapse. Careful patient selection for surgical management is important.

Solitary rectal ulcer syndrome

Solitary rectal ulcer syndrome is an uncommon but distressing problem. It usually affects young adults, and is more common in women. Typically, patients present with passage of blood and mucus per rectum. While the bleeding is usually slight and intermittent, occasionally it is massive and may require transfusions. Some patients experience tenesmus and a feeling of rectal discomfort that is difficult for patients to describe. Many patients habitually strain when passing stools. Rectal prolapse, overt or occult, is present in about one-third of patients. In 25% of subjects, endoscopic and histological features of solitary rectal ulcer syndrome may be present without causing any symptoms.

While the clinical picture of solitary rectal ulcer syndrome may be diverse, its histological appearances are typical and include fibromuscular obliteration of the lamina propria with hypertrophy of the muscularis mucosa. Sometimes biopsy may show cysts caused by displaced but normal mucosa and the retention of mucus, which is often called 'colitis cystica profunda'. The pathology is usually located anteriorly 5–8 cm from the dentate line, although it can be in any site within the rectum.

The solitary rectal ulcer may appear, macroscopically, as ulcerated, polypoid or hyperaemic. Multiple rather than solitary rectal lesions may be present. The ulcers, when present, tend to be shallow and grey in colour with a sharply demarcated and friable wall. The differential diagnosis includes cancer, lymphoma or Crohn's disease. It is important, therefore, to rely on the pathological features for a diagnosis of solitary rectal ulcer syndrome.

Pathogenesis

The aetiology of solitary rectal ulcer syndrome remains unknown. Trauma associated with rectal prolapse or self-digitation in the rectum is contributory in some patients. Anorectal physiological testing suggests that the puborectalis muscle fails to relax during straining in some, but not all, patients. This may result in abrasion of the anterior rectal wall against the contracted puborectalis muscle, resulting in ischaemia and ulceration.

Management

The rectal lesion must be biopsied to establish the diagnosis. Biopsy should be taken from the edge of the ulcer or from the polypoid lesion itself. A defecating proctogram is performed to detect occult prolapse and anorectal physiological testing to evaluate the pelvic floor.

Initially, the patient should be reassured that the condition is benign and the process should be explained. Conservative therapy with bulk laxative and re-education of bowel habit, such as avoidance of straining and biofeedback, leads to improvement or stabilisation of symptoms in 70% of patients. Symptoms may persist despite healing of the rectal lesion. Additional therapies include salazopyrine, steroid enema and sucralfate enema. None of these has been proven to show any additional benefit.

Unacceptable symptoms will persist in one-third of patients. Many of these have rectal prolapse, overt or occult. Ninety per cent of patients with rectal prolapse will improve following surgical repair of the prolapse. If no prolapse is noted, healing with surgical procedures is less reliable. Local excision of the rectal lesion is the simplest surgical procedure and may lead to improvement in symptoms, at least in the short term, in two-thirds of patients. Rectopexy in the absence of rectal prolapse results in healing in only 25% of cases. Other surgical options include low anterior resection or a diverting stoma. Both are associated with a significant morbidity and the surgical outcome is unpredictable.

Solitary rectal ulcer syndrome is an interesting condition. More research into its pathogenesis is necessary to define the most appropriate therapy.

MCQs

Select the single correct answer to each question.

1 Surgery for complete rectal prolapse includes the following EXCEPT:
- **a** abdominal rectopexy
- **b** sigmoid colectomy and rectopexy
- **c** Hartmann's procedure
- **d** perineal proctosigmoidectomy
- **e** Délorme's procedure (mucosal sleeve resection)

2 Full-thickness rectal prolapse is characterised by:
- **a** faecal incontinence in approximately half the patients
- **b** a rare association with uterine prolapse
- **c** a peak incidence in elderly males
- **d** a high incidence of psychotic disorders
- **e** characteristic abnormalities on anorectal manometry

30 Intestinal stomas

Joe J. Tjandra

Introduction

Although the need for permanent stomas has reduced in recent years with technical advances in restorative rectal surgery and sphincter salvage, the abdominal stoma still serves a critical function in the management of benign and malignant gastrointestinal problems. Although the quality of life of most ostomates is near-normal, there are physical and psychosocial limitations as a result of the stoma. The judicious assessment of the need for the stoma, careful surgical technique and skilled enterostomal nursing are essential for a satisfactory outcome. The management of patients with a stoma must begin before the operation, and the key to management of surgical complications is prevention. The main types of intestinal stoma are:

- ileostomy: end, loop, loop-end
- colostomy: end, loop
- caecostomy.

Ileostomy

End ileostomy

An end ileostomy is formed usually from the end of the terminal ileum (Fig. 30.1A). Formerly, a permanent ileostomy was made after a proctocolectomy for

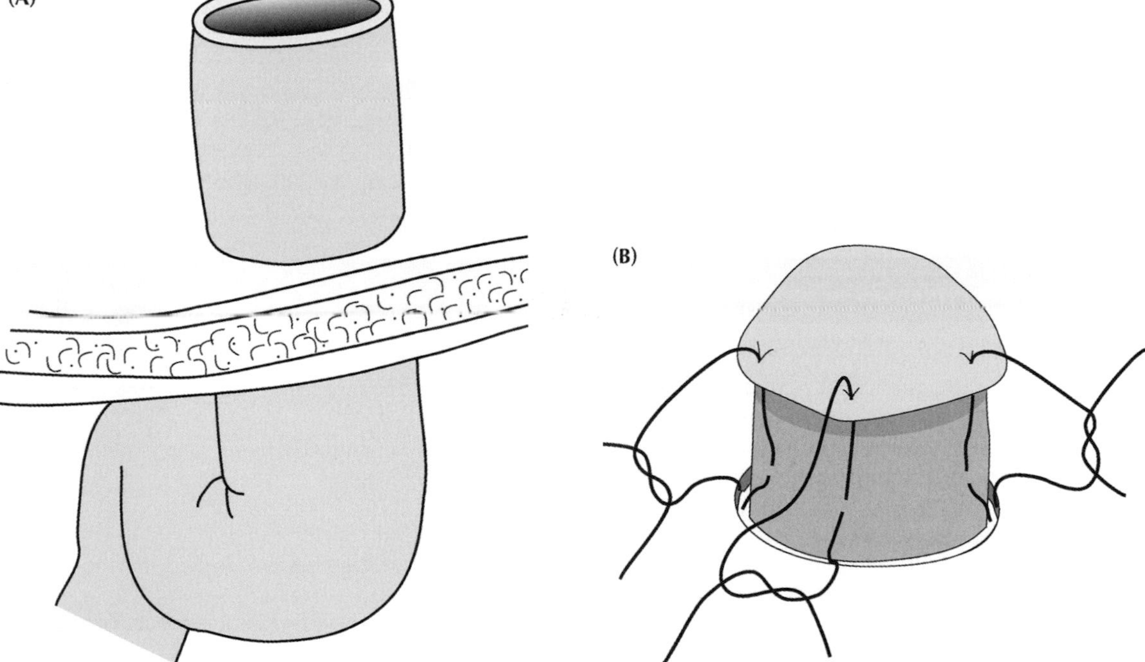

Fig. 30.1 (**A**) Construction of an end ileostomy. (**B**) Eversion and maturation of an end ileostomy.

inflammatory bowel disease or familial polyposis. With the advent of newer sphincter-saving procedures, such as a restorative proctocolectomy, this is now less commonly performed. The ileostomy can be temporary and is potentially reversible when it has been done in conjunction with subtotal abdominal colectomy for toxic colitis, left-sided large bowel obstruction or ischaemic bowel. In the latter situation, diversion is established when the hazards of primary anastomosis between the ileum and the colon or rectum are considered to be unacceptably high, because of bowel ischaemia, severe sepsis or gross nutritional depletion.

The terminal ileum is drawn through an elliptical incision in the right lower quadrant and through a muscle-splitting incision in the rectus muscle. A full-thickness eversion of the bowel is then performed to obtain primary Brooke-type maturation between the distal edge of the ileum and the dermis of the skin (Fig. 30.1B).

The principles of construction of an ileostomy are given in Box 30.1.

Loop ileostomy

This is used temporarily to protect a distal anastomosis such as an ileal pouch–anal anastomosis or a low colorectal anastomosis, or to divert stool from the distal anorectum such as for perianal Crohn's disease, fungating anorectal cancer, severe perineal trauma or sepsis and faecal incontinence. It is formed using a loop of the distal ileum delivered through the abdominal wall, usually in the right lower quadrant as for end ileostomy (Fig. 30.2A). A supporting rod is usually inserted through the mesentery under the apex of the ileal loop to relieve tension on the loop ileostomy. An incision is then made just above the skin level on the efferent (defunctioned) loop of ileum. The afferent (functional end) is then everted to form the larger of the two stomas (Fig. 30.2B). The afferent limb produces the stool output and the efferent limb allows passage of flatus and mucous discharge from the distal defunctioned portion of the bowel. Subsequent take-down and closure of a loop ileostomy can usually be done through a parastomal incision and generally does not involve a formal laparotomy. If done successfully, recovery is rapid and the duration of hospitalisation averages 4–5 days.

The loop-end ileostomy is an alternative to a temporary loop ileostomy when the loop of ileum cannot be delivered beyond the stoma aperture without excessive tension. This ileostomy is matured as a conventional loop ileostomy.

Ileostomy management

The stoma is oedematous immediately post-operatively, but this resolves within a week or so. The normal colour of the mucosa ranges from pink to deep red. The viability of the stoma is examined periodically in the post-operative period.

Intestinal peristalsis usually recommences 2–5 days after surgery. Sometimes there is an early output of watery intestinal content (bowel sweat) before return of bowel function. Oral feeding should be deferred until the paralytic ileus is resolved. Occasionally, the supporting rod of a loop ileostomy causes partial

Box 30.1 The principles of construction of an ileostomy

- Pre-operative marking of the stoma site. It must be visible to the patient, at the summit of the abdominal fat mound and away from bony prominences, skin creases, old or intended incision sites, and damaged skin. It should be sited within the rectus abdominis muscle to minimise parastomal hernia formation.
- Aperture of adequate size in the abdominal wall. If the fascial aperture is too small, obstructive bowel symptoms may occur. If the fascial aperture is too large, parastomal hernia or prolapse may occur.
- Adequate exteriorisation of the bowel.
- Adequate blood supply of the bowel.
- Haemostasis of the parastomal subcutaneous space to avoid haematoma formation. It is important to ensure that the inferior epigastric vessels are not traumatised during formation of the stoma aperture.
- Obliteration of any mesenteric defect between the cut edge of the small bowel mesentery and the anterior abdominal wall to prevent herniation of the small bowel through the defect.
- Stoma education.

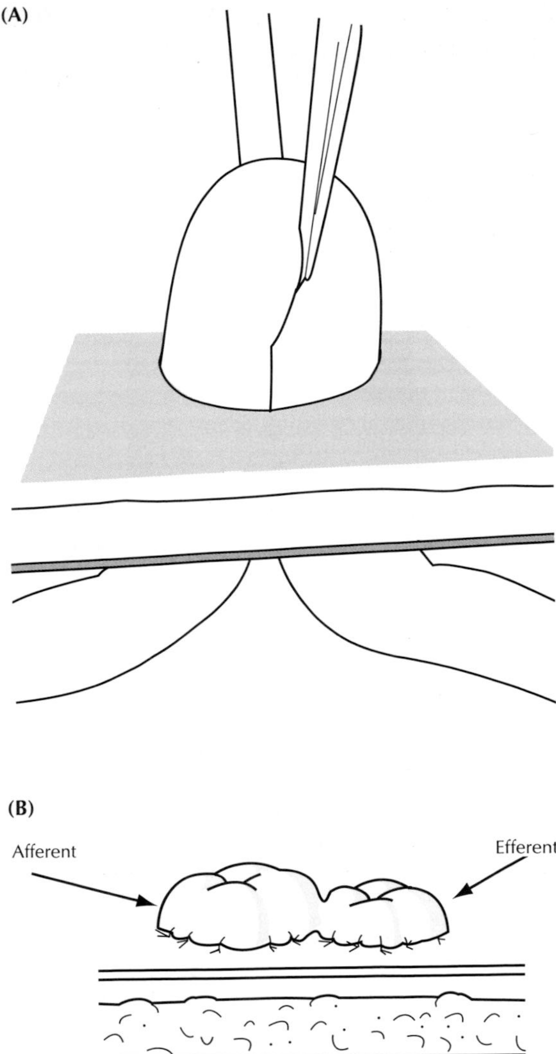

Fig. 30.2 (A) Construction of a loop ileostomy. (B) Loop ileostomy.

obstruction at the fascial level. The rod is usually removed after 4–5 days when sufficient adhesion has formed between the loop of bowel and the stoma aperture to prevent retraction of the stoma. The normal ileostomy output ranges between 500 and 1000 mL. Higher outputs may result in dehydration. Low output may indicate an obstruction. A partial bowel obstruction may, paradoxically, be associated with a high output of watery intestinal content.

Education on stoma care commences pre-operatively and continues post-operatively. As oedema subsides, the stoma is remeasured for new appliances about 4 weeks after construction. A properly fitting stoma appliance is important to avoid leakage of small bowel content, with resultant skin excoriation.

About 50% of patients experience some dietary restrictions post-operatively. Initially, a low-residue diet is recommended but within a few weeks other foods may be introduced. Foods that commonly affect ostomates are nuts, popcorn, corn, string vegetables, cabbage, oranges or fruit peels.

With a well constructed stoma and good stoma education, most ostomates achieve a good quality of life and the majority enjoy a normal life or experience only minor restrictions.

Complications

Complications after the creation of an ileostomy may be due to technical error, recurrent disease or poor stoma care (Box 30.2). Overall about 30% of patients experience a stoma-related complication.

About 20% of patients require revisional surgery to the ileostomy; such revisional surgery is more frequent in patients with Crohn's disease because of recurrence of disease. With recurrent Crohn's disease, treatment is directed towards the Crohn's disease itself. It may entail a laparotomy, resection of the diseased stoma and the adjacent segment of ileum, and formation of a neo-ileostomy at the same or another site. Other common indications for revisional surgery are retraction or prolapse of the stoma, and stricture and fistula formation. Some patients may require resiting of the stoma because of problems related to leakage. Unlike the situation with colostomies, parastomal hernia formation is infrequent.

Colostomy

End sigmoid colostomy

This may be temporary or permanent. The end stoma is permanent following abdominoperineal resection of the rectum for malignant disease or for severe faecal incontinence not appropriate for a perineal repair. It may serve as a temporary stoma for faecal diversion in radiation proctitis or following a Hartmann's procedure for resection of the rectosigmoid with benign or malignant disease. Because of the absorptive capacity of the proximal colon, the colostomy effluent is usually solid

Box 30.2 Common complications of ileostomy

- **Ischaemia**. Ischaemia ranges from relatively harmless mucosal sloughing to frank gangrene, which requires urgent laparotomy and refashioning of the stoma. If necrosis is superficial and is above the abdominal wall fascia, this can be managed expectantly. Subsequently, a stricture of the stoma may occur and require revision. A dusky stoma may be due to mesenteric venous engorgement, which will invariably improve with time.
- **Mucocutaneous separation**. This occurs if the mucocutaneous sutures separate. Minor separations will heal spontaneously. Gross separation may lead to serositis and stricture.
- **Parastomal abscess**. In the early post-operative period, a fistula or infected haematoma may be the source of a parastomal abscess. With delayed presentation, recurrent disease such as Crohn's disease with underlying fistula may be present.
- **Fistula**. In the early post-operative period, this usually arises from surgical trauma such as an unrecognised enterotomy or sutures that tear through the bowel. With delayed presentation, this may be a sign of recurrent Crohn's disease.
- **Bleeding**. Bleeding from the edge of the stoma is rarely a problem and, if troublesome, is treated with a simple suture ligation. Most will stop with simple pressure or cauterisation with silver nitrate. Bleeding from the proximal or distal portion of the bowel should be investigated appropriately.
- **High output**. Output from the newly constructed ileostomy is usually high (1–1.5 L) in the first 2 weeks. The average daily output from an established ileostomy is 500–800 mL/day. A high-output ileostomy is one that has an effluent discharge of more than 1 L/day. Patients with an ileostomy are prone to high-output diarrhoea, with resultant water and sodium depletion.
- **Ileostomy retraction**. For an end ileostomy, a 2–3-cm spout is optimal. If the stoma is too short, there is a strong tendency for leakage of ileostomy effluent under the stoma plate, with secondary skin damage. A convex appliance may be sufficient to obviate the commonly associated problem of leakage; otherwise, a surgical revision may be necessary. A local skin-level revision is often successful but sometimes a laparotomy is required to mobilise the small bowel adequately.
- **Parastomal hernia or prolapse**. Factors that predispose to development of hernia or prolapse include obesity, a stoma aperture that is too large or that is placed outside the rectus sheath, or multiple previous incisions in the abdominal wall around the stoma. Major symptomatic hernia or prolapse usually requires a formal laparotomy and stoma relocation. A strangulated parastomal hernia may pose a surgical emergency.
- **Small bowel obstruction**. Intra-abdominal adhesions, volvulus or internal herniation of small bowel through the lateral space may cause small bowel obstruction. Ingestion of high-residue food such as peanuts, string vegetables or corn may precipitate stomal blockage by bolus obstruction.
- **Parastomal ulcer**. Local sepsis, trauma or recurrent prestomal Crohn's disease accounts for most parastomal ulcers. A stoma-plate aperture that is too small may cut into the stoma and cause a linear ulcer on the inferior aspect of the stoma.
- **Skin irritation**. Contact of ileostomy effluent with the parastomal skin may result in skin irritation because it contains pancreatic proteolytic enzymes, bile acids and a high concentration of alkali.
- **Ileostomy stricture**. This may occur as a late complication of ischaemia, parastomal sepsis, recurrent Crohn's disease, previous radiation therapy or an opening in the fascial level of the abdominal wall that is too tight.

and non-irritating. Thus, the colostomy can be made flush with the skin without a spout.

Loop colostomy

Loop colostomy may be constructed using a loop of the transverse or sigmoid colon. It serves as a temporary faecal diversion following a low colorectal anastomosis or for obstruction, inflammation, trauma or perineal wounds. The loop colostomy may be constructed over a supporting rod through the mesocolic window, analogous to a loop ileostomy. An incision is made across the apex of the colon and both the afferent and efferent limbs of the bowel are sutured to the skin. Depending on the mobility of the colon and the body habitus of the patient, the loop of colon may be brought through either the lower quadrant or the right upper quadrant. While most loop colostomies are fully diverting in the first few months after construction, faecal diversion becomes incomplete in about 20% of patients subsequently because of recession of the stoma.

Caecostomy

A tube caecostomy using a No. 30 Fr Foley catheter is usually performed rather than a primary stoma. It is done for either colonic decompression or caecal volvulus. The tube can be removed after 7–10 days and the caecocutaneous fistula should close spontaneously in the absence of a distal obstruction. However, a caecostomy is not fully diverting and is difficult to manage because of dislodgement or blockage of the tube. This procedure is now rarely performed.

Colostomy management

The early management of a colostomy is similar to that for an ileostomy. Pre-operative stoma siting and counselling are as important. These patients tend to have concerns different from those of ileostomates, because they are often elderly and the diagnosis is usually cancer.

Following abdominal surgery, there is an ileus for the first 2–3 days. In contrast to ileostomy, where oral feeding is often delayed until the ileostomy has passed gas and effluent, the colostomy often requires stimulation by ingestion of food before it begins to function. Ischaemia tends to occur more with a colostomy than with an ileostomy because of the poorer vascular supply of the colon.

Function through a descending colostomy is similar to normal bowel function and may be susceptible to constipation. Bulking agents may help regulate the stoma. Some patients with an end colostomy may wish to try daily colostomy irrigations with lukewarm water. While the irrigation procedure takes 1–2 hours and the patient has to be motivated, there will be no soiling of stool throughout the rest of the day and a cap may be worn.

Complications

Complications associated with a colostomy are similar to those with an ileostomy (see Box 30.2), but they differ in frequency. Parastomal hernia (Fig. 30.3) and stoma prolapse are common because of the larger stomal aperture, especially with a loop stoma. Stricture also occurs more frequently because of the more tenuous blood supply. Food bolus obstruction and skin irritation are less common than that found in ileostomates.

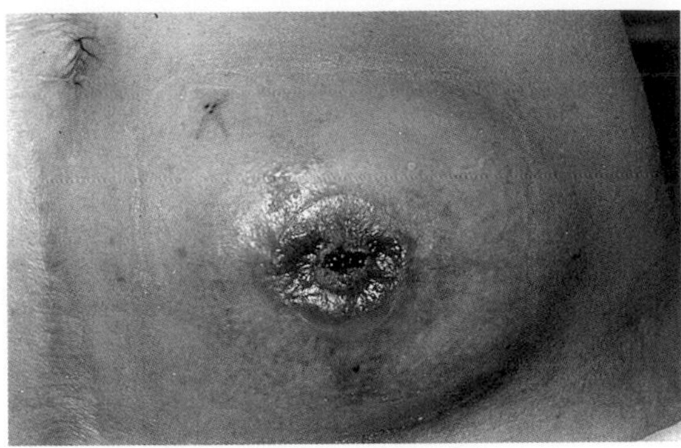

Fig. 30.3 Paracolostomy hernia with a colostomy stricture.

MCQs

Select the single correct answer to each question.

1 Complications of ileostomy include the following EXCEPT:

a ileostomy prolapse
b skin irritation around stoma site
c ileostomy retraction
d food bolus obstruction
e peptic ulcer

2 Which of the following is INCORRECT concerning stoma management?

a pre-operative stoma siting and counselling are important
b further measurements for new stoma appliances are performed approximately 4 weeks after surgery
c dietary restrictions are necessary
d sexual activities are to be avoided because of the stoma
e the enterostomal therapist is an integral member of the management team

31 Anal and perianal disorders

Leslie Bokey, Pierre Chapuis and Joe J. Tjandra

Anal fissure

Definition

An anal fissure is a linear tear or superficial ulcer of the anal canal, extending from just below the dentate line to the anal margin (Fig. 31.1). It usually occurs in the midline posteriorly, or sometimes anteriorly in females, particularly after a pregnancy.

Aetiology

Although the precise aetiology is unknown, it is usually related to constipation and trauma to the anal canal from a hard stool. Hypertonia of the internal anal sphincter with an associated raised anal resting pressure is common.

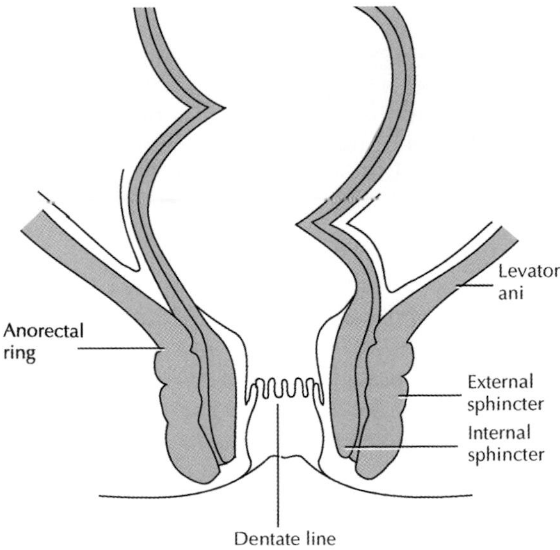

Fig. 31.1 Anatomy of the rectum and anal canal.

Symptoms

The cardinal symptoms are severe anal pain during and immediately after defecation and anal outlet bleeding. The pain is so intense that the patient is afraid of and consequently avoids opening the bowels. The pain has been attributed to spasm of the internal sphincter.

Diagnosis

The diagnosis is readily made on inspection. Anal fissure may be acute or chronic. Chronic anal fissure is associated with a sentinel skin tag at the anal margin and a hypertrophied anal papilla at the upper end of the anal canal. If the diagnosis is suspected on history and visual inspection of the anus, then it is important *not* to proceed to digital examination of the rectum: this would cause severe and unnecessary pain.

Inspection is the most important step in the diagnosis of anal fissure. This is performed with the patient in the left lateral position with the buttocks protruding well beyond the edge of the examining table. Good light must be made available. The buttocks are gently stretched apart and, providing the examiner is looking, a fleeting glimpse of the fissure will be obtained before sphincter contraction causes it to be withdrawn from view.

Differential diagnosis

Differential diagnosis includes fissures due to Crohn's disease and neoplastic ulcers. Fissures due to Crohn's disease are usually not in the midline. These fissures are deep, with indolent edges, tend to be multiple and occur at atypical sites; they are relatively pain-free. Anorectal strictures or ulcers and Crohn's proctitis are usually present. Neoplastic ulcers are usually due to squamous cell carcinoma. The ulcer is deep and has heaped-up edges. Other conditions that may have to be considered include sexually transmitted diseases (syphilis and HIV).

Treatment

The principal aim is to relax the internal sphincter, thereby relieving pain (which is due to spasm of that sphincter).

Conservative treatment

Conservative treatment includes the application of topical anaesthetic and hydrocortisone ointment, and a high-fibre diet to increase stool bulk (so that the stool itself dilates the sphincter). The complete healing rate is about 50% after 4 weeks of treatment. Recurrence rate is high, at about 25%. Glycerine trinitrate paste (0.2%) is effective in up to 50% of patients by relaxing the internal sphincter; however, the recurrence rate is high. It may also cause severe headache. More recent examples of chemical sphincterotomy include the use of calcium channel blockers and botulinum toxin.

Surgical treatment

Lateral internal anal sphincterotomy is the procedure of choice for chronic anal fissure or an acute fissure that remains severely symptomatic after a prolonged course of non-operative measures. The aim of surgery is to break the vicious cycle of internal sphincter spasm. The distal internal sphincter, up to but not above the dentate line, is divided under anaesthesia (Fig. 31.2). This procedure offers almost immediate relief of pain. The large sentinel skin tag and hypertrophied anal papilla are excised. After sphincterotomy, the patient should be put on a high-fibre diet. The recurrence rate is less than 3%. Some minor impairment of control of flatus occurs in up to 10% of patients but major faecal soiling is rare. In this regard, sphincterotomy performed through the base of the fissure is best avoided.

Some surgeons have advocated anal dilatation using six or eight fingers instead of sphincterotomy. This technique is imprecise and associated with a high prevalence of incontinence of both faeces and gas. It has no place in the modern management of anal fissure.

Perianal abscess

Aetiology

Perianal abscess is a common condition that is usually due to a blocked anal gland (Fig. 31.3) that subsequently becomes infected (cryptoglandular origin). There are usually no predisposing factors, but patients with diabetes, Crohn's disease or those who are immunocompromised are susceptible. The abscess may discharge spontaneously to the skin, and if a communication to the skin is established then a fistula may result. This may occur in up to 50% of patients.

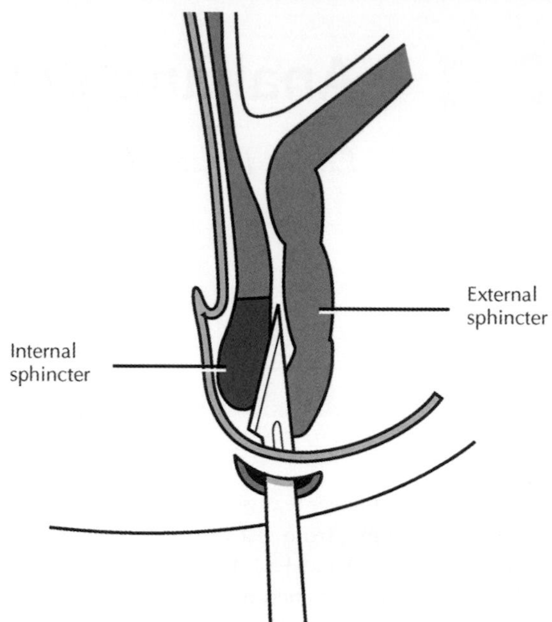

Fig. 31.2 Lateral sphincterotomy for chronic anal fissure.

Classification

Although most abscesses are perianal, sepsis can occur either above or below the levator muscle, in the intersphincteric space, submucosally or in the ischiorectal space (Fig. 31.4). Abscesses that involve the upper portion of the anal sphincters are complex and require specialist management.

Diagnosis

The diagnosis is readily made from a history of throbbing pain and visual inspection, which demonstrates localised swelling, tenderness and redness. A large or a deep-seated abscess, such as an ischiorectal abscess, often presents with systemic symptoms of sepsis and fever.

Investigations

A full blood count and blood glucose level measurement should be performed. Further investigations

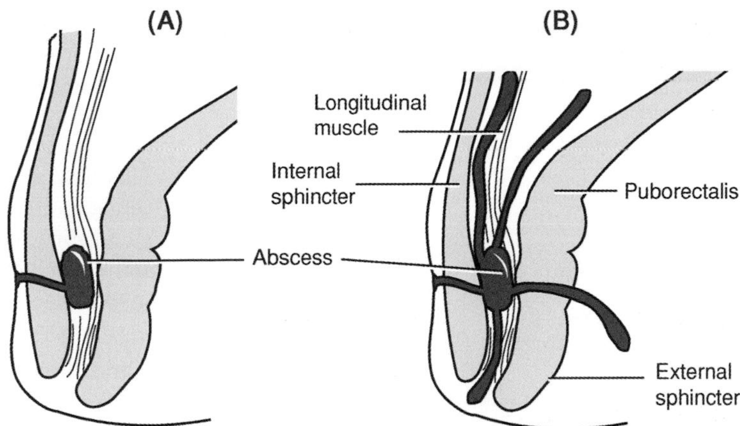

Fig. 31.3 Spread of infection (**A**) from the primary anal gland abscess and (**B**) to the perianal region.

should be performed if associated conditions are suspected as defined under 'Aetiology' above.

Treatment

The most common practice is to incise and drain the abscess under local anaesthesia. Antibiotics are used if the sepsis is extensive or if the patient is immunocompromised. There is little role for antibiotics in the primary management of perianal abscess of cryptoglandular origin. It is usual to leave a small drain or packing gauze in the abscess cavity for a few days postoperatively. Bigger and deeper abscesses, such as an ischiorectal abscess, are drained under general anaesthesia. Perianal abscesses must be drained with optimal preservation of underlying anal sphincters. A sigmoidoscopy to examine the rectal mucosa should be performed in this situation. It is important to recognise these complex or horseshoe ischiorectal abscesses so as not to damage the anal sphincter. Simple drainage will suffice, followed in a few weeks by a more sophisticated test such as an endorectal ultrasound, and a further examination under anaesthesia if discharge persists. Underlying bowel disease such as Crohn's disease must be excluded in these complex situations. Almost 50% of abscesses are associated with a fistula-in-ano and therefore many of these abscesses recur. Should this happen, an examination under anaesthesia should be performed after the abscess has been drained to determine whether a fistula is indeed present.

Fistula-in-ano

Definition

A fistula is an abnormal communication between two epithelial-lined surfaces. A *fistula-in-ano* implies a communication between the anorectum and the perineal skin.

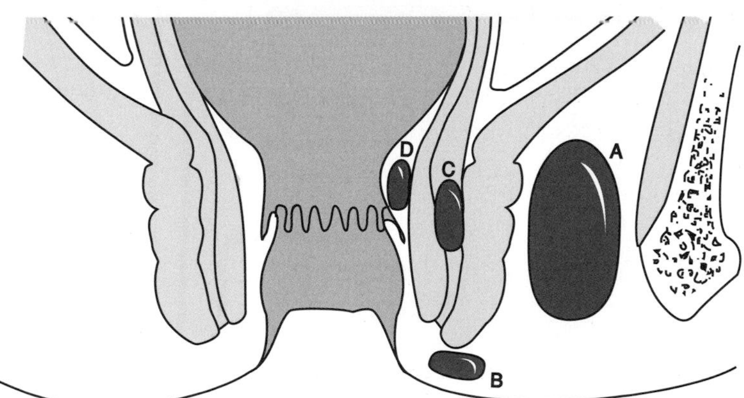

Fig. 31.4 Types of perianal abscess: (**A**) ischiorectal, (**B**) perianal, (**C**) intersphincteric, and (**D**) submucosal.

Box 31.1 Aetiology of fistula-in-ano

- Idiopathic. In most patients the exact cause cannot be determined but is probably related to anal gland infection.
- Anal gland infection. An anal gland abscess may spontaneously track and discharge onto the perineal skin.
- Crohn's disease.
- Iatrogenic. Some fistulas, especially those with a high internal opening, may be caused inadvertently during drainage of a perianal abscess or fistula surgery.
- Carcinoma.
- Trauma, especially obstetric.
- Foreign body. Occasionally a chicken or fish bone may get stuck in the anal canal and cause a fistula.
- Radiation damage.
- Tuberculosis, actinomycosis.

Aetiology

The causes of fistula-in-ano are given in Box 31.1.

Classification

The most important determinant of a fistula-in-ano is whether its internal opening is below or above the anorectal ring (Fig. 31.5). Those below are low fistulas and those with an internal opening above the levator are high fistulas. In general terms, low fistulas tend to be either idiopathic or associated with anal gland infection, and high fistulas have other, more serious aetiological associations.

The line of communication between the internal and external openings is not always direct, and may indeed be very tortuous. Goodsall observed that when the external opening was anterior to the anus, it communicated directly with the internal opening; while when the external opening was posterior to the anus, the internal opening tended to occur in the midline posteriorly. This may produce complex fistulas with a horseshoe configuration with blind tracks on either side communicating with the anus in the midline posteriorly, and probably result from an abscess in the postanal space.

Symptoms

The patient may present with recurrent perianal abscesses or with a bloody and purulent discharge. Pain and discomfort are usual. A careful history may elicit symptoms of inflammatory bowel disease or other conditions.

Diagnosis

The diagnosis is usually confirmed by examination. An external opening is usually readily visible. The track leading to the internal opening is sometimes palpable and, with experience, the internal opening may sometimes be identified on rectal examination. Whenever possible, it is important to determine by examination the level of the internal opening in relation to the levator mechanism. Goodsall's law indicates that fistulas with an anterior external opening drain directly into the anus at the dentate line, and those with a posterior external opening take a curved course to enter the anal canal in the midline (Fig. 31.6). While the majority of fistulas probably conform to Goodsall's law, there are some exceptions.

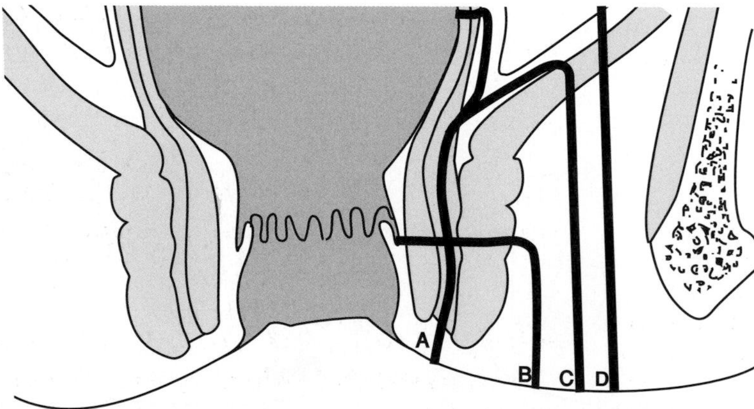

Fig. 31.5 Types of perianal fistulas: (A) intersphincteric, (B) trans-sphincteric, (C) supra-sphincteric, and (D) extra-sphincteric.

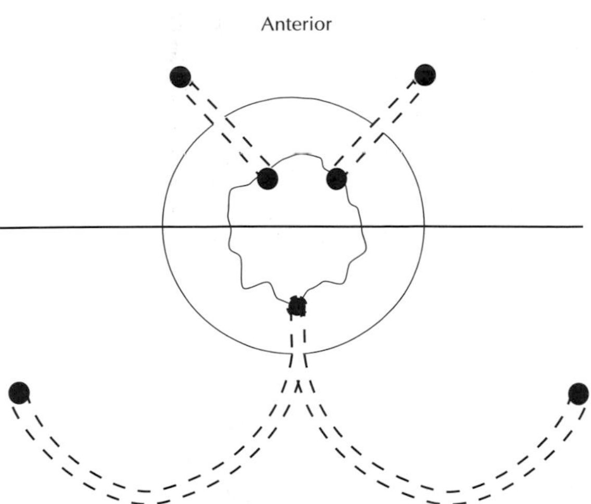

Fig. 31.6 Goodsall's law.

Investigations

Sigmoidoscopy is necessary to examine the mucosa of the rectum to exclude inflammatory bowel disease. If the latter is suspected then colonoscopy and a small bowel series should be performed to determine the extent of the disease.

Examination under anaesthesia is very useful, especially in patients with complex or high fistulas. A fistulogram may be useful in identifying the extent of complex fistulas. Endoluminal ultrasound and magnetic resonance imaging (MRI) are proving very useful in patients with complex fistulas as they clearly demonstrate the relationship of the fistula track to the levator mechanism and anal sphincters.

Treatment

Spontaneous healing of perianal fistula is rare. Surgical treatment is usually required. The key to management includes identification of the fistulous tracts and their relationship with the anal sphincters.

Low fistula

The mainstay of treatment is to identify the internal and external openings and to 'lay open' the intervening track by fistulotomy. This allows the track to heal by secondary intention. Special assessment of the adequacy of the sphincter mechanism should be considered in females who have had several vaginal deliveries because occult injuries to the anal sphincters and pudendal nerve may already be present.

High fistula

Fistulotomy is contraindicated if the internal opening is above the levator mechanism. In these patients fistulotomy would include division of the levator, which would result in incontinence. Caution should be exercised when more than one-third of the external anal sphincter needs to be divided. To avoid this serious complication it is useful to insert a seton between the two openings: silk or silastic tubing is railroaded into the track and loosely tied. The seton may act as a drain and if it is progressively tightened it may gradually divide the muscle while allowing it to heal by fibrous tissue formation. Alternatively, the seton downstages the sepsis and facilitates subsequent repair of the fistula with an advancement rectal flap. Occasionally, with more complex fistulas, a proximal stoma is constructed to divert the faecal stream, in addition to other local surgical manoeuvres.

Anovaginal and rectovaginal fistulas

Special mention is made of anovaginal and rectovaginal fistulas because they are not uncommon and are usually very distressing to the patient.

Aetiology

Obstetrical trauma is the most common cause. This may be related to either a tear during delivery or an inappropriately sited episiotomy (or one that may not have been expertly repaired). Other causes include trauma, radiation injury and inflammatory bowel disease (especially Crohn's disease).

Symptoms

The patient complains of passing flatus or faeces per vaginum. The symptom is socially and sexually embarrassing and some patients only seek advice after several years of social isolation.

Diagnosis

The diagnosis is readily made during examination under anaesthesia.

Treatment

It is usually possible either to directly repair the defect between the anorectum and vagina or to advance a mucosal–submucosal flap of rectum or vagina to cover the defect. This treatment is efficacious even in patients with Crohn's fistulas. Occasionally, a covering (diverting) stoma may be required following repair of a very complex fistula.

Anal cancer

Anal cancer is rare and represents less than 5% of all large bowel cancers. Most anal cancers are malignant epithelial tumours of the anal canal. The majority are squamous cell carcinomas (SCC). There are various additional subtypes, including cloacogenic carcinoma (transitional, basaloid, pleomorphic), adenocarcinoma of anal gland origin and malignant melanoma. The latter represent less than 1% of all malignant tumours of the anorectum. In Queensland with the highest incidence of cutaneous melanoma in the world, anorectal melanoma is the fourth more common site of occurrence after cutaneous, occular and vulval melanomas.

Squamous cell carcinomas of the anal canal occurs commonly in elderly women, while SCC of the anal verge is more often seen in men. The reason for the higher prevalence in women is unclear but it may be due to human papilloma virus (HPV) infection from secondary spread from cervical HPV (genotypes 16 and 18) or from the practice of receptive anal intercourse. Many agents may act as cofactors with HPV to promote epithelial dysplasia into invasive cancer including carcinogens (tobacco); other viral infections (HIV, herpes simplex II); immunodeficiency; and sexually transmitted diseases (syphilis, lymphogranuloma venereum, chlamydia). Also, Bowen's disease and extra-mammary Paget's disease are important premalignant skin conditions that may give rise to an invasive cancer of the anal verge. Anal cancer is now commonly seen in male homosexuals often in association with AIDS-related illnesses.

Classification of anal cancer

A knowledge of the different epithelia that line the anal canal is helpful in understanding the origin and classification of the various tumour types that may arise from the anus and adjacent perianal skin (Fig. 31.7). The dentate or pectinate line (Fig. 31.8) is a circumferential landmark which, at the bases of the anal columns, unites the anal valves covering the anal crypts containing the openings of the anal glands (Fig. 31.9).

The epithelium lining the upper third of the canal is known as the 'anal transitional zone' (ATZ). It has a variable proximal extension into the lower rectum that is age-dependent (broader in the elderly) and represents the remnant of the cloacal membrane in the foetus. It consists of a mixture of stratified squamous, stratified columnar and cuboidal epithelium (so-called transitional epithelium), which blends with the typical simple columnar epithelium of the rectum. Between the dentate line and the anal verge is the pecten, which is lined by stratified squamous non-keratinised epithelium that lacks skin appendages and has few sweat glands. Below this is true skin composed of stratified squamous keratinised epithelium with sweat glands and hair follicles.

It is important to distinguish between cancer of the anal canal from that arising from the anal verge, because their treatment and prognosis are different.

Diagnosis

Anal cancer typically presents with bleeding or symptoms of pruritus ani, such as moisture, perianal itch, a burning sensation or pain after defecation if the tumour is ulcerated and infected. It is often difficult to be certain of the diagnosis on clinical examination alone and a high level of suspicion is necessary when examining this area.

Clinical features

Cancer of the anal canal is indistinguishable from rectal cancer and usually presents as an ulcer with typical rolled edges (Fig. 31.10). Cancer of the anal verge also presents as an ulcer or chronic fissure. Occasionally, the perianal tissues may show a superficial palpable, irregular brownish eczematoid plaque. The diagnosis must always be confirmed by incisional biopsy. In this context, any haemorrhoidectomy specimen should always be labelled separately and sent for histological examination if cancer is suspected. In melanoma, those arising from the rectum are far less common than those arising from the ATZ.

Tumour spread

Anal canal cancer grows predominantly by upward spread along the line of least resistance. Distal spread

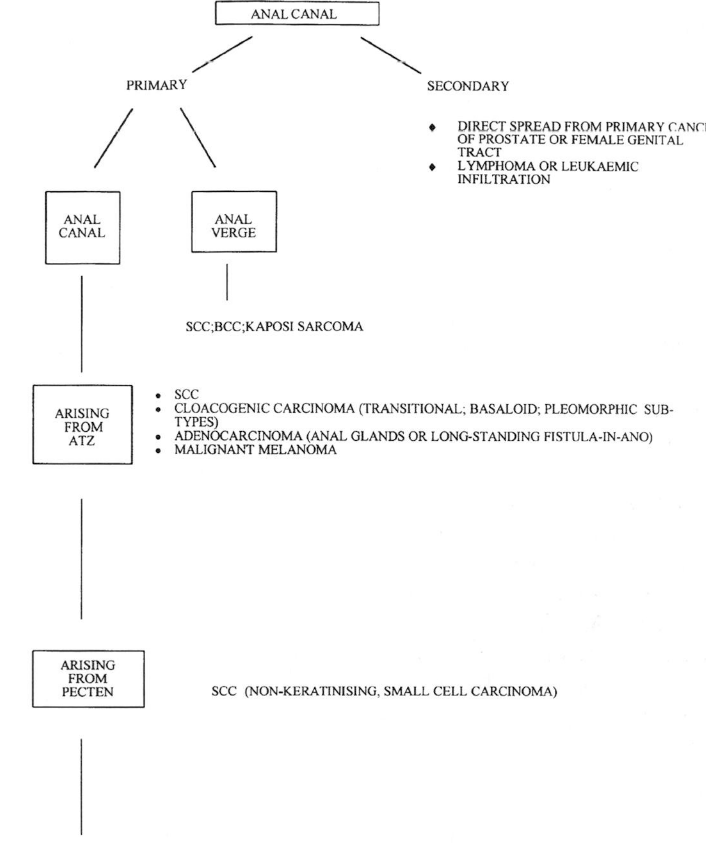

Fig. 31.7 Origin and classification of anal canal tumours.

is limited as the dentate line is relatively fixed to the underlying internal anal sphincter. As it arises in the ATZ or watershed area, it may then spread via

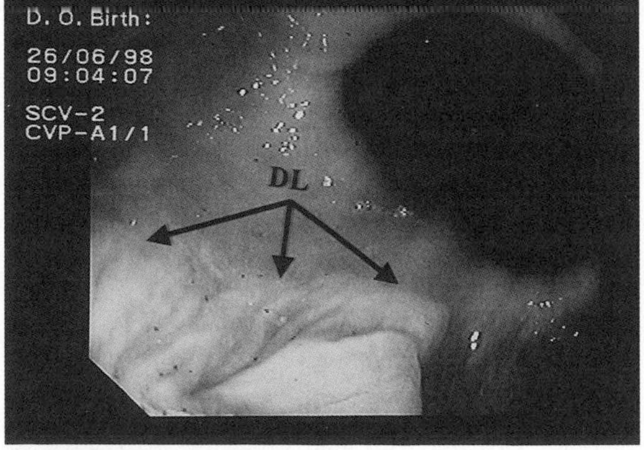

Fig. 31.8 Anal canal. DL, dentate line.

lymphatics accompanying the superior and middle rectal arteries and has a tendency to present at an advanced stage. Cancer of the anal verge is likewise slow growing and may metastasise along lymphatics that accompany the inferior rectal artery to superficial inguinal lymph nodes.

Treatment

Treatment depends on location, size and extent of local spread of the tumour. Pretreatment evaluation depends on careful clinical examination. This usually implies examination under anaesthesia with biopsy of the tumour. Transanal ultrasonography will accurately determine the level of direct spread into surrounding tissues and an abdominopelvic computed tomography scan is useful in detecting distant spread prior to planning treatment.

Cancer of the anal verge is usually treated by a wide local excision with clear margins. Skin grafting may

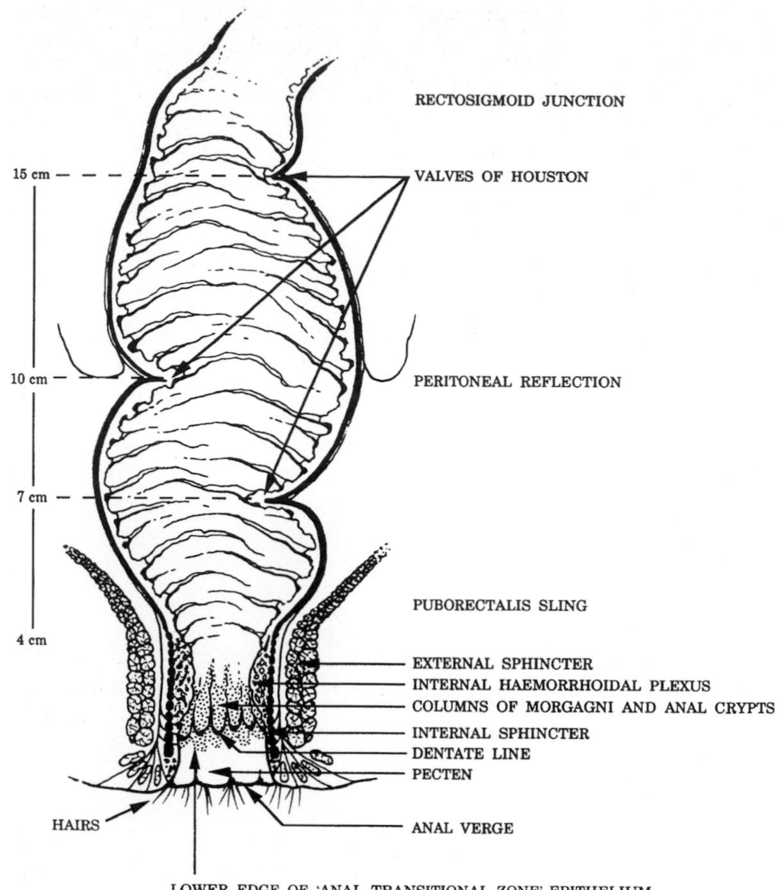

Fig. 31.9 Anal canal and rectum.

be necessary to cover the defect. A large SCC ($\geq$2 cm) occasionally may require chemoradiotherapy. Excision of the rectum and anus (abdominoperineal excision [APE]) may be necessary for a large tumour that extends into and involves the anal canal.

Cancer of the anal canal is primarily treated by chemoradiotherapy. This now is considered the treatment of choice as such tumours have an extensive lymphovascular drainage area and local relapse is high if treated by APE alone; they are radiosensitive tumours; chemoradiotherapy ensures preservation of a functioning anus in the majority of patients; and often such patients are elderly and have associated comorbidity, placing them at a high risk for surgery. Chemoradiotherapy is still based on the original regimen developed by Dr Norman Nigro (Box 31.2). This protocol uses a small dose of external beam radiotherapy, which has remarkably low toxicity when combined with chemotherapy. After treatment, patients are followed closely for at least 5 years. Salvage APE is offered to selective patients who develop local recurrence or such patients may receive additional chemoradiotherapy. Up to 25% of patients will present with clinically involved inguinal lymph node metastases at the time of initial consultation. Any suspicious node must be biopsied. If involved, mobile nodes are usually treated by block dissection of the groin, while fixed nodes are better treated by radiotherapy.

The treatment of anal melanoma is controversial but usually involves APE, often with radiotherapy.

Results

Anal cancer is commonly staged using a modified TNM classification (Box 31.3) developed by the Union Internationale Contre le Cancer (UICC). Importantly, prognosis for patients with anal canal SCC is related to

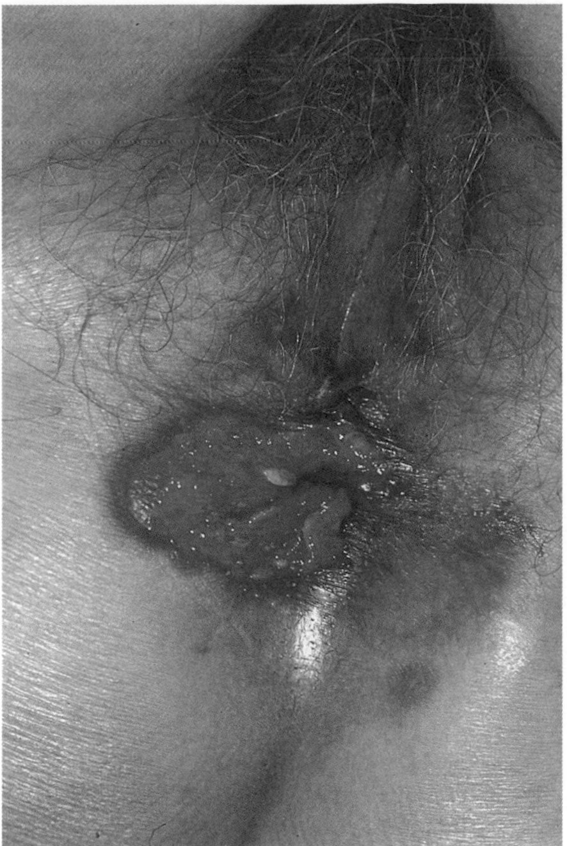

Fig. 31.10 Squamous cell carcinoma of the anal verge.

tumour size, histological grade, the extent of local spread and the presence of regional lymph node metastases. Cell type is not a prognostic factor; survival rates for SCC and cloacogenic carcinoma are the same. After local excision with tumour-free margins patients generally have a good prognosis, with more than 80% surviving 5 years. Patients who show an initial complete response to chemoradiotherapy can expect up to 80% 5-year survival on completion of such treatment. The results of treatment for melanoma are poor, varying from 7% to 20% overall 5-year survival.

Box 31.2 Nigro's regimen

External beam radiotherapy
30 Gy delivered to the pelvis in 15 fractions beginning on day 1

Chemotherapy
Systemic 5-FU as continuous infusion on days 1–4
Mitomycin-C given as intravenous bolus on day 1
5-FU repeated 4-day infusion on day 28

Box 31.3 Modified TNM staging for anal cancer

T_1	Tumour $\leq$ 2 cm in greatest dimension
T_2	Tumour > 2–5 cm
T_3	Tumour > 5 cm
T_4	Tumour invades adjacent organ (vagina, urethra, bladder)
N_0	No regional lymph node metastases
N_1	Perirectal lymph node metastases
N_2	Unilateral internal iliac/inguinal
N_3	Perirectal and inguinal/bilateral internal/inguinal
M_0	No distant metastases
M_1	Distant metastases

Stage grouping

Stage I	T_1 N_0 M_0
Stage II	T_2 N_0 M_0; T_3 N_0 M_0
Stage III	T_{any} N_1 M_0
Stage IV	T_{any} N_{any} M_1

Pilonidal sinus

Pilonidal sinus is an acquired, chronic inflammatory condition in which hair becomes embedded in a midline pit or track, usually between the buttocks around the coccygeal region. It mainly affects young hirsute males and is almost never seen in prepubescent subjects. The sinus may consist of a single track, but commonly there may be subsidiary lateral tracks extending on either side to the buttocks. The sinuses are usually filled with hairs. Pilonidal sinuses can also occur between fingers and in the neckline posteriorly.

Presentation

The presentation of pilonidal sinus can vary.

- Asymptomatic. This is found incidentally during physical examination.
- Abscess formation. This occurs with local pain and swelling, and systemic effects.
- Chronic sepsis with discharge and discomfort. There are occasional episodes of abscess formation.

Diagnosis

The diagnosis is readily made by simple observation of the sinus with or without evidence of sepsis.

Treatment

Conservative

Providing there is no sepsis, some patients may be treated conservatively by careful hair control using depilatory creams, regularly shaving the natal cleft and proper hygiene. Antibiotics are prescribed for acute exacerbations. The acute episode may sometimes settle simply by removing the hair.

Surgery

Patients with an abscess should, in the first instance, have it drained. Some surgeons advocate injection of the track with a solution of phenol with the aim of obliterating it. Phenol is very irritating and it is important to protect the surrounding skin with petroleum jelly. Excision is the most commonly practised procedure. The principal track and subsidiary sinuses are excised. The resulting defect is then either left open to heal by secondary intention or is primarily sutured. If the defect is very large, as is occasionally the case, then a flap may be rotated to close it. Occasionally a split skin graft may also be used to close the defect.

Pruritus ani

Pruritus ani is an unpleasant yet common condition; however, it is poorly understood and often poorly managed. The patient complains of varying degrees of discomfort and itching around the anal area. No amount of scratching gives relief to the patient, who is often left anxious and frustrated. Symptoms are often more acute at night, exacerbated by the local warmth of bed clothing. Itch leads to repeated scratching with skin trauma, and further scratching leads to secondary infection and further itch.

Aetiology

The causes of pruritus ani are given in Box 31.4. A common exacerbating factor is said to be coffee, which acts as an irritant. Other predisposing conditions include diabetes, immune deficiency syndromes (HIV in particular) and, occasionally, psychological disorders. Diarrhoea of any cause can contribute to pruritus ani. However, causative or precipitating factors are identified in only 25% of patients.

Box 31.4 Aetiology of pruritus ani

- Idiopathic
- Poor hygiene
- Haemorrhoids
- Fissure-in-ano
- Drug hypersensitivity and allergies
- Anal warts
- Fungal infection
- Parasites
- Faecal incontinence
- Anal cancer
- Premalignant conditions (e.g. Bowen's disease)
- Systemic disease (e.g. renal failure, diabetes mellitus)

Diagnosis

A careful history and physical examination are required to exclude predisposing and associated conditions. Flexible sigmoidoscopy and proctoscopy are necessary to identify common anorectal conditions. When fungal infections are suspected, skin scrapings should be obtained for microscopic examination.

Treatment

Coexistent and contributing conditions, such as diabetes, should be treated and managed first. The patient should be reassured that there is no sinister underlying pathology. Advice regarding personal hygiene is crucial. It is important that although the perineum should be clean, patients should not wash excessively lest the skin become too dry. After defecation, soft tissue or moist cotton wool pads should be used to wipe the anal area. The patient should avoid rubbing with harsh toilet paper. Cotton underwear is better than that made of synthetic material and tight clothes should be avoided. Whenever possible, hot humid conditions should be avoided. Medicated soaps should be not be used because they may exacerbate the irritation. Local application of zinc-based creams has been found to be useful, especially when the skin is very inflamed. A simple acid pH ointment, such as calamine lotion, helps to reduce the contact of the irritant with the perianal skin. Steroid-based creams may be used very sparingly in severe chronic cases, but should not be applied on a long-term basis because of toxicities with skin atrophy and superinfection. Disordered defecation such as anismus or mucosal prolapse may cause 'after-leak' following a bowel movement and may respond to specific treatment for these conditions.

Hidradenitis suppurativa

Hidradenitis suppurativa is a chronic, debilitating inflammatory condition of the apocrine glands. The axillae, groin, perineum and perianal skin are primarily involved. Apocrine glands begin to function at puberty and their secretions are thick and foul-smelling. It is thought that an endocrine disorder (elevated levels of androgen) leads to abnormal keratin production and obstruction of gland ducts.

Pathology

Abnormal keratin plugging obstructs the ducts of the apocrine glands, which then become secondarily infected. The histopathology of hidradenitis suppurativa is usually non-specific.

Symptoms

The onset of disease usually coincides with puberty and mimics Crohn's disease. Clinically, the disease begins as a small, firm, subcutaneous nodule that subsequently becomes tender. The infected glands are painful and discharge malodorous fluid. The disease is characterised by remission and relapse, and is associated with significant scarring and consequent social isolation. Ultimately, the condition results in multiple subcutaneous tracks and fibrosis around the anus, and may mimic a complex fistula-in-ano (Fig. 31.11). Only the distal one-third of the anal canal that contains apocrine glands is involved. Other regions should always be examined, including the axillae, groins and perineum, to ensure adequate treatment.

Differential diagnosis

Differential diagnosis includes:
- lymphogranuloma venereum
- tuberculosis
- actinomycosis
- pilonidal sinus
- fistula-in-ano
- Crohn's disease
- squamous cell carcinoma.

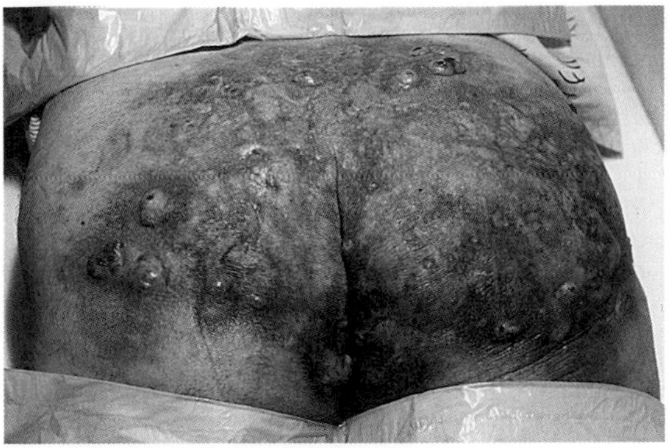

Fig. 31.11 Hidradenitis of the perineum and perianal region.

Evaluation of the patient includes inspection of all apocrine gland-bearing areas. Sigmoidoscopy is done to determine the extent of anal disease and to rule out Crohn's disease. If the diagnosis is in doubt, biopsy of the involved tissue is performed.

Treatment

Acute

Broad-spectrum antibiotics such as augmentin are useful. Acute abscesses are drained. Long-term antibiotics do not alter the likely chronicity of the course of illness.

Chronic

The treatment of choice is an *en bloc* excision of the involved skin-bearing apocrine glands. Minor defects may be closed primarily. However, more radical surgery usually results in a wide defect that needs to be grafted. Alternatively, incision and drainage of subcutaneous abscesses without radical excision may be done for very extensive disease. Repeated sessions may be needed to lay open all the tracks. Very occasionally, with very severe perineal disease, preliminary faecal diversion by loop colostomy may be helpful.

Perianal warts

Perianal warts, also known as condylomata acuminata, are sexually transmitted. They are most often seen in adult homosexual males and less frequently in the heterosexual population. About two-thirds of patients with perianal warts also have warts within the anal canal. Perianal warts are caused by HPV, and genotype 6 is most frequently seen. There is an association between warts, receptive anal intercourse and anal cancer. Perianal warts may become locally invasive without invasion of lymphovascular structures. These are the so-called giant condylomata.

Squamous metaplasia and *in situ* carcinomatous changes within the perianal warts may occur. Sometimes they become malignant and result in invasive SCC.

Treatment

Treatment involves the combination of diathermy fulguration of small clusters of warts or warts within the anal canal and scissor excision of more extensively involved areas. Topical application of 25% podophyllin in benzoin tincture has a role in small isolated clusters of perianal warts but may cause pain. Several sessions may be needed to clear recurrent warts. Warts may also disappear spontaneously, presumably due to the development of some degree of immunity.

Levator syndrome

The cause of levator syndrome is obscure. Patients describe a sudden onset of severe perineal pain that is self-limiting, lasting from only a few minutes to less than half an hour, often after sexual activity or awakening from sleep (also called proctalgia fugax). It mainly affects young men and tends to regress spontaneously in later life. The majority of patients are anxious. A large number of patients also present with a ball-like rectal pressure radiating from the rectum toward the coccyx and sometimes into the buttock. This is usually aggravated by sitting and is relieved by ambulation or lying down. This occurs more frequently in women. The term *levator syndrome* is used to describe this entity but more often it encompasses a generalised diagnostic group with obscure causation. It is important to exclude other organic causes that may cause perineal or anal pain (Box 31.5). Proctalgia or levator syndrome pain should not be confused with coccygodinia, which implies pain due to a coccygeal injury. Computed tomography scan, magnetic resonance imaging as well as transanal ultrasonography are all useful techniques to investigate patients with chronic pain; however, in the majority of patients the aetiology remains obscure and is commonly explained on the basis of idiopathic, self-limiting painful spasm of the pelvic floor muscles (levator ani, puborectalis).

Box 31.5 Causes of anal pain

- Inflammation: anal fissures, perirectal abscesses or haematomas, strangulated haemorrhoids
- Anorectal neoplasm
- Post-operative (e.g. haemorrhoidectomy)
- Orthopaedic: coccygeal, neurogenic
- Pelvic floor disorders and levator syndrome

Treatment is empirical and patients should be reassured that they have no sinister pathology. Massage of the puborectalis sling, local heat, muscle relaxants, galvanic muscle stimulation and biofeedback have all been claimed to alleviate pain. Reassurance is often sufficient to deal with most of the symptoms. Management is difficult and recurrence rates are substantial owing to psychogenic reasons.

Anorectal manometry

Anorectal manometry is a method of measuring anal canal pressure. It may be useful in the investigation of patients with faecal incontinence and obstructed defecation. In most patients with anorectal disorders, however, anorectal manometry is not essential.

A small balloon mounted at the end of a catheter that is connected to a pressure transducer is passed into the anal canal and slowly withdrawn. Resting pressures are measured at 1-cm intervals. This permits an estimation of the length of the anal canal and measures the resting pressure, which reflects the function of the internal sphincter. The patient is then asked to contract the sphincter muscle, and the maximum squeeze pressure is measured. This is a function of the external sphincter. Sophisticated computerised equipment has been developed to provide longitudinal and circumferential pressures along the entire length of the anal canal.

When the rectum is filled with faeces, the internal sphincter should relax (the rectoanal inhibitory reflex). This does not occur in conditions like Hirschsprung's disease. To test this reflex, a second, longer catheter-mounted balloon is passed into the rectum and slowly inflated, at the same time measuring the resting pressure in the anal canal. This pressure should decrease as the rectal balloon volume increases.

Anorectal manometry ascertains coordination of the pelvic floor and anal sphincters during straining at stool and simulated defecation in a laboratory setting. Paradoxical contraction of the puborectalis muscle with straining (anismus) can be demonstrated by pressure and electromyographic study of the anal canal.

Endoluminal ultrasound

During the past decade, intrarectal and intra-anal ultrasound probes have been developed to obtain accurate and detailed views of the five layers of the rectal wall and the pararectal tissues. The examination is rapid, well tolerated by the patient and accurate. Endoluminal ultrasound can be used to accurately assess the degree of invasion of tumours through the bowel wall. It is especially useful in assessing patients with villous tumours of the rectum and can assess whether a rectal cancer has invaded adjacent organs. It is less accurate in determining whether metastases to lymph nodes have occurred. Ultrasound-guided biopsies of adjacent structures can also be performed with remarkable accuracy. Endorectal ultrasound is particularly useful for pre-operative staging of low rectal tumours in determining whether patients should have abdominoperineal excision or a transanal local excision with preservation of anal sphincters. It also helps select those lesions that might benefit from pre-operative adjuvant therapy. Endorectal ultrasound is also invaluable in the evaluation of a pararectal mass because it helps define its relationship with the rectal wall.

Endorectal ultrasound is emerging as a potentially useful tool for the surveillance of patients after surgery for rectal cancer. The test may detect extrarectal recurrence or enlarged pararectal lymph nodes in the preclinical stage, at a time when therapeutic intervention may have a beneficial effect. It may also help to confirm a local recurrence when clinical examination and other tests, such as computed tomography scan, is equivocal.

Endo-anal probes are available to provide a clear view of the anal sphincters, the pelvic floor and perianal tissues. Indications for this test include the evaluation of complex or recurrent anal fistulas, faecal incontinence and anal carcinoma. An occult intersphincteric abscess (causing anal pain) may also be identified using endo-anal ultrasound (Fig. 31.12).

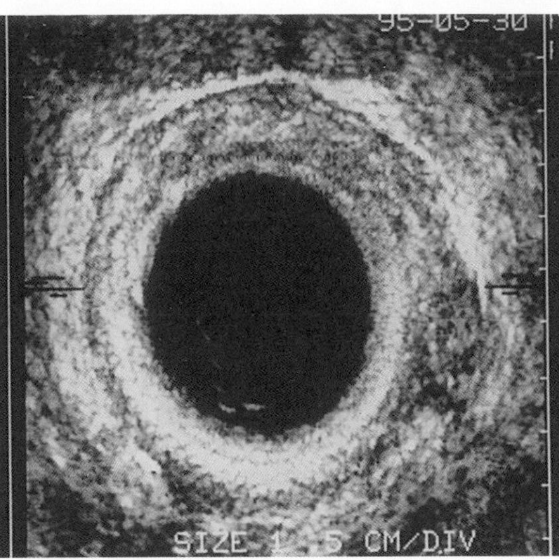

Fig. 31.12 Endo-anal ultrasound showing a left-sided intersphincteric abscess.

Further reading

Fazio VW, Tjandra JJ. The management of perianal disease. In: Cameron JL, ed. *Advances in Surgery*. Vol 29. Philadelphia: Mosby-Year Book Inc; 1996:59–78.

Orsay C, Rakinic J, Perry WB, et al. Practice parameter for the management of anal fissures. *Dis Colon Rectum*. (In press).

Tjandra JJ, Fazio VW. Perianal disease. In: Cohen AM, Winawer SJ, eds. *Cancer of the Colon, Rectum and Anus*. New York: McGraw-Hill; 1995:1007–1012.

Wong S, Gibbs P, Chao M, Jones I, McLaughlin S, Tjandra JJ. Carcinoma of the anal canal: a local experience and review of the literature. *Aust NZ J Surg*. 2004;74:541–546.

Tjandra JJ, Lubowski D. Anorectal physiological testing in Australia. *Aust NZ J Surg*. 2002;72:757–759.

Schraffordt SE, Tjandra JJ, Eizenberg N, Dwyer PL. The anatomy of the pudendal nerve and its terminal branches: a cadaver study. *Aust NZ J Surg*. 2004;74:23–26.

MCQs

Select the single correct answer to each question.

1 The preferred treatment of an ischiorectal abscess is:

a a prolonged course of antibiotics to abort the infection
b incision and drainage under general anaesthesia
c needle aspiration under local anaesthesia

d warm salt baths
e fistulotomy

2 The aetiology of anal fistula includes:
a anal gland infection
b ulcerative colitis
c ischaemic colitis
d anal syphilis
e levator syndrome

3 Painful perianal conditions include:
a Bowen's disease
b second-degree haemorrhoids
c perianal haematoma
d anal warts
e ulcerative colitis

4 Complications of haemorrhoidectomy include the following EXCEPT:
a severe anal pain
b urinary retention
c anal stricture
d pyelonephritis
e rectal bleeding

5 Anal fissure is characterised by the following EXCEPT:
a severe anal pain during and immediately after defecation
b bleeding on defecation
c a sentinel anal skin tag
d a relapsing history
e a patulous anus

Breast Surgery

32 Breast surgery

Joe J. Tjandra and John P. Collins

Introduction

Management of breast disease has become increasingly specialised. A multidisciplinary and integrated approach is used, involving surgeons, radiologists, pathologists, oncologists and breast counsellors. A substantial component of the workload includes differentiation of benign breast disease from a breast cancer and allaying the patient's anxiety about breast cancer.

Anatomy of the adult breast

The breast is invested with the superficial fascia that divides into two layers. The anterior layer separates the relatively small subcutaneous fat lobules and the larger lobules of mammary fat. The posterior layer of superficial fascia abuts against the deep fascia derived from the pectoralis major and serratus anterior. Between the two layers of superficial fascia, there are condensations of fibrous tissue (suspensory ligaments of Cooper) that divide the breast into lobes.

The main blood supply is via the second perforating branch of the internal mammary and lateral thoracic branches of the axillary artery. Lesser supply is via the thoracoacromial and subscapular arteries. A rich subareolar venous plexus drains via the intercostal, internal mammary and axillary veins.

The distribution of major lymphatics follows the blood supply. About 75% of the lymphatic vessels drain to the lymph nodes in front of and below the axillary vein. These axillary nodes are divided into three groups according to their relationship to the pectoralis minor muscle (Fig. 32.1): level 1, nodes lying below the pectoralis minor; level 2, nodes lying behind the pectoralis minor; level 3, nodes lying above the pectoralis minor. Most lymph drains from nodes at level 1 sequentially to those at levels 2 and 3, and a small amount drains in retrograde fashion to the subscapular and interpectoral groups of nodes. The latter becomes significant when there is extensive nodal metastasis in the axilla. A small amount of lymph drains from the superior aspect of the breast directly to the apical nodes in level 3, bypassing nodes in levels 1 and 2. About 25% of lymph (mainly from the medial half of the breast) drains to the internal mammary nodes in the second, third and fourth intercostal spaces.

Benign breast disease

Many so-called diseases of the breast are aberrations of the processes of development, cyclical change and involution (ANDI). Benign breast disease refers to more severe disorders. In general, there is a poor correlation between clinical, pathological and radiological features.

The symptoms of benign breast disease are summarised in Box 32.1.

Mastalgia

Mastalgia is a common breast symptom; however, mastalgia does not imply any specific pathological process and the condition is not well understood. Mastalgia can be cyclical, varying with the menstrual cycle, or non-cyclical where there is no such relationship.

Cyclical mastalgia

Cyclical mastalgia is the most common type of breast pain affecting premenopausal women. The median age of presentation is 35 years. The breast discomfort lasts for a varying period prior to menstruation and relief of the pain comes with menstruation. The pain is

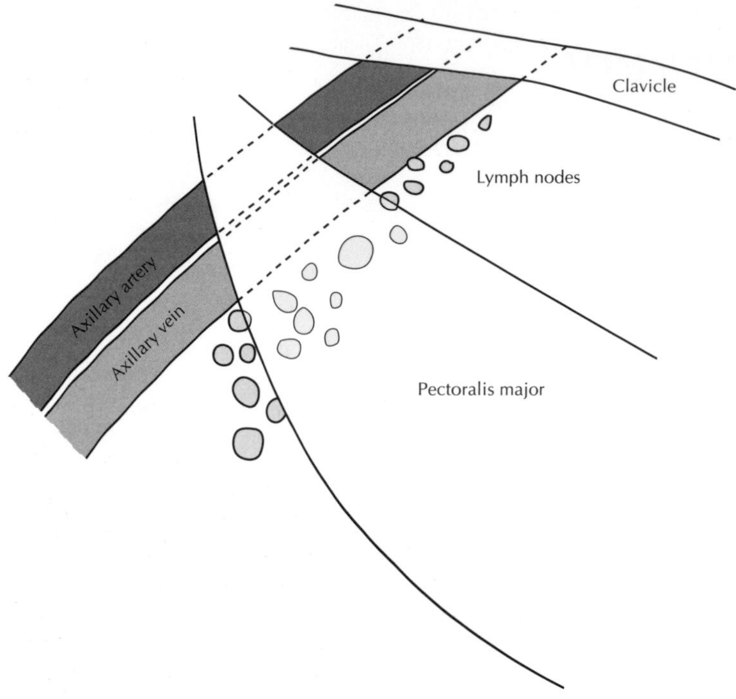

Fig. 32.1 Right axilla.

commonly in the upper outer quadrant of both breasts and radiates into the axilla and the medial aspect of the arm.

Box 32.1 Symptoms of benign breast disease

Mastalgia
- Cyclical
- Non-cyclical

Breast lumps
- Nodularity
- Cysts
- Fibroadenoma
- Mammary duct ectasia
- Sclerosing adenosis
- Fat necrosis
- Lipoma

Disorders of the peri-areolar region
- Discharge
- Retraction

Mastitis
- Lactational
- Non-lactational

Aetiology

As symptoms of cyclical mastalgia vary with menstrual cycle, there is probably a hormonal basis in the aetiology. The precise pathogenesis is, however, poorly understood. Possible factors may include abnormal prolactin secretion, fluid retention, excessive caffeine ingestion, inadequate essential fatty acid intake and psychoneurosis.

Treatment

More than 80% of women require no treatment other than reassurance that there is no cancer.

Drug treatments are described in Table 32.1. These drugs have a potential for side effects. The initial treatment is usually with evening primrose oil and a reduction of caffeine intake including tea, coffee, chocolate and cola drinks. Natural or treatment-induced remissions are common, but recurrence of mastalgia does occur.

Second-line treatment with low-dose tamoxifen, danazol or bromocriptine is reserved for severe refractory symptoms. The use of these drugs is limited by their side effects. Second-line treatment has a lower response rate.

Table 32.1 Drug treatments for cyclical mastalgia

Drug	Action	Response rate (%)
Evening primrose oil (6 capsules/day)	Essential fatty acid replacement	50
Oral contraceptives	Correct luteal insufficiency	50
Tamoxifen (10 mg/day)	Anti-oestrogen	80
Norethisterone (5 mg/day)	Progestogen	60
Danazol (200 mg/day)	Suppress FSH, LH	70
Bromocriptine (2.5 mg b.d.)	Dopamine agonist, correct hyperprolactinaemia	50

FSH, follicle-stimulating hormone; LH, luteinising hormone.

Non-cyclical mastalgia

The breast pain has no relationship to the menstrual cycle. It tends to be unilateral, more chronic and sometimes has a well localised 'trigger spot'. It affects both pre- and postmenopausal women and the median age at presentation is 45 years.

Management

Any primary pathology of the breast and of adjacent structures should be excluded by a careful clinical evaluation and appropriate imaging (see the following section). Treatment involves reassurance that there is no underlying pathology but drug treatment is generally unrewarding. Treatment principles similar to those for cyclical mastalgia are used. However, the response rate is worse and averages about 50%. The use of evening primrose oil is particularly disappointing in this subgroup. Occasionally, surgical excision of the painful trigger spot may alleviate the symptoms.

Benign breast lumps

More than half the women attending a breast clinic have a benign breast lump. Clinical history includes the nature and duration of the lump and its relationship to the menstrual cycle. Any changes in the lump and a similar past history are important. Risk factors for breast cancer are sought, including age, family history, use of hormone replacement therapy or oral contraceptives. The age at first pregnancy and the number of children are also of interest.

A careful examination is performed to determine whether the lump is truly present or whether it is within the spectrum of normality or an area of nodularity (thickening). The lump, if present, should be carefully examined to note for features of malignancy. Diagnosis now follows a structured algorithm (Fig. 32.2), following the development of diagnostic aids such as mammography (Fig. 32.3), ultrasonography and fine-needle aspiration cytology (FNAC).

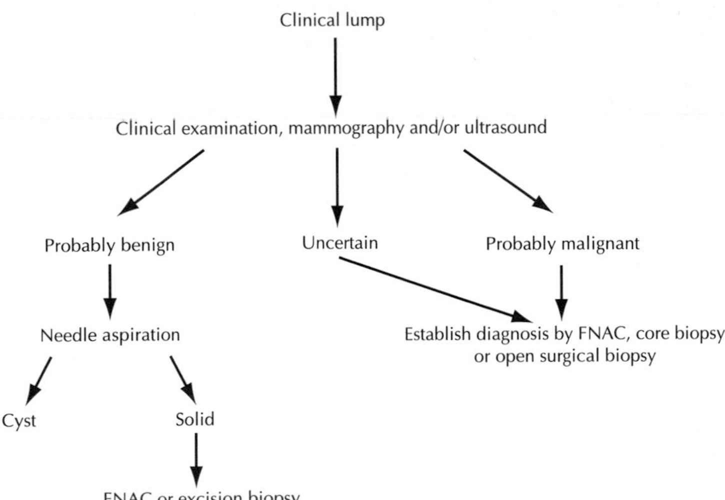

Fig. 32.2 Management of palpable breast lumps. FNAC, fine-needle aspiration cytology.

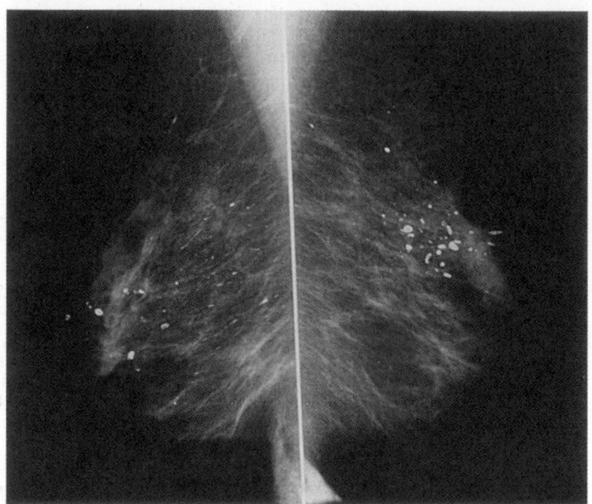

Fig. 32.3 Bilateral mammography showing coarse calcifications consistent with benign breast disease.

If FNAC is inconclusive or if any doubt of a malignancy remains, then surgical biopsy is indicated. A discrete solid breast lump in women over the age of 30 years is best removed, especially in the presence of a strong family history of breast cancer and other risk factors.

Fibroadenoma

Pathology

Fibroadenoma is a benign breast tumour in young women between 15 and 25 years. It consists of a fibrous connective tissue stroma and epithileal proliferation, usually with low cellularity. It is very occasionally seen in association with lobular carcinoma. The incidence falls markedly after menopause, when the breast lobules undergo involution.

The fibrous stroma of a fibroadenoma may surround a duct circumferentially (pericanalicular pattern) or compress adjacent ducts to become slit-like structures (intracanalicular pattern). With a benign fibroadenoma, the fibrous stroma has low cellularity. Epithelial hyperplasia may be present but has no prognostic importance. Coarse calcification may also occur.

A locally invasive variant (phyllodes tumour) also occurs (see later).

Clinical features

Fibroadenoma is smooth and very mobile (breast mouse). It measures about 2 or 3 cm in diameter. Some patients have multiple fibroadenomas at presentation. Others have multiple recurrent fibroadenomas.

Investigations

A clinical examination is usually adequate in young women up to 25 years old. In women older than this, an ultrasound with either fine-needle aspiration cytology, core biopsy or excisional biopsy, confirming a benign fibroadenoma is required. Mammography has little place.

Management

Fibroadenomas have a tendency to slowly increase in size. Most of the growth phase is within the first 12 months. Following that period, fibroadenomas remain the same size or may, occasionally, gradually reduce in size.

In women under 25 years, the lump may be left alone unless the patient wants it removed. In older women, pathological confirmation with FNAC or core biopsy or removal of the lump is recommenced.

Giant fibroadenoma

Giant fibroadenoma occurs in the very young (about 16 years old) or in the perimenopausal age group (about 50 years old). It is characterised by its rapid growth to a large size, and treatment is by surgical enucleation. This is a benign tumour.

Phyllodes tumour

Pathology

Phyllodes tumour has a wide spectrum of activity, ranging from almost benign to locally invasive. Histologically, the fibrous stoma is hypercellular with cellular atypia and mitoses.

Clinical features

Phyllodes tumours occur in premenopausal women and clinically resemble a fibroadenoma, but they grow quite rapidly. They rarely spread to the axilla.

Treatment

This entails a wide local excision with a clear margin of normal breast tissue. Local recurrence is common (25% at 10 years) and if the tumour is aggressive, then total mastectomy may be required.

Breast cysts

Pathology and incidence

Breast cysts are very common, with up to 10% of women developing a clincal breast cyst during their lifetime. Many women have subclinical breast cysts measuring 2–3 mm identified on ultrasound and most occur in the peri-menopausal age group, but they may occur at any age. Breast cysts are often multiple. The pathogenesis of breast cysts is not clear. The breast cyst may be lined by an apocrine or a simple cuboidal epithelium. There may be multiple cysts in a breast.

Clinical features

Breast cysts often appear suddenly and can be quite large. This is because the subclinical flaccid cyst accumulates a small amount of fluid and becomes tense and painful menstruation.

On clinical examination, the cyst is smooth and firm but not as mobile as a fibroadenoma. It is situated deep in the breast, and it may feel quite nodular.

The diagnosis of a breast cyst is confirmed by cyst aspiration, and cytological examination of the cyst fluid is generally unhelpful unless the fluid is blood stained. A breast cyst is usually well shown on ultrasound (Fig. 32.4), and imaging, mammography or ultrasound are only performed to exclude underlying breast cancer.

Treatment

Palpable breast cysts are treated by simple aspiration, in the consulting room, without any anaesthesia. If a mass persists, further investigations are required to define the cause of the mass.

Surgical excision is indicated if a non-traumatic aspirate is blood stained (because of the risk for intracystic cancer) or if the cyst continually recurs. A significant number of women develop further cysts which require repeat aspiration. Detection of breast cancer in this group is slightly more difficult, and they require regular surveillance mammograms.

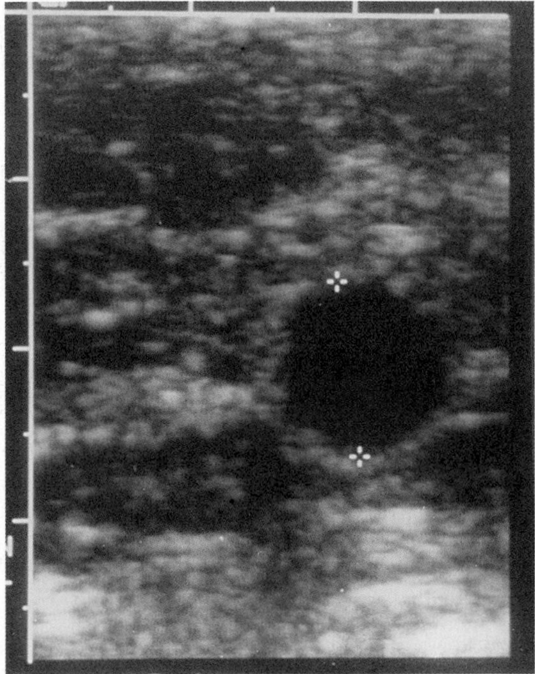

Fig. 32.4 A breast ultrasound showing a well-defined breast cyst.

Mammary duct ectasia and periductal mastitis

Clinical features

Mammary duct ectasia and periductal mastitis have a diverse clinical spectrum. The aetiology is unclear but involves the accumulation of secretions in the duct and inflammation of the surrounding tissues leading to inflammation, sometimes secondary infection, a thick nipple discharge and nipple retraction. Secondary infections can sometimes follow and inflammatory masses in the peri-areola region can form abscesses and mammary fistulae between the ducts and the skin at the areola margin.

Treatment

The inflammatory phase is treated with antibiotics, for example metranidazole or surgery of the major ducts, including local incision and drainage of abscess or major duct excisions for more chronic cases.

Box 32.2 Causes of nipple discharge

- Physiological (pregnancy, lactation)
- Duct ectasia
- Galactorrhoea
- Duct papillomas
- Fibrocystic disease
- Carcinoma
- Idiopathic

Nipple discharge

Clinical features and investigation

Nipple discharge is a common problem and the causes are outlined in Box 32.2. Investigations include mammography and ultrasound with cytology of the discharge, ductography and ductoscopy. These investigations are often disappointing and may be confusing.

Galactorrhoea

Galactorrhoea may be a primary physiological process, occurring during menarche, menopause or secondary to drugs that stimulate dopamine activity.

Duct papillomas

The discharge may be serous but is often blood stained and arises from a single duct. The solitary papillomas are benign and do not have malignant potential. The risk for malignancy is slightly raised in the unusual circumstance of multiple papillomas affecting several ducts.

Management of nipple discharge

Clinical history should include use of drugs (haloperidol, metoclopramide), menstrual history and risk factors for breast cancer. Examination should determine the presence of lumps and imaging with ultrasound or mammogram if over 35 years old.

If a breast lump is present, management is directed to the lump itself. If a lump is not present, management depends on the nature of the discharge and the results of breast imaging by ultrasound and mammography.

Box 32.3 Relationship between benign and malignant breast disease

Moderately increased risk (4–5×)
- Atypical ductal hyperplasia
- Atypical lobular hyperplasia
- Radial scar

Slightly increased risk (1.5–2.0×)
- Moderate or florid hyperplasia
- Multiple papilloma

No increased risk
- Cysts
- Fibroadenoma
- Duct ectasia
- Mild hyperplasia
- Sclerosing adenosis
- Apocrine change

Relationship of benign breast disease to breast cancer

Benign breast disease is a risk for cancer (Box 32.3), although the literature is confusing.

Gynaecomastia in males

About one-third of adult males and more than half of normal pubescent boys have some degree of gynaecomastia (Box 32.4, Fig. 32.5). Physiological gynaecomastia occurs in the neonate because of circulating

Box 32.4 Causes of gynaecomastia in males

Physiological

Pathological
- Drug-induced (e.g. hormone supplements, alcohol, cimetidine, digoxin, phenothiazines, tricyclic antidepressants, some antihypertensive agents)
- Increased oestrogen production (e.g. hepatoma, testicular and adrenal tumours or paraneoplastic syndrome)
- Reduced production of testosterone (e.g. Klinefelter's syndrome, mumps orchitis)
- Testicular feminisation syndrome

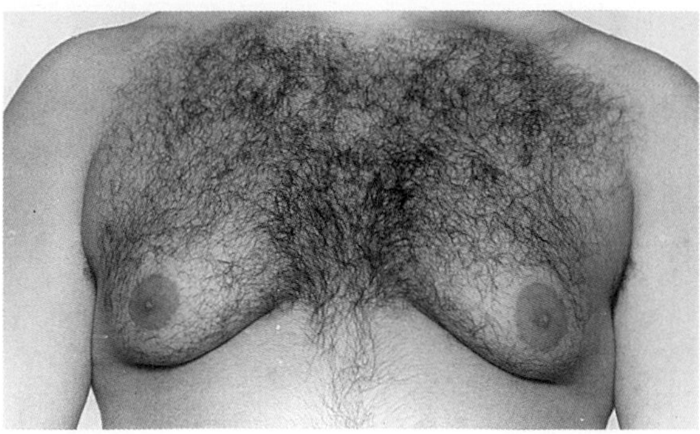

Fig. 32.5 Bilateral gynaecomastia in a man.

maternal sex hormones, at puberty because of a high serum oestradiol to testosterone ratio, and in the elderly because of reduced testosterone production. With significant gynaecomastia causing social embarrassment, surgical excision of the breast plaque is recommended. This is done through an incision at the margin of the areola to minimise the cosmetic effect.

Breast cancer

Introduction

Breast cancer is a heterogeneous disease with a varying propensity for spread. The disease tends to be slow growing, with pre-invasive phases that may extend over a number of years. Breast cancer may recur many years after surgery, indicating the need for prolonged monitoring.

Incidence

Breast cancer is common and the incidence is increasing. The lifetime risk for breast cancer in an Australian woman is 1 in 13, but is lower in Asian countries. About 1 in 25 women die of breast cancer. The incidence of breast cancer rises with age, and the disease is more common in women of higher socioeconomic class.

Risk factors

Several interrelated factors are associated with an increased risk for developing breast cancer (Box 32.5).

Box 32.5 Factors associated with an increased risk for developing breast cancer

- Sex. Breast cancer is 100 times more common in women than in men.
- Increasing age. Breast cancer is uncommon in women under 30 years. The mean age at diagnosis is 60 years.
- Past history of breast cancer. The development of a second cancer may be part of the multifocal origin of the first cancer or an entirely new cancer.
- First-degree relatives (mother, sister or daughter) with breast cancer, especially if they were under 50 years of age when the cancer developed.
- Previous history of benign proliferative disease with cellular atypia, multiple papillomatosis, atypical ductal and lobular hyperplasia or lobular carcinoma *in situ*.
- Other factors (e.g. nulliparity at 40 years, previous breast irradiation, younger age of menarche). The data on the cancer risk with hormone replacement therapy is conflicting, but short duration (<5 years) appears safe. The oral contraceptive pill does not seem to be associated with any increased risk.

Spread of breast cancer

The rate and extent of spread varies between individuals because of the heterogeneous nature of the cancer. In some patients, regional nodal and distant metastases occur rapidly, even if the primary breast cancer is small, while in others the tumour remains largely localised in the breast.

Local invasion

This occurs by direct infiltration of the breast parenchyma, overlying skin or underlying fascia, giving rise to the characteristic stellate appearance of breast cancer. Invasion along the ducts may also occur (Pagetoid spread). Local lymphovascular spread indicates a worse prognosis.

Regional spread

The axillary lymph nodes are the most important and most common site of regional spread. Clinical assessment of axillary nodes is unreliable and the false positive and false negative rates are about 30%. Axillary nodal metastases are more common with larger tumours and are the most important prognostic factor.

The incidence of axillary nodal metastases is less than 20% in tumours smaller than 2 cm but rises to more than 50% in tumours larger than 5 cm. A high number (>4) of nodes involved is associated with a particularly bad prognosis. Internal mammary lymph nodes lie in the anteior intercostal spaces adjacent to the internal mammary vessels and spread to the internal mammary nodes is usually associated with axillary node metastasis and carries a poor prognosis. Supraclavicular nodal metastases are also associated with a poor prognosis.

Distant metastases

The most common sites of disease are the bone, liver and lung. Other sites include the brain, skin and peritoneum. Micrometastases in the bone marrow may occur in up to one-third of patients who have breast cancer apparently confined to the breast.

Staging of breast cancer

Staging is an attempt to classify breast cancer according to the extent of the disease and thus stratify the prognosis. However, this is somewhat simplistic because of the large number of prognostic variables and the heterogeneity of the disease. The Manchester system is a simple clinical staging system, while the TNM classification provides a more accurate assessment and is useful in clinical trials (Table 32.2).

History

A thorough clinical history should be taken, including menstrual, obstetric, family and medication history, and the interview will establish a sound professional association with the patient.

Common symptoms include:

- a lump that may be firm or hard with a varying degree of fixity to surrounding tissues, overlying skin and underlying pectoral muscles. While pain is an uncommon symptom, the cancerous lump may have increasing discomfort, especially prior to menstruation. In neglected cases, a foul-smelling malignant ulcer may arise in the breast
- changes to the breast that include distortion, puckering of skin and nipple retraction
- a blood-stained nipple discharge may arise from an intraductal cancer and is typically unifocal
- rarely, regional or distant metastases may be the cause of symptoms such as a lump in the axilla or neck and bone pain or dyspnoea.

Table 32.2 Staging systems for breast cancer

Manchester system	
Stage I	Tumour confined to the breast with skin involvement less than the size of the tumour
Stage II	Tumour confined to the breast with palpable mobile axillary lymph nodes
Stage III	Locally advanced breast cancer with skin fixation larger than the tumour. Cutaneous ulcers or fixity to pectoralis fascia may be present. Peau d'orange or satellite chest wall nodules. Fixed axillary nodes, supraclavicular nodal involvement
Stage IV	Distant metastases
TNM classification	
Tumour categories	
T_x	Primary tumour cannot be assessed
T_{is}	Carcinoma *in situ*
T_1	Tumour size <2 cm
T_2	Tumour size 2–5 cm
T_3	Tumour size >5 cm
T_4	Any tumour size with fixation to chest wall or skin
Nodal categories	
N_x	Regional lymph nodes cannot be assessed
N_0	Axillary lymph nodes not involved
N_1	Ipsilateral axillary nodal metastases (mobile)
N_2	Ipsilateral axillary nodal metastases (fixed)
N_3	Ipsilateral supraclavicular or internal mammary nodal metastases
Metastasis categories	
M_x	Presence of distant metastases cannot be assessed
M_0	No distant metastases
M_1	Distant metastases

Clinical examination

Clinical examination can be normal, especially in screen-detected cancers, or in patients with small (<1 cm) lumps. Larger lumps may be firm to hard, irregular and have skin attachment or distort the breast shape. More advanced cancers can have Peau d'orange or even skin inflammation. If the tumour ulcerates, it becomes foul smelling.

Paget's disease of the nipple presents with an eczema of the nipple itself and is associated with underlying intraductal carcinoma, often with an invasive component.

Both breasts, axillae and supraclavicular fossae are examined for signs of local spread of the breast cancer. Clinical assessment of the axilla is inaccurate and lymph node metastases can only be determined by histological examination.

Systemic examination looking for metastatic disease should be carried out.

Investigations

Most cancers can be accurately diagnosed with a combination of mammography, ultrasound, fine-needle aspiration and core biopsy. It should be remembered however that negative imaging does not completely rule out breast cancer particularly and invasive lobular cancer.

Mammography

Mammography has a higher level of accuracy in detecting breast cancer, and its specifity increases with the age of the patient. Classic mammographic features include a mass, tissue asymmetry and microcalcification (Fig. 32.6). Mammography detects impalpable cancers and, in clinically palpable cancers, helps assess the extent of the disease and so helps planning of treatment.

Breast ultrasound

This is most useful to evaluate:

- a dense breast parenchyma (as in younger women) where mammography may fail to demonstrate the tumour clearly
- an equivocal mammographic abnormality
- a palpable lump (solid vs. cystic), especially in pregnant or lactating breast
- and guide a needle or core biopsy.

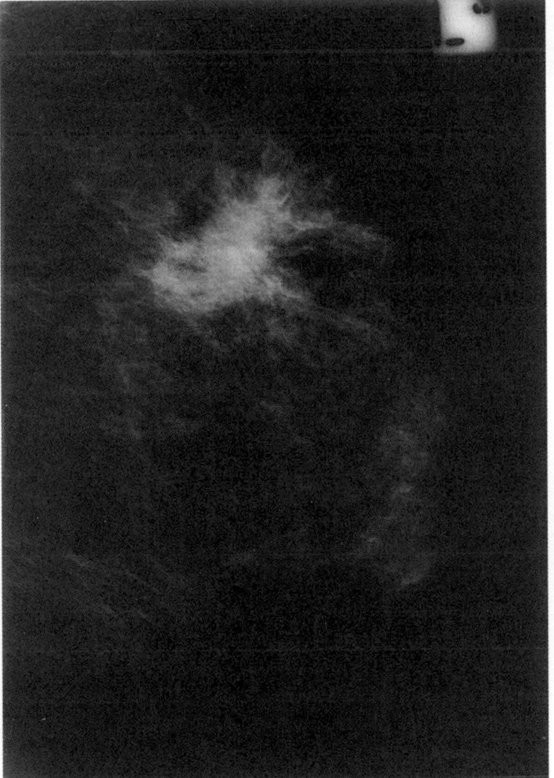

Fig. 32.6 Mammogram showing a stellate mass with irregular margins, consistent with a breast cancer.

Fine-needle aspiration cytology

Fine-needle aspiration cytology (FNAC) guided by either ultrasound, mammography, manually or palpation yields cells which are diagnostic of cancer. It is not possible to distinguish *in situ* from invasive cancer. False negatives arise from sampling errors or a cellular cancer; false positives also occur but are most unusual. Core biopsy, which provides histology and differentiates *in situ* from invasive, is progressively replacing FNAC. Diagnostic biopsy followed by definite surgery; for example Mastectomy with axillary clearance is now avoided.

Core biopsy

This is performed using a 14- or 16-gauge wide-bore needle under local anaesthesia and is replacing FNAC as it has a higher sensitivity and specificity.

Open surgical biopsy

This is performed as a day procedure under general anaesthesia in the following cases:

- if FNAC or core biopsy is inconclusive and has not been helpful and there is a clinical suspicion of malignancy
- the patient is anxious
- there is a discrete lump which is increasing in size (e.g. fibroadenoma).

Impalpable lesions require pre-operative localisation with a needle or carbon or radio isotope and the lesion is carefully oriented for the pathologist.

Frozen section histology

This may be used to confirm a pre-operative cytological diagnosis of malignancy or to provide an immediate diagnostic report when the open biopsy is performed as an independent procedure.

Frozen section histology should not proceed to immediate mastectomy unless there has been discussion with the patient and agreement about the procedure to be followed, which will depend on the outcome of the frozen section. Frozen section has a false positive rate of 1%, because of confusion with sclerosing adenosis, nipple adenoma and mastitis.

Selective tests

Specific staging tests for breast cancer include:

- full blood examination, urea and electrolytes, liver function tests, bone scan, liver ultrasound and chest and abdomnial CT scan.

These tests are usually performed after surgery when the nodal status fo the patient has been established, that is node positive patients. Sometimes these tests are performed to reassure the patient; however, they have significant false positive rates and often cause considerable confusion.

Pathology features

Pathological examination is essential in confirming the diagnosis and complete excision of the lesion. It also provides useful prognostic information (Box 32.6). Breast cancer may be invasive or non-invasive (*in situ*) and may arise from the duct or the lobule. Most tumours arise from the terminal ductules, with mixed features of ductal and lobular components.

Box 32.6 Major prognostic determinants of breast cancer

- Axillary nodal status
- Tumour size
- Histological grade
- Hormone receptor status
- Others (e.g. vascular invasion, menopausal status, HER2 overexpression)

Ductal carcinoma *in situ (DCIS)*

This is a pre-invasive breast cancer and is characterised by proliferation of malignant breast epithelium that is confined to the duct system and has not yet invaded through the basement membrane. The entity is associated with microcalcification on mammography. Since the introduction of screening, ductal carcinoma *in situ* has risen from 2% of breast cancers to now around 20 to 25%. This condition is premalignant and often multicentric in the breast. A less severe form, atypical ductal hyperplasia, exists which has a four times increased risk for developing breast cancer.

Lobular carcinoma *in situ*

Lobular carcinoma *in situ* (LCIS) is asymptomatic and mammographically occult. It is often multifocal and bilateral and is an increased risk factor for breast cancer (relative risk × 10) but it is not pre-malignant in itself. This is in contrast to DCIS. LCIS does not require radical excision but careful follow-up of the patient.

Less severe changes, called atypical lobular hyperplasia, carry a four times higher risk for developing breast cancer.

Invasive ductal carcinoma

'Invasive' ductal carcinoma refers to cancer which has invaded the basement membrane of the duct and invaded the surrounding tissue. The majority of these have no histological characteristic and are classified according to their differentiation as low-, intermediate- or high-grade.

Special types exist, including medullary, tubular, mucoid and inflammatory cancer, which are recognised as special behavioural types.

INFLAMMATORY CARCINOMA

This tumour has a very poor prognosis and is associated with tumour emboli in the dermal lymphatics and increased vascularity, producing a reddening of the skin.

Invasive lobular carcinoma

Classical lobular carcinoma has the histological feature of single files of malignant cells (Indian files). All the cells are similar and it is difficult to grade. It is often multifocal, meaning ductal carcinoma, and has a better prognosis.

Screen-detected breast cancer

Early detection of breast cancer by mammographic screening has been shown to improve survival. Whether this is truly cost-effective for the community is yet to be determined.

Early trials of breast cancer screening in Sweden, Holland, United States and Canada have confirmed the value of screening in early detection of tumours and, in particular, in increasing the rate of breast preservation. Screening has also detected an increased number of ductal carcinomas *in situ*, and this has improved the overall survival rate of breast cancer by including more favourable tumours in the treated group.

National Breast Screening programs have been established in many countries around the world, including Australia. In Australia, women aged 40 to 70 are screened at 2-year intervals. Patients have a two-view mammogram performed and if an abnormality is identified, they are recalled to an assessment clinic. The majority of abnormalities, greater than 90%, detected in the screening are benign and the patient is discharged. These assessment clinics are staffed by a multi-disciplinary team consisting of a surgeon, radiologist, radiographer, pathologist, breast care nurse and counsellor. To be effective, screening requires high participation rates and high-quality mammography and reporting.

Treatment of breast cancer

There has been a major change in the philosophy of the treatment of breast cancer because of an understanding of the systemic nature and heterogeneity of the disease. Surgery is now less radical and adjuvant therapy is now used more often.

The management of breast cancer involves a coordinated and multidisciplinary approach involving surgeons, radiologists, radiation oncologists, medical oncologists, pathologists and breast care nurses. Patient education, counselling and informed consent play an increasing role in the overall management.

Breast surgery

The principle of surgery in early breast cancer is to remove the tumour and have a clear margin of tissue around it. In many cases, particularly in screen-detected cancers, surgery will be curative.

Total mastectomy

This involves complete excision of the breast and nipple with preservation of the underlying pectoral muscles. Pectoralis fascia is usually removed as well. This is usually combined with excision of axillary lymph nodes. This used to be the standard therapy for all breast cancers but is now reserved for:

- a cancer that is large relative to the size of the breast
- cancer that involves the nipple or overlying skin (breast conservation surgery might still be possible in selected cases)
- multifocal disease or extensive intraductal carcinoma involving the surgical margins
- prior breast irradiation
- women who choose not to have breast conservation.

Breast reconstruction is offered to most women after a total mastectomy.

Breast conservation surgery

This involves complete local excision of the primary breast tumour with a rim of macroscopically normal breast tissue on all sides. The overlying skin may be included, if necessary. The incision must be carefully planned and the specimen oriented.

Breast conservation surgery is routinely followed by radiotherapy. This reduced the local recurrence rate to between 1 and 2% per year compared with 0.5% per year following a total mastectomy. Breast conservation and radiotherapy has now become the standard procedure for patients with breast cancer and is performed on greater than 70% of all patients. Many trials have now confirmed that breast conservation is as safe as total mastectomy with regard to overall survival, and the cosmetic and psycholgical result is far superior. Breast conservation is however time-consuming and expensive, and radiotherapy is not easily available for all patients.

INDICATIONS

The indications for breast conservation surgery have gradually broadened. Now as long as you can achieve a reasonable cosmetic result and obtain clear margins on the tumour, breast conservation should be offered.

The patient does require counselling about the decision for breast conservation and the need for radiotherapy as well as the long-term swelling and discomfort which occurs in the breast.

CONTRAINDICATIONS

Relative contraindications include multicentric disease, a second breast cancer in the same breast or multifocal disease. Pregnant patients pose a particular problem, as do patients with connective tissue diseases, where radiotherapy may be contraindicated.

Axillary dissection

Axillary dissection aims to:
- remove metastatic disease within the axillary lymph nodes
- assess nodal status for prognosis
- assess nodal status to determine adjuvant systemic therapy.

Traditionally axillary surgery involves removal of all 3 levels of axillary nodes. More recently the lower axilla, in particular level 1 and level 2, nodes have been removed. More recently a new procedure called a sentinel node biopsy has been introduced where the specific lymph node draining the tumour is removed after being labelled as a radio isotope and marked with a blue dye.

This reduction in axillary surgery has been made possible because patients presenting with smaller tumours are less likely to metastasise in axillary lymph nodes. Whilst large tumours 50 mm or greater have a 60% node-positive rate, small tumours 10 mm or less have only an 8% lymph-node-positive rate.

In the future, it is likely that the sentinel node only will be removed and the axillary dissection will only be performed if the sentinel node is positive or if the axilla is clinically involved with tumour. If any axillary node is involved, then axillary dissection is required.

Box 32.7 Main risks for breast surgery

Mastectomy
- Breast haematoma
- Wound infection
- Seroma of the skin flap
- Psychological effects on body image and self esteem

Axillary dissection
- Seroma of axilla
- Pain and numbness of the upper medial aspect of the arm and the chest wall below the axilla as a result of division of the intercosto-brachial nerve
- Limitation of shoulder movement (especially abduction and elevation)
- Lymphoedema of the arm. The risk is about 5% but is increased substantially if radiation therapy is also given to a surgically dissected axilla

Currently the sentinel node procedure is being evaluated in a number of clinical trials around the world and its eventual role is being determined.

Complications of surgery

Breast surgery has few complications (Box 32.7). Lymphoedema of the arm requires special care because of a high risk for infection. Trauma to the arm should be avoided.

Breast reconstruction

Breast reconstruction can be performed both with patients having total mastectomy and breast preservation surgery.

In general, breast reconstruction is carried out either using the patient's own tissue and taking muscle flaps from the back or lower abdomen or by using prostheses made from a cohesive silicone gel. Currently, only about 10% of Australian women have breast reconstruction following mastectomy, but this incidence is slowly rising.

Radiotherapy

After breast conservation surgery

Breast irradiation is indicated following breast-conserving surgery after complete excision of the tumour and clear margins have been obtained.

A subgroup of women in whom breast irradation can be omitted. There is no doubt that while breast irradiation reduces the risk of recurrence, it can probably be omitted in a subgroup of women, especially if they are elderly (older than 70), where the tumour is small (less than 10 mm), has low histologic grade and has abundant hormone receptors. Radiotherapy is not really available in a number of rural areas of Australia. This influences some women from rural areas to opt for a mastectomy, where breast conservation would have been a reasonable treatment.

After mastectomy

There is an increasing role for adjuvant radiotherapy following total mastectomy. In selected patients, particularly those with large tumours, large numbers of axillary lymph nodes are involved, the risk of local recurrence is significantly reduced. The value of radiotherapy in reducing overall survival however is more contentious, and further studies are awaited.

Complications

The complications following radiotherapy vary with the total dose, the number of fractions and the arrangement of the radiation fields. Recent improvements in delivery techniques have significantly reduced the complications.

Local effects which occur in the first 2 to 6 weeks include redness, soreness and ulceration of the skin. Discomfort and swelling of the breast occur early and often persist for a number of years and continue to improve over several years. It is not possible to breast feed from the radiated breast.

Cardiac damage particularly in patients with left sided tumours is reported however modern techniques should reduce this. Lymphoedema of the arm occurs in a small but significant number of patients following surgery and radiotherapy.

Adjuvant systemic therapy

The aim of this therapy is to eradicate micrometastases in order to ultimately improve survival. There is no evidence that adjuvant systemic therapy will maintain local control in women with a high risk of loco-regional relapse. Adjuvant systemic therapy with tamoxifen, with combination cytotoxic chemotherapy or, in premenopausal women, ovarian ablation, reduces the risk of recurrence and death after treatment for node-positive and node-negative breast cancer. Combinations of various adjuvant systemic treatments may confer additional benefits and are currently being evaluated in clinical trials.

With systemic therapy, the risk for recurrence within 10 years of surgery with node-positive breast cancer will be reduced from 60 to 42%, and with node-negative breast cancer reduced from 25 to 15%.

Thus adjuvant systemic therapy is recommended for all women with involved axillary lymph nodes. Use of adjuvant systemic therapy in node-negative breast cancer is controversial and is considered if there are poor prognostic features, such as tumour size more than 2 cm, oestrogen and progesterone receptor negativity, poor differentiation or lymphovascular invasion. In contrast, a small screen-detected tubular cancer has such a good prognosis that adjuvant systemic therapy is unnecessary. The choice of the type of systemic therapy varies with the nature of the tumour, and the age, general health and preferences of the woman (Table 32.3). Hormonal manipulation with tamoxifen

Table 32.3 Schema for systemic adjuvant therapy

Menopausal status	Adjuvant therapy
Node-positive	
Premenopausal	Combination chemotherapy withr doxorubicin and cyclophosphamide (CMF) (4 cycles). In receptor-positive women, ovarian ablation may be an alternative
Postmenopausal	Receptor-positive: tamoxifen for 5 years. In fit women with poor prognostic features, chemotherapy before tamoxifen may have additional benefit
	Receptor-negative: combination chemotherapy
Node-negative	
Premenopausal	Combination cytotoxic chemotherapy if there are poor prognostic features
Postmenopausal	Receptor-positive: tamoxifen for 5 years
	Receptor-negative: tamoxifen for 5 years. Note risk of endometrial cancer. If poor prognostic features are present, consider combination chemotherapy in younger patients

or ovarian ablation is less valuable in women with oestrogen receptor (ER)-negative cancers.

Cytotoxic chemotherapy

Adjuvant cytotoxic chemotherapy gives a survival advantage for all node positive women 70 years old or younger. The value of the chemotherapy increases with decreasing age and increasing nodal involvement. In those negative women, adjuvant cytotoxic chemotherapy also conveys a survival advantage but of lesser proportions and is reserved for poor prognosis tumours, such as large high-grade tumours which lack estrogen receptor.

Commonly used regimens include adreomycin and cyclophosphamide, methotrexate and 5-fluorouracil and other combinations of these drugs for a period of approximately 6 months. The toxicities of cytotoxic chemotherapy, which include nausea, vomiting, lethargy, alopaecia and early menopause, have been significantly reduced in recent years, by carefully planned drug regimens.

Adjuvant cytotoxic chemotherapy has become much more commonly accepted in early breast cancer.

Tamoxifen

Adjuvant tamoxifen is associated with an improvement of 6% at 10 years in both disease-free survival and overall survival. It is effective at all ages but most effective in women with ER-positive tumours. The value of tamoxifen adjuvant therapy in truly ER-negative tumours is uncertain but is probably minimal. Tamoxifen may also reduce the risk of cancer in the contralateral breast.

The optimal duration of treatment is 5 years, at a dose of 20 mg/day.

Side effects of tamoxifen include hot flushes, vaginal discharge and an increased incidence of endometrial cancer in postmenopausal women. This endometrial cancer risk is about 1 in 1000 women per year and is far outweighed by its beneficial effect. Annual gynaecological review is sometimes recommended, and abnormal vaginal bleeding shoud be promptly investigated.

Ovarian ablation

Ovarian ablation in premenopausal women is associated with an improvement of 10% at 15 years in both recurrence-free and overall survival. The beneficial results are greater in women with positive oestrogen receptors and may confer additional effectiveness even in the presence of cytotoxic chemotherapy. Ovarian ablation is not indicated after menopause.

Ovarian ablation is achieved by surgical oophorectomy, ovarian irradiation or by using luteinising hormone–releasing hormone (LHRH) analogues such as goserelin. The LHRH agonists produce a medical oophorectomy that is usually reversible on cessation of therapy. Their use and efficacy in breast cancer is currently being studied. The safety of oestrogen replacement therapy in women who have had treatment for breast cancer is still not clear.

Counselling

The manner in which the diagnosis of breast cancer is communicated may have an important impact on the woman's ability to cope with the diagnosis and treatment. There are individual differences in women's views about and needs for information, options and support.

Women with breast cancer and their families will need further counselling to allow assimilation of information and should be given repeated opportunities to ask questions. Women with good emotional support from family and friends tend to adjust better to having breast cancer. Doctors, nurses, breast cancer support services and other allied health professionals are all important sources of support. Many specialist breast centres have a dedicated, well-trained breast counsellor to help coordinate the care with the doctor (the team approach).

Breast cancer support services are available in all states in Australia. They are staffed by trained volunteers who have had breast cancer or who have a broad perspective of the disease. Appropriate counselling has the potential to improve the quality of life.

Follow-up

With the multidisciplinary approach in the care for breast cancer, it is important that follow-up is coordinated so that patients are not subjected to an excessive number of visits. The rationale of follow-up is outlined in the following sections.

Detection of local recurrence

The local recurrence rate after breast conservation surgery and radiotherapy is 10–15% and less after mastectomy. Most recur within the first 3 years. Clinical examination of the skin flap, axilla and neck is performed after mastectomy, supplemented by mammography after breast conservation surgery.

Detection of distant recurrence

Intensive follow-up confers no survival benefit over a minimal follow-up regimen, because distant metastases are not curable.

Screening for a new breast primary

The risk of a new contralateral breast primary cancer is 1% per year. Annual mammography is recommended.

Management of treatment-associated toxicities

These include problems after axillary dissection (shoulder stiffness or lymphoedema), or with adjuvant chemotherapy (e.g. premature menopause) or anthracyclines (e.g. delayed cardiac toxicity). Gynaecological symptoms should be sought in women taking tamoxifen because of a relative risk of 2–5 times of endometrial cancer.

Psychosocial support

Anxiety and depression are common following diagnosis and treatment. Often there are difficulties with sexual image and adjustment.

Pregnancy and breast cancer

Women should be advised not to get pregnant during treatment for breast cancer because of the effect of the toxicities of treatment on the foetus and the additional physical demand of pregnancy on the women. The changing hormone levels with pregnancy may also induce progression of breast cancer. However, there is no evidence that pregnancy is harmful after completion of treatment.

Treatment of breast cancer in a pregnant woman is complex. The prognosis may be impaired because of hormonal and immunological changes. Surgery is best performed during the second or third trimester. Radiotherapy and chemotherapy should, whenever possible, be avoided and deferred until the second trimester.

Metastatic breast cancer

Breast cancer tends to be slow growing and has a tendency to recur many years after apparently successful treatment. However, once metastasis has become evident it is associated with a poor outcome, with a median survival of 16 months. The most important prognostic factor in metastatic disease is disease-free interval after diagnosis of the primary breast cancer. Where recurrence is within 1 year, there is a much worse outcome than in those with recurrence more than 5 years after initial diagnosis.

Loco-regional (Fig. 32.7) or bony metastases also tend to have a better outcome than liver or cerebral metastases. The tumour burden, in terms of the extent of metastases, is also an important prognostic indicator.

Examination and investigation

A full clinical assessment and investigative staging are performed to determine the full extent of metastatic spread. This includes chest radiography, computed tomography (CT) scan of the chest and abdomen, and bone scan. A CT scan of the brain is performed only if there are relevant symptoms. A full assessment helps to determine prognosis and to plan appropriate therapy.

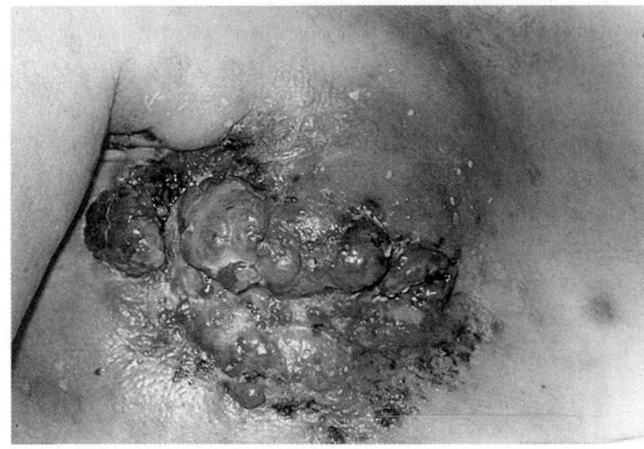

Fig. 32.7 A fungating local recurrence after mastectomy.

The main aim of therapy is to palliate symptoms and demands a multidisciplinary approach. Counselling is particularly important. None of the plethora of new therapeutic options has reliably improved survival. Patients with tumours positive for oestrogen and progesterone receptors are more likely to respond to endocrine manipulation, so receptor status should be determined.

Treatment of metastases

Systemic therapy with endocrine manipulation or cytotoxic chemotherapy is the basis for treatment.

Endocrine therapy

The response to endocrine therapy is of the order of 50% in patients positive for oestrogen receptors.

Tamoxifen

The anti-oestrogen tamoxifen is the agent of choice in postmenopausal women and has side effects. Younger patients are more prone to hot flushes and weight gain with such treatment. Failure to respond is an indication to abandon endocrine therapy and to pursue treatment with cytotoxic chemotherapy.

Relapse after an intial response to tamoxifen can be treated with LHRH progestogens. In premenopausal women, such relapses may be treated with LHRH agonists such as Zoladex administered subcutaneously monthly.

Oophorectomy

An alternative is surgical oophorectomy, which may be performed by laparoscopic techniques with few complications or, if perimenopausal, by radiotherapy.

Progestogens

Progestogens are as active as tamoxifen as a first-line treatment but because of their side effects, particularly weight gain, fluid retention and nausea, they are more commonly used as the second-line treatment after failure of response to tamoxifen. However, the response rate to such second-line treatment is only half that seen with first-line treatment.

Non-steroidal aromatase inhibitors

Letrozole (Femara) or anastrozole (Arimidex) can markedly inhibit oestrogen synthesis within the breast cancer and is now used as second- or third-line treatment for advanced breast cancer after initial response to endocrine treatment. The treatment is fairly non-toxic.

Chemotherapy

The response rate to chemotherapy in previously untreated metastatic breast cancer is about 60%, but few obtain complete resolution of disease. The median duration of response is 1 year. Chemotherapy is the treatment of choice for visceral metastases, such as those in the liver and lung.

Combination therapy with cyclophosphamide, methotrexate and 5-fluorouracil is the most popular regimen. Replacement of methotrexate with adriamycin is associated with an increased response rate but with more side effects. Newer agents such as taxanes are evolving and are constantly being tested in clinical trials.

Radiotherapy

External beam radiotherapy has particular application for cerebral or painful bony metastases. Systemic agents often fail to cross the blood–brain barrier to treat cerebral metastases effectively, and radiotherapy is the treatment of choice. Rapid pain relief is usual after treatment with radiotherapy.

Surgery

Surgery has a limited role and is reserved for the treatment of troublesome metastases, such as excision of a symptomatic local recurrent skin nodule or full surgical clearance of an axillary relapse where no previous surgery has been undertaken, surgical fixation of pathological fractures, and pleurodesis for treatment of persistent pleural effusion. Surgery has a small role in the treatment of acute spinal cord compression.

Supportive treatment

Hypercalcaemia may complicate bony metastases and requires treatment with rehydration, forced diuresis with frusemide and, sometimes, use of steroids to enhance excretion of calcium in the urine. Resistant cases require treatment with the diphosphonates or mithramycin.

Adjuvant pain control with adequate analgesia, and sometimes support braces, can be used for a painful bony metastasis.

Patients with metastatic breast cancer often are anaemic, malnourished and suffer from complications of therapy. These co-morbid factors must be corrected.

Prevention of breast cancer

Genetic factors account for breast cancer in less than 10% of cases. Most other breast cancers are sporadic. Until the causation of breast cancer is understood, attempts at its prevention are somewhat ineffective.

Chemoprevention with tamoxifen for 'high-risk' subjects is currently on trial. However, there are concerns about the risk of endometrial cancer following long-term use of tamoxifen.

Prophylactic mastectomy with or without breast reconstruction is occasionally performed for very-high-risk individuals who demand it.

MCQs

Select the single correct answer to each question.

1 A 48-year-old woman presents with thick greenish nipple discharge from both breasts. There is no palpable breast lump, although both nipples are slightly retracted. The patient does not take any medication. Mammogram and ultrasound do not show any evidence of cancer. The most likely diagnosis is:

a galactorrhoea
b duct papilloma
c mammary duct ectasia
d fibroadenoma
e lobular carcinoma *in situ*

2 A 42-year-old woman presents with a 2-cm breast lump, detected 2 weeks ago. The lump is discrete but soft. There is no past history of breast disease. The initial management includes:

a repeat clinical examination in 4 weeks' time to detect any changes
b bilateral mammogram with or without breast ultrasound
c fine needle aspiration cytology of the lump as breast imaging is unnecessary in this age group
d excision biopsy
e unilateral mammogram and ultrasound of the breast with the lump

3 Mammography screening programmes:

a reduce mortality of breast cancer, especially in women aged between 40 and 50 years
b detect smaller cancers with a lower incidence of axillary nodal metastases than in the unscreened population
c show a higher incidence of lobular but not ductal carcinoma *in situ*
d include quality assurance targets of attendance rates higher than 50% and recall rates lower than 50%
e involve radiologists as the primary personnel responsible for diagnosis and management

4 A 39-year-old woman has a 5-cm, grade III breast cancer. Twelve of 16 lymph nodes contain metastases. The oestrogen receptor is negative, although the progesterone receptor is positive. There is no evidence of systemic metastases on chest X-ray and bone scan. Following a total mastectomy and axillary clearance, the MOST likely follow-up management would be:

a regular review, with reservation of chemotherapy for recurrent disease
b adjuvant tamoxifen
c adjuvant chemotherapy
d adjuvant radiotherapy
e oophorectomy

5 Correct statement concerning ductal carcinoma *in situ* (DCIS):

a it is associated with microcalcification on mammography
b DCIS is less commonly found in women undergoing routine mammographic screening
c comedo subtype is rarely multicentric
d there is a high risk for lymph node metastasis with the papillary subtype
e the risk for progression to invasive cancer is smaller than with lobular carcinoma *in situ*

Endocrine Surgery

33 Thyroid

Leigh Delbridge

Introduction

The thyroid gland lies in the anterior triangle of the neck. Thyroid follicular cells arise from the foramen caecum in the tongue, and during embryological development the gland descends in the midline to the level of the larynx, where it buds laterally. A contribution of neural crest cells arising from the fourth branchial cleft and the ultimobranchial body gives rise to the C-cells of the thyroid as well as to a small projection from the postero-lateral surface (the Tubercle of Zuckerkandl). The thyroid comprises two lateral lobes, an isthmus and a pyramid. The function of the follicular cells is to produce, store and release the thyroid hormones thyroxine (T4) and tri-iodothyronine (T3). The function of the C-cells is to produce the calcium-lowering hormone calcitonin.

Diseases affecting the thyroid gland can generally be grouped into disorders of thyroid function (including hypothyroidism and thyrotoxicosis) or disorders affecting thyroid structure (including nodular goitre and thyroid neoplasms). Disorders of both function and structure coexist and, from the surgical point of view, thyroid disease can be considered in the following groups:

- Disorders of embryological development
- Benign thyroid nodules
- Multinodular goitre
- Thyroid cancer
- Thyrotoxicosis
- Thyroiditis

Disorders of the thyroid gland

Disorders of embryological development

Pathology

As the thyroid gland descends during embryological development, remnants of thyroid tissue may be left behind anywhere along the thyroglossal tract. Occasionally some respiratory epithelium may be included in the remnant, resulting in a thyroglossal duct cyst. A non-cystic benign thyroid nodule, or even thyroid cancer, may also develop anywhere along the tract. Embryological descent may also continue into the anterior mediastinum, giving rise to a thyrothymic thyroid remnant.

Clinical presentation

Thyroglossal duct cysts most commonly present either in childhood or adolescence. The usual clinical presentation is that of a midline swelling that moves with protrusion of the tongue. Inflammation may give rise to an abscess or a fistula. Thyrothymic thyroid remnants usually remain asymptomatic unless other pathology, e.g. nodular change, develops – in which case they may present as an intrathoracic goitre.

Investigations

The diagnosis of a thyroglossal duct cyst is usually self-evident on clinical examination. Fine-needle aspiration cytology (FNAC) will confirm the nature of the cyst contents, although this may precipitate inflammation.

Treatment

The only treatment is surgical excision through a skin-crease incision. In order to prevent recurrence, the cyst and the thyroglossal tract must be removed, which involves excision of the mid-portion of the hyoid bone and tracing of the tract to its upper limit. Thyrothymic thyroid remnants which are symptomatic require surgical excision.

Benign thyroid nodules

Pathology

Between 30 and 40% of clinically single thyroid nodules will represent a dominant nodule in a multinodular goitre. Of the remainder, the majority will be benign nodules, either simple thyroid cysts, solitary colloid nodules, or benign follicular adenoma. Approximately 7% will be a thyroid cancer and a further small group will represent an area of nodularity within thyroiditis.

Clinical presentation

The most common presentation of a single thyroid nodule is that of an asymptomatic swelling in the neck. The characteristic clinical feature of a thyroid nodule is that it moves on swallowing. Benign thyroid nodules may also present with local pressure symptoms. These include dysphagia from oesophageal pressure, a persistent cough or stridor from tracheal pressure, a hoarse voice from pressure on the recurrent laryngeal nerve, or superior vena cava (SVC) obstruction from a large single nodule obstructing the thoracic inlet. A toxic nodule will present with symptoms of thyrotoxicosis.

Investigations

Thyroid function tests (TFTs), including thyroid stimulating hormone (TSH), free T4 and free T3, should be performed in all patients, especially the elderly, in order to exclude subclinical thyrotoxicosis, or to diagnose a toxic nodule or an autonomously functioning nodule. In the latter case, a suppressed TSH will be seen in association with normal free T4 and free T3 levels. Fine-needle aspiration cytology is the definitive investigation, and the possible cytological reports are categorised in Table 33.1. It is important to note that an atypical report indicates the presence of a follicular neoplasm, but cannot differentiate between a benign follicular adenoma and a follicular carcinoma. This diagnosis can only be made by the finding of either capsular or vascular invasion on histology. Ultrasound scans have limited value in the investigation of thyroid nodules, although FNAC is best performed with ultrasound guidance. The role of nuclear medicine scans is now limited to the investigation of patients with thyrotoxicosis or thyroiditis.

Table 33.1 Classification of fine-needle aspiration cytology reports

Category	Cytology	Pathology	Interpretation
Inadequate	Insufficient cells or excess blood		Needs to be repeated
Cystic	Cyst fluid and degenerate cells	Simple thyroid cyst or colloid cyst	Repeat if cyst recurs
Benign (benign follicular pattern)	Normal follicular cells and abundant colloid	Colloid nodule or macrofollicular adenoma	Conservative management if asymptomatic
Atypical (suspicious; atypical follicular pattern; follicular neoplasm)	Microfollicles and scant or absent colloid	Microfollicular adenoma or follicular carcinoma	Surgery required because a follicular carcinoma cannot be excluded
Malignant	Cells consistent with the specific histology	Papillary, anaplastic or medullary carcinoma, lymphoma	Surgery appropriate to the specific type of cancer
Thyroiditis	Inflammatory cells and colloid	Hashimoto's thyroiditis, de Quervain's thyroiditis	Therapy specific to the type of thyroiditis

Treatment

Asymptomatic thyroid nodules that are benign on FNAC do not generally require treatment. Indications for surgery include the presence of obstructive symptoms, thyrotoxicosis, or the finding of either malignancy or atypical changes on FNAC. The minimal surgical procedure is a lobectomy, removing all thyroid tissue on the side of the lesion. Thyroxine suppression is generally ineffective in decreasing the size of single thyroid nodules.

Multinodular goitre

Pathology

Multinodular goitre occurs as the result of repeated cycles of hyperplasia, nodule formation, degeneration and fibrosis occurring throughout the gland. It occurs either in response to iodine deficiency or else, in iodine-replete areas, as the result of intrinsic heterogeneity of TSH receptors. The latter has a high familial incidence. A dominant nodule within a multinodular goitre is most likely to be either a hyperplastic or colloid nodule. However, the incidence of malignancy in a dominant nodule is approximately the same as for a single nodule (7%). Multinodular goitre has a high familial incidence, and is also common in areas where iodine is deficient in the diet.

Clinical presentation

Most multinodular goitres present as an asymptomatic mass in the neck. They may also present with local obstructive symptoms to the trachea, oesophagus, recurrent laryngeal nerve or SVC. Thyrotoxicosis is also common, especially in the elderly with large goitres. An otherwise asymptomatic retrosternal multinodular goitre may present as a mass on a chest X-ray or computed tomography (CT) scan.

Investigations

Thyroid function tests must be performed on all patients. FNAC of the dominant nodule or nodules will exclude malignancy and a CT scan will assess retrosternal extension or tracheal compression. An ultrasound adds little to the clinical examination. Nuclear medicine scan only serves to confirm the presence of multinodular change and has little value.

Treatment

Indications for surgical treatment of a multinodular goitre include the presence of obstructive symptoms, thyrotoxicosis, suspicious or malignant changes on FNAC, a strong family history of thyroid cancer, the presence of retrosternal extension, or a past history of head and neck irradiation. In a young patient with a large multinodular goitre who is otherwise asymptomatic, thyroidectomy may also be considered for cosmetic reasons. The only effective treatment is surgical excision. If surgery is undertaken, total thyroidectomy is the preferred option, because it removes all tissue likely to cause symptoms and avoids the possibility of later recurrence, which is of the order of 30%. Lifelong thyroxine replacement is required after total thyroidectomy.

Thyroid cancer

Pathology

Thyroid cancer can arise from the follicular cells, the C-cells, or other cells such as lymphocytes or stromal cells, each giving rise to a different form of thyroid cancer. Papillary thyroid cancer accounts for about 85% of thyroid cancers, tends to occur in a younger age group (20–40 years), is often multifocal, spreads predominantly to local lymph nodes and has a relatively good prognosis, with 10 year survival rates of at least 90%. Follicular cancer occurs in an older age group (40–60 years), arises as a single tumour, metastasises by the bloodstream, and has a worse prognosis than papillary cancer, with 10 year survival rates around 75%. Anaplastic, or undifferentiated, thyroid cancer occurs in the elderly, often presents as a rapidly enlarging diffuse mass, spreads locally, and has a terrible prognosis, with 5-year survival rates of less than 1%. Malignancy arising in C-cells gives rise to medullary carcinoma of the thyroid. This tumour secretes calcitonin, and may be part of a familial multiple endocrine neoplasia syndrome (MEN IIA), occurring in association with phaeochromocytoma and hyperparathyroidism. Ten-year survival is around 35%. Lymphoma of the thyroid is thought to arise in lymphocytes, often in association with pre-existing Hashimoto's thyroiditis. Miscellaneous thyroid malignancies include squamous cancer, sarcoma and metastases, but are all rare presentations. Follicular-derived thyroid cancer has an association with previous exposure to ionising radiation.

Clinical presentation

Thyroid cancer commonly presents as either a single thyroid nodule or a dominant nodule in a multinodular goitre. Thyroid cancer may also present as metastatic disease, such as bony metastases from follicular cancer, or lymphangitic lung involvement from papillary cancer.

Investigation

Depending on the presentation, the most useful investigation is FNAC, but CT scanning is of value in determining extent of tumour and lymph node involvement. Serum calcitonin levels may be raised in medullary tumours.

Treatment

The treatment of all but very-low-risk differentiated thyroid cancer (follicular or papillary) is total thyroidectomy, with local removal of involved lymph nodes. Subsequent treatment involves the administration of radioactive iodine (^{131}I), which allows for both the detection and ablation of metastatic disease and lifelong thyroxine suppression. Low-risk papillary cancer includes young patients with small, often incidentally discovered tumours. Minimally invasive follicular thyroid cancer with capsular penetration alone is also regarded as a low-risk cancer. Both of these may be adequately treated with lobectomy and long-term thyroxine suppression.

Medullary thyroid cancer requires total thyroidectomy and a central lymph node dissection, with lateral neck dissection and mediastinal clearance for node positive patients. Medullary carcinoma does not respond to radioiodine ablation. Surgery for thyroid lymphoma should be limited to biopsy only, because the tumour responds well to external beam radiotherapy and/or chemotherapy. Surgery should be avoided for anaplastic cancer, although pre-operative multimodal chemoradiotherapy may well make such tumours operable.

Thyrotoxicosis

Pathology

Thyrotoxicosis can occur in diffuse hypersecretory goitre (Graves' disease), toxic multinodular goitre (Plummer's disease), toxic follicular adenoma or in the initial stages of thyroiditis. Rarer causes include a TSH-secreting pituitary tumour or struma ovarii. Graves' disease is an autoimmune condition associated with antibodies to the TSH receptor. Toxic nodular goitre results from autonomous activity in a neoplastic nodule.

Clinical presentation

Thyrotoxicosis will present with signs and symptoms of thyroid overactivity, including tachycardia, heat intolerance, sweating, weight loss and anxiety. In addition, Graves' disease may be associated with exophthalmos and pre-tibial myxoedema. Toxic nodules may also present with local pressure or obstruction.

Investigation

The diagnosis of thyrotoxicosis will be confirmed by TFTs with an elevated free T4 and/or free T3, in association with a suppressed TSH. Clinical examination may well indicate the aetiology, demonstrating a diffuse goitre, a multinodular goitre or a single thyroid nodule. Thyroid nuclear scans will confirm the diagnosis, as well as the aetiology.

Treatment

Initial treatment is to render the patient euthyroid by administration of antithyroid medication in the form of propylthiouracil or carbimazole, both of which prevent coupling of iodotyrosine. Patients with Graves' disease are generally treated with medication for 12–18 months. Alternative treatments are ablation with radioactive iodine, usually reserved for patients more than 40 years of age because of the theoretical teratogenic risk, or total thyroidectomy. Graves' disease is treated by surgery if there is relapse following initial medical treatment (about 50% of the time) or non-compliance with such treatment, or if ophthalmopathy is present, in which case radioiodine ablation is contraindicated. Toxic multinodular goitre and toxic adenoma are best treated surgically once the patient is rendered euthyroid by antithyroid medication.

Thyroiditis

Pathology

Thyroiditis is classified as lymphocytic (Hashimoto's), subacute (de Quervain's), acute (bacterial) or fibrosing

(Reidel's). Of these, the two most common are lymphocytic, which is an autoimmune condition often forming part of a spectrum with Graves' disease, and subacute, which is a post-viral phenomenon.

Presentation

Lymphocytic thyroiditis may present with hyperthyroidism (early phase) or hypothyroidism (late phase), or it may present with a nodular or diffuse goitre. Subacute thyroiditis usually presents with an exquisitely tender, enlarged, firm thyroid gland, often with systemic symptoms of headache, malaise and weight loss.

Investigation

Thyroid function tests will determine the level of thyroid activity. A nuclear medicine scan is often diagnostic, showing patchy uptake in lymphocytic thyroiditis and no uptake at all in subacute thyroiditis.

Treatment

Subacute thyroiditis usually responds to high-dose steroids and aspirin therapy, although it may take 3–6 months to fully resolve. Lymphocytic thyroiditis may respond to thyroxine suppression. Surgery may be required for lymphocytic thyroiditis with persistent or suspicious nodules, or for pressure symptoms, although surgery is difficult because of the solid, nonpliable nature of the gland.

Operative management: thyroidectomy

Indications

Thyroidectomy (Box 33.1) is indicated for relief of local obstructive symptoms, for the diagnosis and treatment of thyroid cancer, for the control of thyrotoxicosis, or for cosmetic considerations.

Complications of thyroidectomy

The complications of thyroidectomy include all the general complications of any operation, such as bleeding, wound infection, and reaction to the anaesthetic agent. In addition, there are specific complications, including:

- Damage to the recurrent laryngeal nerves
- Damage to the external branch of the superior laryngeal nerves
- Damage to the parathyroid glands

Box 33.1 Timing of suture removal

Types of thyroid operations

- Total thyroidectomy. This involves the removal of the entire thyroid gland. The procedure is carried out for thyroid cancer, multinodular goitre, and Graves' disease.
- Hemithyroidectomy (thyroid lobectomy). In this procedure all of one thyroid lobe is removed. This procedure is performed for a single thyroid nodule.
- Minimal-access thyroidectomy. Minimal-access approaches to the thyroid include endoscopic, video-assisted and mini-incision techniques. For the present they should still be confined to feasibility studies only.

Unilateral recurrent nerve palsy leads to a hoarse voice that, if permanent, can be treated by procedures such as vocal cord medialisation. Bilateral damage may require a tracheostomy because the cords adopt the medial position. If the external branch of the superior laryngeal nerve is affected, the patient may lose the ability to sing, shout or project their voice. Permanent damage to the parathyroid glands will cause permanent hypoparathyroidism. Temporary damage or oedema, which is much more common, will require short-term administration of oral calcium and 1,25-dihydroxyvitamin D for several weeks. These complications are avoided by understanding the surgical anatomy of the thyroid gland (Fig 33.1) and by the technique of capsular dissection, carefully avoiding the parathyroid glands and their blood supply, and the recurrent laryngeal nerves.

MCQs

Select the single correct answer to each question.

1 Thyroid follicular cells arise primarily from:
  a the laryngeal cartilage
  b the second bronchial arch
  c the oesophagus
  d the base of the tongue
  e the neural crest

2 FNAC can reliably diagnose all types of thyroid cancer *except*:
  a follicular thyroid cancer
  b papillary thyroid cancer

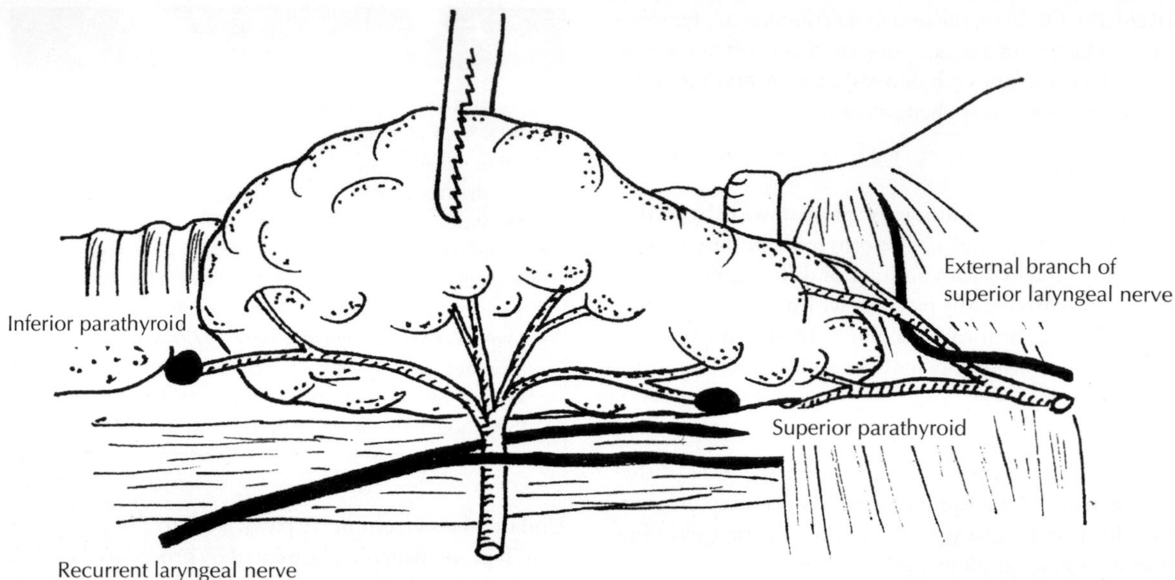

Fig. 33.1 Surgical anatomy of the thyroid gland. The left lobe of the gland is elevated exposing the recurrent laryngeal nerve, the external branch of the superior laryngeal nerve, the Tubercle of Zuckerkandl, and both parathyroid glands, with their blood supply arising from the inferior thyroid artery.

c anaplastic thyroid cancer
d medullary thyroid cancer
e metastases from renal cell cancer

3 The type of thyroid cancer with the worst prognosis (5-year survival <1%) is:
a papillary thyroid cancer
b follicular thyroid cancer
c anaplastic thyroid cancer
d medullary thyroid cancer
e thyroid lymphoma

4 Thyroiditis presenting following a viral infection with an exquisitely tender, enlarged, firm thyroid gland, and with systemic symptoms of headache and malaise is generally due to:
a Hashimoto's thyroiditis
b de Quervain's (subacute) thyroiditis
c Reidels thyroiditis
d acute bacterial thyroiditis
e non-specific thyroiditis

5 Damage to one recurrent laryngeal nerve during thyroidectomy generally leads to:
a the need for a tracheostomy
b an inability to sing high notes
c inability to project the voice to the back of a hall
d a falsetto voice
e a hoarse voice

34 Parathyroid

Leigh Delbridge and Gordon Clunie

Introduction

There are four parathyroid glands, two on each side, having a postero-lateral relationship to the lateral lobes of the thyroid gland. The two superior parathyroid glands arise from the fourth pharyngeal pouch and ultimobranchial body, and migrate medially early in foetal development along with the C cells to meet the developing thyroid gland. They are generally very constant in position in relation to the lateral lobe or to the Tubercle of Zuckerkandl. The two inferior parathyroid glands arise from the third pharyngeal pouch and then descend into the anterior neck along with the thymus. They often are very variable in position and may be found in relation to the inferior pole of the thyroid gland, within or adjacent to the thymus, or in the anterior mediastinum. Ectopic or supernumary parathyroid glands are common, being found in over 10% of the population. They may be located in a variety of positions such as the pericardium, or within the carotid sheath. If parathyroid glands enlarge, they may migrate from their original location. Superior parathyroid glands, as they enlarge, often move down along the oesophagus, presumably aided by peristalsis, and can end up in the posterior mediastinum. Enlarged inferior glands may be found in the anterior. The course of the recurrent laryngeal nerve acts as a marker to the location of the parathyroid glands with abnormal superior glands usually located posterior, and abnormal inferior glands located anterior, to the nerve. The normal parathyroid gland weighs 30–35. The glands derive their primary blood supply from branches of the inferior thyroid artery although superior glands may receive branches from the superior thyroid artery.

The parathyroid glands secrete parathyroid hormone (PTH), an 84–amino acid peptide, which has a half-life of about 5 minutes, which is rapidly broken down into N-terminal and C-terminal fragments in the reticulo-endothelial cells of the liver. PTH acts on bone to promote calcium by stimulation of osteoclast activity, leading to bone resorption. PTH also acts on the kidney to increase calcium resorption in the proximal convoluted tubule and inhibit resorption of both phosphate and bicarbonate. An additional renal effect is the production by the proximal tubule of 1,25-dihydroxy vitamin D, which results in calcium absorption by the small intestine.

Diseases affecting the parathyroid glands result essentially in disorders of function, either excess or reduced PTH secretion. They include

- Primary hyperparathyroidism
- Secondary and tertiary hyperparathyroidism
- Hypoparathyroidism

Disorders of the parathyroid glands

Primary hyperparathyroidism

Pathology

Primary hyperparathyroidism is due to a parathyroid adenoma, either single or multiple in more than 90% of cases. It may also be due to parathyroid hyperplasia or, rarely, parathyroid carcinoma. It may occur as a sporadic phenomenon, or may be associated with one of the familial endocrine syndromes including MEN I, MEN IIA, or familial hyperparathyroidism. Hyperparathyroidism is also associated with a history of previous exposure to ionising radiation.

Clinical presentation

Primary hyperparathyroidism occurs predominantly in women, with the highest incidence being in the fifth to sixth decades. The commonest presentation is in apparently asymptomatic individuals who are found to have hypercalcaemia during routine blood testing, or who present for routine bone mineral density testing and are found to have osteopoenia or osteoporosis. Symptoms specifically associated with primary hyperparathyroidism include neuropsychological manifestations such as tiredness, lethargy and depression, musculoskeletal manifestations such as bone pain and muscle weakness, renal stones, abdominal pain from constipation or peptic ulceration, polyuria and polydipsia.

Investigations

The diagnosis of primary hyperparathyroidism is confirmed by the finding of an elevated serum calcium level in association with an inappropriately raised PTH level. The PTH may well be in the normal range despite the presence of primary hyperparathyroidism, for with all other causes of hypercalcaemia (eg metastatic malignancy), an elevated serum calcium will be associated with a suppressed PTH level. Measurement of 24-hour urinary calcium secretion must also be performed to exclude the rare but confounding genetic disorder of familial hypocalciuric hypercalcaemia, in which an elevated serum calcium may be associated with a marginally raised PTH level.

A careful family history will generally exclude an association with one of the familial endocrine syndromes. If the patient has MEN I, tumours of the pituitary and pancreatic islet cells need to be excluded, whereas if they are part of an MEN IIA family, serum calcitonin and urinary catecholamines need to be measured to exclude medullary thyroid carcinoma and phaeochromocytoma.

Once a diagnosis of primary hyperparathyroidism has been confirmed, and there are no exclusion criteria for minimally invasive parathyroidectomy, for example family history, then parathyroid localisation studies should be undertaken. A sestamibi parathyroid scan will demonstrate uptake in a single parathyroid adenoma in more than 70% of cases, with neck ultrasound providing valuable additional information.

Treatment

The only successful treatment for primary hyperparathyroidism is parathyroidectomy. Current NIH guidelines argue that asymptomatic patients may be treated by observation subject to a set of strict criteria; however there is increasing evidence that even "asymptomatic" patients obtain significant benefit in relation to improvements in non-specific neuropsychological symptoms following normalisation of serum calcium levels after surgery. As such most patients, unless there are specific contraindications to surgery, are now offered parathyroidectomy as initial therapy.

Secondary hyperparathyroidism

Pathology

Secondary hyperparathyroidism is the result of prolonged hypocalcaemia and is usually due to chronic renal failure, although vitamin D deficiency and gluten-sensitive enteropathy must be excluded as causes. The prolonged hypocalcaemia results in chief cell hyperplasia and PTH secretion. In chronic renal failure, this appears to be due to difficulties with excretion of phosphate with secondary hyperphosphataemia and hypocalcaemia, and increases in PTH result in osteodystrophy much greater than that normally seen in primary disease.

Clinical features

The osteodystrophy of secondary hyperparathyroidism causes bone and muscle pain and may lead to pathological fractures. There may be deposition of calcium in soft tissues resulting in skin itch, and even necrosis and severe conjunctivitis.

Investigations

Secondary hyperparathyroidism is characterised by hypocalcaemia, hyperphosphataemia (due to failure of excretion) and an elevated PTH level. Significant bone disease is indicated by elevation of serum alkaline phosphatase. Hypercalcaemia may occur secondary to vitamin D treatment. Radiology demonstrates much grosser changes in the skeleton than is usual in primary hyperparathyroidism in the modern context, with irregular bone density loss and subperiosteal absorption of bone. This produces the classical appearance of the "pepperpot skull", the "rugger jersey" spine and the less dramatic but more frequent loss of the outer third of clavicle and scalloping of the radial side of the middle phalanges. Metastatic calcification can be seen around vessels and in the capsules of joints.

Treatment

Secondary hyperparathyroidism occurs to some degree in all patients with chronic renal failure but the symptoms can usually be controlled by calcium supplementation and the administration of 1,25-dihydroxyvitamin D at the time of dialysis if there is progression to end-stage renal failure. Phosphate binders may also be used to reduce intestinal absorption of phosphate although he use of binders containing aluminium must be avoided to prevent the development of aluminium bone disease and an irreversible dementia. Although the treatment of secondary hyperparathyroidism is therefore largely medical in nature, 20% of patients will not achieve satisfactory symptom or biochemical control. Indications for surgery include the development of hypercalcaemia, because this is likely to lead to metastatic calcification and persistent elevation in alkaline phosphatase, which is an indication of continuing major bone disease. Clinical indications include intractable itch or bone pain. These patients should be treated by total parathyroidectomy with or without parathyroid autotransplantation.

Tertiary hyperparathyroidism

Tertiary hyperparathyroidism results from the hyperplasia of secondary hyperparathyroidism when the glands become autonomously hyperfunctioning rather than responsive to the original stimulus. This is most clearly seen after a successful renal transplant has been performed where the restoration of normal renal function and the appropriate production of 1,25-dihydroxyvitamin D could be expected to restore normal calcium balance. Most patients should receive active medical treatment in an attempt to avoid end-organ damage, and will usually show a return to normal calcium metabolism within a period of 6 months. In the small number of patients whose symptoms are not controlled or in whom the hypercalcaemia persists in spite of adequate treatment and normal renal function, the glands must be assumed to have developed some degree of autonomy and parathyroidectomy is required. The extent of surgery is dictated by the operative findings, with either subtotal or total parathyroidectomy with autotransplantation being undertaken depending on the number of glands involved in this process.

Hypoparathyroidism

Hypoparathyroidism may be due to congenital absence of the parathyroid glands, idiopathic autoimmune failure of the parathyroid glands or, most commonly, due to surgical removal or damage to the parathyroid glands after total thyroidectomy. Temporary hypoparathyroidism is common after total thyroidectomy, especially if devascularised parathyroid glands have been autotransplanted during the procedure. Such patients may be asymptomatic or may present with paraesthesiae in the limbs and around the mouth. This is easily managed by replacement therapy with oral calcium and 1,25-dihydroxyvitamin D for several weeks awaiting recovery of the autotransplanted glands.

Operative management

Parathyroidectomy

Patients with primary hyperparathyroidism and concordant localisation to a single site can undergo minimally invasive parathyroidectomy. Patients with primary hyperparathyroidism where localisation has not been successful are more likely to have multiple gland disease and should undergo open parathyroidectomy and four-gland exploration. Patients with secondary and tertiary hyperparathyroidism require either subtotal parathyroidectomy or total parathyroidectomy with or without forearm autotransplantation. Successful detection and removal of the involved parathyroid tissue will occur in 98% of patients. In the small percentage of patients in whom the gland is not detected at the time of primary surgery, it is likely to lie in an ectopic position, e.g. pericardium or middle mediastinum and additional, localisation studies such as CT scanning and selective venous sampling will be required prior to a second operation.

Complications of parathyroidectomy

The complications of parathyroidectomy include all the general complications of any operation, such as bleeding, wound infection, and reaction to the anaesthetic agent. In addition, there are specific complications, including:

- damage to the recurrent laryngeal nerves and to the external branch of the superior laryngeal nerves
- failure to locate abnormal parathyroid tissue
- hypoparathyroidism

Recurrent nerve palsy leads to a hoarse voice that usually recovers but may require procedures such as vocal cord medialisation. If the external branch of the superior laryngeal nerve is damaged, the patient may lose the ability to sing, shout or project their voice. Failure to locate abnormal parathyroid tissue may be due to the adenoma being in an ectopic site such as the mediastinum. Further localisation studies and surgery will be required. If more than one parathyroid gland is involved, subtotal parathyroidectomy may lead to hypoparathyroidism, which may require short-term administration of oral calcium and 1,25-dihydroxyvitamin D for several weeks.

MCQs

Select the single correct answer to each question.

1 The parathyroid glands arise from:
- **a** the third and fourth branchial pouches
- **b** the base of the tongue
- **c** the first branchial pouch
- **d** the thyroid parenchyma
- **e** a tracheal diverticulum

2 Parathyroid hormone (PTH) has a half-life of:
- **a** 7 seconds
- **b** 5 minutes
- **c** 1 hour
- **d** 2 days
- **e** 5 weeks

3 Primary hyperparathyroidism is due, in 90% of cases, to:
- **a** metastatic cancer
- **b** parathyroid cancer
- **c** parathyroid hyperplasia
- **d** multiple parathyroid tumours
- **e** a single parathyroid adenoma

4 The diagnosis of primary hyperparathyroidism is usually confirmed by the following biochemical results:
- **a** raised serum calcium, suppressed PTH
- **b** raised serum calcium, raised or normal PTH
- **c** normal serum calcium, raised PTH
- **d** normal serum calcium, suppressed PTH
- **e** low serum calcium, raised or normal PTH

5 The most common cause of hypoparathyroidism is:
- **a** congenital absence of the parathyroids
- **b** autoimmune parathyroid failure
- **c** parathyroid cancer
- **d** surgical removal of the parathyroids at total thyroidectomy
- **e** acute bacterial infection

35 Tumours of the adrenal gland

Leigh Delbridge

Introduction

The adrenal glands lie superomedial to the upper poles of both kidneys. Each adrenal gland comprises a medulla and a cortex, and each component has a distinct embryological origin. The adrenal cortex is of mesodermal origin, whereas the adrenal medulla arises from neural crest cells along with the sympathetic ganglia. The adrenal medulla produces catecholamines, including adrenaline, noradrenaline and dopamine and is under the control of the sympathetic nervous system. The adrenal cortex produces glucocorticoids (cortisol, corticosterone), mineralocorticoids (aldosterone) and sex steroids (oestrogen, testosterone, dihydroepiandrosterone). The adrenal cortex is under the control of adrenocorticotropic hormone (ACTH), a hormone produced by the pituitary gland.

Adrenal and neural crest tumours

Adrenal masses are common, affecting 3–7% of the population. Tumours can arise from both the adrenal cortex and the adrenal medulla as well as from neural crest structures. Tumours of either origin may be benign or malignant, functioning or non-functioning, and solitary or multiple. Adrenal tumours can be considered in the following groups:

- Tumours of the adrenal medulla/neural crest (phaeochromocytomas and paragangliomas)
- Adrenocortical tumours
- Adrenal incidentalomas

The clinical features and investigation of adrenal tumours are summarised in Table 35.1.

Table 35.1 Clinical features and investigations for adrenal tumours

	Syndrome or tumour	Hormones secreted	Symptoms
Adrenal medullary or neural crest tumours	Phaeochromocytoma Paraganglioma	Adrenaline Noradrenaline Dopamine	Sweating, palpitations, hypertension (intermittent or sustained)
Adrenocortical tumours	Cushing's syndrome	Glucocorticoids	Central obesity, buffalo hump, abdominal striae, hypertension, peripheral weakness, plethoric facies
	Conn's syndrome	Aldosterone	Hypertension, hypokalaemia
	Virilising/feminising tumours	Sex steroids	Virilisation in females, feminisation in males
Adrenal incidentaloma	Benign adrenocortical adenomas Adrenal cysts Adrenal lymphomas Schwannomas Myelolipomas Metastases	Non-secreting	Asymptomatic (picked up on incidental CT scan or ultrasound)

Phaeochromocytoma and paraganglioma

Pathology

Phaeochromocytoma and paraganglioma are tumours arising from the adrenal medulla or neural crest. Although the classification has been confusing in the past, a consensus is now emerging (Table 35.2). All such tumours are thought to ultimately be of neural crest origin. Adrenal phaeochromocytomas are of sympathetic origin. Extra-adrenal tumours may be of sympathetic origin and are located anywhere from the cervical ganglia to the urinary bladder. They are classified as extra-adrenal phaeochromocytoma, although they have also been labelled as paraganglioma in the past. Extra-adrenal tumours may also be of parasympathetic origin, comprising mainly head and neck tumours such as carotid body tumours.

The majority of adrenal phaeochromocytomas are benign and functioning, but between 10 and 20% are malignant. This diagnosis may be difficult to make on histological examination, as with most endocrine tumours, and may not become apparent until the appearance of distant metastases during follow-up. Such tumours have a tendency to grow along the adrenal and renal veins and may extend into the inferior vena cava. Approximately 10% of phaeochromocytomas are bilateral within the adrenal glands.

The majority of extra-adrenal phaeochromocytoma are also functioning, but a greater percentage are malignant compared to adrenal tumours. True paragangliomas only rarely function, and the rate of malignancy is very low.

Phaeochromocytomas and paragangliomas may occur sporadically, or in association with a familial disorder such as multiple endocrine neoplasia IIA (MEN IIA – medullary carcinoma of the thyroid, phaeochromocytoma and hyperparathyroidism) or von Hippel–Lindau syndrome (retinal, cerebellar, spinal and medullary hemangioblastomas, renal cysts and carcinoma, pancreatic cysts, phaeochromocytoma and papillary cystadenoma of the epididymis).

Clinical presentation

Phaeochromocytomas present a rare but curable cause of hypertension, with varying combinations of paroxysmal or sustained hypertension (0.5% of patients with hypertension have a phaeochromocytoma), headache, sweating and palpitations. Loss of weight is a common symptom. Up to one third of cases may be asymptomatic.

Investigation

The clinical diagnosis of phaeochromocytoma is confirmed on the basis of elevated catecholamine levels (adrenaline, noradrenaline, dopamine) in the plasma or urine. Once a biochemical diagnosis is established, the tumour can usually be localised with by CT scan, or by MRI. A nuclear medicine scan performed with metaiodo-benzyl-guanidine (MIBG) is

Table 35.2 Classification of adrenal medullary and neural crest tumours

Origin	Tumour site	Pathology
Sympathetic tissue	Adrenal gland Extra-adrenal	Adrenal phaeochromocytoma Extra-adrenal phaeochromocytoma • Zuckerkandl remnant • Filum terminal tumour • Urinary bladder tumour • Thoracic paravertebral tumour • Cervical ganglia tumour
Parasympathetic tissue	Extra-adrenal	Paraganglioma • Carotid body tumour • Vagal paraganglioma • Jugulotympanic paraganglioma • Laryngeal paranganglioma • Aorticopulmonary paraganglioma

useful to confirm the functional status of a tumour, and may detect an extra-adrenal phaeochromocytoma, or demonstrate small lesions within the adrenal gland that are not apparent on other forms of imaging.

Treatment

Phaeochromocytoma and paraganglioma are treated by surgical excision. Careful pre-operative preparation is required in order to prevent an intra-operative hypertensive crisis, due to the massive release of catecholamine with tumour handling, or profound post-operative hypotension and massive fluid requirements resulting from the fluid shifts that follow catecholamine control. Pre-operative preparation is best undertaken with administration of alpha-adrenergic blocking agents, such as phenoxybenzamine.

Adrenocortical tumours

Pathology

These tumours may be non-functioning, or may secrete glucocorticoids, aldosterone or the sex steroids. They may occur sporadically, or as part of an hereditary syndrome such as Li–Fraumeni syndrome, Beckwith–Weidmann syndrome, Carney's complex or MEN I. The majority of glucocorticoid-producing adrenocortical tumours are benign but up to 20% may be malignant. As with other endocrine tumours, a diagnosis of adrenocortical carcinoma is based on the finding of capsular or vascular invasion, but again may not be made until the later appearance of distant metastases. These tumours may reach a very large size before diagnosis, and as the size increases the risk of malignancy also rises.

Mineralocorticoid-producing adrenal tumours are almost always small (<1 cm) and virtually always benign. Bilateral nodular hyperplasia may be difficult to distinguish from a single aldosterone-producing adenoma. The majority of sex steroid–producing tumours are malignant at presentation. Adrenocortical carcinomas are rare and 70% are associated with hormonal hypersecretion.

Clinical presentation

GLUCOCORTICOID-PRODUCING TUMOURS

Most patients present with features of glucocorticoid excess (Cushing's syndrome), which includes central obesity, peripheral weakness, abdominal striae, buffalo hump, hirsutism, plethoric facies and hypertension. Occasionally a large tumour may present with local symptoms, such as pain or fullness in the flank. A number of hormone-secreting tumours are diagnosed incidentally, on the basis of a CT or ultrasound scan, (adrenal incidentaloma), although many such tumours have now been shown to be associated with subclinical Cushing's syndrome (pre-Cushing's syndrome). This syndrome is associated with hypertension, diabetes, obesity and osteoporosis but without the full biochemical manifestations of Cushing's syndrome. Often all that is demonstrated on investigation is loss of the diurnal rhythm of cortisol secretion and suppression of function of the contralateral gland.

ALDOSTERONE-PRODUCING ADENOMAS (CONN'S SYNDROME)

Most of these tumours present during the investigation of hypertension but may be suggested by symptoms such as polyuria, polydipsia and muscle weakness due to the associated hypokalaemia. While hypokalaemia has been used as a screening test for Conn's syndrome in the past, there is increasing evidence that up to 50% of mineralocorticoid-producing tumours may be associated with normal levels of serum potassium.

SEX STEROID–PRODUCING TUMOURS

Clinical features will be specific to the type of hormone produced, with either virilisation in females or feminisation in males. Many of these patients also have palpable masses and 50% have metastatic tumour at the time of presentation.

Investigations

The initial test used to diagnose Cushing's syndrome is measurement of serum cortisol and 24-hour urinary free cortisol levels. A dexamethasone suppression test may be required to confirm true glucocorticoid excess. The presence of an adrenal tumour as the cause of the glucocorticoid excess, rather than a pituitary tumour or an ectopic ACTH-secreting tumour, can generally be made by measuring plasma ACTH levels and performing an abdominal CT scan. Bilateral nodular hyperplasia may occasionally be difficult to differentiate from a single small adrenal tumour.

A low serum potassium level will often suggest the possibility of an aldosterone-secreting tumour although more than 50% of patients are now known to be normokalaemic. Measurement of the ratio of plasma renin and plasma aldosterone (PRA ratio) will confirm the diagnosis of hyperaldosteronism, as primary hyperaldosteronism is characterised by low plasma renin activity. A CT scan may detect an adrenal tumour but, because many of these tumours are very small, selective adrenal vein sampling for aldosterone may be required to localise the tumour.

Measurement of the sex hormones as well as the 17-ketosteroids will confirm the diagnosis of a sex steroid–producing tumour. These tumours are often large and should be detected on CT scanning.

Treatment

Surgical excision (adrenalectomy) is the only treatment for an adrenocortical tumour. For large or potentially malignant tumours, wide local excision and local lymph node dissection may be required.

Adrenal incidentalomas

Pathology

Any tumour arising in the adrenal gland can present as an adrenal incidentaloma, including adrenocortical tumours, adrenal medullary tumours, Schwannomas, myelolipomas, adrenal cysts, adrenal lymphomas and adrenal metastases from other malignancies, particularly breast cancer. Incidental benign adrenocortical adenomas are very common and can be found at postmortem in up to 10% of the normal population.

Clinical presentation

By definition, an adrenal incidentaloma will present as an incidental finding, usually on a CT scan or ultrasound. They will not be associated with local symptoms, nor with any of the syndromes of hormonal excess.

Investigation

The tumour will already have been demonstrated by imaging. Hormonal secretion must be excluded by measurement of 24-hour urinary free cortisol, PRA ratio, adrenal sex steroids and urinary catecholamines. A nuclear medicine scan using seleno-cholesterol may help to determine whether the tumour is arising from the adrenal cortex, and whether or not there is suppression of hormone secretion from the contralateral side.

Treatment

Incidental adrenal tumours that do not secrete hormones are not associated with local symptoms and are less than 4–5 cm in diameter, can be treated conservatively, although there are increasing data to suggest that the potential risk for malignancy may require that cut-off to be lower, for example 3 cm. A follow-up CT scan should be performed after 6 months to make sure there is not a progressive increase in size, which would suggest malignancy. Large tumours, or those that demonstrate an increase in size, should be removed surgically because of the increased risk of malignancy.

Operative management: adrenalectomy

Adrenalectomy can be performed either as an open procedure, as a laparoscopic procedure with hand assist devices, or solely as a laparoscopic procedure. Increasingly, the accepted philosophy is to tailor the surgical approach to the tumour size and clinical situation. The open approach to the adrenal gland is either anteriorly through the peritoneal cavity (now used only for large and probably malignant lesions), or via an extraperitoneal approach, either posteriorly through the bed of the 12th rib or postero-laterally, or combined as a thoraco-abdominal procedure. These procedures should be used for very large tumours, or those known to be malignant.

Laparoscopic adrenalectomy is associated with reduced post-operative pain, and allows the patient to leave hospital after 2 or 3 days. The procedure is ideally suited to small benign adrenal tumours, such as those commonly found in Conn's syndrome, but is also indicated for phaeochromocytoma, including bilateral tumours.

Complications of adrenalectomy include all the general complications of any open abdominal adrenal operation or laparoscopic procedure such as bleeding, wound infection and ileus. The particular anaesthetic complications of phaeochromocytoma surgery have already been discussed. Surgery for glucocorticoid-secreting tumours, and occasionally for incidentalomas with sub-clinical hormone secretion, may be associated with post-operative Addisonian crisis, because of suppression of the contralateral adrenal gland. This will require steroid administration until the remaining gland recovers, which may take 4–6 weeks.

MCQs

Select the single correct answer to each question.

1 Adrenal masses occur in:
- **a** <1% of the population
- **b** 3–7% of the population
- **c** 10–20% of the population
- **d** 40–50% of the population
- **e** >66% of the population

2 Conn's syndrome is due to a tumour of the adrenal cortex secreting excess:
- **a** cortisol
- **b** adrenaline
- **c** noradrenaline
- **d** aldosterone
- **e** sex steroids

3 Paragangliomas arise from:
- **a** the adrenal cortex
- **b** the adrenal medulla
- **c** the carotid bifurcation
- **d** the foregut
- **e** parasympathetic tissue arising from the neural crest

4 The initial test used to diagnose Cushing's syndrome is measurement of:
- **a** serum cortisol and 24-hour urinary free cortisol levels
- **b** serum ACTH
- **c** serum cortisol after a dexamethasone test
- **d** plasma renin/aldosterone ratio
- **e** serum catecholamines

5 Adrenal "incidentalomas" should be removed when they are:
- **a** >25 cm
- **b** >10–15 cm
- **c** >3–5 cm
- **d** >1 cm
- **e** any size at all

36 Endocrine tumours of the pancreas

Gordon J. A. Clunie

Physiology and pathology

Endocrine tumours of the pancreas are rare in comparison with tumours of the exocrine pancreas (see Chapter 15). Such tumours may be benign or malignant, single or multiple, functioning or non-functioning.

The islets of Langerhans contain at least five cell types:

- alpha cells, which produce glucagon
- beta cells, which produce insulin
- gamma cells, which produce somatostatin
- F-cells, which produce pancreatic polypeptide
- enterochromaffin cells, which produce serotonin.

However, it is important to note that individual islet cells are capable of producing more than one hormone and that these hormones may include peptides that are not normally associated with the pancreas, including gastrin, adrenocorticotropic hormone and vasoactive intestinal peptide.

Although the majority of cases occur sporadically, approximately 10% of patients with islet cell tumours are members of families demonstrating multiple endocrine neoplasia type I (MEN I; see Chapter 34).

Clinical features

Islet cell tumours may be functioning or non-functioning.

Non-functioning tumours

Non-functioning tumours, which form approximately 20% of islet cell tumours, produce symptoms related to their site and size, and in many ways are comparable to the more common adenocarcinoma of the pancreas. Most present in the head of the pancreas and most are malignant, so investigation and treatment is similar to those for adenocarcinoma. The differential features that declare these to be 'APUDomas' (APUD: amine precursor uptake and decarboxylation) are their capacity to take up radioactive iodine–labelled metaiodo-benzylguanidine (MIBG) and immunohistochemical staining for neurospecific enolase.

Functioning tumours

Functioning tumours produce a wide range of peptides as already defined. Rare forms are the glucagonoma, which produces the diabetes-dermatitis syndrome, the 'VIPoma' (VIP: vaso-active intestinal peptide), which stimulates cyclic AMP production by the gut leading to massive watery diarrhoea (pancreatic cholera), and the somatostatinoma, which produces diabetes and steatorrhoea.

The most common forms of functioning tumours of the islet cells, although themselves still rarities, are insulinoma and gastrinoma.

Insulinoma

These are the most common forms of islet cell tumour of the pancreas. Seventy-five per cent of lesions are single adenomas, 10% are multiple and 10% are primarily malignant. The remaining 5% represent nesidioblastomas (diffuse micro-adenomatosis or nesidioblastosis hyperplasia of the B cells).

CLINICAL FEATURES

Patients usually present in middle age with Whipple's triad:

- Symptoms of confusion and bizarre behaviour, visual disturbance or transient motor defects following fasting, with the associated sympathetic discharge resulting in palpitations, sweating and tremor.
- Blood glucose levels during these episodes of less than 45 mmol/L.

• Rapid relief of symptoms and signs by the administration of glucose either orally or intravenously.

It is important to note that the neurological effects of hypoglycaemia are easily confused with a number of other conditions, including psychoses, and it is not unusual for there to be a significant delay in diagnosis if the classical features are not recognised.

INVESTIGATIONS

Diagnosis can be established by fasting, with estimation of blood glucose levels and immunoreactive insulin every 6 hours. In the presence of an insulinoma, fasting stimulates hypoglycaemia and the presence of inappropriately high levels of insulin. The fasting is continued until either symptoms or hypoglycaemia result, although this may not occur for up to 72 hours. Very rarely, even such prolonged fasting will not result in hypoglycaemia, but vigorous exercise after 72 hours' fasting will invariably produce hypoglycaemia.

The tumours may be multiple and therefore localisation is necessary. Abdominal ultrasound, MRI and computed tomography (CT) scanning are all of value, but because the lesions are usually less than 2 cm in size at the time of diagnosis, the tumours are demonstrated in only 50% of cases. Recent studies have shown that endoscopic ultrasound may help in localisation of small tumours. As the tumours are hypervascular, arteriography will demonstrate tumours in half of the patients where the lesion has not been demonstrated by CT scanning. The most accurate technique for preoperative localisation is transhepatic portal venous sampling with measurement of insulin levels progressively at points along the portal vein. This technique demonstrates the site of the lesion in 95% of cases.

TREATMENT

Acute hypoglycaemic episodes are easily treated by the administration of glucose, either intravenously or orally. Normal blood glucose can be maintained by frequent small meals.

Once the diagnosis has been established and the tumour localised, the treatment is surgical. Approach may be laparotomy or by laparoscopy. Localisation of the tumour is confirmed by the use of intra-operative ultrasound, using either technique.

Single tumours are removed by enucleation. If multiple tumours or nesidioblastomas are present, all involved tissue is removed as far as possible, usually with retention of the head of the pancreas to preserve both exocrine and endocrine function. This may still result in the development of diabetes. Where lesions are malignant, radical surgery, which may include resection of hepatic metastases, should be undertaken because of the difficulty of controlling hypoglycaemia in the presence of a large tumour burden. Diazoxide and long-acting somatostatin analogues may be used to inhibit the production of insulin when there is residual malignancy and the tumours themselves can be treated by a combination of streptozotocin and 5-fluorouracil directed against the tumour, although the effect of these drugs is temporary and both have significant toxicity.

Gastrinoma

This is the second most common form of islet cell tumour, with the gastrin secretion resulting in Zollinger–Ellison syndrome. This is still a rare condition, with peptic ulcer disease being caused by a gastrinoma in less than 0.1% of patients with such ulcers. The lesions are most commonly single, in the form of either adenoma or carcinoma, with a small percentage resulting from multiple microadenomas or hyperplasia. Sixty per cent of the lesions are malignant and 40% benign. Ninety per cent of tumours are found in the 'gastrinoma triangle' (Fig. 36.1) Rarely, the lesions are in the submucosal region of the first or second parts of the duodenum. Lesions at that site are usually benign.

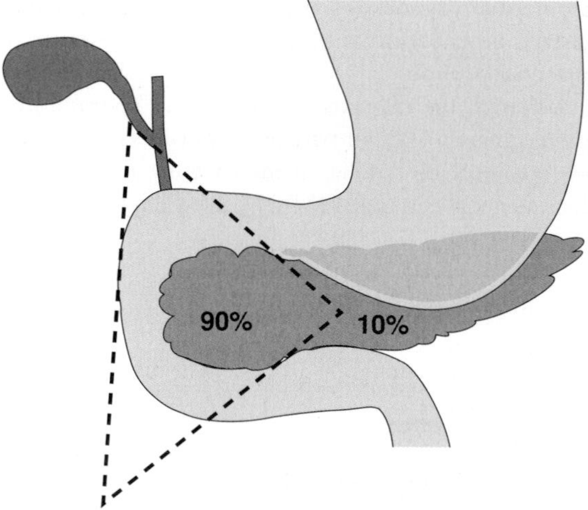

Fig. 36.1 Gastrinoma triangle bounded by the cystic duct and the common bile duct, junction of the head and neck of the pancreas, and the second and third part of the duodenum. Ninety per cent of gastrinomas are found in this area.

CLINICAL FEATURES

Three-quarters of patients present in a sporadic fashion, with the remaining 25% showing the features of MEN I. The diagnosis is suggested by the aggressive behaviour of peptic ulcers, with failure to respond to standard forms of medical therapy or rapid relapse after cessation of medical therapy for peptic ulcer. The gastric hypersecretion as a result of the inappropriate gastrin production may lead to profuse watery diarrhoea and indeed 5% of patients present with diarrhoea alone and no evidence of peptic ulcer disease.

INVESTIGATIONS

Patients presenting with the features described should have serum gastrin measured. Very high levels of gastrin suggest malignancy. To distinguish other causes of hypergastrinaemia a secretin test should be performed, as secretin acts as a stimulant for gastrin release from gastrinoma, while having little effect on other conditions. It is not necessary to carry out measurement of gastric acid levels, as was once thought to be important.

Upper gastrointestinal endoscopy will demonstrate the presence of an ulcer or ulcers that may be in unusual sites, such as the second part of the duodenum or in the jejunum after previous gastric surgery. Again endocopic ultrasonography may assist in detecting small tumours.

Dynamic CT scanning will demonstrate 80% of tumours, and because the tumours are not as vascular as insulinomas, arteriography has little additional role. Transhepatic portal venous sampling for measurement of gastrin levels after intra-arterial calcium gluconate injection may assist in tumour localisation.

TREATMENT

There is now little role for extensive gastric surgery, including total gastrectomy, partly because medical therapy is now much more effective and partly because preoperative and intra-operative localisation of tumours has led to a much greater success rate for direct surgery to control the gastrinoma. Where tumours are small, localised and readily acccessible by open laparotomy or minimally invasive surgery, they should be removed, since this offers the only chance of cure.

Following recurrence after surgery or where surgery is not applicable, medical treatment should be undertaken.

This requires lifelong administration of H_2-receptor antagonists or omeprazole to control acid secretion. However, because the risk of malignancy is relatively high, it is now usual to attempt cure of the syndrome. At laparotomy, intra-operative ultrasound is of major value, as it is with insulinomas, and this together with the pre operative CT scanning should allow detection of most lesions. Single lesions or multiple small adenomas can be enucleated but, as with insulinoma, all involved tissue should be removed as far as possible. Again it is usual to leave the head of the pancreas, in an attempt to maintain endocrine and exocrine function. If no lesion is detected at operation, the duodenum should be opened to search for submucosal lesions, which although rare are easily treated by excisional surgery.

Unresectable or metastatic gastrinoma is compatible with long survival, with either repeated resection of metastases or the administration of combined streptozoticin and 5-fluorouracil. These agents appear to be more effective with gastrinoma than with insulinoma, and although they may produce side-effects of nausea and vomiting, and renal and hepatotoxicity, their administration may produce several years of life of reasonable quality.

MCQs

Select the single correct answer to each question.

1 The most common form of functioning tumour of the pancreatic islet cells is:
- **a** gastrinoma
- **b** insulinoma
- **c** somatostatinoma
- **d** vipoma
- **e** glucagonoma

2 The Zollinger–Ellison syndrome can be controlled by administration of:
- **a** omeprazole
- **b** folic acid
- **c** methotrexate
- **d** atenolol
- **e** atorvastatin

3 The islets of Langerhans contain all these types of cells except:
- **a** alpha cells
- **b** beta cells
- **c** gamma cells
- **d** delta cells
- **e** enterochromaffin cells

Head and Neck Surgery

37 Eye injuries and infections

J. E. K. Galbraith

Visual acuity

The visual acuity of all patients with an ocular injury must be measured using a Snellen chart, and recorded. Eye injuries caused by an accident or personal violence are often the subject of litigation. The visual acuity on presentation can then be of importance, especially if there is a delay in reaching specialist care.

Visual acuity testing

The Snellen chart consists of rows of letters of decreasing size. The number on each line shows the distance at which a person with normal sight should be able to read the line.

- Stand the patient 6 m from the chart with the palm of the left hand covering the left eye, but not pressing on the eye.
- Instruct the patient to read the letters on the chart from the top down. Each line is numbered. The number represents the distance in meters at which a person with normal sight can read the line.
- The last line the patient reads is recorded: e.g. 6/18. The top line represents the distance from the chart, and the bottom line the distance from the chart at which a person with normal sight would read that line. Thus 6/18 is not a fraction; the patient reads at 6 m the line a normal person would read at 18 m. The patient now covers the right eye and repeats the test.
- If no letters on the chart can be seen, bring the chart closer until the top letter can be identified. If this occurs at 2 m the acuity is recorded as 2/60 (the top letter on the chart can be seen by a person with normal sight at 60 m).
- If the top letter cannot be identified at any distance, then wave a hand in front of the eye (with the other eye covered). If the movement is perceived, it is recorded as HM (Hand Movements).
- If hand movements cannot be seen, shine a light into the eye. If it is seen, this is recorded as LP (light perception). Shine the light into the eye from different directions and instruct the patient to point to the light. If this is performed accurately, the acuity is recorded as "LP with accurate projection."
- If a bright light cannot be seen, the acuity is recorded as NLP (no light perception).

Eye injuries

Eye injuries may be caused by a concussive blow, by perforation of the eye, and by chemical or thermal damage.

Always identify the causative mechanism as this has predictive value in determining both investigations and treatment. For example, an eye with visual loss from an accident using a hammer and cold chisel may harbour a retained intra-ocular foreign body, and indicate the need for a CT scan.

History and examination

Take a careful history of the cause of the injury, and then examine the eye.

Always use the same routine in examining an eye.

Face – note any abnormality in the lids or eyes in relation to the rest of the face

Lids – check lid movement

Conjunctiva and sclera – the white of the eye should be white

Cornea – the cornea should be clear

Pupil – should be black and moving

Eye movements – up to the right and left, down to the right and left, and from side to side.

Concussive injuries

Injuries such as a punch or a blow by a tennis ball may produce a peri-orbital haematoma (black eye), which requires no specific treatment provided that intra-ocular derangement has been excluded. Check the visual acuity.

Blow-out fracture of the orbit

An object larger than the orbital opening will compress the orbital contents and may produce a blow-out fracture of the orbital floor into the maxillary antrum or, less commonly, of the medial wall into the ethmoidal air cells. These are the thinnest of the orbital walls and are most likely to be damaged.

The patient will complain of *diplopia* owing to entrapment of the fascia around the inferior rectus muscle in the fracture in the floor of the orbit. (See Fig. 37.1) Because of damage to the infra-orbital nerve in the floor of the orbit the upper teeth and part of the gum and cheek will be *anaesthetic*. Because of prolapse of orbital fat into the antrum, the eye will be *enophthalmic*, as it sinks back into the orbit.

The treatment is surgical with release of the entrapped tissues from the fracture site.

Hyphaema

A hyphaema is a haemorrhage into the anterior chamber of the eye (between the cornea and iris).

The visual acuity will be decreased. The pupil will usually not respond to light. Check the intra-ocular pressure by *gently* palpating the eye as one would to assess fluctuance. Compare with your own eye.

When blood completely fills the anterior chamber, the pressure may rise acutely to a level sufficient to occlude the central retinal artery, and cause permanent blindness. Immediately commence treatment with Acetazolamide 500 mg initially, and 250 mg three times a day. The patient must be referred immediately for specialist treatment.

Where the hyphaema occupies less than three quarters of the anterior chamber, treat with bed rest and sedation; the blood will absorb in a day or two. A hyphaema may be complicated by intra-ocular damage, which will not be apparent on presentation. Therefore refer for specialist examination to exclude intra-ocular damage

Traumatic mydriasis

Following a blow on the eye, the iris muscles may be paralysed, producing a fixed dilated pupil, which may recover within a few days. Small tears in the lid margin may involve the sphincter and cause permanent pupil dilatation.

Retinal oedema

The retina at the posterior pole of the eye may become oedematous and pale, with decreased acuity due to macular involvement. Recovery will take several days and may be incomplete.

Choroidal rupture

Rupture of the choroid occurs in an arc concentric with the optic nerve. It results in disruption of the overlying nerve fibers and hence produces a permanent visual field defect. If the rupture occurs between the disc and the macula the central vision is permanently lost.

Contusion deformity of the chamber angle

The intra-ocular pressure is controlled by a balance between the rate of formation of aqueous humour, and its rate of removal from the eye via the trabecular meshwork in the angle between the cornea and the iris. Damage to this structure can cause glaucoma up to 10 years after the injury.

Perforating injuries

Perforating injures are caused by laceration of the cornea or sclera – commonly by glass in motor vehicle accidents, by knives, and in industrial accidents such as the shattering of a tool when using a capstan lathe.

Examination

Where the suspicion of a perforating injury exists, examine the eye carefully, after the instillation of two or three drops of local anaesthetic. Ask the patient to open the eyes. If this is not possible, assist by pressing on the brow and cheek and gently pulling the lids apart, taking care to apply no force to the eye. If the lids are swollen and they cannot be easily pulled apart, use a retractor made from a bent paper clip which may be hooked under the lid margins and the lids pulled apart, or examine the eye under a general anaesthetic.

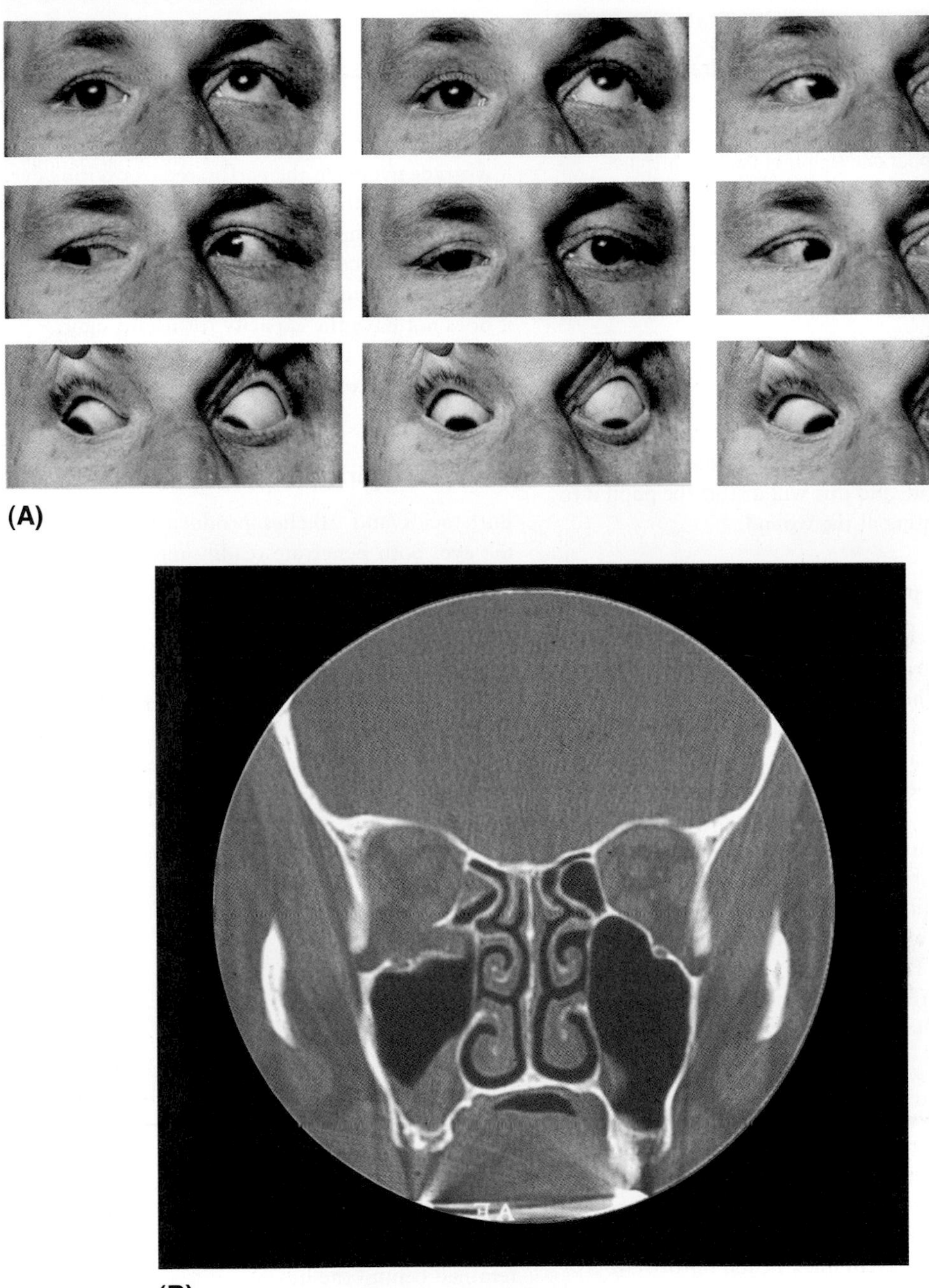

Fig. 37.1 (A) This patient has a blow-out fracture of the right orbit, and shows absent elevation in that eye. (B) CAT scan of the orbit reveals the blow-out of the floor of the orbit.

> **Box 37.1 Protective cone**
>
> From stiff card, cut a circle piece about the diameter of a saucer (14 cm). Cut out a segment of card, the base of which occupies about one eighth of the circumference. Staple the edges together.
>
> Place the cone over the eye so that its edge rests on forehead and cheek. Any inadvertent force applied to the cone will then be transferred to the bone.

Examine the cornea with a good light. A small perforation is often overlooked, but can be detected by examining the pupil – the iris is usually trapped in the perforation as the aqueous humour gushes from the eye through the wound, and this will distort the pupil into a pear shape pointing at the wound.

Transporting the patient

Instill chloramphenicol eye drops, and apply an eye pad – using two strips of transparent tape passing from the forehead on the opposite side to the cheek on the same side. Apply a protective cone over the pad, held with transparent tape. (see Box 37.1)

Instruct the patient to keep the head above the level of the heart during transport to specialist care, to prevent increase in intra-ocular pressure with subsequent loss of intra-ocular contents.

There may be air inside a perforated eye and expansion of the air at altitude may cause internal derangement of the eye. Therefore aerial evacuation of a patient with a perforating ocular wound may exacerbate the injury when the intra-ocular air expands.

Principles of treatment

- Replace the layers of the eye in their normal relationship to each other. Administer antibiotics locally and systemically to control infection.
- Administer steroids topically to control the reparative process and prevent intra-ocular fibrosis. Microsurgical techniques are used to repair the eye, and good results are often obtained.

Sympathetic ophthalmitis

This complication of perforating injury is rare nowadays, thanks to improvements in the surgical repair of perforating wounds. The exact aetiology of the condition is unknown, but is usually regarded as an autoimmune reaction to uveal pigment or antigen or both. Today, repeated retinal surgery causes more sympathetic ophthalmitis than do penetrating injuries. The antigen is thought to be retinal in origin. It causes a low-grade uveitis in the perforated or exciting eye, and also in the healthy sympathising eye. It develops about 2 weeks after the injury but may occur up to 30 years later. It can be completely avoided by removing a perforated eye during the first week after injury, if by then it does not have the capacity for useful sight.

The disease is treated with systemic and topical steroids and many cases recover with aggressive treatment.

Chemical injuries

Both acids and alkalies produce serious damage to the eye. Both penetrate readily into the eye, resulting in corneal opacification, inflammation, and cataract. Long-term complications include retinal detachment and glaucoma. Acids and alkalis also cause thrombosis of the circum-corneal blood vessels which supply nutrients to the cornea, resulting in corneal ischaemia and opacification.

The most important aspect of treatment is first aid, both at the site of injury and in hospital.

First aid

Irrigate the eye immediately by holding the victim's head in a stream of water from a tap or a hose. The victim should then be transported to specialist care rapidly.

Irrigation

On arrival at a hospital instill local anaesthetic drops into the eye. Then insert a giving set into a flask of normal saline. Hold the eyelids open with a speculum and wash the eye and conjunctival sac for 20 minutes. Instill more local anaesthetics as required. Evert the upper and lower lids to ensure that no solid matter is retained behind the lids.

Patients with chemical injuries are usually admitted to hospital for intensive treatment with antibiotics and steroids.

Surgical repair

Chemical injuries have a poor prognosis. The cornea is always damaged, and may require corneal grafting to restore sight. Because of ischaemia of surrounding tissues corneal grafting is often unsuccessful.

Thermal injuries

Thermal injuries cause burns to the eyelids. The management of the skin burn follows the usual principles, but particular care must be exercised to protect the cornea.

Shrinkage of the eyelids in the healing phase puts the cornea at risk from exposure and drying.

Care of the eye

Protect the cornea by the instillation of antibiotic ointment (chloramphenicol) every hour to provide a layer of grease, which would delay the evaporation of tears. If this is insufficient to prevent corneal drying, the eyelids must be sutured together (tarsorrhaphy).

Alternatively, cover the eye with transparent plastic film. A piece large enough to cover the orbit reaching from the forehead to the cheek is held in position by applying a layer of Vaseline to the skin around the orbit to which the plastic film adheres.

Corneal foreign body

The commonest eye injury is probably a foreign body on the cornea. The patient complains of a scratching sensation in the eye, and with a good light and magnification, the foreign body can usually be seen easily.

If it is not immediately obvious, stain the cornea with fluorescein – moisten a fluorescein strip with local anaesthetic and touch the inner surface of the lower eyelid. Ask the patient to blink to spread the dye, and then illuminate with the blue filter in the ophthalmoscope. The site of the foreign body will glow bright green.

The foreign body may be adhering to the deep surface of the upper lid – a sub-tarsal foreign body. Evert the upper lid and wipe off the foreign body. (see Box 37.2)

Box 37.2 Tarsal eversion

1 Tell the patient to look down, then grasp the lashes and pull down the upper lid.
2 Push down and back on the upper edge of the tarsal plate.
3 Fold the lid margin up and the tarsal plate rolls over.
4 Hold the lid averted by resting a finger on the lid margin.

Corneal foreign body removal

- Lie the patient down
- Instill local anaesthetic drops – two drops every minute for three minutes
- Use a focused bright light to illuminate the eye
- Lift off the foreign body with a cotton-tipped applicator or needle
- Instill antibiotic drops and apply an eye pad.

It is helpful to use a magnifying lens to facilitate foreign body removal.

Instill antibiotic drops (chloramphenicol) every 2 hours until the cornea heals and the eye is comfortable.

If the foreign body is hot and for example was from using a grindstone, a rust ring may be left in the cornea after its removal. Instill chloramphenicol ointment in the eye four times a day for 2 or 3 days. The rust ring can then be lifted off with a fine needle.

Eye infections

The main defence mechanisms against infection in the eye are the tears, which contain lysozyme, and the corneal epithelium. Once these are breached, an infection can be established and will progress rapidly.

Extra-ocular infections

Conjunctivitis

Acute conjunctivitis is common, usually due to a staphylococcus and responds rapidly to the instillation of eye drops every 2 hours. The most commonly used antibiotic is chloramphenicol. Even untreated, most acute conjunctivitis resolves in about 3 days.

Trachoma

Of more concern in rural and underdeveloped communities is trachoma. This recurrent conjunctivitis is caused by the organism *Chlamydia trachomatis*. The organism replicates intra-cellularly in the conjunctival epithelium. It is a mild infection but after each attack, scarring occurs at the site of the follicles in which the organism replicated. After probably 30 or 40 attacks the

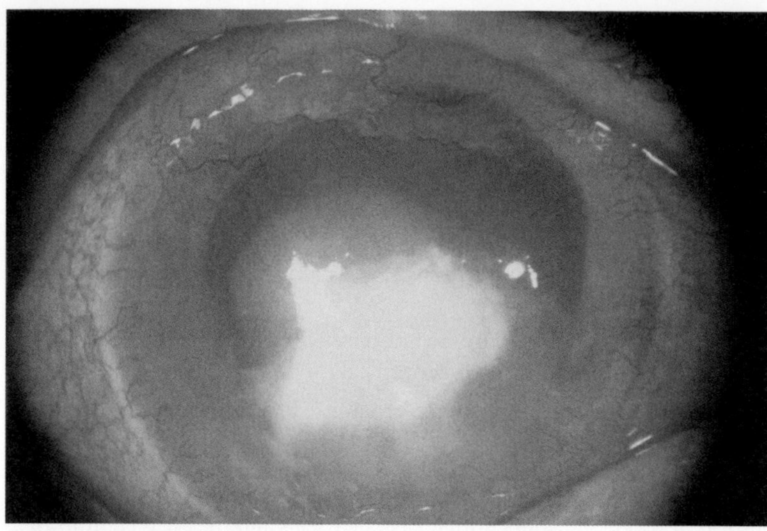

Fig. 37.2 Corneal abscess. The pathological process is visible because of the transparency of ocular structures.

scarring becomes serious and causes inversion of eye lashes and subsequent damage to the cornea, causing blindness.

The control of trachoma requires attention to the following:

- Surgery to the inverted eye lids
- Antibiotic treatment with azothromycin
- Fly eradication – the commonest vector
- Environmental upgrade.

This is the SAFE strategy devised by the World Health Organization.

When trachoma is diagnosed all members of the family are treated with a single dose of azithromycin. Children and young mothers are most commonly infected.

Intra-ocular infection

The management of intra-ocular infection follows the principles of management of any infection:

- Identify the organism
- Treat it with the appropriate antibiotic.

If the infection is a corneal abscess (Fig. 37.2), the scrapings should be taken from the surface of the ulcer for culture, and smeared on a slide for Gram staining, and sent to the laboratory for culture and investigating the sensitivities.

If the organism is Gram-negative, commence treatment with gentamycin drops; if Gram-positive, commence treatment with cephalosporin drops. These are not available commercially as they have a short shelf life of a few days only, but can be prepared in a pharmacy by adding the antibiotic to artificial tear drops to produce a 5% solution.

If no organism can be seen on Gram staining, use both antibiotics. When the results of culture and sensitivities are available the treatment may be modified.

The commonest organisms causing ocular infection are:

- *Staphylococcus epidermidis*
- *Staphylococcus aureus*
- *Pseudomonas pyocyaneus*

The treatment regime is important, and topical treatment must continue around the clock, combined with systemic antibiotics:

- Hour 1: 2 drops every 15 minutes.
- Next 4 hours: 2 drops every 30 minutes.
- Then: 2 drops every hour, day and night.
- If both antibiotics are being used, alternate them.

Intra-ocular infections require specialist treatment and must be referred.

MCQs

Select the single correct answer to each question.

1 The Snellen visual acuity in a patient is noted to be 6/60 in the right eye and 6/18 in the left eye. Which of the following statements is correct?

a the Snellen acuity in the right eye is better than the left eye

b the denominator expresses the distance acuity in the tested eye
c the numerator expresses the near vision in the tested eye
d Snellen acuity compares a tested eye to a normally seeing eye

2 Which of the following is most likely to be found in a patient with an orbital blow-out fracture?
a proptosis
b horizontal diplopia
c anosmia
d upper gum anaesthesia

3 The preferred treatment for an intra-ocular infection is:
a intravenous steroids
b intensive antibiotic drops
c intensive antibiotic drops combined with intravenous antibiotics
d intravenous antibiotics

38 Otorhinolaryngology

Stephen O'Leary and Neil Vallance

Otology

Otologic surgery aims to eradicate aural disease and restore hearing in the ear, or gain surgical access to the skull base. The proximity to the brain, major vessels, and the facial nerve demands skill in microsurgery of bone, soft tissues, and nerve. Surgical treatment of the hearing apparatus requires a good working knowledge of auditory physiology and pathophysiology.

Surgical anatomy of the ear

The tympanic membrane (TM) and the ossicles (malleus, incus, and stapes) collect sound and deliver them to the inner ear (the labyrinth). The space behind the TM is in continuity with a system of air cells extending posteriorly into the mastoid, and together these constitute the middle ear cleft. Aeration of the middle ear cleft is maintained by the eustachian tube (ET), which runs from the nasopharynx to the anterior tympanic cavity (Fig. 38.1). The middle ear cleft is lined with respiratory epithelium (mucosa). The external ear canal and external surface of the TM are lined by skin. The facial nerve traverses the middle ear and mastoid.

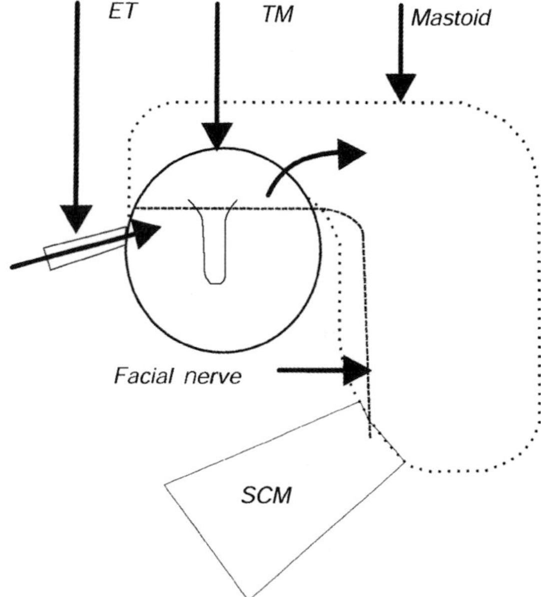

Fig. 38.1 Schematic anatomy of the ear. ET – eustachian tube; TM – tympanic membrane; SCM – sternocleidomastoid muscle, which attaches to the mastoid tip. The mastoid is a system of air cells within the temporal bone. The dotted arrows depict the flow of air through the eustachian tube into the middle ear and mastoid.

Chronic otitis media

Chronic otitis media (COM) is an ear disease requiring surgical treatment. It presents as aural discharge with or without hearing loss.

Pathophysiology

Most cases of COM is a consequence of ET dysfunction. The ET's role is to aerate the middle ear cleft (Fig. 38.1). Inadequate aeration of the middle ear leads to negative pressure with respect to the atmosphere behind the ear drum. There is a tendency for the TM to become retracted and the mucosal lining to exude a serous or mucoid discharge. Infection may ensue if bacteria are present in the middle ear cleft, frequently leading to perforation of the TM. In the presence of chronic ET dysfunction, the TM perforation will tend not to heal. An infected discharge follows, associated with chronic changes to the middle ear mucosa and a low-grade osteitis of the temporal bone.

Cholesteatoma

This is an important manifestation of COM. Acquired cholesteatoma is the invagination of the TM into the middle ear cleft. This occurs where the drum is weakest, usually in its postero-superior segment. Although causes of cholesteatoma may vary, most often the invagination is secondary to the negative middle ear pressure accompanying ET dysfunction. The invaginated skin continues to desquamate, but the squames become trapped in the retracted pocket of skin. It is at this stage that the retraction pocket is no longer self-cleaning and is, by definition, a cholesteatoma. The desquamated skin within the retraction pocket will usually become infected, with the development of an aural discharge. The cytokines liberated erode surrounding bone, with expansion of the cholesteatoma into the mastoid, the ossicles and/or the labyrinth. Complications of this disease can be serious and include facial nerve palsy, loss of labyrinthine function and intracranial sepsis.

Clinical findings

Expect a history of aural discharge, hearing loss and sometimes otalgia or tinnitus. Vertigo suggests erosion of the labyrinth and warrants urgent surgical treatment. Examination of the TM in non-cholesteatomatous COM is associated with a central perforation of the TM, where the edges of the perforation are visible and are bounded by a rim of drum (Fig. 38.2A). A marginal perforation is the hallmark of cholesteatoma, where a perforation extends beyond the edge of the drum and 'disappears' behind the postero-superior wall of the ear canal (Fig. 38.2C). Always examine the facial nerve and test the hearing clinically and audiometrically. Both ears must be examined. A computed tomography (CT) scan of the temporal bone, at 2-mm slices with bony windows, helps to define the extent of disease.

Treatment

Cholesteatoma is an absolute indication for surgery, unless the patient is elderly, when regular aural toilet may suffice. Chronic otitis media is a relative indication for surgery, particularly when medical treatments (such as aural and/or oral antibiotics) and keeping the ear dry have failed to settle recurrent aural discharge. However, the condition of the contralateral ear must be considered. A better hearing ear is a relative contraindication, due to the risk of sensorineural deafness at surgery. Restoration of hearing is another indication for surgery. The overall aim of surgery is to produce a disease-free and hence non-discharging ear. The surgical principles include the preservation of vital structures, including the facial nerve and inner ear, the eradication of disease and the reconstruction of the TM and hearing. Eradication of disease involves the removal of diseased bone and mucosa, and cholesteatoma if it is present.

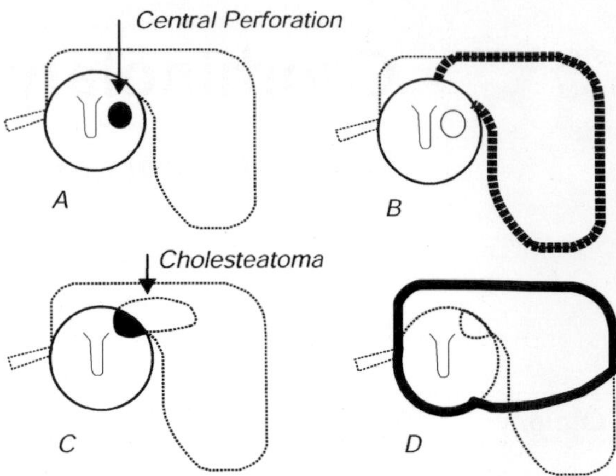

Fig. 38.2 Chronic otitis media and surgical treatment. (**A**) Chronic otitis media with a central perforation of the TM. (**B**) A canal wall up mastoidectomy. The mastoid air cells have been removed, as indicated by the thick, dashed line. (**C**) Cholesteatoma, presenting as a 'marginal' perforation of the TM. The cholesteatoma extends beyond the TM into the mastoid. (**D**) A canal wall down mastoidectomy. The limits of the mastoid cavity, created by removing the mastoid air cells and taking down the posterior and superior canal walls is indicated by the thick, solid line.

The appropriate operative procedure depends on the extent of the disease and the surgeon's estimate of ET function. If disease is confined to the middle ear and ET function is only moderately impaired, then grafting the TM (myringoplasty) may be all that is required. If the mastoid is also infected, exenteration of the mastoid air cell system is combined with myringoplasty (a 'canal wall up' mastoidectomy; Fig. 38.2B). The mastoidectomy both removes the disease and reduces the surface area of the middle ear cleft, thus decreasing the work done by a compromised ET. For cholesteatoma, or failed canal wall up mastoidectomy, a modified radical mastoidectomy is performed. This involves performing a mastoidectomy, removing the posterior and superior (ear) canal walls, and grafting the TM (a 'canal wall down' mastoidectomy; Fig. 38.2D). Following this operation, the mastoid cavity is exteriorised so that it is now part of the external ear and is lined with skin.

Hearing impairment

Pathophysiology

Hearing impairment is classified as either conductive or sensorineural. A conductive loss results from an interruption of sound transmission through the TM and the ossicles. It may arise from an effusion of the middle ear ('glue ear') or a TM perforation. Sound transmission through the ossicular chain may be interrupted if the ossicles are no longer in continuity or if the ossicular chain is fixed. Ossicular discontinuity usually arises from ossicular erosion following COM. The most common cause of ossicular fixation is otosclerosis, where the bone of the labyrinth is abnormal and the stapes footplate becomes fixed to surrounding labyrinthine bone. Sensorineural hearing loss is due to cochlear, or rarely retrocochlear, pathology. The most common causes of sensorineural loss are hereditary, meningitis, ototoxic, trauma and progression of unknown aetiology. A TM perforation will lead to a mild-to-moderate conductive hearing loss (20–30 dB). Ossicular chain discontinuity will lead to an additional 20–30 dB loss. Ossicular chain disruption behind an intact drum leads to a 60-dB hearing loss. A 'mixed' hearing loss has both conductive and sensorineural components.

Treatment

Hearing loss is treated when it impedes an individual's ability to communicate. Surgery is indicated when a hearing aide is not helpful or is unacceptable to the patient. Hearing restoration surgery will also be performed with operations for COM as discussed above. However, it is usually not possible to reconstruct the ossicular chain if there is a co-existent TM perforation. A better approach is to repair the drum first, and perform an ossicular chain reconstruction as a staged procedure. For this reason, ossicular chain reconstruction is usually a second-stage procedure following surgery for COM.

Conductive hearing loss is amenable to surgical treatment. Glue ear may be treated by performing a myringotomy and placing a ventilation tube within the TM. A perforated TM may be grafted ('myringoplasty'). When the ossicles are disrupted, reconstruction aims to re-establish a stable link between the TM and the stapes footplate. The configuration of the reconstruction depends upon which ossicle(s) remain intact. These procedures do not restore anatomical normality, and this is not required to achieve good hearing.

Cochlear implantation

Severe-to-profound sensorineural hearing loss is characterised by a loss of clarity of speech, which is not overcome by the amplification of sound with a hearing aide. Eventually, amplification ceases to aide communication, and, under these circumstances, a cochlear implant may be of more benefit. A cochlear implant is also indicated for congenitally deaf children, provided that the operation is performed before the child is 5 years of age. Up until this age a child may learn to comprehend speech with the implant, even though he or she has no previous auditory experience. Children implanted before the age of 3 may learn to speak. The younger the child at the age of implantation the better the speech and language outcomes, and it is preferable to implant before the child's second birthday.

The operation for a cochlear implant involves implanting a prosthesis, the 'receiver–stimulator', which electrically stimulates the auditory nerve within the cochlea. The receiver–stimulator is fixed to the parietal bone. Its electrode array passes through the mastoid and middle ear into the cochlea. The receiver–stimulator is entirely subcutaneous. It communicates via a radiofrequency link with an external device called the speech processor. The speech processor translates speech into the pattern of electrical stimulation to be delivered to the auditory nerve.

Tumours of the ear

The most common type of malignant neoplasm of the ear is a squamous cell carcinoma of the pinna or external ear canal, followed in incidence by melanoma. Symptoms include otalgia, aural discharge or hearing loss if the external ear canal is occluded. Treatment is radical surgical excision and radiotherapy.

Rhinology

Nasal polyps

Nasal polyps are translucent pedunculated swellings arising from nasal and sinus mucosa. They are often allergic in origin and result in nasal obstruction and discharge. They usually require surgical excision via an endoscopic approach, with clearance of polyps from the ethmoid sinus being most common, but also from other paranasal sinuses as required.

Septal deviation

Deviation of the nasal septum from the midline may be traumatic or congenital. The deviation may involve the cartilaginous or bony septum. It results in turbulence of nasal airflow and hence a sensation of obstruction. Symptomatic septal deviation is treated surgically. The corrective procedure, septoplasty, involves elevating mucosal flaps and removal of the deviated segment of cartilage or bone.

Rhinorrhoea

Rhinorrhea is continuous discharge of fluid from the nose. It is most commonly due to vasomotor rhinitis, which in turn is usually secondary to allergy or coryza. Rarely, a clear discharge from the nose may be cerebrospinal fluid. This is usually post-traumatic and may originate from a breach of the cribriform plate, a paranasal sinus (ethmoid, frontal or sphenoid sinus) or from the middle ear space via the ET. The fluid will test positive for beta-transferrin. Treatment is initially conservative, with elevation of the head and rest for 2 weeks, but if the leak persists surgical repair will be necessary.

Epistaxis

Epistaxis is dealt with in Chapter 75.

Sinusitis

Acute sinusitis is a bacterial infection of the paranasal sinus secondary to obstruction of the sinus ostium. The obstruction is usually due to a viral swelling of the nasal mucosa, but may also follow dental infection or dental work, nasal allergy, facial fractures and barotrauma. It is usually due to aerobic organisms and manifests as pain, facial swelling and mucopurulent nasal discharge. Treatment requires antibiotics and topical nasal decongestants. Systemic corticosteroids may also be needed to settle a severe attack. Occasionally, drainage of the sinus via trephination or endoscopic antrostomy may be required.

Chronic sinusitis may follow poorly treated acute sinusitis, or will occur in situations of chronic sinus obstruction (e.g. secondary to nasal allergy or polyps). In this situation anaerobic organisms play a significant role. Treatment with long-term antibiotics targeting anaerobic organisms is often successful. Drainage and aeration of the sinus is of paramount importance; hence, most cases of chronic sinusitis require endoscopic sinus surgery to achieve this.

Nasal tumours

Benign tumours

Inverted papillomas, squamous papilloma and juvenile angiofibroma may all result in obstruction, sinusitis and bleeding. Diagnosis is made following imaging of the paranasal sinuses (CT or MRI scan) and, unless a juvenile angiofibroma is suspected, a transnasal biopsy. (Angiofbromas are not biopsied due to a risk of bleeding.) Benign tumours are best treated with surgical excision, performed either transnasally or via an external transfacial approach.

Malignant tumours

Squamous cell carcinoma of the maxillary sinus is the most common paranasal sinus malignancy. The most common cancer of the ethmoid sinus in Australia is adenocarcinoma, which occurs more commonly in people employed in the hardwood industry. Other cancers of the nasal complex include adenoidcystic carcinoma, sinonasal undifferentiated (small cell) carcinoma, transitional carcinoma and malignant melanoma. Diagnosis is made on radiological and histological grounds and treatment involves surgical excision with adjunctive radiation therapy and/or chemotherapy.

Oral cavity, oropharynx and larynx

Tonsil and adenoid disease

The tonsils and adenoids are the commonest area of infection in the head and neck. They belong to a collection of lymphoid tissue called Waldeyer's ring which also comprises an aggregate of lymphoid tissue at the base of the tongue called the lingual tonsil and lymphoid tissue around the opening of the eustachian tube called the tubal tonsil. The adenoid tissue usually atrophies over the second decade of life and is not a common cause of disease after childhood. Tonsillectomy and adenoidectomy is performed if the tonsils become recurrently infected. In childhood, tonsils and adenoids may become large enough to interfere with the airway and can cause significant obstruction with the interference and intermittent cessation of breathing overnight (obstructive sleep apnoea). This necessitates the removal to reestablish a normal airway and breathing pattern.

Tonsillitis may become complicated by an abscess formation in the peritonsillar space, which is commonly referred to as quinsy. This results in severe pain, toxicity and trismus and usually a large unilateral tonsillar swelling. The abscess must be drained by an incision in the upper half of the tonsil pillar followed by admission to hospital and intravenous antibiotics for several days. In a history of recurrent tonsillitis, this is an indication for a tonsillectomy, usually after the acute abscess has settled down.

Epiglottis

Epiglottitis is a peculiar and serious disease often affecting children, and occasionally adults. There is an acute bacterial inflammation of the epiglottis and supraglottic structures with rapid onset and rapid progression such that the airway may be occluded, with death resulting from acute upper airway obstruction. Intubation in an operating theatre environment is the treatment of choice in both adults and children, with the surgeon standing by to perform urgent surgical access to the airway should intubation fail. After the airway is secure, the problem usually settles rapidly with intravenous antibiotics and, on occasion, steroids. *Haemophilus influenzae* is a common casual organism in the paediatric population. The condition is life-threatening and must be treated urgently.

Benign vocal fold lesions

Vocal nodules are common benign bilateral swellings at the junction of the middle and anterior third of the vocal fold. They result from vocal abuse in children and heavy vocal use and abuse in adults. They may be physiological in heavy voice users, such as singers. There is rarely an indication for surgery as almost all cases will improve or resolve completely with voice therapy and re-education of vocal habits.

Benign cysts and polyps are less common conditions and are usually unilateral and require surgical intervention. The lesions are removed with microsurgical techniques via a direct laryngoscopy under general anaesthesia.

Reflux commonly causes hoarseness, throat discomfort and a variety of laryngeal conditions resulting from chronic inflammation due to refluxate in the laryngopharynx. Very commonly, heartburn is absent in laryngopharyngeal reflux. The condition responds to anti-reflux measures and medication, including proton pump inhibitors.

Vocal cord paralysis

Loss of vocal fold movement is caused by loss of function of the recurrent laryngeal nerve. The nerve is a branch of the vagus nerve. The left arises in the thorax looping around the aorta. On the right side, it arises higher in the thorax looping around the right subclavian artery. Both travel in the tracheo-oesophageal groove superiorly to the larynx, where they supply the intrinsic muscles that move the vocal folds. Causes of unilateral paralysis may be tumours of the thyroid, lung or metastatic deposits within mediastinal lymph nodes. Surgical trauma during thyroidectomy may also result in paralysis. The commonest cause of paralysis, however, is idiopathic and the commonest nerve affected is the left, probably because of its greater length. The presentation of unilateral paralysis is hoarseness and breathiness. This may improve as the larynx compensates and other muscles assist in phonation. A common misconception is that the intact vocal cord compensates for the palsy, but this is not true, as the functioning vocal fold can never adduct further than the midline. If both vocal folds are paralysed, the voice is often normal, but the airway can be severely compromised if the vocal folds both lay well towards the midline. Hence the need to assess vocal fold function prior to thyroidectomy to exclude an asymptomatic old palsy and, therefore, exercise diligence in protecting the intact nerve.

Diagnosis of the palsy is made by indirect mirror examination or flexible fibreoptic laryngoscopy. A thorough search to exclude tumour, including CT scan from skull base to thorax, must be made. Treatment is required for unilateral palsy if the voice is poor and sufficient time has elapsed (usually 6 months) to exclude spontaneous recovery. Such operations may be medialisation of the vocal fold via laryngeal framework–type surgery or injection of fat lateral to the fold to medialise it. There is no longer any place for teflon injection of the vocal fold. Bilateral vocal fold paralysis can present an upper-airway emergency that may require tracheotomy. In the long term, endoscopic laser techniques allow the reestablishment of an airway, often with the preservation of good voice.

Cancer of the head and neck

Cancer of the head and neck is relatively uncommon when compared to the frequency of other, more common tumours such as bowel and breast cancer. Nonetheless, because of the significance of functional impairment and the potential for disfigurement, it is an important management problem. Significant advances have seen improvements in survival and outcomes for patients. These tumours are best treated via a multidisciplinary surgical approach in departments, which can make the best use of advances in tumour biology, imaging modalities, radiotherapy and chemotherapy and conservation and organ preservation techniques. A recent advance in endoscopic laser surgical techniques has also seen an improvement in outcomes and organ preservation for laryngeal and hypopharyngeal cancers. Reconstructive techniques and the use of free flaps is well established and continues to provide better outcomes.

Squamous carcinomas of the upper aerodigestive tract

Pathogenesis

Most malignant tumours of the upper aerodigestive tract are squamous cell carcinomas. Up to 80% of these cancers can be attributed to a combination of cigarette and alcohol abuse. Their effects are believed to be synergistic, resulting in widespread changes in the mucosa and the potential for multiple tumours (estimated at between 15 and 20%). Other aetiological factors may include human papilloma virus in laryngeal cancer.

Pathology

Most head and neck squamous cancers will metastasise to cervical lymph nodes and this factor bears the most significance in terms of prognosis. It is generally accepted that the survival rate of head and neck cancer is halved when a positive neck node is present. Head and neck cancer surgeons refer to neck nodes in terms of different levels, I through V. Level I are the uppermost nodes in the submental and submandibular triangles. Levels II, III and IV correspond to the upper, middle and lower cervical lymph nodes respectively and Level V represents the nodes in the posterior triangle. On this basis, it is now possible to tailor neck dissection according to the site of primary tumour and the levels of nodes involved. Neck dissections are now almost exclusively of a selective nature rather than the older-style radical neck dissection, which sacrificed the sternomastoid muscle, the internal jugular vein and the accessory nerve. It is rare now to sacrifice the accessory nerve in neck dissection as this often produces significant morbidity with denervation of the trapezius muscle and resulting shoulder droop. Prognostic variables include the T stage of the primary tumour (Table 38.1); the N stage of the neck; the presence of extracapular spread in cervical lymph nodes; perineural, lymphatic and vascular invasion and the depth of tumour invasion. The differentiation of the primary cancer does not appear to have prognostic significance, with the possible exception of the oral tongue.

Clinical presentation and investigation

Clinical presentation is dependent on the anatomic subsite of the disease. In the oral cavity and the oropharynx, for example, common symptoms include

Table 38.1 Tumour staging in squamous carcinoma

Regional lymph nodes	
Nx	Regional lymph nodes cannot be assessed
No	No regional lymph node metastasis
N1	Metastasis in a single ipsilateral lymph node, 3 cm or less at greatest dimension
N2a	Metastasis in single ipsilateral lymph node, more than 3 cm but not more than 6 cm at greatest dimension
N2b	Metastasis in multiple ipsilateral lymph nodes, none more than 6 cm at greatest dimension
N2c	Metastasis in contralateral lymph nodes, none more than 6 cm at greatest dimension
N3	Metastasis in lymph node greater than 6 cm at greatest dimension
Primary tumour	
Tx	Primary tumour cannot be assessed
To	No evidence of primary tumour
Tis	Carcinoma *in situ*
T1	Tumour 2 cm or less at greatest dimension
T2	Tumour more than 2 cm but not more than 4 cm at greatest dimension
T3	Tumour more than 4 cm at greatest dimension
T4	Tumour invades adjacent structures

a mass or an ulcer with pain and difficulties with speech and swallowing. Painful swallowing (odinophagia) is a serious symptom which indicates the presence of a cancer until otherwise proven. Likewise, pain referred to the ear is a serious symptom. Vocal fold cancers frequently present with hoarseness which does not resolve with adequate treatment after 2 or 3 weeks. Cancers in the hypopharynx may be more subtle in presentation and can reach a significant size before the primary tumour presents problems for the patients. These lesions frequently present with a painless, enlarging, lump in the neck which represents a metastatic node.

Thorough clinical evaluation is essential to exclude a cancer in a site not readily seen, such as the tongue base or hypopharynx. Thorough endoscopic evaluation and fine-needle aspiration cytology (which has not been found to cause recurrent neck disease) should be used to investigate these lesions before open biopsy or surgical removal.

Modern CT scanning and MRI are invaluable for the accurate assessment and staging of head and neck cancer disease. It is well demonstrated that they are more sensitive than clinical examination in detecting metastatic neck disease. CT scanning is beneficial in the detection of bone disease and spread of laryngeal disease beyond the laryngeal framework. MRI is particularly useful for investigation of the tongue and soft tissue extension of disease, including involvement of the nerves and brain.

A relatively new imaging technique, positron emission tomography (PET) is an imaging technique which looks at the metabolic behaviour of the tumour and images this characteristic rather than an anatomical mass.

Guidelines for diagnostic and pre-operative workup of a patient with a suspected head and neck malignancy are given in Box 38.1.

Box 38.1 Diagnostic and pre-operative workup of the patient with head and neck squamous carcinoma

1 Confirm diagnosis by biopsy of primary lesion and/or fine-needle aspiration cytology of cervical nodes.
2 Clinical staging of disease by TNM classification.
3 Investigate with CT, MRI, PET scan for selected cases.
4 Endoscopic evaluation under anaesthesia for more accurate staging and to exclude a second primary.
5 For cervical node with unknown primary, full endoscopic evaluation and, if no primary found, proceed to open biopsy with frozen section and neck dissection if squamous cell carcinoma is confirmed.

Treatment

The goals of treatment in head and neck cancer are:
- Eradication of disease
- Restoration of function, particularly speech and swallowing
- Minimal cosmetic deformity

The following general points are relevant.
- For early disease, particularly in the larynx, cure rates of radiotherapy and surgery are equivalent.
- Chemotherapy on its own has little role to play in the treatment of squamous cell cancer of the head and neck other than in a palliative sense, but is used as an adjunct to the use of radiotherapy.
- The emphasis in treatment is now on organ preservation, particularly with respect to the larynx. There has been a shift away from radical surgery, such as total laryngectomy, to the use of protocols involving the use of chemo-radiation for relatively advanced tumours. Partial laryngectomy, particularly with endoscopic laser surgery, often provides organ sparing and successful outcomes. It should be remembered, however, that the preservation of a crippled larynx which does not function and aspirates is a poor outcome.
- The combination of surgery and radiotherapy in advanced disease is superior to single modality therapy.
- In planning treatment, it is vital to consider general patient factors such as general health and medical condition, fitness for either surgery or a challenging course of radiation, nutritional status, which is often poor in these patients, and may need attention pre-treatment.

MANAGEMENT OF THE PRIMARY TUMOUR

Surgical resection is a better option in the following situations:
- Small tumours where the surgical defect is minimal and functional restoration assured.
- Large tumours with spread beyond the primary site to involve bone or cartilage. These tumours rarely, if ever, respond to radial radiotherapy. Modern reconstructive techniques and the use of free flaps

have allowed many of these tumours to be successfully resected and reconstructed in a single-stage procedure. This has allowed a more rapid transition to post-operative radiotherapy, which is essential if all the benefits of multimodality therapy are to be achieved.

- Salvage of lesions unresponsive or recurrent after radiotherapy. Reconstructive techniques involving free flaps which bring a better blood supply to the area have allowed better healing in previously irradiated tissues where the blood supply has been diminished by radiation.
- Endolaryngeal and hypopharyngeal disease is now being successfully treated with endoscopic laser techniques where previously external partial procedures, and even total laryngectomy, may have been considered.

Radiotherapy is considered for the following situations:

- As a single-modality treatment in early lesions. This was traditionally the case with small tumours of the true vocal fold. Cure rates are excellent, as are functional outcomes. The disadvantage is a 5-week course of therapy. Consequently, laser surgery is tending to replace radiotherapy for these lesions as the outcomes are similar and the treatment involves only a 1- or 2-day stay in hospital.
- In certain advanced hypopharyngeal and laryngeal cancer, where combined radiotherapy and chemotherapy offers organ preservation and good locoregional control without surgery.
- For palliation for recurrent disease or advanced disease not suitable for surgery or organ preservation through chemoradiotherapy.
- Post-operatively and, less commonly, pre-operatively, in disease where it is felt prudent to use multimodality therapy. Whether radiation is used pre-operatively or post-operatively is often determined by the accepted practices in individual cancer treatment units.

Radiation is delivered by external beam in dedicated radiotherapy units. Radiation affects both normal tissue and cancer tissue, and the salivary glands and oral mucosa are particularly affected. Dryness is a common post-radiotherapy complaint. The mandible is commonly devascularised following radiotherapy and very prone to osteomyelitis and necrosis, secondary to dental sepsis. Dental consultation and management of the teeth are therefore essential if the jaw is to be involved in the radiotherapy field.

MANAGEMENT OF THE NECK

Metastatic disease in the neck may be obvious or occult at presentation. Secondary neck disease is a significant factor in determining prognosis and, in general, the presence of neck disease lowers the survival by some 50%. Neck disease is best treated by neck dissection. There are accepted poor prognostic indicators with neck disease. These are multiple levels of nodes involved or spread of tumour beyond the capsule of the lymph node on pathology assessment. In these instances, post-operative radiotherapy is always used in the neck.

The approach to neck dissection has changed over the years. The mainstay in the past was the so-called radial neck dissection. It is apparent now that similar regional control of disease can be achieved by a more selective approach. These modified or selective neck dissections remove node levels which are most likely to contain metastatic disease from the associated primary. Consequently, fewer than the 5 levels of nodes are removed and, inherent in this approach, is the preservation of various non-lymphatic tissues, including the spinal accessory nerve, internal jugular vein and sternomastoid muscle. This has led to better functional outcomes with no sacrifice of disease control.

Tumours of the nasal cavity and paranasal sinuses

These are rare tumours. It is worth noting that a significant aetiological factor is wood-dust. People with a long history of wood-dust exposure (cabinet makers, sawmill operators) are usually common among patients diagnosed with ethmoid cancer. This is usually an adenocarcinoma. Efforts have been made to make the woodworking industry aware of this danger.

Presentation depends on the anatomical subsite but, unfortunately, tumours are often very advanced at diagnosis. It is not unusual to find orbital and anterior cranial fossa involvement on CT and MRI scanning.

The usual treatment principle is surgery combined with post-operative radiotherapy. The prognosis of these cancers is poor, usually because of the advanced state of disease at diagnosis and the proximity of the anterior cranial fossa.

Nasopharyngeal carcinoma

Nasopharyngeal cancer is the commonest tumour seen in certain Asian countries (South China and Southeast

Asian countries with Chinese populations). In Hong Kong and China, it accounts for about 20% of all malignancies. In South China, it comprises approximately 50% of all head and neck cancers.

Pathology

The nasopharynx is the space situated behind the nasal cavity and above the oropharynx. The mucosa is stratified, ciliated, columnar epithelium, with a large aggregate of lymphoid tissue forming part of Waldeyer's ring.

Nasopharyngeal cancer is classified according to the World Health Organisation classification. There are three types: Type 1 – keratinising squamous carcinoma; Type 2 – non-keratinising poorly differentiated carcinoma and Type 3 – undifferentiated carcinoma. Type 3 is by far the more common sub-type in endemic Asian areas. Type 1 is more common in developed countries.

Aetiology

Epstein–Barr virus is implicated in the pathogenesis of nasopharyngeal carcinoma. An elevation of viral titres can precede the onset of disease. Titres are useful as tumour markers following treatment. Genetic markers have also been investigated because of the ethnic predilection of the tumour. An increased incidence is seen in patients with certain major histocompatibility complex profiles (HLA). The ingestion of preserved foods, especially salted fish, duck eggs and salted mustard green, have also been implicated in nasopharyngeal cancer.

Presentation and management

Nasopharyngeal cancer often presents late and frequently as a lump in the neck. It is a very infiltrative cancer with often very little in the way of mucosal changes. It frequently invades the base of the skull, causing cranial nerve involvement and palsies. It is one of the few cancers of the head and neck with a predilection to distant metastases with the bone, lung and liver, the preferred sites. MRI scan is the investigation of choice and, universally, radiotherapy with concomitant chemotherapy is the treatment of choice. The tumour is usually radiosensitive and, due to the inaccessibility of the site, surgery with clear margins is usually not possible. Neck nodes are always irradiated with the primary site.

MCQs

Select the single correct answer to each question.

1 Which modality of treatment is most useful for nasopharyngeal carcinoma?
- **a** chemotherapy
- **b** radiotherapy
- **c** surgery
- **d** immunotherapy
- **e** hormonal therapy

2 Which of the following statement concerning nasopharyngeal carcinoma is INCORRECT ?
- **a** keratinising SCC is most common in developed countries
- **b** examination of the nasopharynx is usually positive
- **c** in 90% of patients, cervical nodes were involved
- **d** there are known aetiological factors
- **e** the tumour tends to infiltrate widely

3 Which of the following statement concerning parotid gland tumours is INCORRECT ?
- **a** a cystic lesion in the lower pole is likely to be benign
- **b** a long-standing tumour that enlarges and becomes painful suggests malignancy
- **c** bilateral tumours in elderly men are usually benign
- **d** facial nerve palsy suggests malignant disease
- **e** needle aspiration cytology of parotid tumours is contraindicated

39 Tumours of the head and neck

Rodney T. Judson

Introduction

The concentration of anatomical structures and the rich traversing lymphatic system, bearing drainage from all parts of the body, explains the diversity of primary and secondary tumours found in the head and neck region. Exposure of the skin to ultraviolet B radiation results in 85–90% of cutaneous carcinomas, the most common human malignancy occurring in the head and neck area. Excluding cutaneous tumours, 90% of head and neck tumours are squamous cell carcinomas arising from the epithelium of the upper aero-digestive tract. These tumours are predominantly the result of the carcinogens released from tobacco, either due to smoking or chewing. Primary tumours, malignant and benign, can arise from all other structures; glandular, vascular, lymphatic, neural, muscular, bony or of connective tissue origin.

Metastatic tumours to the head and neck are predominantly due to lymphatic spread. Metastatic lymph nodes characteristically firm to hard and matted which are confined to the upper third of the neck are most commonly the result of tumour spread from a primary squamous carcinoma of the upper aero-digestive tract. Metastatic lymph nodes confined to the lower third of the neck are less commonly from an aero-digestive tract origin and more likely from primary sites such as skin, thyroid or a malignant focus below the clavicle. Rare blood-borne metastases are seen in the parotid gland from colon, kidney, breast and lung and in the thyroid from lung and kidney.

The common mode of presentation of head and neck tumours is that of a painless neck mass or swelling. The approach to solving the problem of a neck swelling is dealt with in detail in Chapter 67.

An understanding of the characteristic features of the common head and neck tumours and of the anatomy of the region should guide the clinician as to the likely diagnosis based on clinical assessment (see Table 39.1). Treatment planning, however, requires a detailed assessment including endoscopy, accurate anatomical localisation with CT or MRI and pathological appraisal utilising the least invasive technique applicable. Needle aspiration cytology, either free hand for accessible masses or ultrasound guided for deeper tumours usually provide diagnostic material. Core biopsy or carefully considered open biopsy may be required if cytology is inconclusive.

Characteristics of common tumours

Squamous cell carcinoma

The commonest head and neck malignancy is squamous cell carcinoma rising from the upper aero-digestive tract. Full details of this problem are covered in Chapter 38.

Cutaneous squamous cell carcinoma

The lips, forehead and ear are the commonest sites for squamous carcinoma of the head and neck due to their exposure to sunlight. Lesions vary from an area of crusting through to ulceration and induration. Squamous cell carcinoma (SCC) of the upper lip has a higher propensity for lymph node metastasis than SCC arising at other sites. SCC of the temple and ear may metastasise to the pre-auricular intra-parotid lymph nodes. Such metastasis may appear some time following successful local excision of the primary tumour. Involvement of the facial nerve from intra-parotid metastasies carries a very poor prognosis. Metastatic lymph nodes from a cutaneous SCC, like those from an aerodigestive tract origin, often undergo cystic degeneration. Rapid growth, redness of the overlying skin and clinical fluctuance can lead to the mistaken diagnosis of

Table 39.1 Tumours of the head and neck

Tissue of origin	Benign/ malignant	Tumour type	Clinical site	Common clinical feature
Upper aerodigestive tract mucosa	Benign	Squamous papilloma	Oral cavity mucosa	Solitary papillary lesion
	Malignant	Carcinoma *in situ*	Oral cavity larynx - pharynx	White or red mucosal patch
		Squamous cell carcinoma	Mucosa of upper aerodigestive tract	Ulcerated, infiltrative lesion with raised edges
		Lympho-epithelial carcinoma	Nasopharynx	Ulcerated lesion, frequent nodal metastases, nasal symptoms
Salivary gland	Benign	Pleomorphic adenoma	Parotid commonest	Painless, slow-growing firm mass
		Oncocytic tumour (Warthin's tumour)	Parotid grand	Soft to firm, occasionally bilateral, mass
	Malignant	Mucoepidermoid carcinoma	Parotid commonest	Slow-growing firm mass
		Adenoid cystic	Minor salivary glands commonest	Slow-growing submucosal nodule in the upper aerodigestic tract
		Acinic cell tumour	Parotid gland	Slow-growing nodule
		Adenocarcinoma	Minor salivary gland	Submucosal lump
Thyroid	Benign	Follicular adenoma	Thyroid	Slow-growing smooth thyroid nodule
		Hurtle cell adenoma	Thyroid	Slow-growing smooth thyroid nodule
	Malignant	Papillary carcinoma	Thyroid gland +/− nodes	Slow-growing nodule. 50% children have associated nodal metastases
		Follicular carcinoma	Thyroid	Slow-growing smooth thyroid nodule
		Anaplastic carcinoma	Thyroid	Rapidly growing infiltrating mass often arising within a pre-existing goitre
		Medullary carcinoma	Thyroid +/− nodes	Firm thyroid nodule, may be associated with multiple endocrine adenoma syndrome
Parathyroid cells	Benign	Parathyroid adenoma	Parathyroid glands (Impalpable)	Commonest cause of primary hyperparathyroidism
	Malignant	Parathyroid carcinoma	Parathyroid +/− nodes	Progressive hyperparathyroidism. Nodule may be palpable
Neuroendocrine	Benign	Paraganglionoma	Carotid body Glomus jugulare Glomus intravagale	Mass in region of upper carotid sheath. Occasional symptoms resulting from noradrenaline secretion

Table 39.1 *(Continued)*

	Malignant	Olfactory neuroblastoma	Olfactory mucosa in nasal vault	Bimodal age distribution occurring in adolescents and adults. Epistaxis and nasal obstruction
Adipose	Benign	Lipoma	Commonest in subcutaneous layer	Mobile superficial soft mass
	Malignant	Liposarcoma	Neck, larynx, pharynx	Rare head and neck tumour. Occurs in elderly patients
Vascular	Benign	Haemangioma	Face, scalp, neck	Seen in childhood. Compressible red to purple mass
		Lymphangioma	Neck	Soft, occasionally translucent neck mass in children
	Malignant	Angiosarcoma	Skin of scalp or face	Ulcerating cutaneous nodule occurring in elderly white males
Fibrous tissue	Benign	Fibromatosis	Commonly in neck	Slow-growing mass in young females
		Dermatofibroma	Skin	Small plaque in skin
	Malignant	Fibrosarcoma	Face, neck, scalp and paranasal sinus	Painless growing mass in adults
		Malignant fibrous histocytoma	Deep tissues of head and neck	Infiltrating mass in elderly males. Commonest post-irradiation tumour
Neural tissue	Benign	Schwannoma	Cranial nerves VIII, IX, X, XI and XII	Lateral neck mass
		Neurofibromas	Peripheral nerve sheaths	Isolated subcutaneous neck nodule, or multiple nodules and large plexiform benign neuromas in familial neurofibromatosis
	Malignant	Malignant schwannoma	Cranial and cervical nerve roots	Fixed mass. Metastases possible
Muscle cell	Malignant	Rhabdomyosarcoma	Orbit, nasal cavity and paranasal sinuses	Commonest soft tissue sarcoma seen in children
Bone	Benign	Osteoma	Bony skeleton of face	Smooth mass occurring in paranasal sinuses; multiple osteomas associated with Gardner's syndrome
	Malignant	Osteosarcoma	Mandible or maxilla	Painless enlarging bony swelling
Skin	Malignant	Squamous cell carcinoma (SCC)	Sun-exposed skin	Crusting ulcerating lesion
		Basal cell carcinoma (BCC)	Skin of central face	Translucent nodular lesion. Rarely a deeply ulcerating or erosive lesion.
		Malignant melanoma	Skin of face. Mucosa of nasal cavity	Pigmented skin lesion or polypoid nasal mass

Continued

Table 39.1 *(Continued)*

Tissue of origin	Benign/ malignant	Tumour type	Clinical site	Common clinical feature
Lymphoid tissue	Malignant	Lymphoma	Lymphatic tissue, salivary glands, thyroid	Rubbery, discrete, multiple neck nodes
Dental tissue	Benign	Ameloblastoma Squamous ontogenic tumour Ondontoma Ondontogenic fibroma	Usually intra-osseous but may involve the gingiva	Expanding mass arising in association with mandible. Rarely malignant

a suppurating lymph node. Thorough clinical assessment noting the absence of pain and the presence or history of a primary lesion coupled with aspiration cytology should avert the disaster of inappropriate incisional drainage. Management of cutaneous SCCs involves full clinical assessment of the tumour and draining lymph nodes aided by fine cut CT scanning if deep tissue or nodal involvement are suspected. Localised small lesions are cured by excision with clear surgical margins. Larger lesions may necessitate extensive surgical resection involving underlying tissues and a planned lymph node clearance. Elaborate reconstructive procedures may be necessary especially for areas of the face to restore function and attain acceptable cosmesis. Cutaneous SCCs are radio-sensitive. Radiotherapy as primary treatment, owing to its protracted treatment time, is reserved for small primary tumours in difficult anatomical sites. Radiotherapy is used as adjuvant therapy post-operatively in the management of advanced, infiltrative tumours, especially with multiple lymph node metastases or perineural tumour spread.

Cutaneous basal cell carcinoma

The most common site for BCC of the head and neck is the central face. The most common clinical variant is a translucent nodule made clinically more apparent by stretching the skin around the lesion. Most tumours run a slow protracted course and nodal metastases are rare. Tumours in areas of embryonal fusion lines may burrow deeply, making surgical clearance difficult. Local surgical excision is the usual form of treatment.

Salivary gland tumours

Introduction

Salivary tissue is found not only in the three pairs of major salivary glands (the parotid, the submandibular and the sublingual glands) but also in small submucosal glands known as the minor salivary glands, which are scattered throughout the upper aerodigestive tract. The parotid glands are host to a variety of tumours both benign and malignant, primary and secondary.

Anatomy

The parotid glands, so named because of their anatomical proximity to the ear, are the largest salivary glands and produce a high volume of serous saliva. The most important anatomical relationship of the parotid gland is the facial nerve. This enters the posteromedial aspect of the gland as a single trunk and divides within its substance to emerge at the anterior border as the five main branches. In so doing, the facial nerve, for descriptive purposes, divides the gland into the larger superficial lobe covered by skin, platysma in part, and parotid fascia, and the smaller deep lobe, which lies in the parapharyngeal space and through which passes the posterior fascial vein and external carotid artery. Saliva drains from the gland via the parotid duct, which crosses the masseter muscle, and enters the buccal cavity opposite the upper second molar teeth.

The submandibular glands lie close to the inner aspect of the mandible lying on the mylohyoid muscle. The larger superficial lobe is covered by skin, platysma and deep cervical fascia, with the mandibular branch of the facial nerve on its way to supply the depressor anguli oris crossing its upper border. The posterior aspect of the submandibular gland is wrapped around the posterior-free border of the mylohyoid muscle, and the deep lobe of the gland passes forward deep to the mylohyoid lying on the hypoglossus muscle. The submandibular duct drains from the deep lobe, running a long course in the floor of the mouth to open at a papilla in the anterior floor of mouth just lateral to the lingual frenulum. The deep lobe of the gland and the duct are closely related to the lingual nerve, which may be involved in pathological processes and damaged during surgical treatment of the gland. The deep lobe is inferolaterally related to the mylohyoid and supramedially covered only by the oral mucosa in the floor of the mouth, thus being easily assessed clinically by bimanual palpation. Using the gloved left index finger placed in the floor of the mouth and the right fingers applied externally, submandibular glandular swelling may be differentiated from lymph node swellings.

The sublingual glands, predominantly mucus-secreting, lie submucosally in the anterior floor of the mouth, supported by the mylohyoid muscles. These glands drain by multiple small ducts opening directly into the floor of the mouth along the sublingual folds.

Assessment of salivary gland disorders

The diagnosis of salivary pathology can be determined in a high proportion of cases by a thorough history, clinical examination and the judicious use of special tests.

Clinical history

A history of a slowly growing lump suggests a benign tumour. The rapid growth of a lump with the development of pain would strongly suggest a malignant process.

Clinical examination

Clinical examination, including intra-oral and manual examination noting the site, size, shape, texture, tenderness, fixation, involvement of surrounding anatomical structures and the state of the regional lymph nodes, should not only define involvement of the salivary gland but also suggest the most likely pathological process. Deep lobe parotid masses may be detected by a diffuse bulge in the root of the soft palate or tonsillar fossa region and also may be palpable manually. Facial nerve function must be assessed with all parotid lesions. Tongue sensation should be tested in the presence of submandibular problems.

Special tests

Computed tomography

Computed tomography (CT) scans are useful to clarify anatomical detail in suspected malignant processes.

Magnetic resonance imaging

Magnetic resonance imaging (MRI) scans are indicated if cranial nerve involvement is suspected in malignant processes, especially those involving the parotid gland.

Fine-needle aspiration cytology

Cytological assessment of clinically suspected tumours of the salivary glands produces useful information in treatment planning. This is a safe procedure that is not associated with tumour dissemination or seeding.

Parotid tumours

The parotid gland is not only the commonest site of primary salivary neoplasms but is also affected by a wide variety of infiltrative and inflammatory processes. From a clinical point of view, it is easier to consider the presentation of either diffuse parotid swelling or a mass within the region of the parotid.

Any mass arising within the region of the parotid (i.e. from the zygomatic arch superiorly, the upper neck inferiorly, the anterior border of the masseter anteriorly and the mastoid process posteriorly) should be suspected as arising from within the parotid gland and treated accordingly. An isolated mass within the parotid is most commonly due to a parotid tumour. Eighty per cent of all salivary tumours occur within the parotid gland, and approximately 80% of parotid tumours are benign.

Pleomorphic adenoma (mixed salivary tumour)

Approximately 65–75% of mass lesions arising within the parotid gland are a benign, slowly growing, firm, smooth, usually asymptomatic tumour called pleomorphic adenoma. It is so named because of its histological appearance of a variable mix of glandular and stromal elements, both of which are thought to arise from myoepithelial cells. While the peak incidence is in the fifth decade with a slight female preponderance, this tumour can occur from childhood to old age. Malignant transformation is uncommon and rarely reported in those tumours present for less than 10 years' duration. While initially a smooth lump, with time multiple bosselations may develop. Rapid growth with pain and facial nerve involvement are the hallmark of advanced malignant change. Given the relentless growth pattern, the chance of malignant change and the inability to differentiate this benign tumour clinically from slow-growing malignant parotid tumours, all parotid tumours are best treated by complete surgical excision.

Usually no pre-operative investigation is necessary after establishing that the mass is mobile within the parotid gland. Cytology may help treatment planning by deciding the urgency and timing of surgery. Radiological assessment with CT scanning is only necessary when malignancy is suspected. Treatment consists of excision of the lesion with an intact capsule and preservation of the facial nerve. Incomplete excision or capsular rupture at the time of excision predisposes to local recurrence, which may be multinodular and exceedingly difficult to eradicate. Complete excision is associated with a very low local recurrence rate (usually <2%). The surgical technique involves identification of the main trunk of the facial nerve, which is then traced through the gland while the tumour with the surrounding parotid tissue is excised. This is known as a superficial parotidectomy. For deep tumours, the superficial lobe is excised first. The facial nerve and branches are then fully mobilised to allow removal of the deep lobe, either between or below the facial nerve. With careful surgical technique, the risk of permanent facial damage is low, but some degree of temporary facial weakness due to neuropraxia is not uncommon.

Adenolymphoma (Warthin's tumour)

Approximately 6–10% of parotid masses are due to a benign, softer tumour, more commonly found in males and arising in the inferior pole of the parotid, called an adenolymphoma. This tumour is so called because of the dense lymphocytic infiltration. The exact origin of this lesion is uncertain. Approximately 10% of cases are bilateral. The cytological picture is usually diagnostic. Surgical excision in the form of parotidectomy is usually recommended, except in the frail and elderly, in whom clinical observation may be more appropriate.

Malignant parotid tumour

Approximately 15–20% of parotid tumours are malignant. In Australia, the most common malignancy involving the parotid is metastatic squamous cell carcinoma from a skin primary arising in the head and neck region. Such tumours tend to spread to intraparotid lymph nodes. These lesions are often characterised by rapid growth due to tumour necrosis producing a cystic lesion within the parotid. Treatment of metastatic squamous cell carcinomas involve parotid resection, often in association with a neck dissection and post-operative radiotherapy. The parotid is uncommonly the site of metastases from other tumours, but kidney, thyroid, lung and breast cancers may all spread to the parotid and mimic primary parotid tumours.

PRIMARY PAROTID MALIGNANCIES

- Mucoepidermoid carcinoma

  The most common primary malignancy of the parotid is mucoepidermoid carcinoma, which can occur from childhood onwards, with a peak incidence in the fifth to sixth decades. Approximately 75% of mucoepidermoid carcinomas are of low-grade histological type and present with a slowly growing parotid mass. High-grade tumours have a more rapid growth pattern and a poorer prognosis. Lymph node metastasis is uncommon.
- Adenoid cystic carcinoma

  Adenoid cystic carcinoma, formerly known as cylindromas, also present with a slowly growing asymptomatic parotid mass. These tumours are characterised by early perineural spread and have a propensity for late recurrence, often to bone or lung, even up to 20 years following an apparent cure.
- Acinic cell tumour

  Acinic cell tumour is another low-grade malignancy arising from the reserve cells of the terminal ducts and seen more commonly in females.
- Malignant pleomorphic adenoma

  Malignant pleomorphic adenoma is a more aggressive tumour that can arise either *de novo* or from a pre-existing pleomorphic tumour.

• Adenocarcinoma

Adenocarcinoma, otherwise unspecified, may also arise in the parotid and displays a more aggressive growth pattern.

Treatment of malignant parotid tumours

Treatment decisions are based on the biological and histological features of the tumour. Slow-growing, clinically discrete, low-grade lesions are usually cured by complete surgical excision with sparing of the facial nerve. For those tumour demonstrating more aggressive histological features, parotidectomy with facial nerve sparing may be followed by radiotherapy. Clinically aggressive tumours with facial nerve involvement will require radical surgery with sacrifice of the facial nerve and radiotherapy. Primary nerve grafting using the sural nerve if possible is performed. Lymph node dissection is usually only performed for clinically or radiographically detected nodal metastasis.

Submandibular tumours

Unlike the parotid gland, tumours of the submandibular gland are relatively uncommon. However, a higher proportion (approximately 40%) of submandibular tumours are malignant. Pleomorphic adenoma is the most common tumour affecting the gland. As with the parotid, most submandibular tumours present as a slowly growing asymptomatic lump. The diagnosis is usually suspected clinically and based on bimanual palpation. Differentiation from submandibular lymph node pathology can usually be confirmed by aspiration cytology. Submandibular tumours are treated by total gland excision. Malignant lesions with local spread beyond the submandibular gland may require sacrifice of the underlying lingual and hypoglossal nerves followed by radiotherapy to effect a cure.

Sublingual tumours

Primary tumours of the sublingual gland are rare. Of those that do occur, 60% are malignant and only 40% are benign.

Paraganglionomas

The extra-adrenal paraganglia of neural crest–derived cells can be the site of tumours known as paraganglionomas. These, usually benign, tumours may release neurotransmitters and produce intermittent hypertension and facial flushing. Tumours are named according to the neurovascular structure with which they are associated. The common sites for these uncommon tumours are the carotid body, the jugular bulb and the vagus nerve. Whilst most tumours occur sporadically, 10% represent an autosomal dominant inherited condition often associated with multiple paraganglionomas.

Carotid body tumour

The carotid body paraganglion is a chemoreceptor situated in the adventitia of the carotid bifurcation. Tumours present with a slowly growing, painless, smooth, firm, deep, lateral upper neck mass with limited supero-inferior mobility. Transmitted pulsation may be evident but tumours, although vascular, are not truly pulsatile. The intense contrast enhancement on CT scanning with splaying of the carotid bifurcation and the typical clinical presentation are usually diagnostic. Surgical excision in the subadventitial plane with preservation of the carotid vessels is curative for benign small tumours. Occasionally vascular reconstruction may be necessary for excision of larger and malignant tumours.

Glomus jugulare

Glomus jugulare tumours arise from the jugular bulb at the skull base. These deeply placed tumours are not clinically apparent until their growth impinges on surrounding cranial nerves IX, X, XI and XII or the internal auditory canal. Presenting symptoms include tinnitus, hearing loss, voice and swallowing problems. If bone erosion of the hypotympanum occurs a vascular mass may be clinically apparent medial to an intact tympanic membrane. A combination of contrast-enhanced CT scanning and MRI should demonstrate the degree of bony erosion and the relationship of the tumour to the surrounding cranial nerves. The optimal treatment of these tumours is unresolved. Complete surgical excision with sparing of the facial and lower cranial nerves may be difficult to achieve. Post-surgical recurrent and persistent disease of 7% and 8%, respectively, are usually reported. Radiotherapy leading to tumour fibrosis produces similar imperfect results and carries its own morbidity.

Glomus intravagale

Glomus Intravagale tumours arise from the paraganglionic tissue within the perineurium of the vagus nerve. These tumours are usually situated at the level of the inferior vagal ganglion. The usual clinical presentation is that of a neck mass near the origin of the sternocleidomastoid muscle with an associated vocal cord palsy. Multiple cranial nerve neuropathies may develop with progressive tumour growth. Contrast CT scanning demonstrates a vascular tumour within the carotid sheath displacing the vessel anteriorly. Other neural tumours of the vagus nerve form the differential diagnosis. Malignant transformation is commoner with glomus intravagale tumours than other parapharyngeal tumours with pulmonary metastases present in 20% of cases. Treatment consists of either radiotherapy or surgical excision based on an assessment of the tumour size and associated cranial nerve involvement. Although surgical resection necessitates sacrifice of the vagus nerve, more than 50% of the cases present with an established vocal cord paralysis.

Neural tumours

Schwannomas

50% of the solitary well encapsulated tumours arising from the schwann cells of peripheral nerve sheaths occur within the head and neck. Within the head and neck the common nerves of origin are the acoustic nerve and vagus nerve and less commonly from VII, IX, XI and XII. These tumours expand the nerve from which they arise and surgical excision with preservation of the nerve can occasionally be achieved. The clinical presentation is of a slow-growing, painless, lateral neck mass with limited mobility. Neurological signs suggesting the nerve of origin are unusual. Radiological examination demonstrates a well-circumscribed mass with some but not marked contrast enhancement. MRI may demonstrate an associated neural structure suggesting the diagnosis. Tumours arising from a cervical nerve root may extend through the intervertebral foramen, producing a dumb bell tumour with a cervical and spinal component. Aspiration cytology with its benign spindle cell pattern is usually inconclusive. Treatment is determined by tumour extent and the clinical picture. Slow-growing, small tumours in elderly patients may be observed. Tumours arising peripherally in the neck may be separated from the associated nerve with minimal morbidity. Surgical excision of large tumours or those in surgically less accessible sites or contiguous with important neurological structures such as the brachial plexus is associated with the risk of significant neurological morbidity.

Malignant schwannomas

Less than 5% of schwannonas are malignant. These tumours infiltrate locally, may extend intracranially or intravertebrally and can metastasise to the lungs. Aggressive surgical resection is advocated.

Neurofibromas

Neurofibromas are tumours arising from the peripheral nerve sheaths and present commonly as rubbery, fusiform subcutaneous nodules. Multiple neurofibromas and plexiform neurofibromas are found along with café au lait spots, skeletal, C.N.S. and ocular lesions in the autosomal dominant inherited disorder of neurofibromatosis. Surgical excision, with sacrifice of the associated nerve is definitive treatment for isolated lesions.

Soft tissue sarcomas

Soft tissue sarcomas are tumours of mesenchymal origin that display a wide spectrum of clinical and biological behaviour. Less than 10% of these uncommon tumours arise in the head and neck. A number of genetic abnormalities have been identified. Many of these clonal abberations have the potential to be applied to the differential diagnosis, in these, often difficult to categorise, tumours. Most tumours present as a painless neck mass. Tumours arising from the tissues of the upper aerodigestive tract or the deep tissue spaces may present with a variety of symptoms such as epistaxis, otalgia, visual disturbance or cranial nerve palsies resulting from local tumour infiltration. A thorough clinical examination including intra-oral, neurological and endoscopic examination of the upper aerodigestive tract often forms an impression of the extent of the tumour. High quality CT scanning and MRI allow accurate anatomical assessment. Fine needle aspiration cytology is simple and safe for accessible tumour and is helpful in differentiating sarcomas from other more common tumours but is usually unhelpful in the precise diagnosis of tumour type and grade. Core needle biopsies, radiologically directed, usually provide adequate tissue for pathological assessment. Tumours are staged according to their size, whether superficial or deep and histological grading based on differentiation, cellularity, density of the stroma, vascularity and the degree of necrosis.

Malignant fibrous histiocytoma (MFH)

MFH is the commonest soft tissue sarcoma in adult. Less than 3% involve the head and neck, with the upper aerodigetive tract being favoured and less commonly neck and salivary glands. Five-year survival for these aggressive tumours is approximately 50%.

Dermatofibrosarcoma protuberans

Dermatofibrosarcoma Protuberans, which accounts for approximately 7–15% of soft tissue sarcomas, usually presents as an elevated, firm, solitary, slowly growing, painless mass in the scalp or neck. Metastases are uncommon and an excellent outcome is achieved if histologically clear margins are obtained following local excision.

Angiosarcoma

Over half of all angiosarcomas present as an ulcerating, nodular or diffuse dermal lesion of the scalp or face in elderly white males. They are uncommon tumours, accounting for only 0.1% of all head and neck tumours.

Rhabdomyosarcoma

Rhabdomyosarcoma is the most common paediatric soft tissue sarcoma. This malignant tumour of striated muscle cell origin arises in the nasal cavity, paranasal sinuses, orbit, nasopharynx and middle ear. Early metastases both regional and distant are common. Treatment usually involves chemotherapy and irradiation with an overall survival of approximately 50%.

Bone tumours

Bone tumours may affect the mandible, maxilla or cervical vertebrae, presenting usually as painless swellings. Tumours are classified according to the matrix produced by the tumour cells into condro sarcomas if cartilagenous, osteo sarcomas if osteoid and fibro sarcomas if they lack a distinct matrix. Surgical excision with clear margins is associated with survival rates of 40–80% independent of the anatomical sites of origin. Distant metastases are infrequent.

Metastatic tumours

The management of neck metastases is outlined in Chapter 67. An understanding of the pattern of lymphatic drainage should direct the clinician to the likely site of the primary lesion. Primary tumours in the tongue base and the tonsil, occasionally small and hidden within the tissue convolutions, may thwart attempts at detection. Melanoma may also present with metastatic nodes in the absence of a detectable primary lesion, which may be amelanotic or have undergone spontaneous regression. Definitive treatment of the primary tumour and neck metastases arising from squamous cell carcinoma of the upper aerodigestive tract may be achieved with radiation often followed by surgery. Palliative radiotherapy may have a role in reducing the local devastating effects of uncontrolled neck disease arising from a distant incurable primary tumour.

MCQs

Select the single correct answer to each question.

1 The commonest tumour of the head and neck area is:
- **a** pleomorphic tumour of the parotid gland
- **b** squamous cell carcinoma of the larynx
- **c** squamous cell carcinoma of the skin
- **d** basal cell carcinoma of the skin
- **e** carcinoma of the thyroid gland

2 The most common paediatric soft tissue sarcoma in the head and neck area is:
- **a** angiosarcoma
- **b** malignant fibrous histiocytoma
- **c** dermatofibrosarcoma protuberans
- **d** rhabdomyosarcoma
- **e** chondrosarcoma

3 The highest propensity for lymph node metastasis occurs in squamous cell carcinoma of the:
- **a** ear
- **b** scalp
- **c** upper lip
- **d** nose
- **e** lower lip

[illegible] the pathological assessment [illegible] staged according to the size, whether superficial or deep and histological grading [illegible] cellularity, [illegible] stroma, vascularity and the degree of necrosis.

Malignant fibrous histiocytoma (MFH)

MFH is the commonest soft tissue sarcoma in adults. [illegible]

Dermatofibrosarcoma protuberans

[illegible]

Angiosarcoma

[illegible]

Rhabdomyosarcoma

[illegible]

Bone tumours

[illegible]

Metastatic tumours

The management of [illegible] neck metastasis is outlined in Chapter [illegible]. An understanding of the pattern of lymphatic drainage [illegible]

MCQs

[illegible]

Hernias

40 Hernias

David M. A. Francis

Introduction

A hernia is an abnormal protrusion of a viscus or part of a viscus through a defect either in the containing wall of that viscus or within the cavity in which the viscus normally is situated. In abdominal hernias, the 'wall' refers to the anterior and posterior muscle layers of the abdomen, the diaphragm, and the walls of the pelvis. Hernias are either external or internal.

External hernias

External hernias are common and present as an abnormal lump which can be detected by clinical examination of the abdomen or groin. The relative occurrence and gender distribution of external abdominal hernias are shown in Tables 40.1 and 40.2.

Internal hernias

Internal hernias are rare, and occur when the intestine (the 'viscus') passes beneath a constricting band or through a peritoneal window (the 'defect') within the abdominal cavity or in the diaphragm. They present as

Table 40.1 Relative occurrence of external abdominal hernias in adults

Hernia	Percentage
Inguinal	80
Incisional	10
Femoral	5
Umbilical	4
Epigastric	<1
Other	<1

Table 40.2 Sex distribution of abdominal hernias

	Male (%)	Female (%)
Inguinal hernia	96	45
Femoral hernia	2	39
Umbilical hernia	1	15
Other	1	1

- Acute intestinal obstruction, with or without intestinal ischaemia, perforation and peritonitis, or
- Chronic recurrent abdominal pain and vomiting due to incomplete and intermittent intestinal obstruction.

Sites of internal herniation include (i) the paraduodenal and paracaecal fossae, (ii) the lesser sac through the epiploic foramen (foramen of Winslow) or a defect in the transverse mesocolon, (iii) beneath congenital bands or adhesions, (iv) through defects in the small bowel mesentery, (v) between the lateral abdominal walls and intestinal stomas, and (vi) through defects in the diaphragm (hernias of Bochdalek and Morgagni). Treatment consists of laparotomy, removal of the distended bowel from the hernial orifice and resection if strangulation has occurred. Closure of the defect is required to prevent recurrence.

Components of a hernia

Hernias are composed of a sac, the parts of which are described as the neck, body and fundus (Fig. 40.1), and the hernial contents. The sac consists of peritoneum which protrudes through the abdominal wall defect or 'hernial orifice', and envelopes the hernial contents. The neck of the sac is situated at the defect. Hernias with a narrow or rigid neck are more likely to obstruct and strangulate (see below). The body is the widest part of the hernial sac, and the fundus is the apex or furthest

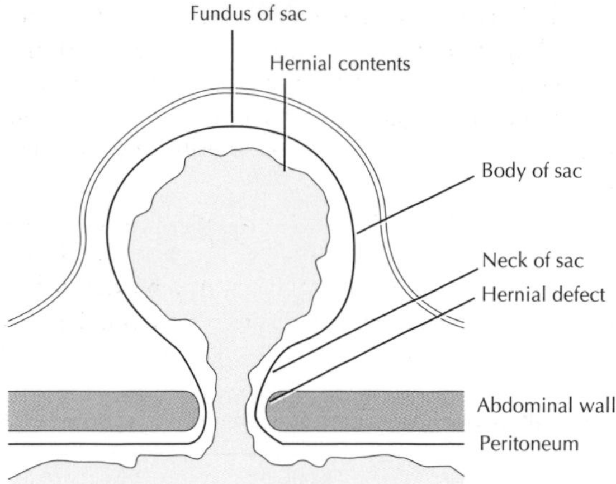

Fig. 40.1 Components of a hernia.

extremity. Viscera most likely to enter a hernial sac are those normally situated in the region of the defect and those which are mobile, namely the omentum, small intestine and colon. Some hernial contents have been ascribed generic names.

Richter's hernia

Only part of the circumference of the bowel (usually the anti-mesenteric border) is trapped within the hernial sac (Fig. 40.2). The herniated part may become ischaemic. Because the lumen of the bowel is not occluded, intestinal obstruction does not occur, and there are few symptoms until the ischaemic part perforates.

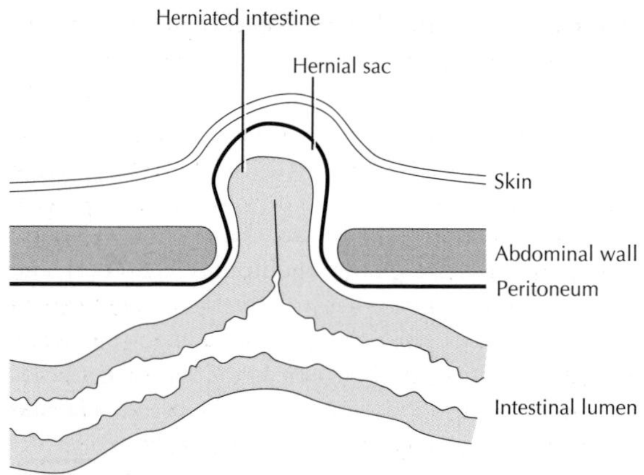

Fig. 40.2 Richter's hernia.

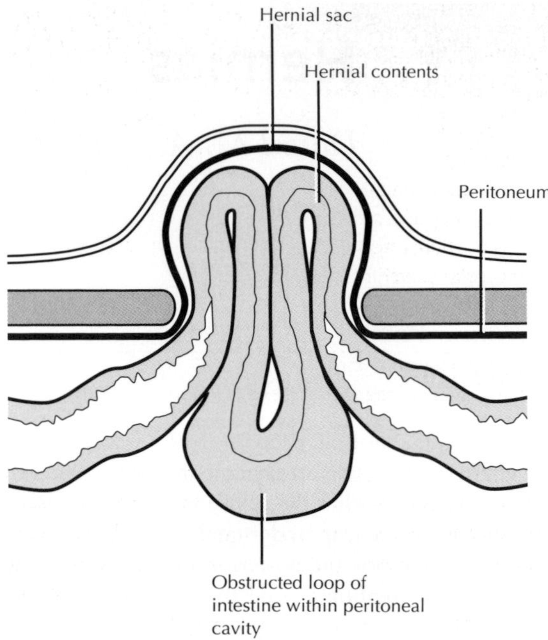

Fig. 40.3 Maydl's hernia.

Littre's hernia

A Meckel's diverticulum lies within the hernial sac. Littré's hernia occurs most commonly in a femoral or inguinal hernia (see below).

Maydl's hernia

The hernial sac contains two loops of intestine (Fig. 40.3). The loop of intestine within the abdominal cavity may become obstructed or strangulated, and this may not be recognised unless the hernial contents are inspected and returned to the abdominal cavity ('reduced') completely.

Predisposing factors

A hernia occurs because of (a) weakness or defect in the abdominal wall, and (b) positive intra-abdominal pressure (IAP) (which is often raised) forces the viscus into the defect.

Sites of weakness in the abdominal wall

Weaknesses in the abdominal wall may be:

Box 40.1 Causes of sudden or sustained increases in intra-abdominal pressure

- Coughing
- Vomiting
- Straining during urination or defecation
- Pregnancy and childbirth
- Occupational heavy lifting or straining, and strenuous muscular exercise
- Obesity
- Ascites
- Continuous ambulatory peritoneal dialysis (CAPD)
- Gross organomegaly

- Congenital (i.e. present at birth) – e.g. patent processus vaginalis or canal of Nuck, posterolateral or anterior parasternal diaphragmatic defect, patent umbilical ring in children.
- Where a normal anatomical structure passes through the abdominal wall – e.g. oesophageal hiatus, umbilical ligament in adults, obturator foramen, sciatic foramen.
- Acquired – e.g. surgical scar, site of an intestinal stoma, muscle wasting with increasing age, fatty infiltration of tissues because of obesity.

Increased intra-abdominal pressure

Raised intra-abdominal pressure (IAP) stretches the abdominal wall vertically and horizontally, thereby increasing the circumference of any defect. Also, high IAP forces abdominal contents through a defect. Sudden or sustained increases in IAP are due to several causes (Box 40.1).

Complications

Most hernias are uncomplicated at presentation. The three important complications of hernias are, in order of progression, irreducibility, obstruction and strangulation.

Irreducibility

A hernia is 'irreducible' when the sac cannot be emptied completely of contents. Irreducibility is caused by (i) adhesions between the sac and its contents, (ii) fibrosis leading to narrowing at the neck of the sac, or (iii) a sudden increase in IAP that causes transient stretching of the neck and forceful movement into the sac of contents, which cannot subsequently return to their original location.

Generally, irreducible hernias should be operated on soon after presentation. Although irreducibility is not an indication for urgent operation, it is the step before obstruction supervenes. In addition, irreducible hernias are usually painful.

Obstruction

A hernia becomes obstructed when the neck is sufficiently narrow to occlude the lumen of the intestine contained within the sac. Obstructed hernias are nearly always irreducible and, if not treated, may become strangulated. Often, there is a history of a sudden increase in IAP that has pushed intestine or other contents into the sac. The patient presents with symptoms and signs of intestinal obstruction (abdominal colic, vomiting, constipation, abdominal distension) (see Chapter 19), together with a tender irreducible hernia. Failure to examine the hernial orifices in a patient with intestinal obstruction may lead to the wrong operative approach being undertaken. It may be difficult to distinguish obstruction from strangulation on clinical grounds, and therefore obstructed hernias should be treated as a matter of urgency.

Strangulation

Strangulation means that the blood supply of the contents has ceased due to compression at the hernial orifice. Initially, lymphatic and venous channels are obstructed, leading to oedema and venous congestion but with continued arterial inflow. When the tissue pressure equals arterial pressure, arterial flow ceases and tissue necrosis ensues. Strangulation is a serious complication and, if the intestine is involved, leads to peritonitis (see chapter 65) which can be fatal. A strangulated hernia is both irreducible and obstructed, and is very tense and usually exquisitely tender. Erythema of the overlying skin is a late sign. Strangulated hernias must be operated on urgently. A strangulated Richter's hernia is not preceded by intestinal obstruction and there may be few local signs.

Principles of treatment

Uncomplicated hernias require either no treatment, support with a truss, or operative treatment, whereas complicated hernias always require surgery, often urgently.

No treatment

No treatment may be advised in debilitated patients who are not medically fit for surgery and who have uncomplicated hernias with minimal symptoms. Few patients fall into this category. Most external hernias can be successfully repaired surgically under regional or local infiltration anaesthesia with minimal morbidity. If a patient refuses treatment, then the full implications of this decision must be explained.

Truss or abdominal binder

A truss or some form of hernia support may be used to provide symptomatic relief for large uncomplicated hernias in elderly unfit patients and those who decline surgery. After the hernia has been reduced, the truss presses on the hernial orifice to prevent protrusion. However, it frequently does not prevent prolapse of the hernia and simply presses on the hernial contents, and is uncomfortable to wear.

Reducing raised intra-abdominal pressure

Causes of increased IAP should be corrected. Stopping smoking, investigation and treatment of prostatism and constipation, weight reduction, and effective management of ascites should be attempted where indicated. Changes in occupation and physical exercise also may have to be considered.

Operation

Operation is indicated for all other patients because of symptoms and the risk of complications. Surgery aims to (i) reduce the hernial contents, (ii) excise the sac (herniotomy) in most cases, and (iii) repair and close the defect, either by approximation of adjacent tissues to restore the normal anatomy (herniorrhaphy), or by insertion of additional material (hernioplasty). The site of the hernia must be marked clearly on the skin during consultation with the patient before induction of anaesthesia so that no mistake is made about its location.

Urgent operation

Urgent operation is indicated when obstruction or strangulation is suspected. Resuscitation with intravenous fluids, antibiotics, analgesia and nasogastric aspiration is required before surgery.

Attempted reduction of a hernia

When a patient presents with an apparently irreducible hernia, it is reasonable to make some attempt to reduce it, unless strangulation is suspected. The foot of the bed is elevated, the patient is kept warm, and given intramuscular opiate analgesia. After 20–30 minutes, firm manual pressure is applied to the hernia. Manual reduction may not be successful if adhesions have developed between the contents and the sac, or if the hernial orifice is narrow. Attempts at reducing a hernia should not be prolonged. Patients should be observed after successful reduction.

Inguinal hernia

Inguinal hernia is the commonest hernia, and is approximately 10 times more common in males than females (Tables 40.1 and 40.2). Two types of inguinal hernia (IH) are recognised (Fig. 40.4), indirect (IIH) and direct (DIH), but they can occur together.

Importance of the integrity of the inguinal canal

The inguinal canal passes through the abdominal wall between the deep (internal) and superficial (external) inguinal rings. It carries the spermatic cord to the scrotum in the male, or the round ligament of the uterus to the labium majora in the female, together with the ilioinguinal nerve. The canal is a site of weakness and therefore potential herniation.

In addition to the presence of a patent processus vaginalis in an IIH, both IIH and DIH result from failure of normal mechanisms that maintain the integrity of the inguinal canal, including:

(i) 'shutter mechanism' around the deep inguinal ring – during straining, a U-shaped condensation of transversalis fascia which passes under the cord is pulled upward and laterally, closing the deep ring around the cord and increasing the obliquity of the inguinal canal.

(ii) 'shutter action' of the internal oblique and transversus abdominis muscles – contraction of these muscles draws them downwards so that the

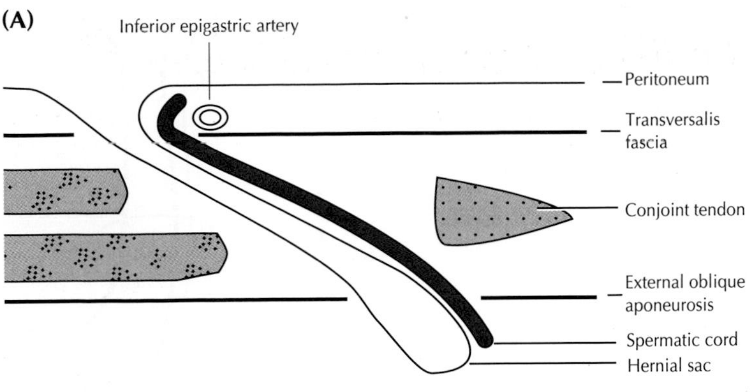

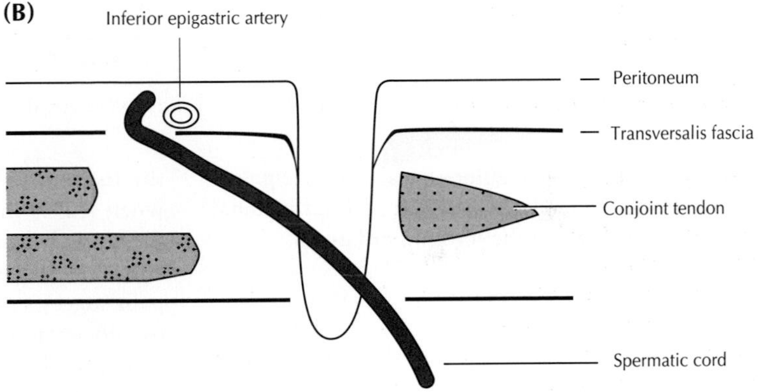

Fig. 40.4 Types of inguinal hernias (right side). (**A**) Indirect inguinal hernia; (**B**) direct inguinal hernia.

inguinal canal tends to close and become more oblique.

(iii) integrity of the posterior wall of the inguinal canal – weakness of the conjoint tendon reduces the strength of the posterior wall of the inguinal canal and reduces support behind the superficial inguinal ring.

(iv) oblique direction of the inguinal canal – if the deep and superficial inguinal rings enlarge, they may almost overlie each other and obliquity of the canal is lost.

Indirect inguinal hernia

The hernial sac of an IIH is a patent processus vaginalis, and the neck of the sac is situated at the deep inguinal ring, lateral to the inferior epigastric artery. The sac accompanies the spermatic cord along the inguinal canal towards the scrotum for a varying distance (see below). The sac lies in front of the cord and is enclosed by the coverings of the cord. Except in children and infants, the essential cause of an IIH is (a) failure of the processus vaginalis to become completely obliterated to form the ligamentum vaginale, which normally occurs within a few days after birth, and (b) loss of integrity of the inguinal canal (see above). Even though the sac of an IIH is congenital, herniation may not occur until later in life, when there is failure of the normal mechanisms that maintain the inguinal canal.

The incidence of IIH is approximately 800–1000 per million male population. Indirect IHs are approximately four times more common than DIH, occur at any time during life, and have a male to female ratio of about 10:1.

Classification of indirect inguinal hernias

Indirect IHs are classified according to the length of the hernial sac (Fig. 40.5).

- Bubonocele – the sac is confined to the inguinal canal.
- Funicular – the sac extends along the length of the inguinal canal and through the superficial inguinal ring, but does not extend to the scrotum or labium majora.

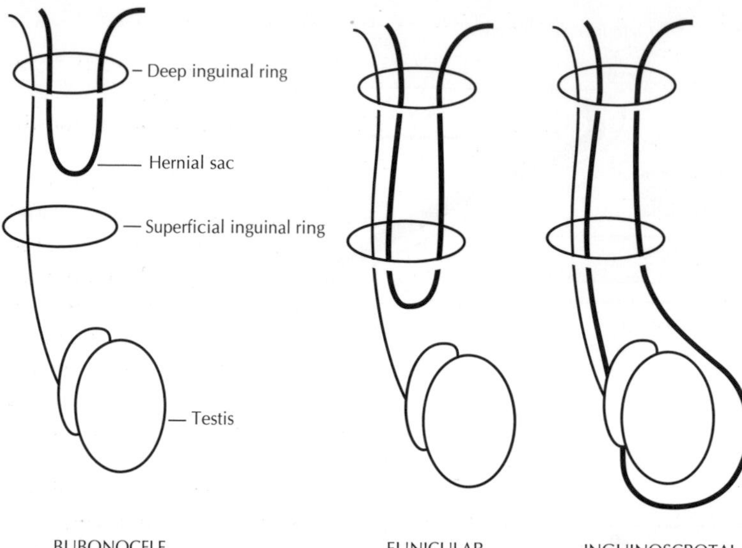

Fig. 40.5 Types of indirect inguinal hernias.

- Complete, scrotal or inguinoscrotal – the sac passes through the inguinal canal and superficial inguinal ring and extends into the scrotum or labium.

Direct inguinal hernia

A DIH protrudes directly through the posterior wall of the inguinal canal, medial to the inferior epigastric artery and deep inguinal ring. The essential fault with a DIH is weakness of the inguinal canal, and is invariably associated with poor abdominal musculature. Herniation occurs at a site where the transversalis fascia is not supported by the conjoint tendon or the transversus aponeurosis, an area known as Hesselbach's triangle. The neck of a DIH is usually larger than the body and so strangulation is rare. The hernia passes forwards as it enlarges, stretching muscle and fascial layers. It rarely reaches a large size or approaches the scrotum. Occasionally, the inferior epigastric vessels straddle the hernia which is then known as a 'pantaloon hernia'.

Direct IH is rare in females and does not occur in children. It is more common on the right side after appendicectomy, suggesting that damage to the ilio-hypogastric and ilio-inguinal nerves with subsequent weakness of the internal oblique and transversus abdominis muscles is an aetiological factor.

Clinical features of inguinal hernias

Inguinal hernias present with inguinal discomfort, with or without a lump. Discomfort is due to stretching of the tissues of the inguinal canal and occurs typically when IAP is increased. Pain may also be referred to the testis because of pressure on the spermatic cord and ilio-inguinal nerve. Severe inguinal or abdominal pain suggests obstruction or strangulation. A lump is usually obvious to the patient, is often precipitated by increasing IAP, and may reduce completely with rest and lying down.

The patient initially is examined standing to demonstrate the lump and possible cough impulse, and then lying down to allow the hernia to be reduced. An IIH protrudes along the line of the inguinal canal for a variable distance towards the scrotum or labia; a DIH appears as a diffuse bulge at the medial end of the inguinal canal. The significance of a 'cough impulse', or sudden bulging of the inguinal region with coughing, must be interpreted carefully. A generalised weakness in the inguinal region will result in a diffuse bulge appearing with coughing, but this condition (known as a Malgaigne's bulge) is not the same as a hernia in which the cough impulse is discrete and confined to the area of herniation. Abdominal examination is performed to detect organomegaly, a mass or ascites.

Indirect or direct inguinal hernia?

An IIH is prevented from appearing by applying pressure over the deep inguinal ring (which lies just above the midpoint of the inguinal ligament) because an IIH protrudes through the deep inguinal ring. A DIH protrudes through the posterior wall of the inguinal canal medial to the deep ring. IIH and DIH may be distinguished by firstly reducing the hernia by gently pushing it upwards and laterally. Then, the index and middle fingers are placed firmly over the surface marking of the deep ring and the patient is asked to cough. If the hernia is controlled by pressure over the deep ring, then it is presumed to be indirect. If the hernia appears medial to the examiner's two fingers, then it is direct.

Accurate distinction of an IIH from a DIH may not be possible because of slight variation in the position of the deep inguinal ring. However, an attempt should be made to distinguish between the two because IIHs are more likely to develop complications and should be repaired sooner rather than later.

Sliding inguinal hernia

A sliding inguinal hernia is a variant in which part of a viscus (usually the colon) is adherent to the outside of the peritoneum forming the hernial sac beyond the hernial orifice. Thus, the viscus and the hernial sac, which may contain another abdominal viscus, lie within the inguinal canal (Fig. 40.6). Sliding hernias are more common on the left side (where they contain part of the sigmoid colon) than on the right (where they contain part of the caecum). Sliding hernias occasionally contain part of the bladder or an ovary and ovarian tube. A sliding hernia may be indirect or direct. They are nearly always found in males. A sliding hernia should be suspected if the neck of the hernia is bulky, or if the hernial sac does not separate easily from the cord at operation.

Inguinal hernias in infants and children

Inguinal hernias are always indirect in infants and children and are due to a patent processus vaginalis. Ninety per cent occur in males and more commonly on the right side, presumably due to the slightly later descent of the right testis. Approximately 10–20% are bilateral. If the contralateral side is also explored in a child undergoing unilateral inguinal hernia repair, a patent processus is found in approximately 50% of cases. Irreducibility is common and occurs in about 50% of hernias presenting within the first year of life. Strangulation appears to be rare. Testicular infarction can occur if a large irreducible hernia severely compresses the spermatic cord, and is more common than infarction of the hernial contents.

Inguinal hernias in children should be repaired surgically. The hernial sac is very thin and, because the superficial and deep inguinal rings are almost superimposed upon one another in children, the sac can be mobilised and ligated through the superficial inguinal ring. Herniotomy is all that is required.

Treatment of inguinal hernias

As with other external hernias, the precipitating cause of the hernia must be identified and treated. A truss may be useful for uncomplicated hernias in elderly debilitated patients and in those who decline surgery, but is rarely effective in controlling the hernia. Inguinal hernias are best treated surgically.

Inguinal hernia repair can be undertaken under general, regional or local infiltration anaesthesia, often

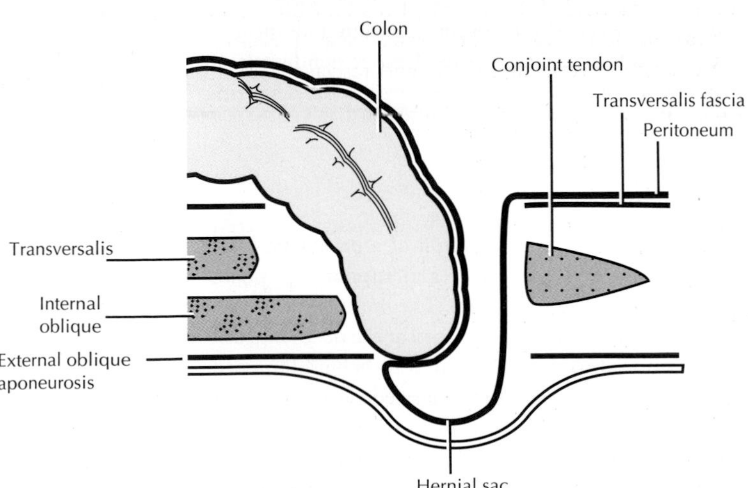

Fig. 40.6 Section through sliding inguinal hernia.

as a day procedure in fit patients who have adequate home support. Open repair is performed through a skin crease incision centred over the inguinal canal. The sac is dissected carefully from the cord, opened and the contents returned to the abdominal cavity. In an IIH, the sac is ligated at the deep inguinal ring and excised (herniotomy), whereas in a DIH the sac is formed from layers of the posterior wall of the inguinal canal and so it is not excised. A procedure to strengthen the posterior wall of the inguinal canal is performed (herniorrhaphy or hernioplasty).

Herniorrhaphy

'Herniorrhaphy' refers to repair of the posterior wall of the inguinal canal behind the spermatic cord by one of several methods, together with repair of the external oblique aponeurosis in front of the cord. Strong non-absorbable sutures are used.

- Shouldice repair – The weakened transversalis fascia is incised along the line of the inguinal canal and repaired in an overlapping fashion. The deep inguinal ring is closed snugly around the cord. The internal oblique and transversus are approximated to the deep aspect of the inguinal ligament.
- Bassini repair – The conjoint tendon is sutured onto the inguinal ligament. A J-shaped incision, known as a 'Tanner slide', is made in the anterior rectus sheath to enable the conjoint tendon to 'slide' down towards the inguinal ligament without tension.
- Nylon darn repair – The weakened transversalis fascia is plicated from the pubic tubercle to the deep ring. A second continuous nylon suture is inserted as a loose darn from the inguinal ligament below to the anterior aspect of the conjoint tendon and aponeurosis of the internal oblique above, extending from the pubic tubercle medially to beyond the deep ring laterally.

Hernioplasty

'Hernioplasty' refers to insertion of a prosthetic mesh (e.g. polypropylene) to cover and support the posterior wall of the inguinal canal. The mesh is cut to size, with two limbs encircling the cord at the deep ring, and is then sutured to the posterior wall behind the cord. Alternatively, the mesh can be inserted via an extraperitoneal approach and placed deep to the defect in the posterior wall.

Laparoscopic hernia repair

Laparoscopic repair is performed under general anaesthesia, using either a transperitoneal or extraperitoneal approach. The technique is not appropriate for large or irreducible hernias. The sac is separated from the spermatic cord and excised, and a mesh is inserted to strengthen the posterior wall, with or without a small plug of synthetic material being inserted into the deep ring. Advantages of laparoscopic hernia repair include reduced post-operative pain and earlier return to work. Disadvantages include increased risk of femoral nerve and spermatic cord damage, risk of developing intraperitoneal adhesions with the transperitoneal procedure, and greater cost and duration of the operation. Initial experience indicates that recurrence rates are similar to those associated with open operations.

Management after inguinal hernia repair

Patients require analgesia for the first few days. They should avoid straining and lifting for about 4 weeks after surgery, and avoid very heavy physical work for about 6–8 weeks. The average length of stay off work is approximately 2–4 weeks after open repair and 1–2 weeks after laparoscopic repair.

Potential complications of inguinal hernia repair

In addition to the complications of any surgical procedure (haemorrhage, haematoma, wound and chest infection, deep vein thrombosis, pulmonary embolus, anaesthetic complications) there are a number of potential complications specific to inguinal hernia repair.

- Urinary retention – Elderly male patients are particularly susceptible to retention of urine. Prostatic symptoms should be identified and treated before the hernia is repaired.
- Scrotal swelling and haematoma – Oedema, swelling and bruising of the scrotum are common (especially with bilateral repairs) and resolve spontaneously. Scrotal support may bring symptomatic relief. Large haematomas require operative drainage.
- Wound infection – A deep wound infection which does not settle with antibiotocis requires removal of the prosthetic mesh.

- Recurrent hernia – Recurrence is related to surgical technique and expertise, experience of the operator, postoperative infection and haematoma, and failure to correct factors predisposing to hernia formation. Also, failure to examine the spermatic cord for the presence of an indirect inguinal sac when repairing a DIH may lead to an apparent 'recurrence'. Recurrence rates should be less than 2%. About 50% of recurrences appear within 5 years after the initial repair, and approximately 50% of recurrences are indirect hernias. A first recurrence is treated along the principles outlined in the previous section. Subsequent hernia recurrence requires mesh repair by an extraperitoneal approach, or complete closure of the inguinal canal by sutures after excision of the cord and testis.
- Nerve injury – injury to the ilio-inguinal nerve, which lies below the spermatic cord in the inguinal canal and passes out through the superficial inguinal ring, occurs in 10–20% of inguinal hernia repairs, resulting in paraesthesia or numbness below and medial to the wound over the pubic tubercle and proximal scrotum. The lateral cutaneous nerve of the thigh and the femoral nerve are at risk during laparoscopic repair.
- Persisting wound pain – This is uncommon, and results from nerve entrapment or damage, neuroma formation, osteitis pubis if sutures have been inserted into the pubis, displacement of a mesh repair, or pressure on the spermatic cord. Pain may be a symptom of recurrent herniation. Local anaesthetic or phenol injections may help, and surgical exploration is indicated for severe or persistent pain.
- Testicular ischaemia and atrophy – interruption of the testicular arterial supply (testicular artery and indirectly from the cremasteric artery and the artery of the vas deferens) can occur during dissection of an indirect sac from the cord. Ischaemia produces testicular pain, tenderness and swelling. Testicular atrophy is observed in 1–5% of males.
- Hydrocele – a long-term complication probably resulting from the repair being too tight or scarring, with subsequent compression of lymphatics of the cord.
- Injury to the vas deferens – a rare complication, is most likely to occur when a recurrent hernia is repaired and with laparoscopic repair.
- Visceral injury – viscera in a sliding hernia are at risk for injury when the sac is being dissected away from them.

Femoral hernia

A femoral hernia occurs when the transversalis fascia which normally covers the femoral ring is disrupted, so that a peritoneal sac and hernial contents pass through the femoral ring into the femoral canal. The femoral canal is the most medial compartment of the femoral sheath, medial to the femoral vein. Femoral hernias are 2–3 times more common in females than males, and occur in the older age group, often after a period of weight loss. Femoral hernias are never congenital, and are twice as common in parous as in non-parous females. Inguinal hernias are more common than femoral hernias in females (Table 40.2). Approximately 60% of femoral hernias are on the right, 30% on the left, and 10% bilateral. A femoral hernia is the commonest site for a Richter's hernia (Section 2.1).

Aetiological factors in femoral hernia formation are:

- localised weakness at the femoral ring.
- factors which increase intra-abdominal pressure (Box 40.1).

Presentation

A femoral hernia presents as either discomfort in the groin together with a lump, or as intestinal obstruction with or without strangulation. A small hernia may be difficult to palpate, especially in the obese patient. The hernia is frequently irreducible and may not have a cough impulse.

On examination, the bulge of a femoral hernia appears in the region of the saphenous opening. The neck of the sac is always located below the line of the inguinal ligament, even though the fundus may appear to be above the ligament. This is because once within the femoral canal, the hernial sac is prevented from continuing inferiorly down the thigh with the femoral vessels because the femoral sheath (which encloses the femoral vessels and the femoral canal) becomes narrow and tapers to a point around the vessels. The hernia is therefore directed forwards through the fossa ovalis, and is quite superficial at this point (Fig. 40.7). It cannot continue down the thigh in a subcutaneous plane because the superficial fascia of the thigh is attached to the lower border of the fossa ovalis and is firmer than the superficial fascia above the level of the foramen ovalis. As the hernia enlarges, it turns upwards into

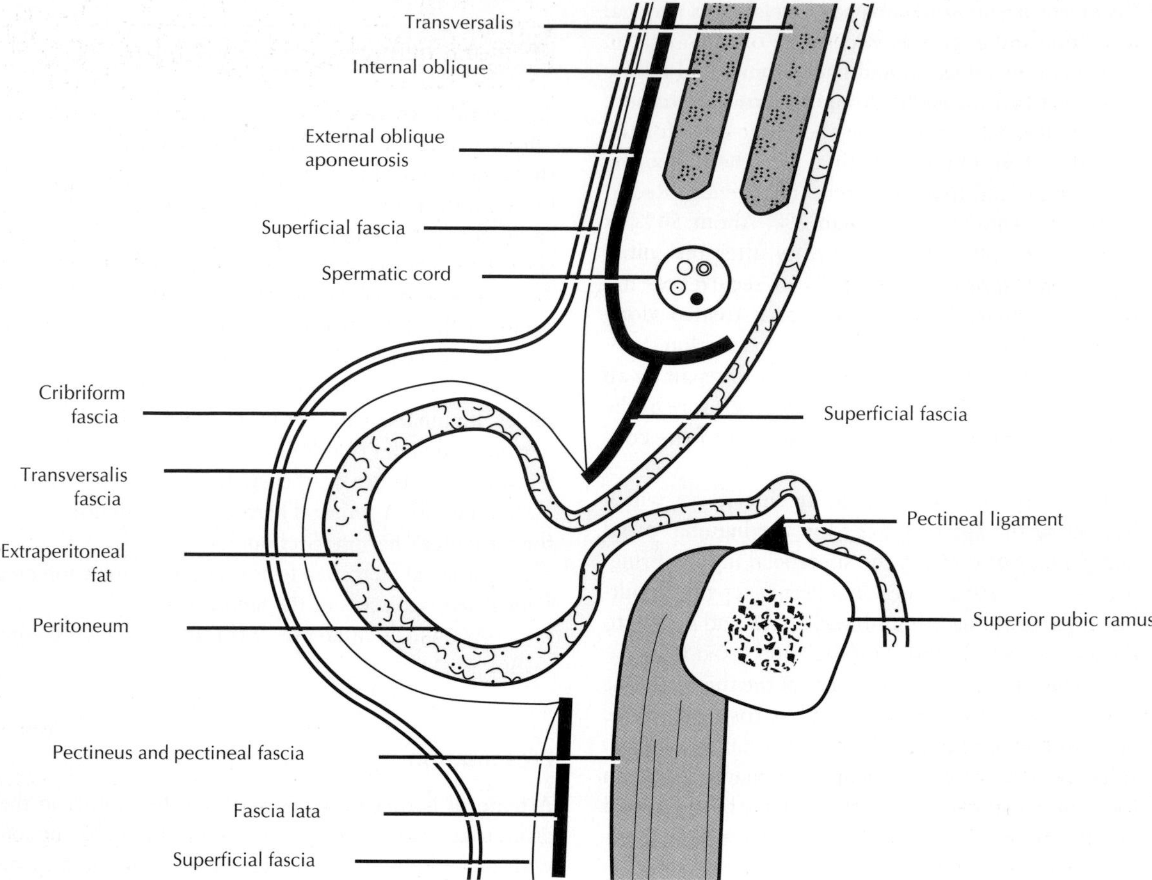

Fig. 40.7 Sagittal section of a femoral hernia.

the looser areolar tissue beneath the skin of the groin crease and may be confused with an inguinal hernia.

Thus, the direction taken by a femoral hernia is initially downwards through the femoral canal, then forwards through the fossa ovalis, and then upwards in the loose areolar tissue of the upper thigh. Therefore, in attempting to reduce the hernia, pressure is applied in the reverse order, that is, initially downwards, backwards and then upwards.

Inguinal or femoral hernia?

Inguinal and femoral hernias are distinguished by their positions relative to the inguinal ligament and pubic tubercle. The inguinal ligament is identified by palpating the anterior superior iliac spine and the pubic tubercle; an imaginary line drawn between the two points is the line of the inguinal ligament. The neck of an inguinal hernia is above the inguinal ligament and pubic tubercle, and the hernia protrudes initially from above the ligament even though it may descend into the scrotum. The neck of a femoral hernia is below the inguinal ligament and lateral to the pubic tubercle, and the hernia protrudes initially from below the ligament.

Treatment

Surgical treatment of a femoral hernia should always be advised because of the risk of obstruction and strangulation. A truss cannot prevent herniation through the femoral ring and has no place in the management of femoral hernia.

Surgery involves opening and emptying the sac, and performing a herniorrhaphy to prevent recurrence. Herniorrhaphy aims to reduce the size of the femoral ring and is performed by inserting several sutures between the inguinal and pectineal ligaments, thereby effectively closing off the femoral canal. One of two operative approaches is used:

- A 'low' or subinguinal approach is used for small uncomplicated femoral hernias by making an incision over the hernia below the level of the inguinal ligament.
- The 'high' or supra-inguinal approach is used for large or complicated femoral hernias in an emergency situation. The extraperitoneal space between the peritoneum and abdominal wall muscles is accessed through an abdominal incision. The sac is identified and opened to inspect the contents. The intestine is resected if necessary, and the sac is excised. The femoral ring is repaired from this intra-abdominal approach.

Incisional hernia

An incisional hernia is a protrusion of the peritoneum (the sac) and abdominal contents into the subcutaneous plane through a defect at the site of a scar following an abdominal operation. The true incidence is difficult to ascertain, but is in the order of 5% at 5 years and 10% at 10 years. There is a higher preponderance in males. Patients present with nagging discomfort and a bulge at the site of a previous incision. Incisional hernias increase in size with time and frequently become irreducible.

The main predisposing factors for an incisional hernia are poor surgical techniques, local wound complications, impaired wound healing, and increased intra-abdominal pressure (Box 40.2).

Box 40.2 Aetiological factors in incisional hernias

1 *Poor surgical techniques*
- Angulated incision
- Parallel incisions
- Devitalised tissue in wound
- Tightly sutured wound
- Poor technique of abdominal wound closure
- Absorbable sutures of short duration

2 *Local wound factors*
- Infection
- Haematoma
- Foreign body
- Wound edges not in apposition

3 *Impaired wound healing*
- Malnutrition
- Corticosteroids, anti-proliferative and immunosuppressive drugs
- Uraemia
- Jaundice
- Diabetes
- Anaemia

4 *Raised intra-abdominal pressure (Box 40.1)*

Treatment

Incisional hernias should be repaired because (a) they increase in size with time and may be very difficult to repair when large, (b) they are at risk of becoming irreducible, obstructed and strangulated, especially if the neck is narrow, and (c) patients request repair because of discomfort and unsightly appearance. Pre-operative weight reduction in obese patients aims to facilitate the repair, and to reduce post-operative respiratory problems and likelihood of recurrence. With massive incisional hernias, pre-operative progressive pneumoperitoneum for 1–2 weeks may be considered to facilitate replacement of viscera into the abdominal cavity and abdominal wall closure. An abdominal support or binder may be helpful in very large hernias or in patients unfit for surgery.

Operation involves defining the sac and neck, returning the contents to the abdominal cavity, and repairing the hole in the abdominal wall. If the omentum is within the hernial sac, it is excised. The intestine should be handled as little as possible to minimise post-operative ileus. If the edges of the defect can be apposed without tension, the defect is closed directly with strong non-absorbable sutures; if not, the defect is covered with prosthetic mesh (e.g. polypropylene or polytetrafluoroethylene 'Goretex' dual mesh) sutured to the edges of the defect. Prophylactic antibiotics are used in cases of mesh repair.

Epigastric hernia

An epigastric hernia is a protrusion of extraperitoneal fat, with or without a small sac of peritoneum through a defect in the linea alba anywhere between the xiphisternum and the umbilicus. The defect is characteristically small, often about 1 cm in diameter. Patients are frequently fit young males who present with epigastric pain, which may be confused with peptic ulceration or biliary disease. Patients should be examined in both standing and lying positions. The hernia is usually easier to feel than to see, and is diagnosed by palpation of a small, often very tender, lump in the linea alba. Ultrasound may be helpful when a hernia is suspected but cannot be palpated. Epigastric hernias are usually irreducible and may be multiple.

Treatment

Surgery is undertaken to relieve symptoms. The hernia is marked pre-operatively because it may reduce with anaesthesia and the defect may be too small to palpate. If there are multiple hernias, the linea alba is exposed through a vertical incision, the extraperitoneal fat is excised, and each defect is repaired. A 'keel' repair of the linea alba is then performed by inserting two or more layers of sutures into the linea alba and anterior rectus sheath, each successive layer covering the previous layer so that the repaired tissue resembles the keel of a boat (Fig. 40.8). If a single defect is present, a transverse incision is usually made, and the defect is repaired with a 'Mayo' repair (Fig. 40.9), in which the upper and lower edges of the defect are overlapped with interrupted sutures ('pants over vest' repair).

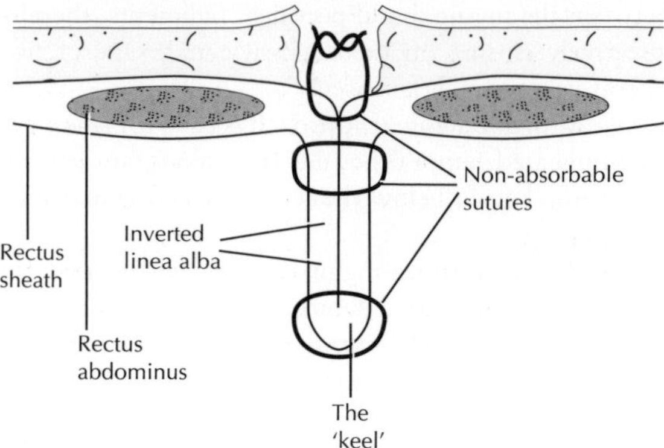

Fig. 40.8 Keel repair.

Umbilical hernia in children

An umbilical hernia in a child is a congenital defect in which a peritoneal sac protrudes through a patent umbilical ring and is covered by normal skin. Approximately 5–10% of Caucasian infants have an umbilical hernia at birth. About one-third of hernias close within a month of birth, and they rarely persist beyond the age of 3–4 years. The hernia is noticeable whenever the child cries, coughs or vomits, and is a cause of

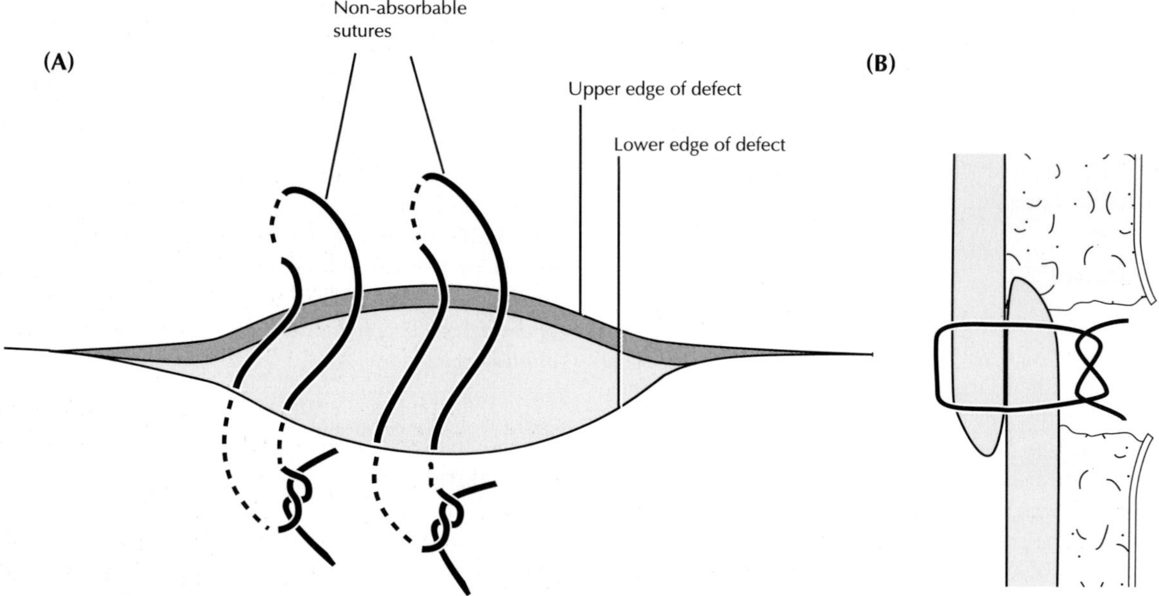

Fig. 40.9 Mayo repair. (A) Insertion of two sutures through upper and lower edges of hernial defect. (B) Sagittal section of linea alba after repair.

concern for parents. Umbilical hernias in children rarely become irreducible or strangulate.

Umbilical hernia is a separate entity from exomphalos (omphalocele). Exomphalos is a rare congenital condition in which the midgut fails to return to the abdominal cavity during the first trimester, with subsequent failure of the abdominal wall to close at the umbilicus. At birth, the intestine protrudes into the base of the umbilical cord and is covered by a thin opaque sac of amnion, not normal skin.

Treatment

An expectant approach can be adopted as nearly all hernias close or greatly reduce in size. Repair is recommended for unusually large hernias or if the hernia is still present at school age. A short transverse subumbilical incision is made, the sac is excised, and the defect is closed by either edge-to-edge apposition or a Mayo repair (Fig. 40.9). The umbilical cicatrix is preserved. Recurrence is rare.

Para-umbilical hernia in adults

A para-umbilical hernia in an adult is an acquired condition and quite distinct from the umbilical hernia of childhood. A para-umbilical hernia protrudes through one side of the umbilical ring, while the umbilicus still retains its fibrous character within the linea alba, although it becomes effaced by the pressure of the hernial contents and has an eccentric 'half-moon' or crescentic furrow. Para-umbilical hernias initially contain extraperitoneal fat but, as the hernial orifice enlarges, omentum enters the sac. The contents typically adhere to the sac so that the hernia becomes loculated and irreducible. Para-umbilical hernias occasionally become very large and contain transverse colon and small intestine.

Treatment

Para-umbilical hernias are treated surgically because of the risk of obstruction, strangulation and, rarely, excoriation and ulceration of the skin overlying the hernia. The classic operative procedure is a Mayo repair (Fig. 40.9), but repairs with mesh are performed increasingly.

Hernias related to intestinal stomas

A hernia may occur through the abdominal wall at the site of an intestinal stoma (see Chapter 30). The surgically created defect through which the stoma is fashioned enlarges due to raised IAP and allows protrusion of the peritoneum (the hernial sac) through the defect to lie adjacent to the stoma (Fig. 40.10).

Para-stomal hernias eventually occur in about 10–30% of patients with colostomies and ileostomies. Correct surgical technique when fashioning intestinal stomas is of paramount importance in prevention. For example, stomas should be brought out through the aponeurotic part of the abdominal wall, not the muscular part, and they should not be sited in the main abdominal wound or the umbilicus.

Treatment

Surgery is required if the bulge of the hernia causes poor fitting of the stoma appliance and consequent leakage from beneath the appliance. Also, intestinal obstruction and strangulation may occur. Operation involves reducing the size of the stomal orifice by closing the abdominal wall tissues around the stoma, but this method

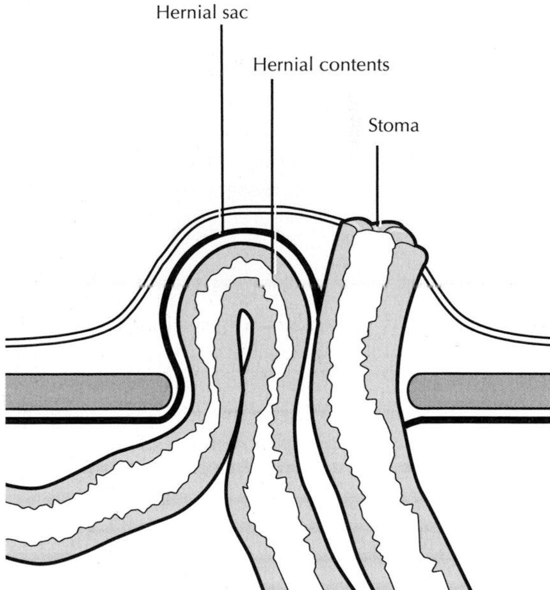

Fig. 40.10 Para-stomal hernia.

has a high recurrence rate. Insertion of prosthetic mesh in an extraperitoneal or extraparietal plane to cover the defect in the abdominal wall generally provides a good repair but runs the risk of infection of the mesh. Relocation of the stoma and complete closure of the previous stoma site provides the best chance of cure.

Spigelian hernia

Spigelian hernias are rare. A Spigelian hernia occurs through the transversus abdominis aponeurosis of the anterior abdominal wall, usually below the level of the umbilicus. The vertical curved line at which the transverse abdominis muscle becomes an aponeurosis is the semilunar line, and it extends from the costal margin to the pubic tubercle. The transversus abdominis aponeurosis extends medially from the semilunar line to the lateral edge of the rectus sheath. A Spigelian hernia usually occurs at the widest and weakest point of the aponeurosis, which is about halfway between the umbilicus and the inguinal ligament.

Clinically, the diagnosis of a Spigelian hernia may be difficult. The patient, who typically is a middle-aged female, presents with diffuse aching pain in the area of the hernia, which is small and may not be palpable. Pain is often present during the day but may recede at night if the hernia reduces, and may be made worse by raising the arm on the affected side. If a lump is not palpable, the diagnosis may be confirmed by ultrasound or computed tomography scanning. The hernia usually contains omentum but may contain small or large bowel. A Richter's hernia may occur, and obstruction and strangulation are well-recognised complications.

Treatment

Spigelian hernias should be treated surgically because of the severity of symptoms and the risk of complications. A skin crease incision is made over the hernia, the sac is excised and the defect in the transversus abdominis aponeurosis is closed with non-absorbable sutures.

Lumbar hernias

Lumbar hernias are rare. They occur typically in individuals with poor muscle tone, either spontaneously, or following trauma, surgery, or paralysis of paravertebral muscles secondary to poliomyelitis. Differential diagnosis includes a lipoma, lumbar abscess or haematoma.

Lumbar hernias occur through two triangular sites of weakness in the lumbar region of the abdominal wall.

- Inferior lumbar triangle hernia (triangle of Petit) – herniation occurs between the iliac crest inferiorly, the posterior edge of external oblique muscle anteriorly, and the anterior edge of latissimus dorsi posteriorly. The 'floor' of the triangle through which the hernia protrudes is formed by the internal oblique and transversus abdominis muscles.
- Superior lumbar triangle (triangle of Grynfeltt–Lesshaft) – the hernia occurs between the lowermost edge of serratus posterior inferior muscle and the twelfth rib superiorly, the anterior border of internal oblique muscle anteriorly, and the lateral edge of erector spinae muscle medially. Grynfeltt's triangle lies superior to Petit's triangle, and the 'floor' is formed by the quadratus lumborum muscle. The hernia is covered by the latissimus dorsi.

Treatment

Treatment of lumbar hernias is difficult because of their anatomical boundaries, their size, the type of patient in whom they occur, and because they are bounded in part by muscle rather than tough aponeurotic tissue. Prosthetic mesh repair is required.

Obturator hernia

An obturator hernia is rare. It protrudes through the obturator canal or foramen, which is a normal anatomical structure between the obturator groove on the inferior aspect of the superior pubic ramus and superior border of the obturator membrane. The obturator canal carries the obturator nerve and vessels. When large, the hernial sac passes between the pectineus and adductor longus muscles and protrudes forwards to produce a diffuse bulge in the femoral triangle, where it can be mistaken for a femoral hernia. It is more common on the right side.

The hernia occurs most often in elderly females, particularly in those who have become debilitated and lost weight rapidly. Usually, the patient presents with intestinal obstruction of unknown cause, and the hernia is diagnosed at laparotomy. Patients may complain of diffuse pain in the groin together with pain in the medial side of the thigh and knee because of pressure on the obturator nerve. The hernia may be felt in the femoral triangle and also on vaginal examination. A Richter's hernia may occur with strangulation of the entrapped part of the intestinal wall.

Treatment

Laparotomy is performed and the entrapped segment of bowel is released. The hernial defect is often found to be small. Care is taken not to damage the obturator nerve when either closing the defect or covering it with prosthetic mesh.

Sciatic hernias

Sciatic hernias are very rare and occur when a peritoneal sac enters the greater (gluteal hernia) or lesser sciatic foramina. Pain caused by pressure on the sciatic nerve or a palpable swelling and tenderness in the buttock suggests the diagnosis. Most commonly, sciatic hernias are discovered at laparotomy for intestinal obstruction. The sac is excised, but attempts to close the defect run the risk of sciatic nerve damage.

Further reading

Cheek CM, Black NA, Devlin HB, Kingsnorth AN, Taylor RS, Watkin DFL. Groin hernia surgery: a systematic review. *Ann R Coll Surg Engl.* 1998; 80:S1–S80.

MCQs

Select the single correct answer to each question.

1 The commonest type of hernia is:
- **a** inguinal
- **b** femoral
- **c** epigastric
- **d** incisional
- **e** umbilical

2 The most serious and urgent complication of a hernia is:
- **a** pressure on the spermatic cord
- **b** irreducibility
- **c** obstruction
- **d** strangulation
- **e** neuralgia

3 Indirect inguinal hernias:
- **a** can hardly ever be distinguished from direct inguinal hernias by clinical examination
- **b** rarely occur in children
- **c** can be treated by herniotomy, herniorraphy and hernioplasty
- **d** should not be treated laparoscopically
- **e** arise beneath the inguinal ligament

4 Femoral hernias:
- **a** may occasionally appear above the inguinal ligament in young children
- **b** should always be repaired surgically
- **c** can be treated with a surgical truss
- **d** are caused by a defect in the cribriform fascia
- **e** may compress the femoral artery

Skin and Soft Tissues

41 Tumours and cysts of the skin

Gordon J. A. Clunie and Peter Devitt

Introduction

The skin has many functions, including the provision of a physical barrier between the body and the environment, and temperature regulation. The skin structure, of epithelium and appendages with the underlying dermis, forms a complex and interactive grouping of tissues and cells to serve these functions. It is not surprising that genetically determined processes and external factors can interact to produce lesions that by their superficial placement are both obvious and deserving of attention. The common lesions of the skin of importance in relation to possible surgical therapy will be dealt with under the headings of cysts, benign tumours, malignant lesions and malignant tumours.

Cysts of the skin

These are common lesions whose only importance is their cosmetic effect and their propensity to become infected.

Epidermal or epidermoid cysts

Epidermal or epidermoid cysts are the most common cysts, and are frequently misnamed sebaceous cysts in the mistaken belief that they arise from sebaceous glands. True sebaceous cysts do occur but are rare. Epidermal cysts are in fact inclusion cysts lined by fully differentiated epidermis. They are filled by laminated keratin, which forms the characteristic, white, unpleasant-smelling content. They occur most commonly on the face, the scalp, the back and the scrotum and may be shelled out under local anaesthesia if uninfected or indeed enucleated through small incisions to provide optimal cosmetic results. Infected cysts should be treated by incision and drainage, with later excision to avoid recurrence.

Milia are tiny multiple epidermal cysts that occur on the face, particularly around the eyes, and can be shelled out for cosmesis.

Dermoid cysts

Dermoid cysts are congenital inclusion cysts that occur at points of fusion, particularly in the face. Their structure differs from epidermal cysts in that they show multiple skin appendages rather than epidermis alone. They can be treated by excision but are less readily enucleated than epidermal cysts.

Post-traumatic dermoid cysts result from implantation of epidermis and appendages under the skin surface by penetrating injury and are most common in the hands and fingers. Such cysts are often densely adherent to the underlying dermis but are readily excised.

Benign epidermal tumours

These are extremely common and arise from the epidermis itself, or more rarely from the skin appendages.

Seborrhoeic keratosis

Seborrhoeic keratoses are the most common of these lesions and occur on the trunk or limbs of the middle-aged or elderly. They develop initially as flat plaques with a waxy surface that progressively thickens, often with pigmentation due to haemosiderin deposition. Exuberant keratin and parakeratin production results from simple proliferation of keratinocytes for unknown cause, without any dermal involvement, so that the lesions are said to have a 'painted on' appearance. Their protruding nature means that the lesions can be traumatised, with subsequent low-grade infection. Such keratoses can be removed under local anaesthesia for this reason or for cosmesis.

Actinic keratosis

Actinic keratosis represents a progressive dysplastic change in the epidermis and the underlying dermis as the result of exposure to UV light. There is a build-up of excessive keratin and parakeratin, while the underlying dermis contains thickened elastic fibres (elastosis) produced by damaged fibroblasts. The lesions occur most commonly on exposed areas, such as the ears in the male, or the nose and the backs of the hands and forearms. They appear as rough crusty areas of thickening that may bleed when traumatised. Actinic keratoses are unquestionably premalignant, in contradistinction to seborrhoeic keratosis. They can be managed by the application of cytotoxic creams or by surgical excision if there is any suspicion that malignant change has already occurred.

Kerato-acanthoma

Kerato-acanthoma is a benign lesion that presents on the cheek, nose, ear or back of the hand in the elderly as a rapidly growing nodule which develops a characteristic central keratin plug. The lesions usually develop to several centimetres in diameter over the course of a few weeks and regress spontaneously and rapidly. They can thus be treated expectantly.

Kerato-acanthomas may occur in patients receiving immunosuppression, such as transplant recipients, and in these circumstances should be treated as squamous carcinoma because they may behave aggressively.

Malignant epithelial tumours

The most common tumours arise from the cells of the epidermis in the form of basal and squamous carcinomas and melanoma, which will be considered with pigmented lesions.

Basal cell carcinoma

Basal cell carcinoma (BCC) is the most common form of skin cancer and occurs almost exclusively in sun-exposed areas of the skin, in the adult white population over the age of 40 years. They are rare in the oriental population and almost never occur in black-skinned races.

Between 75 and 80% of the lesions occur in the head and neck, usually above a line running from the corner of the mouth to the ear, with the remainder being situated on the limbs and a minority on the trunk. Although the cell of origin was presumed to be the basal cell in the epidermis, it is probable that the true progenitor is a potential epithelial cell in pylosebaceous tissue. Exposure to UVB is believed to be the precipitating factor, and there is no clear genetic basis for the disease apart from race, except in some rare conditions such as the naevoid BCC syndrome, where BCC occurs in childhood, often in non–sun-exposed areas and with associated odontogenic cysts of the mandible, medulloblastoma and tumours of the reproductive organs.

Clinical presentation

Basal cell carcinoma presents in a wide variety of forms, but the most common is as a waxy translucent nodule with a thin overlying epithelium and a fine network of vessels traversing the margins, probably the result of tumour-induced angiogenesis. Central regression may lead to depressions in the centre of the lesion, which may progress to ulceration to show the classical 'rodent ulcer' appearance. The tumours may be multifocal and as they grow tend to become infiltrative and may involve deeper tissues. They may thus become locally aggressive but they do not metastasise except in very rare instances.

Treatment

Optimal treatment for nodular BCC depends on size. Lesions less than 1 cm in diameter are rarely deeply invasive and can be treated by electro-desiccation with curettage, by cryosurgery or by excision with a narrow margin in terms of depth and width. Radiotherapy is an alternative form of therapy but not in areas close to cartilage. Lesions greater than 1 cm in size are best treated by excision with peroperative confirmation of the margins of excision, which should not be less than 1 mm.

If treatment has been adequate, recurrence is rare, except in the case of sclerosing BCC, which may require multiple procedures to achieve control.

Squamous cell carcinoma

Squamous cell carcinoma (SCC) is the second most common tumour of the skin. The major aetiological factor is again exposure to UV light. Although such lesions are most commonly seen in the elderly, they are now becoming increasingly frequent in young adults because of excessive sun exposure in childhood. As expected from its aetiology, the lesions are most common in white populations and are seen most frequently on the face and ears, lip, the back of hands and forearms.

Clinical presentation

Clinical presentation is initially as an area of crusting that is clinically indistinguishable from solar keratosis but which on excision shows the cellular atypia that provides the diagnosis of carcinoma *in situ* before the breaching of the basement membrane at the dermoepidermal surface to form frank invasive carcinoma. If the lesions are untreated at this stage, they will progress to form a nodule or plaque that is irregular in shape and may ulcerate with a pink rolled edge. Unlike BCC, SCC can metastasise, usually to the regional lymph nodes but also systemically, although this is unusual unless the lesions are large or neglected. It should be noted that immunosuppression is associated with a much higher incidence of SCC, as for example in renal transplant recipients in whom the normal 4 : 1 ratio of BCC to SCC is reversed; BCC are also more common in such patients than in the normal age- and sex-matched population.

Treatment

Treatment of SCC is primarily surgical with excision to a margin of at least 0.5 cm in depth and laterally, as determined on clinical grounds, although this margin may be reduced in the head and neck because of cosmetic problems. If lesser margins are used, frozen section should be utilised to ensure that complete excision of the lesion has occurred. Tumour thickness is closely related to outcome. Local recurrence is unusual with lesions less than 4 mm in thickness and metastasis is more common in lesions which are greater than 10 mm in thickness (Table 41.1). Adjuvant radiotherapy is only used when the margins of excision are compromised by vital structures. Radiotherapy as a primary treatment is almost as effective as surgery but should be reserved for those patients not fit for surgery. As nodal involvement with cutaneous SCC is unusual, prophylactic lymph node dissection is not used and therapeutic dissection is only indicated when there are enlarged glands that prove on biopsy to demonstrate involvement with tumour. Prognosis is good, with at least 95% disease-free survival at 5 years. Local recurrence is rare as long as surgical excision has been adequate in the first instance.

Table 41.1 Excision margins related to tumour thickness

Thickness of melanoma	Stage (TNM)	Excision margin
In situ	pTis	5 mm
<1.5 mm	pT1, pT2	1 cm
1.5–4 mm	pT3	1–2 cm
>4 mm	pT4	2–3 cm

Pigmented lesions

Pigmented tumours of the skin are common. Their major importance is the propensity of some lesions to progress to the formation of melanoma, or the initial clinical differentiation from primary melanoma. A number of lesions that may become pigmented, such as seborrhoeic keratoses or basal cell carcinoma, have been dealt with previously.

Naevus

The term *naevus* should refer by definition to any congenital lesion of the skin, but by convention is used to describe any congenital or acquired neoplasm of melanocytes.

Acquired naevus

Acquired or naevo-cellular naevi are common. An Australian survey demonstrated 15 such lesions per person in an adult white Caucasian population. They are most common in sun-exposed areas of the body. They are formed by melanocytes that have been transferred from their usual dendritic single-cell position among the basal layers of keratinocytes to form aggregates along the dermo-epithelial junction. This aggregation of cells forms a junctional naevus. The cells of such naevi show little individual change, and mitotic figures are not numerous.

The clinical appearance of each form of naevus is thus important, although it must be understood that clinical interpretation of any skin lesion is not always accurate and such lesions must be subjected to excisional biopsy if there is any uncertainty about their nature. The junctional naevus is impalpable, pale to dark brown in colour and is usually small, rarely being more than 1 cm in diameter. They may appear in childhood but usually become obvious around puberty, growing slowly until the cessation of skeletal growth in late adolescence. In contrast, compound naevi are palpable, because of the size of the collection in the papillary dermis. These naevi are usually darker in colour than junctional naevi. The transitional phase between junctional and compound naevus means that some lesions show the characteristics of both.

Dysplastic naevus (DN)

Dysplastic naevi (BK-moles) occur as large (greater than 5 mm in diameter) flat macules or slightly raised plaques that are present in large numbers all over the body surface but with a particular concentration on the trunk. These naevi, in contrast to the naevi already described, are frequent in non–sun-exposed areas. They commonly have an irregular contour and variable colour, particularly being darker in the centre than on the periphery. Histologically, there is replacement of the normal basal cell layer of the epidermis by naevus cells at the dermo-epithelial junction with elongation of rete ridges. In the majority of cases there is a strong family history of such naevi and sometimes an additional family history of melanoma. Where there is an established family history of melanoma in association with DN, the trait is inherited in an autosomal dominant fashion. DN may be a pleiotrophic manifestation of the Ip36 familial melanoma gene, designated CMM1.

The management of such patients requires excisional biopsy of a typical lesion to establish the diagnosis, with genetic studies where appropriate and regular review with photographs and measurement of lesions for comparison, allowing excision of suspicious lesions at an early stage. Where there is no family history of melanoma, there is a much lesser chance of development of melanoma, and review can be less intense.

Juvenile naevus

Juvenile naevus (Spitz naevus) is most common in children and adolescents but may also occur in adults. It presents as a pink nodule that rapidly increases in size and on excision shows frequent mitoses and cellular pleomorphism which may raise questions of malignancy. Melanoma is comparatively rare in children and it is probable that some cases reported in the past have actually been Spitz naevi, which appear to have no malignant potential. However, this is not to say that melanoma does not occur in children. Indeed when it does occur it may be aggressive in its behaviour and have a poor prognosis.

Melanoma

Aetiology and pathology

Melanomas are made up of malignant cells arising from melanocytes in the skin but can also arise in oral and anogenital mucosa, and in the eye.

Cutaneous melanomas, like naevo-cellular naevi, are a disorder of white-skinned Caucasian populations, with the highest incidence being in white populations living close to the equator who are exposed to UV light during both work and recreation. There has been a rapidly increasing incidence in such populations, and even in susceptible populations in Northern Europe with a much lower regular exposure to sunlight. It is probable that this is a real increase in incidence rather than a process of earlier detection, although public education programmes now lead to much earlier presentation of the disease. The role of UV light is well established, with melanoma being most common in sun-exposed skin such as that of the upper back in males and females and also in the lower leg in females.

Melanoma can be classified into four types: lentigo maligna, superficial spreading, nodular, and acral lentiginous. As noted previously, a melanoma gene has been mapped to chromosome Ip36, and a second, designated CMM2, to chromosome 9p21, with the cell cycle regulator CDKN2A as the candidate gene.

Lentigo maligna

Lentigo maligna occurs in elderly patients, usually more than 70 years of age, and is more common in men than in women. It appears as an extensive melanotic lesion (Hutchinson's melanotic freckle) on the cheek or temple. It is characteristically dark brown in colour and develops over many years as a superficial impalpable lesion unless malignant change occurs. Malignant change is manifested by the development of palpable darker nodules within an irregular edge, and this change is often multicentric. Hutchinson's freckle itself requires no specific treatment apart from regular observation, but lesions demonstrating suspicious changes should be removed by excisional biopsy. If malignant on biopsy, the entire lesion should be widely excised. Prognosis is good, with at least 95% disease-free survival at 10 years. There is a tendency for lateral and superficial spread of tumours long before vertical invasion occurs.

Superficial spreading melanoma

Superficial spreading melanoma is the most common form of melanoma and can occur in any site and at any age, although it is most common in middle age and commonly arises from a pre-existing naevus as already discussed. Characteristically, it is slightly raised above the skin surface, is variegated in colour (often with a dark brown or even black component) and has an irregular edge. Over a variable period, the lesion remains within the epidermis and then involves the reticular dermis. It is rare for metastasis to occur at this phase of radial growth. If untreated, an invasive vertical growth phase supervenes, with progressive involvement of the deeper dermis and underlying tissues and the development of metastatic potential. It is now possible to use a variety of melanoma antigens to discriminate between benign melanotic lesions, *in situ* melanoma, the radial and vertical growth phases of invasive melanoma, and finally metastatic melanoma. These tests give clear indications of differences in cell behaviour at these various phases.

The treatment for superficial spreading melanoma is excisional biopsy with a margin that varies with the size of the primary lesion and subsequent assessment of depth of invasion. This is determined by the use of Clark's levels of invasion, which define six levels in terms of the anatomy of the epidermis and dermis, or by the thickness of the lesion, as described by Breslow. Although Clark's levels have some correlation with prognosis it is clear that the simple measurement of the thickness of the lesion gives an even better correlation. For those with a thickness of less than 0.75 mm, 95% 10-year survival can be expected. This contrasts with only 25% survival at 10 years if the thickness is greater than 4 mm. There has been much controversy about the margins of excision in the past. It had been felt that radical excision with at least a 5-cm margin was necessary for all melanomas, but it is clear that with superficial spreading melanoma, a limited margin is quite adequate.

There is also controversy about the role of elective lymph node dissection (ELND). On present evidence, as nodal metastasis is rare in lesions less than 1 mm in thick, ELND should not be performed in such cases. As patients with invasive lesions more than 4 mm thick are unlikely to survive in any event, the operation is superfluous.

Of particular interest has been the development of lymphotic mapping following intradermal injection of radiolabelled colloids around the primary site, with removal of "sentinel nodes" and histological and histochemical examination with subsequent full node dissection if positive. This procedure is being examined in a large multicentre, international trial and is not standard therapy.

Nodular melanoma

Nodular melanoma presents as its name suggests with a protruding lesion usually arising from a pre-existing naevus, the nodular form being one component of vertical invasion. The nodule may be dark or may be amelanotic. As it is really a particular form of invasive melanoma, it is treated on its merits in terms of thickness by wide local excision with consideration of TLND and adjuvant therapy.

Acral lentiginous melanoma

Acral lentiginous melanoma occurs in all races in non-pigmented areas, such as the palms of the hands, the soles of the feet, the subungual area and on mucous surfaces. They are often pink in colour with little in the way of pigmentation, and there is often delay in diagnosis because of this non-specific appearance. Treatment is as for superficial spreading melanoma, depending on the thickness of the lesion. Late presentation often means that there is a significant invasive element, and wide excision with or without adjuvant therapy may be necessary.

Adjuvant therapy

CHEMOTHERAPY

The benefits of combining surgery with adjuvant chemotherapy are now clear in relation to some cancers. This is undertaken in the belief that metastasis will often have occurred before patients present for primary surgery, although this may not be clinically apparent, and that systemic therapy is most likely to be effective in such patients when the bulk of tumour has been removed by surgery and the residual tumour burden is low.

LIMB PERFUSION

For melanoma of poor prognosis confined to a limb, an additional form of treatment aimed at controlling presumed intransit metastasis is perfusion of the isolated limb at high temperatures through an oxygenated circuit that contains phenylalanine mustard, which is selectively taken up by melanoma cells (at least in theory). The role of isolated limb perfusion (ILP) as an adjuvant to surgical treatment in primary treatment remains unclear until the results of a number of current randomised controlled trials are available.

RADIATION THERAPY

Radiation therapy has no role as an adjuvant to surgery for localised disease that is treatable by wide excision, but it is of value in the treatment of recurrent or inoperable disease with effective local control, particularly of nodal metastases.

IMMUNOTHERAPY

As melanoma is moderately immunogenic, it is reasonable to expect that active or passive immunotherapy might be of value, either as an adjuvant to the primary treatment of melanosis or in the treatment of disseminated disease. However, there is no current evidence from randomised controlled trials of value for such treatment, either alone or in combination with chemotherapy. Biological response modifiers have been investigated, but the only agent which has been shown to provide benefit is interferon-alpha-2b (IFN) in high-risk patients when administered over a 12-month period. IFN has major side effects, and further studies are being undertaken to determine whether lower doses are effective.

MCQs

Select the single correct answer to each question.

1 A 70-year-old man presents with a 1-cm painless nodule on the side of his nose. This has been present for 3 weeks. The centre of the lesion appears to contain a plug of hard skin. What is the most likely diagnosis?
a squamous cell carcinoma
b basal cell carcinoma
c keratoacanthoma
d Merkel cell carcinoma
e seborrhoiec keratosis

2 A 45-year-old motor mechanic presents with a nodule on the tip of his finger. This has been present for 12 months and it bothers him now when he presses on that finger. He seems to remember injuring that finger at work several years earlier. On examination there is a 0.5-cm nodule and the overlying skin is intact. What is the most likely diagnosis?
a dermoid cyst
b epidermoid cyst
c pyogenic granuloma
d dermatofibroma
e cylindroma

3 The parents of a 4-week-old boy are concerned about a lump above the infant's right eye. It has been present since birth and has not changed in size. The skin over the 1-cm lump is intact and the lump appears to be attached to the underlying tissues. What is the most likely diagnosis?
a dermoid cyst
b epidermoid cyst
c cystic hygroma
d branchial cyst
e osteoma

4 A 75-year-old man has what appears to be a 1-cm basal cell carcinoma on the side of his nose immediately below his left eye. What would be the most appropriate treatment?
a radiotherapy
b application of 5-fluorouracil cream
c injection of vinblastine
d excision and split-skin graft
e excision and full-thickness graft

5 A 17-year-old girl presents with a painless swelling on the anterior aspect of her right leg. This has been present for about 6 months and does not bother her much, except that it itches occasionally. The lump is pink and firm, and the overlying skin is intact. What is the most likely diagnosis?
a basal cell carcinoma
b epidermoid cyst
c Bowen's disease
d dermatofibroma
e malignant melanoma

42 Soft tissue tumours

Jonathan W. Serpell

Introduction

Soft tissue tumours are diverse in aetiology and diagnostic possibilities. The commonest cause is a simple lipoma, the majority of which will not require surgical excision. However, there is a rare group of tumours of soft tissue, referred to as soft tissue sarcomas, all of which are individually rare but which need to be diagnosed and treated appropriately, and which therefore must be distinguished from the common lipoma. The key management issues therefore, for a patient presenting with a soft tissue tumour, are the diagnosis of the underlying lump and then its appropriate management, so that the rare but important soft tissue sarcoma is recognised and treated appropriately.

Incidence

Soft tissue sarcomas are rare and occur in roughly the same degree of frequency as testicular cancers. They represent slightly less than 1% of all malignant tumours and occur at a rate of 2 cases per 100,000 population per annum. There are approximately 1200 new cases per annum in the United Kingdom, 6000 in the United States and about 200 in Victoria.

Apart from a small peak in infancy, soft tissue sarcomas are progressively more common with age, most occurring in patients older than 50. There is a slight male preponderance in incidence.

The childhood soft tissue sarcomas should be considered as a separate group as their behaviour and treatment is markedly different from other soft tissue sarcomas. The tumour most commonly affecting infants is the rhabdomyosarcoma, which usually occurs in the head and neck or the retroperitoneum. Unlike other soft tissue sarcomas, this tumour is sensitive to chemotherapy.

However, there is a diverse range of benign soft tissue tumours that may mimic soft tissue sarcomas and collectively these tumours are relatively common. Because of this the diagnosis of soft tissue sarcoma may be unsuspected at the time of presentation and an inappropriate biopsy performed.

Classification

Benign soft tissue tumours

Overwhelmingly the simple lipoma is the commonest tumour occurring in any site.

Other common soft tissue benign tumours include non-neoplastic lesions such as hamartomas, sebaceous cysts, inclusion dermoids, haematomas, seromas, fat necrosis, implantation dermoids, fracture callus, granulomata, degenerative cysts and ganglia, gouty tophi, rheumatoid nodules, lipodystrophy and infective cysts.

In addition, there is an extensive range of benign neoplasms which may also present clinically as a soft tissue lump. These can be classified according to tissue of orgin. Common examples in addition to lipomas, include neurofibromas, dermatofibromas and AV malformations, such as haemangiomas and varieties of lymphangioma (Table 42.1)

Intermediate-grade soft tissue tumours

These tumours include the desmoid tumour (aggressive fibromatosis), atypical deep lipomas (well-differentiated lipoma-like liposarcomas), and dermatofibrosarcoma protuberans.

These intermediate-grade tumours warrant separate classification from benign neoplasms and malignant neoplasms. They are analogous to basal cell carcinomas in the skin in the sense that they are locally malignant and recur locally, if inadequately excised. However, they do not metastasise.

Table 42.1 Benign neoplastic soft tissue lumps

Tissue of origin	Tumour
Adipocyte	Lipoma
Fibroblast	Fibroma
Blood vessel	Haemangioma
Lymph vessel	Lymphangioma
Smooth muscle	Leiomyoma
Synovial cell	Giant cell tumour of tendon sheath
Nerve cell sheath	Neurilemmoma Neurofibroma

Malignant soft tissue tumours

Classification

A classification of malignant soft tissue tumours is given in Table 42.2. Approximately 40 histological subtypes of soft tissue sarcomas are currently recognised, but the commonest varieties are liposarcoma, malignant fibrous histiocytoma (MFH), rhabdomyosarcoma, leiomyosarcoma, and synovial cell sarcoma.

Although they occur at all age levels, different histological subtypes predominate at different ages. For example, rhabdomyosarcoma is commonest in childhood and malignant fibrous histiocytoma tends to occur in the elderly.

The anatomical site may dictate the likely histological subtype. For example, liposarcoma is the commonest sarcoma in the thigh. (Fig. 42.1)

Table 42.2 Malignant soft tissue tumours

Soft tissue sarcomas	Liposarcoma Clear cell sarcoma Haemangio-epithelioma Epithelioid sarcoma Extra-skeletal myxoid condrosarcoma Fibrosarcoma Haemangiosarcoma Leiomyosarcoma Malignant haemangio-pericytoma Malignant fibrous histiocytoma Malignant peripheral nerve sheath tumour (MPNST or neurofibrosarcoma) Rhabdomyosarcoma Synovial sarcoma Sarcoma NOS (not otherwise specified)
Malignant soft tissue tumours other than soft tissue sarcomas	Extra-lymphatic soft tissue lymphoma Metastatic melanoma Metastatic carcinoma Extra-skeletal bone tumours

Soft tissue sarcomas develop in mesodermal tissues with a common histogenetic origin, although malignant peripheral nerve sheath tumours and primitive neuro-ectodermal tumours are of ectodermal origin. It is most useful to use a histogenetic classification of soft tissue sarcomas. Pathologists may have differing

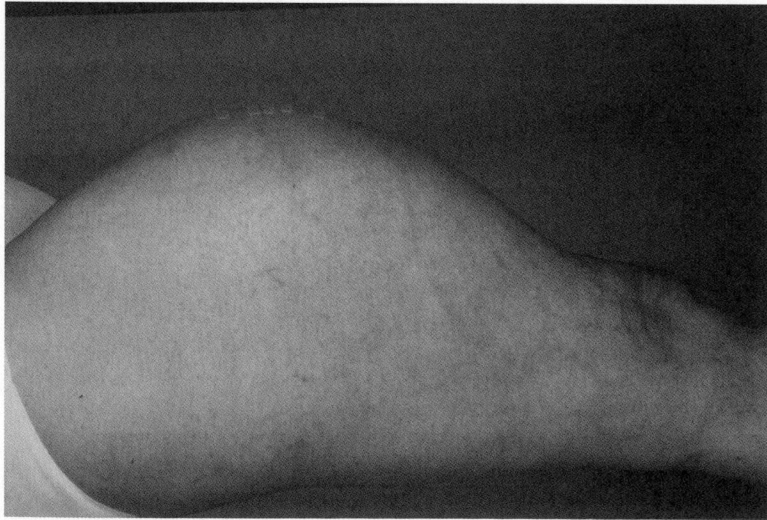

Fig. 42.1 Soft tissue sarcoma of the thigh.

opinions about the exact histological subtype, and it is generally accepted that even in expert hands 10% of tumours are not classifiable histologically. For diagnosing these tumours, immunohistochemistry, electron microscopy and cytogenetics may be helpful.

Soft tissue sarcomas may be usefully defined as malignant neoplasms of supporting connective tissue and muscle other than cartilage or bone, but may arise in any site in the body, excluding tumours of viscera but including tumours of peripheral nerves and rami. The definition therefore excludes, in addition to bone and cartilage, the anatomical sites of sarcomas of lymphoid organs, lymph nodes, viscera and the central nervous system. Also excluded are patients with Kaposi's sarcoma because the clinical presentation and the management of this disorder differs from that of other soft tissue sarcomas. Importantly, soft tissue malignant tumours due to lymphoma, melanoma, metastatic carcinoma such as lung cancer and extra-skeletal bone tumours must always be considered in the differential diagnosis of soft tissue sarcomas.

Site and grade

A number of features of soft tissue sarcoma follow a two-thirds to one-third rule in terms of proportion. Two-thirds of soft tissue sarcomas occur in the limbs and of these two-thirds occur in the lower limbs. Of these, two-thirds occur in the proximal compared to the distal limb. Therefore the commonest site of soft tissue sarcoma is in the thigh. Two-thirds of soft tissue sarcomas in the limbs occur deep to the deep fascia and it is for this reason that any soft tissue mass deep to the deep fascia is more likely to be malignant than benign. Sarcomas occur in the soft tissue compared to bone in the ratio of 2 : 1. Two-thirds of soft tissue sarcomas are of high grade. Various grading systems are employed, but the most useful classification is high-grade versus low-grade. High-grade tumours have a worse prognosis for survival than low-grade tumours. The distinction is also important for treatment. For example all high-grade tumours will usually be treated by surgery as well as radiotherapy; however, for some low-grade tumours radiotherapy may be avoided.

Surgical pathology

Soft tissue sarcomas grow differently to infiltrative carcinomas. They tend to be expansive and form a pseudo-capsule which is partly a fibrous tissue reaction, but partly also surrounding compressed host tissue. The pseudo-capsule, however, always contains malignant cells. Nonetheless, this gives a false impression of a capsule through which a tumour can be enucleated. This should not be undertaken because it always results in tumour cells being left behind. Soft tissue sarcomas tend to infiltrate along the planes of the least resistance and if arising in the centre of a particular muscle, for example, the rectus femoris in the thigh, the tumour will for a considerable time expand within the muscle rather than breaking through the fibrous capsule. For the same reason, the tumour tends to spread along blood vessels and nerves rather than invading them. These macroscopic patterns of growth have important implications for surgery in that if a tumour is confined to one muscle or one compartment in the limb, it is possible by removing that compartment or muscle that a complete excision of the tumour can be achieved. Unfortunately, only 15% of soft tissue sarcomas are appropriately confined to a single muscle or a compartment. The concept of treatment by compartmentectomy is therefore only applicable to about 15% of tumours. Nonetheless, it is a useful concept in understanding the biology of these tumours. Furthermore, vessels and nerves are rarely invaded and therefore vessels and nerves do not need to be sacrificed surgically.

Spread

Soft tissue sarcomas only rarely spread to lymph nodes (less than 5% of cases). Soft tissue sarcomas spread via the haematogenous route, and therefore the commonest site of metastases is pulmonary.

Clinical features

A problem-oriented history and examination are required. The onset and duration of the lump may be important, and a lump which is increasing in size suggests a neoplastic growth. Pain suggests inflammation, but up to one-third of soft tissue sarcomas present with pain. A detailed physical examination is required. There are a number of elements to such an examination.

First, the general features of any clinical lump are noted. These include the site/region, plane or depth, the size in three dimensions, the shape – whether this is regular or irregular, the surface and contour, the edge, the consistency and changes in the overlying skin and underlying fixation.

Second, any special regional features of the lump are noted. For example, distant neurovascular function for a tumour in the thigh.

Third, regional lymph nodes are assessed and finally a complete general examination is always essential.

Features of the commoner soft tissue tumours

Lipomas

Lipomas are the commonest form of benign soft tissue tumour. They are usually subcutaneous and present as soft, fluctuant, lobulated masses which are neither fixed to skin nor deep tissue. The clinical feature of deep fixation is important. The classic feature of a lump deep to the deep fascia in a limb is that it becomes less obvious on contraction of the muscle. The majority of lipoma are small and asymptomatic and will not require removal. Possible indications for removal of a lipoma would include a lipoma which is painful (commonly seen in the variant angiolipoma), an enlarging lipoma, a lipoma causing pressure effects on adjacent structures, a lipoma with any clinical, radiological, cytological or histological feature of concern, a lipoma larger than 5 cm in maximal dimension, and a lipoma deep to the deep fascia. In the limbs, a tumour which occurs deep to the deep fascia is more likely to be malignant than to be benign.

Angiolipomas

Angiolipomas are less common, but typically present with pain and histologically are a mixture of fat and blood vessels.

Dermatofibromas

Dermatofibromas (sclerosing haemangiomas) are characteristic dome-shaped nodules usually found in the upper leg of the middle aged and elderly. They consist of a mixture of mature fibrous tissue, histiocytes and vascular elements. They are benign and require no specific treatment except for cosmetic reasons or if there is doubt about their diagnosis.

Haemangiomas

Haemangiomas are hamartomas and are present at birth, although initially this may not be clinically apparent. Characteristically, enlargement occurs within the first year of life representing proliferation of excessive numbers of mature vessel elements. The endothelial line spaces form either capillary or cavernous lesions according to their size.

In the skin, strawberry haemangiomas have the appearance to be expected by their name, presenting with an irregular pitted surface with protrusions in the form of capillary tufts. Their variant is a more solid, smooth cherry haemangioma.

Cavernous haemangiomas of the skin are more deeply placed, more widely spread and irregular in shape, with a blueish, rather than red, appearance. All three forms blanch with pressure as is expected from their structure. All are self limiting by progressive obliteration and are usually replaced by mature fibrous tissue, sometimes a haemosiderin staining by the age of 6 years. Treatment in the form of surgical excision or obliteration by laser therapy is rarely indicated except for cosmetic reasons in exposed areas or for avoidance of bleeding in areas subjected to frequent trauma.

Lymphangiomas

Lymphangiomas are also hamartomas rather than true tumours and occur in capillary or cavernous forms. The carvernous form is commoner and is seen in the form of cystic hygroma of the neck, axilla or groin. There are usually superficial and deep components without a well defined capsule. Treatment is undertaken for cosmetic or pressure effects, with wide excision being necessary if there is to be no recurrence.

Neurofibromas

Neurofibromas are of diverse lineage including Schwann cells, perineural cells and fibroblasts. They occur sporadically as cutaneous nodules, usually associated with hyperpigmentation of peripheral nerves as solitary lesions. Much more commonly they form a component of neurofibromatosis Type I, a common disorder with an incidence of 1 in 3000, characterised by a strong family history combined with autosomal dominant transmission. The clinical features are multiple neurofibromas throughout the body (including the eighth nerve, pigmented lesions (café au lait spots) and pigmented iris hamartomas (Lisch nodules). The neurofibromas may be plexiform in nature and may grow to an enormous size. Such lesions may undergo malignant transformation, often presenting with rapid growth or major internal haemorrhage. There is an association with other tumours, especially meningiomas, gliomas and phaeochromocytomas.

Desmoid tumours

Desmoid tumours are so named from the Greek term *desmos*, meaning band- or tendon-like appearance of the cut surface of the tumour. Desmoid tumours are locally malignant but do not form a capsule and do not metastasise. They may be multi-centric, but because of their infiltrative nature have a high rate of local recurrence following surgery. The pathogenesis of desmoid tumours has been linked to trauma, sex hormones, particularly oestrogen, and familial adenomatous polyposis (FAP) and Gardner's syndrome.

About 2% of desmoids are FAP associated and patients with FAP are at about 1000-fold-increased risk for developing desmoids compared to the general population. Furthermore, the desmoids seen in FAP are often in the root of the mesentry and here may be termed mesenteric fibromatosis. Mesenteric fibromatosis is now the second most common neoplastic cause of death after colorectal cancer in patients with FAP and is more common than death due to peri-ampullary carcinoma.

Sporadic or non–FAP-associated desmoids are more common in women of childbearing age and are thought to be related to oestrogen hormones. Desmoid tumours are a variety of fibromatosis which are a group of pathologies resulting from proliferation of well-differentiated fibroblasts, which infiltrate and show repeated local recurrence, but are neither malignant nor inflammatory. They are locally malignant but do metastasise. Apart from desmoids, other fibromatoses include palmar fasciitis (Dupuytren's contracture), plantar fascitis, penile fibromatosis and keloids.

Kaposi's sarcoma

Kaposi's sarcoma is of unknown histogenesis, but is usually considered to be a form of angiosarcoma because of its structure: thin-walled, dilated vascular spaces with interstitial inflammatory cells with haemosiderin deposition. Four forms of the disease have been described.

First is the classical form described originally by Kaposi, in the form of pink to purple nodules in the skin of the lower extremities of adult patients of Eastern European origin. The tumours are locally aggressive, but rarely metastasise. The second form, African Kaposi's syndrome, is similar in appearance and behaviour but occurs in children and in young men in Africa. The third form occurs in transplant recipients, is more widespread and more aggressive, both locally and in terms of metastasis. This form of tumour usually regresses on cessation of immunosuppression. The fourth and now most common form of Kaposi's sarcoma is HIV associated and has a wide distribution, including visceral involvement. All four forms respond to cytotoxic chemotherapy with or without alpha-interferon, although HIV patients commonly die of intercurrent infection or develop further malignancies, usually in the form of lymphoma or leukaemia.

Investigation of soft tissue tumours

This will include radiology and biopsy.

Radiology

CT scanning and magnetic resonant imaging (MRI) are useful investigations to determine precisely the anatomical situation of a soft tissue sarcoma. In particular, the precise relationship to vessels and nerves will be well demonstrated by MRI. These studies are essential to the surgical planning of resection of the underlying tumour.

In addition, some tumours (both benign and malignant) have characteristic radiological features. For example, a pure lipoma will have a characteristic CT scan appearance. However, it is important to appreciate that radiology can never determine the underlying histological nature of a soft tissue mass (Fig. 42.2).

Ultrasound will confirm a soft tissue mass and often show the plane the mass is in; however, it is less helpful in determining precise anatomical relationships. It is of most use in obtaining ultrasound guided percutaneous core biopsies of soft tissue masses for histology.

The commonest site of distant metastases for soft tissue sarcomas is pulmonary and for this reason CT scanning of the thorax is essential to stage patients known to have a soft tissue sarcoma.

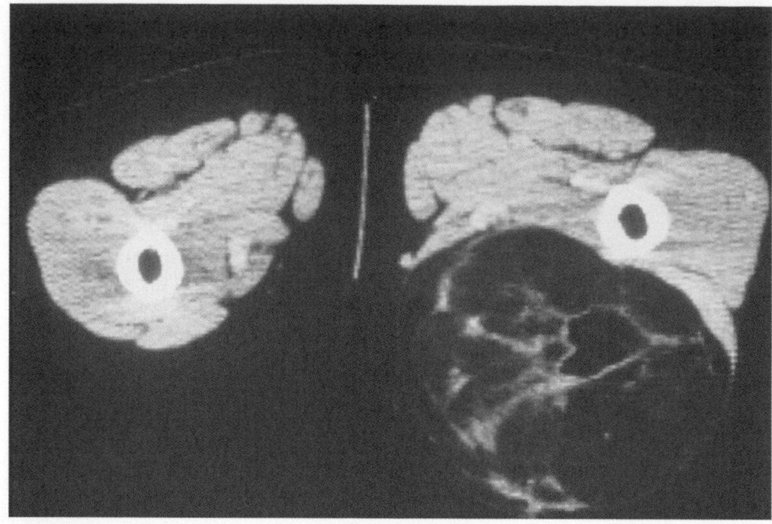

Fig. 42.2 CT scan of thigh, showing a large liposarcoma. There are some features to suggest lipoma; however, the heterogeneous nature of this lesion radiologically suggests the diagnosis of liposarcoma.

Biopsy

It is inappropriate to investigate all soft tissue tumours as if they were soft tissue sarcomas. It is estimated that for each soft tissue sarcoma diagnosed, 100 benign soft tissue lesions will be seen, and the majority of these will be lipomas. However, the differential diagnosis of soft tissue sarcoma versus lipoma must be considered in every case. Therefore, there needs to be a selective policy with regards to which tumours should be biopsied. In general, any tumour with clinical or radiological features of malignancy, a tumour which is growing, a tumour deep to the deep fascia or a tumour greater than 5 cm in size should be biopsied.

Biopsy is essential to obtain a specific diagnosis of the tumour, and for soft tissue sarcomas this will include the histological subtype and grade. This then enables a multidisciplinary planning of treatment and permits some prediction of prognosis.

Pre-operative percutaneous ultrasound guided core biopsies to provide histological diagnosis is becoming a more favoured technique, with the potential to facilitate one-stage surgery.

The principles of management of soft tissue sarcomas

The overall prognosis of soft tissue sarcomas is poor, with a mortality rate of 50% and a local recurrence rate of up to 25%. Nonetheless, with appropriate management many patients will be cured of their disease.

The goals of treatment are to achieve local tumour control, to prevent metastases and to preserve function.

The aim of the local treatment of soft tissue sarcomas is complete resection of the primary tumour with microscopically clear histological margins. Depending on the margin of resection, the recurrence rates vary. Local recurrence rates for amputation alone are 8% and for wide excision alone about 25%. However, when radiotherapy is added to this the local recurrence rates are reduced to rates approaching that following amputation. Therefore, there is no advantage in amputation as the local recurrence rate achieved is similar. When limb preservation function is preserved, a similar local recurrence rate is achieved and there is no difference in long-term survival. It is not currently believed that local recurrence influences overall survival in soft tissue sarcomas. Therefore, limb sparing treatment is usually possible in over 90% of patients with soft tissue sarcomas of the extremities.

Surgical margins following resection of soft tissue sarcomas are categorised as follows (Fig. 42.3). Intracapsular means that the lesion has been removed from within the pseudo-capsule and that gross tumour is seen at the wound margins. A marginal excision means that the tumour has been removed *en bloc* but that there is a significant possibility of tumour cells being left in the surrounding host tissue. A wide surgical margin means the lesion has been removed *en bloc* and that the plane of the resection has been sufficiently peripheral to the tumour to ensure clear histological margins.

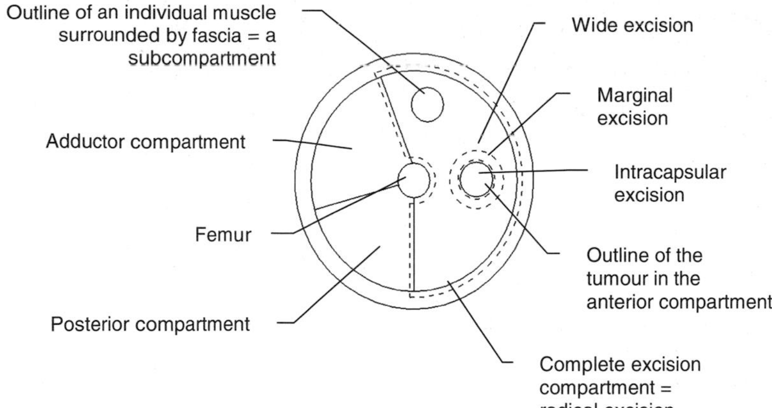

Fig. 42.3 Schematic diagram of surgical margins and compartments, based schematically on a transverse section of the thigh.

A radical resection means that the lesion and the entire compartment which it involves have been removed *en bloc*. The local recurrence rates following these resections are intracapsular 100%, marginal 90%, wide excision 25%, and radical excision 8%. These figures are reduced significantly by radiotherapy.

Therefore, wide excision with at least a 2–3-cm margin, with preservation of vessels and nerves and at least one innervated muscle of the functional compartment to preserve as much function as possible, followed by adjuvant post-operative radiation therapy is the contemporary approach recommended for most extremity soft tissue sarcomas. Desmoid tumours should be treated by a similar wide local excision with a clear 2–3-cm margin to reduce the incidence of local recurrence.

If local recurrence of a soft tissue sarcoma occurs, further surgery is often possible. Distant recurrences in the lungs are on occasion treatable by surgical resection (metastasectomy). Chemotherapy for metastatic soft tissue sarcoma disease may provide symptomatic relief, but has no effect on overall survival.

Desmoid tumours again represent a special group and in addition to surgery there has been some benefit demonstrated by post-operative radiotherapy and the use of agents such as tamoxifen and sulindac.

Prognosis of soft tissue sarcomas

Overall there is a 50% mortality for patients with soft tissue sarcomas, and the vast majority of patients die from metastatic disease. Factors shown to be of importance in predicting survival on multivariate analysis include the grade of the tumour, the size of the tumour, the adequacy of resection, local recurrence and the depth of the tumour.

These factors are, in general, related more to the biology of the tumour itself. Local recurrence will occur in up to 25% of patients, and factors associated with this on multivariate analysis include the adequacy of surgery and the resection margins, previous local recurrence, grade of the tumour and whether or not radiotherapy has been administered.

MCQs

Select the single correct answer to each question.

1 Soft tissue sarcomas are commonest in:
a the abdomen and retroperitoneum
b the head and neck
c the lower limb
d the upper limb
e the thorax

2 The commonest site of metastasis for soft tissue sarcomas is:
a regional lymph nodes
b liver
c bone
d lungs
e brain

3 Which of the following is an indication for removal of a lipoma?
a a 3-cm lipoma in the tibialis anterior

b a 3-cm lipoma in the subcutaneous fat of the anterior abdominal wall
c a 3-cm lipoma in the subcutaneous fat of the buttock
d a lipoma of many years standing which has not changed in size
e a lipoma on CT scanning of homogeneous density

4 Desmoid tumours:
a are increasingly commoner in woman as they age
b occur in the root of the mesentry in association with the FAP syndrome
c cause death by metastasis
d tend not to recur locally
e metastasise to regional lymph nodes

43 Infections of the extremities

David M. A. Francis

Introduction

Infections of the extremities range from common minor problems to unusual life-threatening disorders. Most patients have no serious underlying medical problem, but the possibility of undiagnosed disorders such as diabetes, immunodeficiency and vascular insufficiency must be considered.

Cellulitis

Cellulitis is a common infection of skin and subcutaneous tissues, most frequently caused by *Streptococcus pyogenes* and occasionally *Staphylococcus* species. Infection occurs after the skin is breached (e.g. insect bite, scratching, skin rash, minor trauma). Cellulitis may seem to occur spontaneously, although careful inspection reveals a break in the skin. Lower limb cellulitis is associated commonly with broken skin between the toes due to tinea pedis. Cellulitis may complicate pre-existing limb oedema. After subcutaneous inoculation, streptococci release toxins which permit rapid spread of organisms. The acute inflammatory response results in the clinical features of warmth, pain and tenderness, erythema, and oedema. Severe cellulitis may progress to suppuration and skin necrosis.

Differential diagnosis includes other causes of limb swelling, deep venous thrombosis, rupture of a Baker's cyst, calf haematoma and erythematous skin conditions.

Cellulitis of an extremity is treated by elevation and immobilisation with a splint or plaster 'back slab', and antibiotics. Penicillin (2 million units every 6 hours) or flucloxacillin (1–2 g every 6 hours) is given intravenously for 3–5 days and then continued orally for a further 10 days. Blood levels of penicillin may be increased by oral probenecid, which reduces renal excretion of penicillin. Erythromycin or a third-generation cephalosporin is used in patients with penicillin allergy. Any predisposing cause (e.g. tinea pedis) is treated vigorously. If cellulitis does not resolve rapidly, the antibiotic is increased or changed, a deep collection of pus is sort, and the diagnosis is reviewed.

Lymphangitis

Lymphangitis is associated with bacterial infections of extremities where the inflamed lymphatic vessels appear as several thin, red, tender lines on the slightly oedematous skin progressing towards the regional lymph nodes which are enlarged and tender (lymphadenitis). Lymphangitis usually is caused by streptococci and staphylococci. Chemical lymphangitis may result from irritative compounds used for lymphangiography.

Treatment is the same as for cellulitis, consisting of rest and elevation of the extremity and antibiotics. Rarely, suppurative regional lymph nodes require surgical drainage.

Folliculitis, furuncles and carbuncles

'Folliculitis' refers to infection with pus formation within a hair follicle and is limited to the dermis. It may be extensive if many follicles are infected over a wide area, such as the face.

A 'furuncle' is infection of a small number of hair follicles within a small confined area. A 'carbuncle' is an abscess involving a number of adjacent hair follicles where the infection has penetrated through the dermis and formed a multiloculated subcutaneous abscess between the fibrous septa which anchor the skin to the deep fascia. Furuncles and carbuncles occur most frequently on the back of the neck, lower scalp, and the torso. Abscesses on the upper part of the body are usually caused by staphylococci, while infections below the umbilicus are due largely to aerobic and anaerobic coliform organisms.

Local hygiene is usually sufficient to treat folliculitis, although antibiotics are required for extensive infections. Furuncles and carbuncles require incision and drainage. Fibrous tissue septa must be broken down so that all pockets of pus can be drained completely. Antibiotics are indicated for severe and spreading infections, and in immunocompromised patients.

Hidradenitis suppurativa

Hidradenitis suppurativa refers to infection of apocrine sweat glands, and occurs in the axillae, around the external genitalia, and the inguinal and perianal regions (see Chapter 31). Apocrine sweat glands have tortuous secretory ducts within the skin and produce thick secretions, and infection occurs when ducts become blocked, most commonly during excessive glandular activity at adolescence. Staphylococci or Gram-negative bacilli and anaerobes are causative organisms.

Patients present with multiple small but painful abscesses and sinuses, often bilaterally. Repeated or long-standing infection results in considerable scarring, which hinders resolution. Antibiotic therapy alone is often inadequate, although long-term antibiotic therapy may be useful in suppressing acute infections. Abscesses require incision and drainage. Excision of the affected hair-bearing area and the subcutaneous fat usually is required, and results in good symptomatic relief.

Paronychia

Acute paronychia (Whitlow) is a subcuticular abscess of the nail fold. Infections, usually due to staphylococci, follow minor injury to the nail fold, and begin as cellulitis. Pus forms around the nail fold (Fig. 43.1) and may extend around the whole periphery of the nail, causing pain and inflammation extending proximally from the nail fold towards the distal interphalangeal joint.

Treatment consists of flucloxacillin and, if pus is present, drainage under digital local anaesthetic block using lignocaine without adrenaline and a finger tourniquet. The nail fold is lifted away from the nail to expose the edge of the nail which is excised to allow the pus to drain.

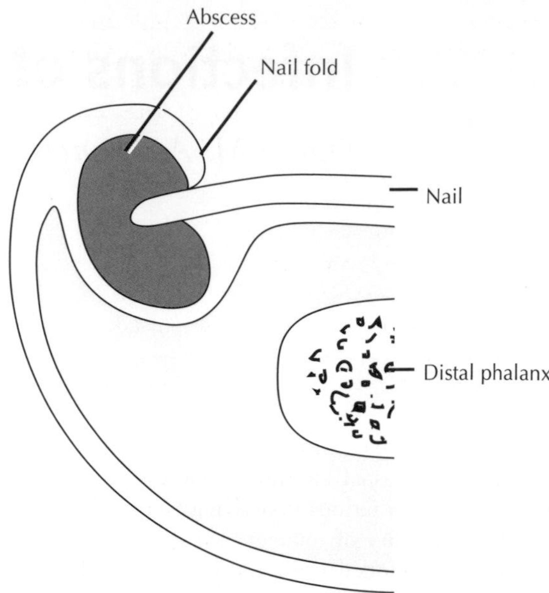

Fig. 43.1 Transverse section of acute paronychia with subungual extension.

Chronic paronychia is a fungal infection of the nail fold. The nail becomes loose and deformed, and ridged or pock-marked. The nail fold is grossly thickened, and the cuticle is absent. Treatment consists of removal of the nail and long-term oral treatment with antifungal medication (e.g. griseofulvin). A subungual amelanotic melanoma may be misdiagnosed as chronic paronychia.

Pulp space abscess

A pulp space abscess (Felon) is a subcutaneous abscess of the pulp overlying the terminal phalanx (Fig. 43.2). It follows a minor penetrating injury (e.g. thorn or pin

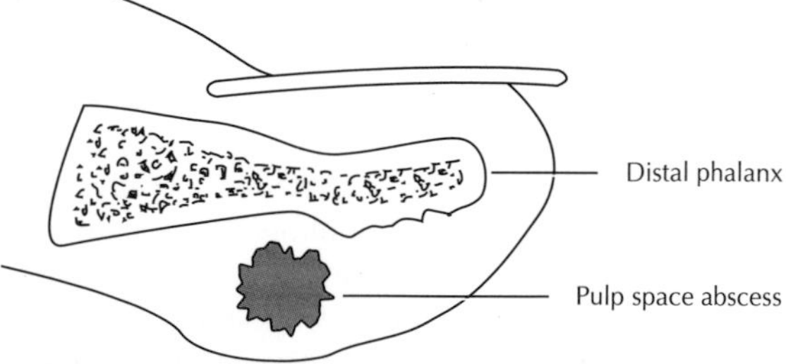

Fig. 43.2 Longitudinal section of the finger tip with a pulp space abscess.

prick), and starts as cellulitis and develops as subcutaneous pus forms. The overlying skin changes from red to a mauve-blue colour, implying imminent necrosis. Sloughing of pulp tissue, lymphangitis, acute suppurative tenosynovitis, and osteomyelitis are potential complications.

Treatment requires antibiotics and drainage of pus. When the abscess is small, an incision is made along the side of the pulp and deepened into the pulp space, breaking down the fibrous septa between the distal phalanx and the skin to ensure complete drainage. When the abscess is pointing to the centre of the pulp, the incision is made over it.

Pyomyositis

Pyomyositis is a purulent infection of skeletal muscle. The infection may complicate a penetrating injury (e.g. needle puncture), blunt trauma close to an infective skin lesion, or a spontaneous bleed into muscle (e.g. in an anticoagulated patient). Severe local pain, fever and inability to move the extremity are characteristic. Pyomyositis requires intensive antibiotic treatment, and aspiration or surgical drainage of pus.

Synergistic gangrene

Terminology

'Synergistic gangrene' refers to a group of soft tissue infections (not necessarily restricted to the extremities) characterised by tissue necrosis and caused by several species of microorganisms acting synergistically. Previous nomenclature (necrotising fasciitis, necrotising erysipelas, Meleney's gangrene, Fournier's gangrene, non-clostridial gangrenous cellulitis) was confusing and attempted to associate a characteristic clinical syndrome with a bacteriological diagnosis.

Clinical features

Synergistic gangrene is caused by micro-aerophilic streptococci acting synergistically with aerobic staphylococci, with or without Gram-negative bacilli. It usually occurs in debilitated patients with other disorders (e.g. diabetes, malnutrition, alcoholism, liver disease, renal failure, malignant disease, immune compromise).

Box 43.1 Treatment of synergistic gangrene

- Wound management – surgical excision of gangrenous tissue, inspect wounds frequently for signs of further tissue necrosis.
- Antibiotics – high-dose, intravenous broad-spectrum antibiotic treatment (penicillin, third-generation cephalosporin and metronidazole), changed according to culture results.
- Supportive therapy – septic shock is treated with oxygen, intravenous fluids, correction of metabolic acidosis, circulatory support, blood transfusion, artificial ventilation, haemofiltration (as required).

Synergistic gangrene presents initially as cellulitis with severe pain which is out of keeping with the minor local clinical signs but consistent with the seriousness of the condition. Infection spreads rapidly along fascial and subcutaneous planes without a severe inflammatory reaction. Bacterial toxins cause tissue and skin necrosis. Crepitus occurs when gas-forming organisms are present. Signs of systemic sepsis and toxaemia occur quickly.

'Fournier's gangrene' is the name given to synergistic gangrene involving the perineum and scrotum. It may be extensive and involve the abdominal wall and buttocks, and is a rare complication of anorectal and perineal surgery, trauma or minor infection.

Treatment

Synergistic gangrene must be treated urgently by debridement of necrotic tissue, antibiotics and general supportive therapy (Box 43.1).

Clostridial infections

Clostridial infections are unusual but serious. They include clostridial myonecrosis and cellulitis, and are not limited to the extremities. 'Gas gangrene' is a confusing term often used to describe infective gangrene with subcutaneous gas production by organisms that are assumed to be clostridial, but in fact most gas-producing infections are not clostridial. Strictly speaking, 'gas gangrene' refers to clostridial myonecrosis and cellulitis with gas formation.

Clostridia are anaerobic, spore-forming Gram-positive bacilli found in soil, manure, marine sediment, decaying plants and animals, and the colon. When a wound is contaminated with clostridia, the likelihood of infection depends on:

- inoculum size
- virulence of the clostridial strain
- conditions within the wound being conducive to clostridial multiplication and tissue invasion (e.g. open fractures, deep wounds, haematoma, ischaemic or devitalised muscle and tissue, foreign bodies especially soil).

Clostridia produce potent exotoxins (haemolysin, collagenase, hyaluronidase, lecithinase and proteolytic enzymes) which cause tissue destruction and facilitate bacterial spread.

Clostridial infections are prevented by adequate initial treatment of contaminated wounds, antibiotics and passive immunisation (Box 43.2). Treatment of established infection is by urgent surgical debridement of the wound, high-dose antibiotics, and supportive therapy with or without hyperbaric oxygen (Box 43.2). Mortality is high (25–40%) and associated with delayed diagnosis and treatment, severity of septic shock, poor medical condition prior to infection, and failure to control infection at the first operation.

Box 43.2 Prevention and treatment of clostridial infections

Prevention

- Adequate initial wound care – excise all devitalised tissue, remove foreign bodies and blood clot, wash with antiseptic solution, leave wounds open, inspect and dress frequently.
- Antibiotics – high-dose, intravenous penicillin (e.g. 10 million units every 4–6 hours) if clostridial infection is considered possible or if patient is at risk for clostridial infection during surgical procedures (e.g. diabetics undergoing amputation for infected gangrene).
- Passive immunisation with polyvalent antiserum (efficacy is unproven).

Treatment

- Urgent wound debridement – excise all necrotic and involved tissue, leave wound open, inspect frequently, repeat debridement as often as necessary.
- Intravenous high-dose penicillin (10 million units every 4–6 hours).
- Supportive therapy.
- Hyperbaric oxygen – efficacy is unproven, hyperbaric therapy must not delay or take precedence over urgent surgical treatment and resuscitation.

Clostridial myonecrosis

Clostridial myonecrosis is a rare, acute infection of muscle. In civilian hospital practice, it occurs in inadequately debrided traumatic wounds and in amputation stumps in diabetics and vasculopaths.

After inoculation, clostridia multiply and release exotoxins which disrupt tissues and increase capillary permeability, and produce profound systemic toxaemia. Infected muscle is initially inflamed, oedematous and friable, and rapidly becomes necrotic. Overlying skin has a marbled mauve appearance and later turns black. Gas may be present in the tissues. The wound discharges a thin, non-purulent fluid with a characteristic sickly sweet smell. The limb is severely painful, and septic shock, haemolysis and jaundice develop rapidly. The incubation period is 1–3 days, but once infection is established, the wound appearance and systemic toxaemia develop over a few hours.

The diagnosis of clostridial myonecrosis must not be delayed because mortality increases dramatically when treatment is not instituted urgently. Diagnosis is made on the clinical setting and appearance of the extremity, and confirmed by urgent microscopy of a wound swab, which reveals numerous Gram-positive bacilli and few leucocytes.

Clostridial cellulitis

Clostridial cellulitis is an infection of subcutaneous or extraperitoneal tissues. It spreads rapidly along tissue planes, causes small vessel thrombosis and tissue necrosis, but does not involve underlying muscle. Subcutaneous gas may form. Wounds have a foul-smelling serosanguinous discharge. Pain, tissue swelling and systemic toxaemia are of moderate severity.

Further reading

Williams JD, Taylor EW, eds. *Infections in Surgical Practice.* London: Arnold; 2003.

Bleck TP. Clostridium tetani. In: Mandell GL, Bennett JE, Dolin R, eds. *Principles and Practice of Infectious Diseases.* Philadelphia: Churchill Livingstone; 1995:2173–2178.

Lorber B. Gas gangrene and other clostridial-associated diseases. In: Mandell GL, Bennett JE, Dolin R, eds. *Principles and Practice of Infectious Diseases*. Philadelphia: Churchill Livingstone; 1995:2182–2195.

MCQs

Select the single correct answer to each question.

1 Cellulitis:

a is occasionally caused by Gram-negative coliforms
b often occurs spontaneously without any apparent cause or organism
c is treated with rest, immobilisation and high-dose penicillin
d frequently requires surgical drainage
e is often complicated by suppuration and skin necrosis

2 Fournier's gangrene:

a is a form of pyomyositis
b occurs mainly in debilitated patients and can be life-threatening
c is usually due to stapylococcal infection
d can be treated by hyperbaric oxygen alone
e is seldom managed surgically

3 Hidradenitis suppurativa:

a is a complication of cystic fibrosis
b rarely occurs in the axillae or groin
c may be associated with pilonidal sinus
d chronic cases are improved by excisonal surgery
e antibiotics have no role in management

4 Clostridial infections:

a are common in domestic gardeners
b can usually be treated expectantly
c are nearly always confined to HIV-positive patients
d advanced infections resolve with hyperbaric therapy alone
e require urgent surgical debridement

44 Principles of plastic surgery

Wayne Morrison

Definition

The term *plastic surgery* is derived from the Greek 'to shape or mould' and refers to that field of surgery which reconstructs defects caused by trauma, cancer removal, burns or disease processes. These deformities may be congenital or acquired, cosmetic or functional. The basis of reconstruction is the science and art of moving tissues, most commonly flaps of skin and subcutaneous tissue, from one site to another. This demands a knowledge of skin and muscle blood supply as well as the skill and experience to anticipate the behaviour of tissues subjected to these processes, especially their laxity, mobility and healing capacities.

History and development of plastic surgery

In approximately 600 BC the Hindu surgeon Shushruta described a technique for nose reconstruction using a long tongue of forehead skin based between the eyebrows that was twisted around to reach the nose tip. Rediscovered during the British occupation of India, it became known as the Indian rhinoplasty. The Italian method of rhinoplasty (Tagliacozzi, 16th century) involved a staged operation where a tube of skin and fat was lifted up from the medial surface of the upper arm and inset into the nasal defect. Development of techniques for reconstruction occurred rapidly from the 19th century onwards. Flaps to the face were described and split skin grafting and full-thickness skin grafts were developed. The need to repair war injuries led to the development of the tube pedicle. The groin flap with its axial vascularisation from a single artery and vein rather than the traditional random pattern was described and paved the way for long, narrow flaps with wide arcs of rotation, which could in many cases obviate the need for a tube pedicle. Microsurgeons who had perfected microvascular anastomosis of small vessels permitting replantation of amputated parts and toe transfers, investigated the microvascular transfer of flaps. The axial vessels feeding such flaps could be isolated, divided and re-anastomosed at the site of the defect. This form of flap transfer became known as a free flap and revolutionised plastic surgery. Musculocutaneous flaps such as the latissimus dorsi and the transverse rectus abdominis myocutaneous (TRAM) flaps were developed and have become the mainstay for breast reconstruction.

Wound healing

Effective wound healing is the basis of all surgery. When wounds do not heal the reason is generally obvious, and is usually associated with inadequate blood supply to the area. Haematoma, excessive tension, foreign body and irradiation all predispose to ischaemic necrosis and wound breakdown. This in turn leads to infection. Reducing infection by the recent innovation of vacuum applied to sponge dressings (vacuum-assisted wound healing) has been shown to dramatically speed healing of contaminated, chronic wounds, such as bed sores, by decreasing oedema, reducing bacterial count, debriding dead tissue and producing a moist environment for epithelialisation.

Recent research is directed towards maximising wound healing and minimising scar formation. Transforming growth factor-β (TGF-β) has been implicated in scar states, such as hypertrophic scar and Dupuytren's contracture. The absence of TGF-β in the early foetus may explain the relative reduction of scarring that occurs in foetal wounds. TGF-β blocking agents are now being developed to reduce adult scarring.

Principles of wound suture

The aim of suturing is to approximate wound edges meticulously in layers so that dead space is eliminated and minimal scar is required to bridge the gap. Damaged skin margins should be resected. Sutures should be placed vertically through the tissues to approximate the full depth of the wound and should be the least number and least calibre required to maintain closure. They should be close to the wound edge and be removed before cross-hatching marks can occur. Subcuticular sutures will avoid cross-hatching, but will not necessarily prevent stretching. More problems occur through removal of sutures too soon than leaving them too long. Elderly people scar less than the young, but are slower to heal, hence sutures should be left in longer. As a general rule, facial sutures should be removed at approximately 1 week and sutures elsewhere at 10 days. Where tissue is missing, suturing under tension may lead to suboptimal scarring, often inducing hypertrophic reaction that will resolve to a wide, stretched scar. Alternatively, tension may result in distortion of local anatomy, especially in the face, causing ectropion or asymmetry. Primary skin grafting or flap repair may obviate the problem, but these techniques create scars in their own right and ultimately it is experience and aesthetic sense that determines the correct procedure.

Placement of incisions

Incisions are used to excise skin lesions and to gain access to deeper structures. In either case their design should be directed towards minimising and disguising scars. Fine scars in or parallel to facial crease lines (Langer's lines), especially in older patients, may be almost imperceptible. Not only do they give the illusion of crease lines, but they remain narrow because they are transverse to the direction of the facial muscles and hence minimise the tension across the scar. Lesions such as naevi, birthmarks and skin cancers should be excised in an elliptical form with their axis in the direction of Langer's lines; that is, the line of least tension or maximum laxity. Although in the trunk and limb Langer's lines are more obscure, the same principle applies.

Incisions should not transgress cavities or flexion creases. Because all linear scars contract, an incision in such sites will heal with webbing and tenting of skin across the hollow and cause contracture or limitation of full extension across joints. Incisions should therefore curve around the concavity or be closed in a fashion that achieves lengthening or relaxation of the line. Such a technique is z-plasty.

The z-plasty closure

Z-plasty closure is most commonly employed to release scar contractures. Along the course of the incision back cuts are made on either side into the adjacent skin at 60° and parallel with each other. The length of the back cuts equals the length of the original incision so that a z-shaped incision now pertains (Fig. 44.1A). The two triangular flaps so created are lifted and interdigitated with each other so that the incision line now forms a new z, with its central axis transverse to the original line of the incision (Fig. 44.1B,D). When used to release contractures, excision of the longitudinal scar along the central line of the z causes immediate springing apart of the incision in a longitudinal direction (Fig. 44.1C). This causes the elevated flaps to automatically transpose into each other's defect, as the axis of the parallelogram lengthens from a transverse to a vertical one. This manoeuvre effectively imports lax tissue laterally into the longitudinal axis and obviously can only work if there is lateral tissue available. Z-plasties not only lengthen scars but also redirect them. This has an important application in camouflaging long scars, especially in the face.

Scars including hypertrophic scars (keloid)

Scars are the trademark of the surgeon. Scars can be minimised but not eliminated. Whenever the skin is breached to the level of the deep dermis there will be a scar forever. The site of the scar determines its nature, rather than how it was created or who repairs it. The eyelid skin may almost leave invisible scars, but rarely elsewhere. The prepectoral region is the worst area in the body for scarring, producing a predictable hypertrophic response commonly seen following midsternal splitting for cardiac surgery. The scar becomes red, raised, hard and welted, and patients complain of intense itch and tearing. The scar base widens and over the course of a year or so gradually softens, flattens, becomes paler and symptom-free, but the patient is left with a permanent, wide, welted scar. This is largely incurable, in that attempts to excise it only reproduce

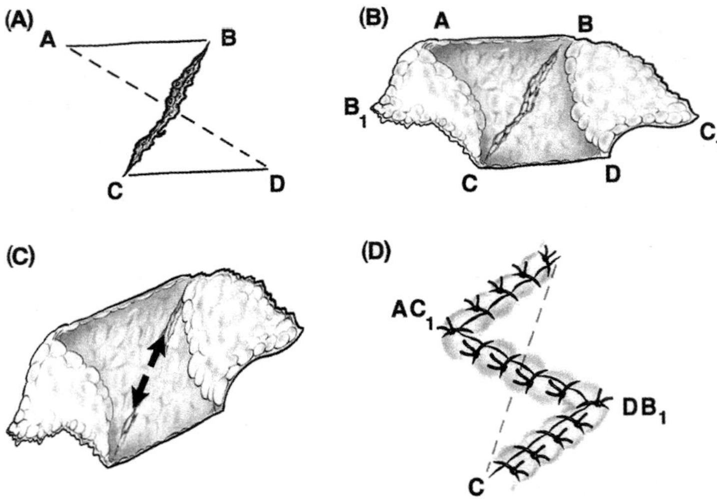

Fig. 44.1 Z-plasty. (A) Design of z-plasty. Length of limbs AB = BC = CD, with BC representing the scar to be reoriented. Angles ABC = BCD = 60° in this design. The AD crosses the scar at 90° and outlines the new central axis of the 'z' following flap transposition. (B) Incisions and elevation of triangular flaps. A parallelogram-shaped defect is formed. (C) With release of the scar contracture, the tension within the skin lengthens the wound at the expense of width. (D) Flaps transpose automatically with release of scar. Scar is now re-oriented perpendicular to originial position.

the circumstances that led to its formation in the first place.

The proper management is to await nature's resolution. Time is a scar's best friend and revisional surgery should be postponed, generally for 6–12 months to assess nature's final result. Silicone gel pressure pads or judicious use of cortisone injection may hasten what nature will eventually do. Cortisone injection is best reserved for symptomatic scars as it risks worsening the cosmetic result by excessive thinning of the scar tissue, leading to transparent, wide, concave scars often with telangiectasia. Scars elsewhere in the body are relatively predictable. The face generally heals with fine scars; neck and ears less so. Ear lobe piercing not uncommonly results in hard, keloid-like lumps often misdiagnosed as cysts. The shoulders and deltoid region, upper back and knees are also notorious for hypertrophic reaction and stretching. The middle and lower back always leave depressingly wide, stretched scars but they are rarely hypertrophic. The upper abdomen frequently passes through a reactive, thickened phase eventually settling to a wide, flat scar; the lower abdomen much less so. Transverse abdominal scars are better than vertical ones. Limb scars are intermediate in their reaction to injury, while hand and foot scars are generally fine. Scars on the sole however can present a unique problem owing to intense hyperkeratotic reaction that can be intractable. This is presumed to be a function of pressure and tension.

Revisional surgery cannot make scars invisible nor can any other technique. All surgery is designed to camouflage the scar so that it is mistaken for a natural line. Theoretically, long scars can be broken up by multiple shorter scars, partly directed into the crease lines by z-plasty (see above). This is particularly useful if the scar crosses natural crease lines. Pigmented, lumpy or wide scars can be excised and sutured to be flatter and narrower, but as stated previously the outcome is related to the site and nature of the skin. Multiple patches of scar can be excised as one and closed in a linear fashion. Stepped, indented and pin-cushion scars can be excised and closed with multiple z-plasties to restore smooth contour. Redness of a scar is worsened by surgery. Time will fade scars, but occasionally laser may speed the process of capillary obliteration.

Tissue transfer

Tissue transfer generally involves skin grafts and flaps to cover a skin defect.

Grafts

A graft is a piece of tissue that is totally detached from the body and after reapplication comes back to life. Its survival depends on revascularisation from its bed. Avascular beds (e.g. bare tendon, bone, ligament, irradiated tissue, ischaemic ulcers) will prevent graft take. Fluid collection between the graft and its bed, such as haematoma, seroma or pus, will prevent revascularisation and traditionally a pressure dressing is applied to the graft to maximise adhesion to the bed. Grafts survive the first few hours by plasmatic imbibition; that is, diffusion of nutrients from the bed. Within hours inosculation occurs, where the transected capillary ends in the graft physically link with those in the bed to achieve end-to-end vascular connections. Blood flow through these is seen by 24 hours. True angiogenesis follows with the establishment of a new vascular pattern and blood flow within the graft.

Classification of grafts

SPLIT SKIN GRAFTS

A split skin graft is shaved with a knife at a dermal level that includes elements of the epidermis and dermis proportional to its thickness. The split skin graft donor site heals spontaneously because dermal elements remain and permit regeneration. The graft quality depends on its thickness, but hair and sweat gland function is not usually transferred. Sensation returns to the graft by ingrowth from its bed. Split skin grafts are indicated where large areas of skin are required, such as burns or degloving injuries or where the graft bed has relatively poor vascularisation, and a thin graft has the best potential for survival. There are several deficiencies of split skin grafts, including graft contracture, poor contour and colour match, and problems with donor site healing. Split skin grafts can be meshed; that is, multiple perforations applied by passing it through a special roller. This allows expansion of the graft for a greater area of cover. Also the perforations permit fluid through the graft to prevent separation from its bed.

FULL-THICKNESS GRAFTS

Full-thickness grafts include all layers of the skin down to the level of the dermal fat. No skin element remains in the bed and therefore the donor defect must be closed. This usually limits the permissible size and sites to regions where there is sufficient loose skin to allow direct suture closure, for example, the groin crease, wrist crease and postauricular region. Full-thickness grafts contract little and retain their colour and texture so that the site can be selected to match the defect. Grafts from behind the ear are particularly valuable in the face for eyelid and nasal bridge reconstruction. Full-thickness grafts revascularise by the same process as split skin grafts.

MUCOSA

Buccal cheek, septal, tongue, vermilion and vaginal tissue can be used as full-thickness grafts for specific reconstruction.

CARTILAGE

Cartilage is normally avascular and survives by diffusion of nutrients. When grafted it generally retains its shape and volume, but is inert. Its surface becomes incorporated into surrounding tissues by vascular ingrowth. It is used for nasal and ear reconstructions and the usual sources include rib, concha and septum.

BONE

Bone grafts act as a scaffold for ingrowth of new bone from the adjacent intact bone bed. Cancellous grafts include stem cells and growth factors, especially bone morphogenic proteins that stimulate osteoblasts. Cortical bone adds strength and stability until living replacement is complete. In long bones, compressive forces then mould the bone stress lines according to Wolf's law, so that strength is restored. Sources of cancellous bone include iliac crest and lower radius; cortical bone grafts are usually fibula or cranial bone.

TENDON

Tendon is essentially avascular and survives grafting almost *in toto*. Finger flexor tendon grafts within their flexor sheath are nourished by synovial diffusion. Blood supply, initially at least, is confined to the repair sites proximally and distally, where capillary ingrowth is accompanied by scar adhesions. Gradually an intrinsic blood supply probably develops within the core of tendon.

NERVE

When a nerve is grafted, the axons are resorbed (Wallerian degeneration) but the Schwann cells, which are the key to axonal regeneration, survive along with the perineurial and endoneurial tubes. The Schwann cell changes phenotype initially to a macrophage-like scavenger cell and then converts to a myelin-producing cell once new axon sprouts appear in the graft. When myelination is complete the Schwann cell reverts to its stable supportive role. Thick nerve grafts, such as nerve trunks, undergo central necrosis when grafted because of insufficient revascularisation. Thin grafts only are clinically useful; for example, sural or medial cutaneous nerve of the forearm. These can be cut into multiple segments and laid side by side to match the volume of larger nerves. They are then known as cable grafts and have been shown to be revascularised within 4 days.

COMPOSITE GRAFTS

Any combination of structures can theoretically be grafted, but the thicker the graft the less likely the vascular bed will be able to penetrate it before necrosis occurs. The most common and most valuable composite grafts include skin and cartilage from the ear for nasal rim repair, and mucosa and cartilage from the nasal septum for eyelid reconstruction.

Flaps

A flap is a piece of tissue, usually skin and subcutaneous fat, which is transferred from one site to another but at all times retains its own blood supply. Unlike a graft it is independent of the vasculature of its bed and it is often indicated for reasons of poor vasculature where skin grafts will not take, for example, over bare tendon or bone, irradiated tissue or chronic scars. Other merits of flaps over grafts, especially in the face, include their close approximation to the qualities of the defect in terms of colour, texture and, particularly, thickness and contour. Cosmetically, therefore, flaps are generally superior to grafts, except for eyelid, inner canthal and nasal bridge defects where full-thickness grafts from behind the ear are ideal. Successful flap transfer is based on a knowledge of skin, blood supply in the various parts of the body and an understanding of the intrinsic properties of the skin with respect to mobility, elasticity and healing potential.

Classification of flaps

ACCORDING TO METHOD OF TRANSFER

Local flaps: For local flaps, tissue immediately adjacent to the defect to be reconstructed is mobilised as a flap and inset into the defect. The secondary defect can usually be closed directly without grafting. These flaps are typically used in the face and head and neck region. They are a single-stage procedure.

Distant flaps: Where no local flap is available, tissue from a distance must be transferred. Flaps from the groin or abdomen are typically used to resurface large skin defects, especially of the hand. The flap is sutured around the circumference of the defect, effectively joining the hand to the abdomen. This posture is maintained until sufficient blood supply has grown into the flap from the periphery on the hand side to allow safe detachment from the abdomen. Usually a minimum of 3 weeks is required before detachment. Other distant flaps include cross finger, cross leg, cross arm and the Tagliacozzi method of nose reconstruction. These are two-staged operations and may include an intermediate delay to reinforce the vascular connection at the recipient site. Where the defect cannot be directly brought to the flap site, such as with head and neck and lower limb defects, the multistaged tube pedicle of Gillies was originally used. Initially, a tube of skin and fat is created on the abdomen and after a period of approximately 2 months one end is detached and joined to the wrist as a carrier. The flap would remain in this position for a further 2 months, when it could be totally detached from the abdomen and transferred to the final destination still attached to the wrist. After a further period of time it could be disconnected from the wrist and inset into the final defect. Because of the impracticality of this today, the free microvascular flap has effectively superseded the tube pedicle.

Free flaps: The flap is totally detached from the body after dissecting out its blood vessel pedicle. The flap is directly transferred to the site of election and the artery and vein are anastomosed to recipient vessels in the region. All flaps that have a single identifiable vascular pedicle supply, namely, axial pattern flaps, myocutaneous or fasciocutaneous flaps (see below) can be transferred as free flaps. Free flaps vastly widen the options of available tissue for a more sophisticated reconstruction. Thin, thick, hair-bearing, innervated or composite flaps can be chosen to better match the defect.

ACCORDING TO VASCULAR BASIS OF THE FLAPS

Random pattern: All small flaps are essentially randomly vascularised, especially in the face, neck and trunk. Larger flaps, particularly if they incorporate the deeper layers, may capture a specific vertically oriented vascular perforator or subfascial horizontally directed vessel that permits much greater flexibility of flap design.

Axial: A known artery (e.g. the superficial circumflex iliac artery of the groin flap) passes along the axis of the flap; similarly, the supraorbital vessels supply the Indian rhinoplasty flap. Such flaps can be developed as island flaps; that is, as an isolated paddle of skin based purely on its blood vessel pedicle, greatly facilitating flap mobility.

Myocutaneous: The skin blood supply is dependent on attachment to its underlying muscle and both the skin and muscle must be raised as a flap to retain its blood supply (e.g. latissimus dorsi and TRAM flaps). These flaps are also commonly transferred as island pedicle flaps.

Fasciocutaneous or septocutaneous: When the blood supply arises from perforators from the deep compartment vessels and emerges via the fascioseptal layers to supply the overlying skin. Limb skin is typically vascularised in this manner.

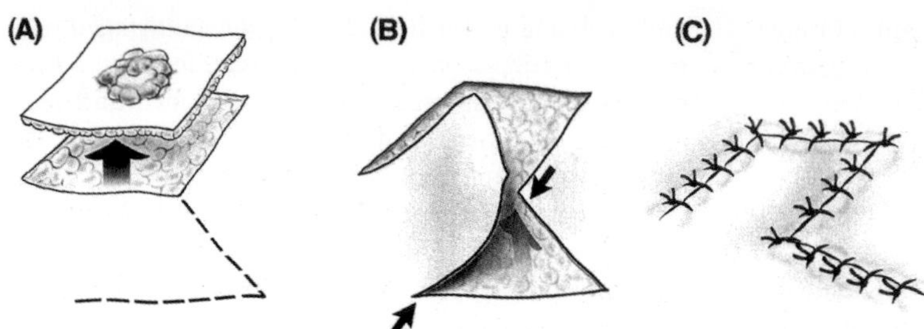

Fig. 44.2 V–Y advancement flap. (A) Design of flap. Triangular flap designed with apex away from defect and in area of laxity. (B) Incision and mobilisation of flap on subcutaneous tissue pedicle. The mobility of this tissue allows advancement of flap into defect. (C) Flap sutured into position and secondary defect closed directly behind the advanced flap.

Prefabricated flaps: Occasionally, large skin flaps are required with unique colour, texture and character to reconstruct specific defects, especially in the face and head and neck region (e.g. nose or forehead). Flaps can be purpose-designed by a process known as prefabrication, using the ability to transfer multiple tissues in stages to create a composite flap.

VARIOUS FLAPS USED FOR CLOSURE OF SKIN DEFECTS

V–Y advancement type flaps are very useful for cheek and forehead defects and can be designed in the axis of crease lines. This flap, which is designed as a V with its apex furthest from the defect, involves cutting circumferentially around it into the fatty tissue (Fig. 44.2A). It survives on perforators coming up through the subcutaneous fat, which is highly mobile tissue, and allows the skin flap to be advanced into the defect (Fig. 44.2B). The secondary defect is pinched together sideways as a Y (Fig. 44.2C). In the temple, preauricular, lateral canthal and neck area, transposition flaps of the Limberg type are most versatile. The defect is marked out as a parallelogram. The shortest diagonal is extended the same length beyond the flap into the area of maximum laxity. The incision is then redirected the same length backwards parallel to the side of the defect (Fig. 44.3A). The flap is transposed into the defect and in so doing the secondary gap closes as this is in the area of laxity (Fig. 44.3B,C). For defects which have no immediate adjacent skin redundancy a rotation flap is required. This is typically used in the scalp. The defect is triangulated and its apex is extended in the form of a large semicircular arc (Fig. 44.4A). This flap is undermined and rotated so that the apex of the flap adjacent to the defect advances to close it (Fig. 44.4B). The secondary deficiency usually closes directly (Fig. 44.4C).

Tissue expansion

Tissue expansion involves progressive stretching of immediate adjacent tissue until enough is created to advance it directly into the defect. Scalp defects are an ideal indication as the technique reproduces the unique hair-bearing skin. It involves implanting one or more tissue expanders, empty silicone balloons, underneath the skin adjacent to the defect to be closed. Progressively over approximately 2 months, the expander, which has a valve port, is injected percutaneously with saline until sufficient volume is obtained. At this point the expander is removed and the redundant expanded skin is advanced to close the defect.

Cosmetic surgery

Operations for correction of cosmetic deformities, both congenital and acquired, have evolved since early in the 20th century. To some extent most plastic surgery includes an aesthetic ideal. Purely cosmetic procedures are technically demanding and successful outcomes

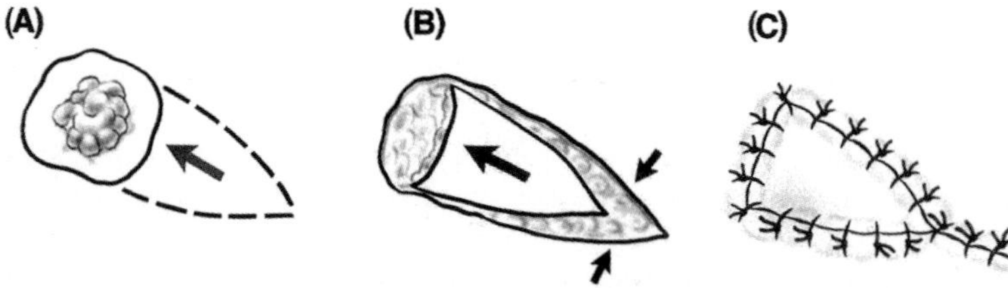

Fig. 44.3 Transposition flap (Limberg flap). (A) Design of flap. Lesion/defect is marked as parallelogram, with flap designed adjacent (see text). (B) Flap elevated and transposed. (C) Flap sutured into defect and secondary defect closed directly.

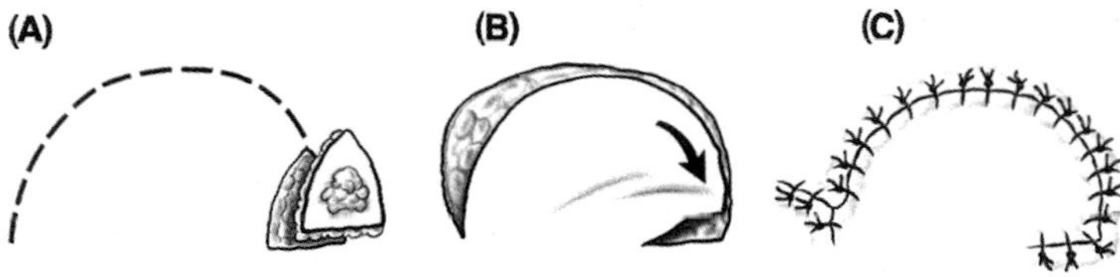

Fig. 44.4 Rotation flap. (A) Design of flap. Lesion/defect triangulated and flap designed as semicircular arc from apex of defect. (B) Flap incised, elevated and rotated into defect. (C) Flap sutured into position with secondary defect closed directly.

require a thorough training in basic plastic surgery principles. Patient's motives and expectations may be unrealistic and not match the technical possibilities that surgery can offer. Alternatively, in this market-driven field, unscrupulous and often untrained practitioners may promote operations in an unrealistic light so that the limitations of surgery are down-played.

The most rewarding, commonly performed cosmetic operation is reduction mammaplasty. Large breasts are a source of physical discomfort, severe back and neck ache, and of psychological embarrassment. Operation is generally predictable and offers dramatic relief of symptoms. Scars, although extensive, are well disguised and accepted by the patient. Other cosmetic operations that can be of great psychological benefit are rhinoplasty, the setting back of prominent ears, augmentation mammaplasty and suction lipectomy for isolated fat reduction. Anti-ageing procedures, such as facelift, blepharoplasty, browlift and laser resurfacing, are in a different age group. Although they can be very beneficial, they are associated with a higher risk for patient dissatisfaction.

MCQs

Select the single correct answer to each question.

1 Which of the following does not predispose to ischaemic necrosis and wound breakdown?
- **a** excessive tension
- **b** foreign body
- **c** application of vacuum
- **d** haematoma
- **e** irradiation

2 Lesions such as naevi, birthmarks and skin cancers can be:
- **a** removed with elliptical excision
- **b** excised perpendicular to Langer's lines
- **c** excised across the line of least tension or maximum laxity
- **d** excised using incisions that transgress cavities or flexion creases
- **e** closed with a z-plasty following all excisions

3 Sutures should:
- **a** be placed horizontally to the wound through the tissues to approximately the full depth of the wound
- **b** be the least number to maintain closure
- **c** be of the greatest calibre to maintain closure
- **d** remain once cross hatching has occurred
- **e** sutures should be left in for longer periods in young patients compared to the elderly patients

4 A graft shaved at a dermal level, which includes elements of the epidermis and dermis:
- **a** is a full-thickness graft
- **b** is used where large areas of skin are required
- **c** is sensate immediately after transfer
- **d** is limited by the donor defect to be closed
- **e** requires 1 week before blood flow is established in it

Trauma

45 Principles of trauma management

Scott K. D'Amours and Stephen A. Deane

General principles

Good trauma management recognises the importance of a number of key issues (Box 45.1).

Trauma as a disease

Injury is a major economic burden to societies such as Australia. The most recent estimates from the late 1990s put the total economic burden on Australia's economy annually at A$13.3 billion, including both direct and indirect costs. Injury is the most frequent cause of death in Australians less than 45 years of age, and is a major cause of death in all age groups. It accounts for more years of productive life lost than cancer and heart disease combined. The major impact of injury deaths and disability is borne by the young adult segment of the population and disproportionately by males. Of injury-related admissions to Major Trauma Services, approximately 30% are road traffic related. These account for approximately 75% of those with serious injury and about 75% of those who die in hospital from injury.

Many of the advances in trauma care in recent years have been derived from experience with injuries suffered in war or with penetrating injuries resulting from interpersonal violence, particularly in the United States. However, the proportion of patients admitted to hospitals in Australia with injuries resulting from gunshot wounds or stabbings is low, varying between 2% and 7%. Even within this population, stabbings predominate and gunshot wounds to the head are often the result of suicide attempts.

Traditionally, much emphasis has been placed on deaths in quantifying the injury problem, and in more recent times there has been a very significant emphasis on injury surveillance and prevention; however, it also needs to be recognised that for every patient who dies from injury, 10 more are admitted to hospital and 2 will suffer significant long-term disability.

Box 45.1 General principles of good trauma management

- The importance of injury as a public health issue.
- The importance of the injury mechanism in predicting actual injuries.
- The differing implications of blunt and penetrating injury.
- The importance of triage.
- The importance to the triage process of:
  - injury mechanism
  - physiological status
  - evident injuries.
- The differing risk exposures and injury patterns in children, young adults and the elderly.
- The patterns of associated injuries that are commonly observed.
- The commonly documented deficiencies in acute injury management.
- The importance of an integrated trauma treatment service in a hospital.
- The importance of a triage-based team approach to acute injury assessment.
- The value of a protocol-directed approach and practice guidelines to acute injury assessment and management.
- The importance of regional trauma care systems that link injury prevention activities, pre-hospital care, acute care hospitals with differing roles, and rehabilitation services.

Trauma system planning

When examining deaths due to injury, there has been a fairly consistent finding worldwide that where systems of trauma care have not been specifically organised, 15–30% of the deaths can be deemed to have been possibly preventable. In addition, approximately two-thirds of deaths in the absence of serious head injury have been deemed to be possibly preventable. Much has been done to improve this situation with respect to education, standardised care, and re-organisation, but more progress is still needed.

Considerable attention has been given internationally in recent years to the appropriate design of regional trauma care systems that enable patients with potentially serious injuries to access a process that minimises the time from injury to definitive care. The aim is to 'get the right patient to the right hospital in the right time'. Implementation of such plans is quite advanced in some parts of Australia. The essential components of such a plan are outlined here.

Pre-hospital triage

Triage is the process of grouping injury victims according to risk of death or other adverse outcome. Pre-hospital care providers can be trained to carry out this process according to a predetermined checklist of criteria or a system of injury severity scoring. This triage of trauma patients usually depends on three simple groups of factors:

- **Physiology**: the vital signs (e.g. pulse >120/min, systolic blood pressure <90 mm Hg, Glasgow Coma Scale score [GCS] <15)
- **Anatomy**: the immediately evident injuries (e.g. fractured long bones, spinal cord injury, penetrating injury)
- **Mechanism of injury**: e.g. fall >5 m, injury to two or more body regions, vehicle crash with ejection

Pre-hospital treatment and transport decisions

On the basis of the triage process, certain predetermined decisions are made, which attempt to direct the transport of patients to the most appropriate hospital. Certain basic life support or advanced life support interventions may also be prescribed on the basis of triage criteria. Sometimes, the most appropriate hospital is not necessarily the nearest hospital as not all hospitals have the resourcing nor expertise to care for all types of injuries. That situation requires that the pre-hospital triage process identify patients that need to bypass the nearest hospital for one that is better able to manage the identified injuries.

Categorisation of hospitals

The role of a hospital within a regional trauma care system is designated by the appropriate health authority. A Major Trauma Service (Level 1) has the facilities and internal organisation to support its role as the most appropriate primary destination for patients with potentially serious injuries, which make up only about 10–15% of the total injured population. The remaining 85% of patients in a local community should be treated within the nearest community hospital. In the semi-rural, rural and remote environments, strategically located 'Regional Trauma Services' (Levels 2–4) are required. These smaller trauma services must have strong links with a Major Trauma Service. Even in remote environments trauma care education, trauma service planning, and strong links with the rest of the regional trauma care network need to be continuously promoted.

Trauma response and trauma teams

Another expression of the planning that helps to ensure efficient initial assessment of trauma patients is an organised trauma response within a hospital. The aim is to minimise the time from injury to definitive care by eliminating the traditional linear sequence of mobilising medical staff of progressively increasing seniority and progressively increasing subspecialty expertise. Such trauma responses or teams have a predetermined multidisciplinary membership, a triage device to trigger mobilisation, predetermined roles for members, and standardised approaches to the performance of primary survey, resuscitation, secondary survey and investigations.

Special circumstances

Certain natural or man-made disasters can result in multiple casualties in the presence of limited resources. Pre-planned disaster responses are essential to ensure that the principles of good injury management are applied to the greatest possible number of casualties using standardised approaches that minimise the stress experienced by medical and paramedical personnel. In situations such as this and in war-time situations, the triage services have to consider not only the severity of injuries and the risk of death for individual victims, but also the limited resources and the chances of achieving good outcomes.

Blunt and penetrating mechanisms of injury

The nature of injuries relates to the mechanisms that cause them. The severity of injuries relates to the amount of energy transferred in the injury process and the amount of the body across which the energy is transferred. Serious injury from blunt trauma is typified by victims of traffic-related injury or by falls from a significant height (greater than 5 m). In these situations, large amounts of energy are often transferred across broad and multiple regions of the body without breaching the walls of the body cavities. Accordingly, certain injury patterns can only be broadly anticipated and, initially, occult injuries are not uncommon. A broader range of investigative tests are often necessary compared with penetrating trauma.

Penetrating injuries are divided into those that result from gunshot wounds and those that result from stabbings. A further small group are patients who suffer impalement. It is important to recognise that the interpersonal violence that results in gunshot wounds or stabbings often results in multiple shots being fired or multiple stab wounds, or accompanying blunt injury (e.g. from a fist or a boot). Possible injuries from stab wounds can often be fairly confidently predicted, and guidelines for the management of stab wounds in particular body regions are generally straightforward. However, gunshot wounds can pose additional difficulties because the missile path may not be predictable. Secondary missiles (e.g. fragments from a shattered bone) can cause gross destruction of surrounding soft tissues, and the physical features of the missile (velocity, size, mass, impact surface) contribute to the amount of energy transferred. Because of the uncertainties posed by these features and the potentially serious nature of possible injuries, a lower threshold usually exists for comprehensive investigation or surgical exploration in the presence of gunshot wounds than with stab wounds.

Goals of assessment and resuscitation

The management of a trauma patient should allow the following aims to be met.

1 Minimise the time from injury to definitive care.
2 Don't allow the obvious injury to distract you from diagnosing other, less obvious injuries.
3 No patient should leave the resuscitation area without a clear management plan.
4 There should be no need for further clinical guesswork after 2 hours from arrival of the patient.

Specific goals

The sequence of goals in the initial assessment of an individual trauma patient are:

1 Save life. This requires knowledge of the causes of death.
2 Prevent major disability. This requires knowledge of the causes of disability.
3 Diagnose and appropriately manage all injuries.
4 Avoid unnecessary investigations or interventions.

Deaths

Deaths from injury can be broadly divided into four groups that link the cause of death to the time from injury to death: death at the scene; death within 'minutes'; death within 'hours'; and death over 'days' (some examples are given in Box 45.2). Many patients in the fourth group are recognised as 'late septic complications' or 'multiple organ failure'. However, the foundations for these late complications are often laid in the first hour or two following injury; they relate to the extent and duration of physiological disturbance. It is therefore clear that they can also relate to the promptness and completeness of early assessment and resuscitation measures. Prevention of death can be linked broadly to the principles in Box 45.3.

Disability

Disability principally relates to:

- cognition
- locomotion
- manipulation skills
- chronic pain.

Box 45.2 Causes of death from injury

Deaths at scene/incompatible with life
- Brain stem transection
- High spinal cord transection
- Decapitation
- Major thoracic vascular injury with free intrapleural bleeding
- Major tracheobronchial disruption
- Liver avulsion
- Cardiac rupture

Death within 'minutes'
- Hypoxia (airway obstruction; tension pneumothorax; open pneumothorax; massive flail chest)
- Major bleeding (external; thoracic [haemothorax]; abdominal [spleen; liver, mesentery, major vessels]; pelvic fracture)
- Pericardial tamponade (cardiac rupture)
- Rapid tentorial herniation (rapid rise in intracranial pressure (ICP))

Death within 'hours'
- Hypoxia (pulmonary contusion; tracheobronchial rupture; diaphragm rupture)
- Sepsis (perforated hollow viscus; e.g. thoracic oesophagus, abdominal viscera)
- Bleeding (external [face, massive wounds]; thoracic aortic rupture; lungs, chest wall [haemothorax]; liver, spleen, retroperitoneum; pelvis fracture; long-bone fractures)
- Brain (increasing intracranial pressure [haematoma, swelling])

Death over 'days'
- Brain (high ICP from brain swelling, no cerebral perfusion)
- Respiratory failure (adult respiratory distress syndrome (ARDS), oedema, septic consolidation)
- Renal failure
- Coagulopathy
- Gastrointestinal failure (especially liver, gut mucosal barrier)
- Sepsis (pulmonary, abdominal, wound)
- Ischaemia (muscle groups, liver, gut)
- Myocardial infarction
- Pulmonary embolus

While definitive care of the actual injuries plays a major role in preventing these categories of disability, it must be recognised that ensuring adequate oxygen delivery to brain and to muscle groups also plays a major role, especially in the first hour or two after injury. As with death, prevention of disability is linked to specific measures (as shown in Box 45.4).

Box 45.3 Prevention of death

General measures
- Optimise oxygenation (A,B)
- Optimise perfusion acutely (C)
- Meticulous continuing fluid management
- Thrombosis prophylaxis
- Adequate nutrition by appropriate route

Local measures
- Arrest or minimise bleeding (C)
- Correct raised ICP (D)
- Control 'leaks' (tracheobronchial, oesophageal, abdominal hollow viscera, pancreas, urinary)
- Decompress or revascularise ischaemic tissue promptly
- Debride dead tissue aggressively
- Debride and clean contaminated wounds

Initial assessment

Efficient initial assessment of a trauma patient derives from the broad principles outlined previously in Box 45.1, a clear understanding of the patterns of death and

Box 45.4 Prevention of disability

General measures
- Optimise oxygenation (A,B)
- Optimise perfusion (C)
- Protect spine (A and following measures)
- Correct raised ICP (D)

Local measures
- Reduce dislocations as soon as possible
- Re-align fractures as soon as possible
- Correct local ischaemia early
- Diagnose and decompress compartment syndromes early
- Prevent secondary damage to nerves (iatrogenic injury, ischaemia, compression, e.g. dislocations)
- Debride ischaemic tissue early
- Debride contaminated wounds early
- Find the 'minor injuries' to ligaments, joints and small bones (tertiary survey)

disability (Boxes 45.2, 45.3 and 45.4) and recognition of the following factors:

- Trauma patient assessment is different from that of the usual patient. The traditional approach of taking a full history, doing a full physical examination, determining a provisional diagnosis and a list of differential diagnoses, and deriving a logical plan for investigation and treatment needs to be laid aside in order to first ensure a patient's survival and then to ensure the smallest possible risk of major complications (see below).
- There is a need to minimise the time from injury to definitive care, particularly so that continuing bleeding is arrested.
- Physiological responses and consequences of injury are often changing and any static set of physiological values (e.g. pulse, respiratory rate, GCS and blood pressure) is of limited value.
- Life-threatening injuries may be occult, multiple life-threatening injuries may coexist in different body regions, and the injuries that appear most dramatic may not be those that pose the most risk.
- The concept of the 'golden hour' is important; a 1–2-hour period during which all opportunities need to be taken to discover injuries that may cause death within minutes and then to discover injuries that may cause death within hours.
- Treating doctors can be under considerable stress and will be assisted by pre-planned protocols or evidence-based guidelines.

Figure 45.1 outlines a well-accepted approach to the first 24 hours of injury management. The term 'initial

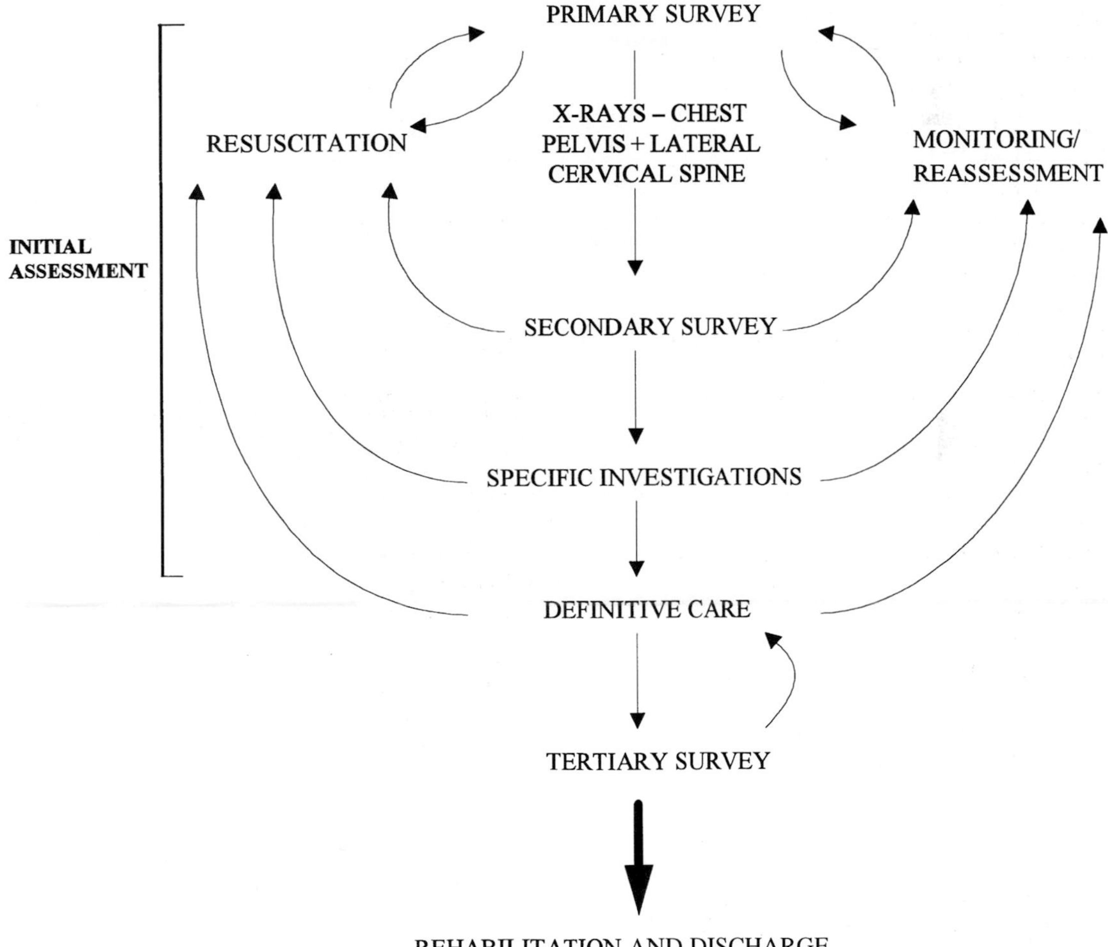

Fig. 45.1 Acute trauma management procedure.

assessment' applies particularly to the elements of primary survey, resuscitation, secondary survey, monitoring/reassessment and specific investigations. The term 'definitive care' relates to specific treatment (operative or non-operative) aimed at establishing the optimal conditions for the healing of specific injuries.

Primary survey and resuscitation

The strategy for primary survey and resuscitation is outlined in Figure 45.2. The ABCDE sequence prioritises the importance of specific injuries and assists clinical performance. Primary survey is the process used to

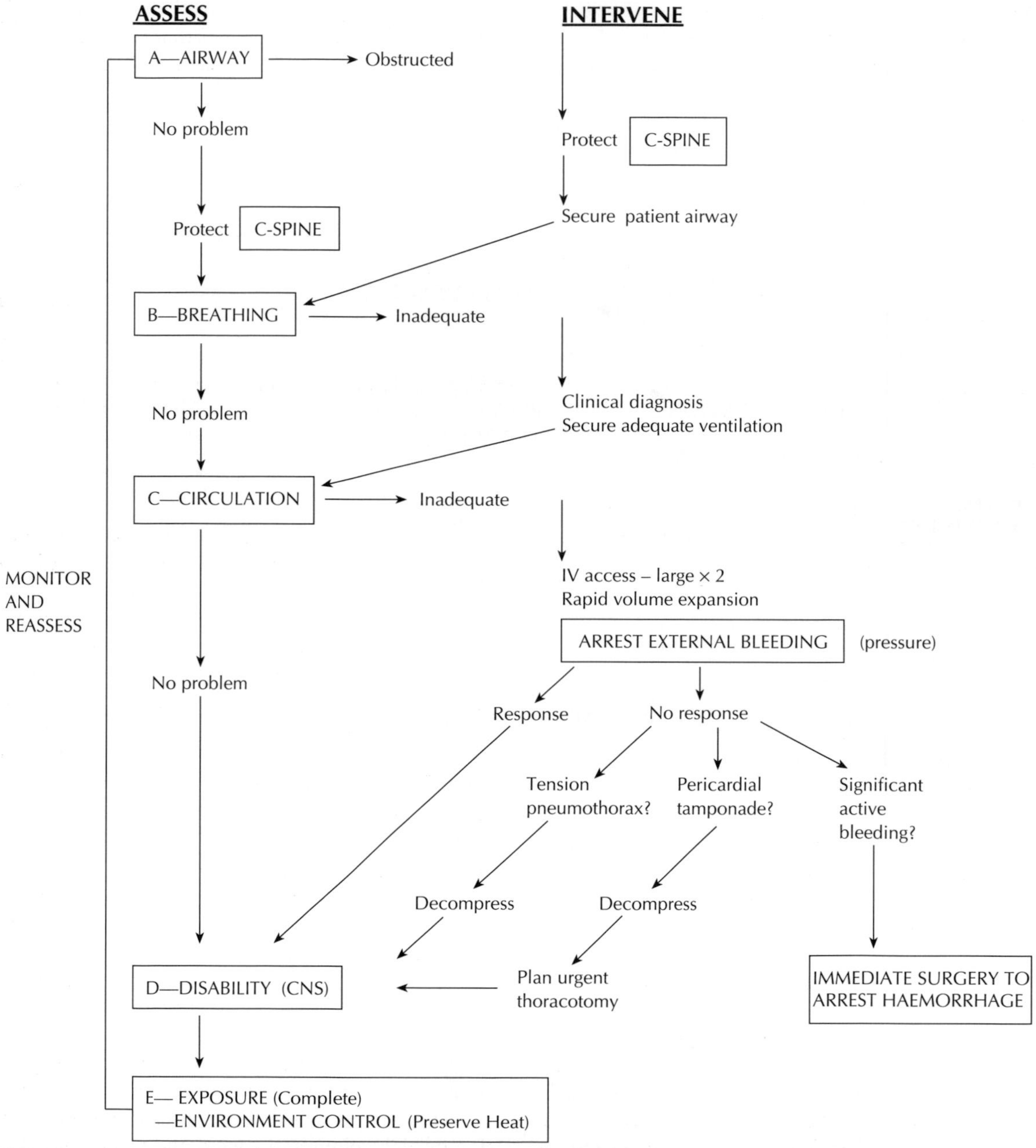

Fig. 45.2 Outline of strategy for primary survey and resuscitation.

assist the recognition of acutely life-threatening injuries and should proceed concurrently with resuscitation. As the primary survey assessment scheme is followed, intervention should be taken immediately to correct the problems that are identified with each step. Note the emphasis given to using simple measures to protect the cervical spine when attending to the adequacy of the airway. External bleeding must be controlled; direct pressure is usually effective.

In a hospital with a major trauma service and an effective trauma-team response there will be enough team members to perform some parts of the primary survey concurrently, together with the necessary resuscitative interventions. However, when resources are limited the framework illustrated in Figure 45.2 assumes even greater importance. Extensive worldwide experience with this approach to primary survey and resuscitation has led to a widespread confidence that even the most apparently difficult trauma scenario becomes readily manageable by following these guidelines.

Table 45.1 provides further detail regarding primary survey and resuscitation. Effective primary survey requires awareness of a limited number of life-threatening entities, rapid and simple systems of physiological assessment, and awareness of a menu of interventions that can be applied to correct the identified problem. Some aspects of care during the primary survey need special emphasis.

X-rays

There are three X-rays that are often considered to be within the scope of the primary survey. The most common of these is a chest X-ray, which should ideally be performed in the upright position although this is frequently not feasible in patients with severe injuries because of haemodynamic instability or potential associated injuries. A lateral cervical spine X-ray is used to screen for injuries in patients where physical examination is unreliable. However, if other measures to maintain in-line immobilisation of the neck are feasible (most commonly with a semi-rigid cervical collar), then the cervical spine X-ray can be delayed until after the completion of the primary survey or later if other injuries or unstable physiology take priority. A pelvis X-ray is commonly performed but is not routinely necessary as part of the primary survey. Its early role is in patients whose physical examination is unreliable and in whom major pelvic fracture is a possible cause of apparent major blood loss.

Shock

A primary goal in minimising death and disability is to ensure adequate oxygen supply to peripheral tissues. The most urgent threat to achieving this is interruption of oxygen supply (airway). The next most urgent threat is interference with alveolar oxygen exchange (breathing). The third most important threat is failure of peripheral delivery of oxygen (via the circulation). The adverse effects of shock occur at the microcirculation level, and early recognition of shock depends upon clinical observations of:

- the microcirculation of the skin (pale, cold, clammy)
- the brain (level of consciousness: confusion, agitation, anxiety etc.)
- the kidneys (timed urinary output via urinary catheter).

The acid–base status of the patient, as manifested in the results of arterial blood gases (ABG), gives an indication of the magnitude of the microcirculatory failure and is an invaluable tool for assessing shock and the response to resuscitation in a critically injured patient.

Cardiac arrest

From time to time, injured patients present in actual or impending cardiac arrest. It is generally agreed that attempted resuscitation of patients who have no vital signs at the scene of injury will not restore life except in some circumstances where hypothermia is extreme.

Victims of blunt trauma who arrive at hospital without vital signs will not be salvaged by the most aggressive resuscitation. However, some patients who have suffered penetrating injury can be salvaged. These patients require aggressive management and a well-organised system to respond quickly.

When patients who have arrived with recordable vital signs deteriorate rapidly so that cardiac arrest is imminent, there is no time even to carry out a rapid systematic primary survey. Management is simplified by rapidly instituting the maximum response to potential problems with airway and breathing and circulation. This involves endotracheal intubation and controlled ventilation with 100% oxygen, insertion of bilateral large-calibre (36F) intercostal catheters with underwater seal drainage, and insertion of two or three large-calibre intravenous cannulas to facilitate pressure infusion of high volumes of colloid and uncross-matched group O blood. External bleeding must be rapidly

Table 45.1 Primary survey and resuscitation

	Problem	Assess	Intervene
Airway	Direct trauma: disruption/oedema Obstruction: Foreign bodies Blood and vomitus Soft tissue oedema Deteriorating consciousness	Cyanosis Tachypnoea Voice Stridor Confusion 'Respiratory distress' Air movement	Gloved finger, light, suction Laryngoscope, forceps Oxygen Chin lift/jaw thrust Oropharyngeal airway Nasopharyngeal airway Orotracheal tube Surgical Airway: Cricothyroidotomy Urgent tracheostomy
C-spine	Unstable fracture	Assume if: Unconscious Head injury Face injury	Semi-rigid collar Sandbags/tape Manual in-line immobilisation
Breathing	Tension pneumothorax Massive haemothorax Open pneumothorax Massive flail Reduction in level of consciousness/poor effort High spinal cord injury	Cyanosis Tachypnoea Confusion 'Respiratory distress' Shallow respiration Poor expansion Asymmetric expansion Hyperinflation Hyper-resonance Breath sounds Tracheal shift Diaphragmatic breathing	Oxygen Ventilation Needle thoracentesis Tube thoracentesis Tracheal intubation Cover open wound
Circulation	Bleeding: External (scene, bed, floor) Chest (chest X-ray) Abdomen (FAST or DPL) Pelvis (X-ray) Femurs (clinical examination) Combination	Pale, clammy, cool Peripheral cyanosis Confusion Tachycardia Low pulse volume Slow capillary refill Neck veins Heart sounds (muffled)	Oxygen Intravenous access (large ×2) Warmed crystalloid/colloid/blood Haemorrhage control (direct pressure or surgery) Pressure infusion Blood warming Gastric tube Surgery (Urinary catheter)
	Heart: Tension pneumothorax Pericardial tamponade Contusion Infarction		Needle/tube thoracentesis Pericardiocentesis
DISABILITY (CNS)	Secondary brain injury Intracranial haematoma	Alert Voice response	A, B, C C-spine protection

Table 45.1 (*Continued*)

	Problem	Assess	Intervene
	Brain Compression Contusion Laceration Swelling	Pain response Unresponsive Lateralising signs Pupils	Hyperventilation
Exposure	Concealed injuries	Prepare for secondary survey	Remove all clothes
Environment control	Hypothermia		Warm fluids Blankets Heating mattress

controlled by direct pressure. External cardiac massage will only be fruitful if restoration of vascular volume can lead to cardiac filling. The components of the usual medical cardiac arrest response may have some role after the initial trauma-orientated response, but will not be successful if instituted as the principal therapeutic approach.

Nasogastric tube

Insertion of a nasogastric tube can be a life-saving manoeuvre if it is used to decompress a full stomach and avoid aspiration of gastric contents. A nasogastric tube should be inserted, usually towards the end of the primary survey in all trauma patients with major abdominal injury, major chest injury, spinal injury, brain injury, major burns and shock. Gastric distension is particularly common in injured children. Patients with a high likelihood of basal skull or cribriform plate fractures should *only* have a gastric tube placed by the oral route.

Urinary catheter

There is no great urgency to insert a urinary catheter but it is helpful if used in patients with potentially serious injury and is inserted at the end of the primary survey. The observation of gross haematuria or documentation of microscopic haematuria may have important diagnostic implications. However, once the bladder is empty, monitoring of the hourly urine output is an important part of assessing the response to intravenous fluid resuscitation. Careful inspection of the perineum and assessment of prostate position (in males) is required before a urinary catheter is positioned to avoid worsening an existing urethral injury.

Secondary survey

The emphasis in secondary survey is on identifying anatomical injuries and providing clinical information that will determine the need for plain X-rays and other special investigations. It is a careful and methodical physical examination from head to toe. It requires close inspection, careful palpation and appropriate auscultation. Common omissions resulting in missed injuries include examination of the entire scalp, careful inspection of the back (often needing a log-roll), inspection of the perineum, inspection of the axillae and digital rectal examination.

Table 45.2 outlines a useful sequence for the execution of the secondary survey. It also indicates the common general abnormalities that may be observed and highlights some simple procedures that assist with pain relief, reduce the risk of infection and lead into the definitive-care phase of early trauma management.

Monitoring

Because injuries may be multiple and occult, and because of the physiological derangements that follow injury, close monitoring is essential, particularly in the first 24 hours following injury. An airway that is patent in a sitting patient with a fractured mandible can become acutely obstructed if the patient lies down. A small pneumothorax can become a life-threatening tension pneumothorax. Apparently small pulmonary contusions can progress to major alterations in pulmonary compliance and oxygen exchange. Small intracranial haematomas can enlarge. Contained vascular disruptions can undergo free rupture. Arterial intimal injuries can lead to thrombosis. Crushed or

Table 45.2 Secondary survey: look! listen! feel!

Head-to-toe	
Glasgow Coma Scale Scalp Ears (including tympanic membranes) Eyes (including pupils, acuity, fundi) Facial bones Mouth (including teeth) Neck (C-spine, soft tissues, trachea) Clavicles Chest: Chest wall Chest movement Lungs Heart	**Seek the following** Tenderness Lacerations (including entry, exit wounds) Swelling (including haematoma) Structural deformity (i.e. bones) Discolouration (e.g. bruising) Crepitus (including subcutaneous) Ischaemia (i.e. limbs) Functional impairment: Visceral (lungs, heart, bowel) Musculoskeletal neurological
Abdomen Pelvis Hips Thighs Knees Legs Ankles Feet Upper arms Elbows Forearms Wrists Hands Fingers	**Proceed with the following** Digital photo (or polaroid) of major wounds Sterile pad on wounds Pressure on bleeding sites Splint fractures Traction splints where indicated Splinting of specific pelvic fractures (open book) Pain relief Tetanus prophylaxis Antibiotics as advised
Back and flanks (log-roll)	
Perineum, genitalia Rectal examination Urinalysis	

reperfused muscles in the extremities can lead to compartment syndromes.

The monitoring strategy varies with the known injuries, co-morbidity and age factors, other anticipated injuries and the potential consequences or complications of the known injuries or their management.

Monitoring of oxygenation (airway and breathing) may include skin colour, level of consciousness, respiratory rate and depth, physical examination of the respiratory system, chest X-rays, pulse oximetry, capnography, arterial blood gases and ventilation pressures.

Monitoring of the circulation may include pulse rate, blood pressure, skin colour and temperature, level of consciousness, urinary output, jugular venous pressure, central venous pressure, pulmonary artery wedge pressure and cardiac output, serial haemoglobin, ABG status, outputs from drains (e.g. chest tube), as well as repeated physical examination of the abdomen and wound dressings.

Monitoring of the central nervous system relies heavily on physical examination and serial head computed tomography (CT) scans where indicated. When CT scans reveal significant injury, placement of an intracranial pressure (ICP) monitoring device is required. Serial documentation of the GCS score is imperative in patients who are not sedated and paralysed.

Early detection and explanation of fever is important in limiting septic complications. Avoidance or detection and reversal of hypothermia are important in limiting its adverse consequences (e.g. coagulopathy).

Repeated physical examination, particularly in regions of known injury, is of great importance in order to detect ischaemia of skin or deeper tissues and adequacy of distal pulses.

Definitive care

Definitive care is the phase of early trauma management when particular injuries receive their specific treatment. Much of this takes place in the operating theatre, and in situations of multiple major injuries a number of surgical subspecialty teams may be involved. Figure 45.1 emphasises the need for resuscitation to be continuing, and for monitoring and re-assessment of a patient's responses to resuscitation to be conducted, throughout this and all other phases of care. Any deterioration in a patient's physiological status should lead to urgent re-assessment of the primary survey priorities and immediate intervention when acutely life-threatening events are identified.

Definitive care continues through any necessary stay in the intensive care unit (ICU) and through early convalescence on the hospital ward. As our systems of trauma care improve, the interface between acute care and rehabilitation should become progressively more invisible.

Tertiary survey

The tertiary survey is a repeat clinical examination along the lines of the primary and secondary surveys. It is performed with the aim of identifying injuries that have been missed during initial assessment. It is best performed after the early phase of definitive care and is most likely to be done if viewed as the first routine clinical task on the morning after admission of the patient to hospital. In addition to clinical examination, all X-rays and CT scans should be reviewed and new X-rays requested as indicated from the physical examination.

Injuries that may be missed during primary survey and that need to be identified during the tertiary survey often have great functional importance and impact the return of the patient to normal occupational, family and social functions. They usually pose little threat to life but often would lead to locomotor or manipulative disability if undetected and untreated. Examples include cervical spine injury without neurological deficit, fractures of small bones in the hands and feet, ligamentous injuries to the knee or ankle, dislocated acromioclavicular joint and peripheral nerve injuries. Review of previous X-rays will sometimes result in a new diagnosis of pneumothorax, widened mediastinum, pelvic fracture or rib fractures that require specific management. Occult visceral injury, in particular small bowel injury, may be suspected at this stage on the basis of increasing pulse rate, increasing temperature and localised abdominal tenderness. Subtle signs of brain injury must be sought.

Outcomes

Prevention of deaths and disability

In accordance with the above strategies, deaths that are avoidable can usually be prevented. Diagnosis of any problems must be early. Surgery must be prompt. Application and extension of the principles outlined for prevention of death will also succeed in minimising disability.

Trauma registries and performance improvement

It is critical that any mature or maturing trauma system establish a computerised trauma registry that incorporates information on injuries sustained and specific criteria of initial assessment and management that can also be used as markers indicating adequate or inadequate care. Additionally, it is important that details of complications and information on outcomes and lengths of stay are included. It is only with this information that objective comparisons can be made and assessments of adequacy of care can be undertaken.

It is only with quality data from a functioning registry that a system of trauma care can be assessed. Performance improvement refers specifically to a process whereby care is objectively assessed and strategies are implemented to either better the process of care or to result in better patient outcomes. This approach requires objective collection of information, a robust system of review or audit, strategies to ameliorate demonstrated deficiencies, and repeated collection of data to assess efficacy of changes. It is only with repeated cycles of assessment and change that better overall results and outcomes can be achieved.

MCQs

Select the single correct answer to each question.

1 The following are critical determinants of patient outcome following injury, EXCEPT:
  - **a** time from injury to definitive care
  - **b** presence of a well-organised regional system of trauma care
  - **c** protocols and guidelines when clinical experience is limited
  - **d** early mobilisation of teams led by doctors to most scenes of injury
  - **e** thrombosis prophylaxis

2 Hypovolaemic shock can result from any of the following, EXCEPT:
  - **a** pulmonary laceration
  - **b** extradural haemorrhage
  - **c** pelvic fracture
  - **d** femur fracture
  - **e** laceration to scalp

3 A restrained 32-year-old male involved in a head-on motor vehicle collision presents with chest pain and the following vital signs on arrival in the emergency department: Heart rate – 120/minute; Blood pressure – 86/50; GCS score – 10; and O_2 saturations of 92%. Which of the following takes first priority?
  - **a** urgent CT scan of the head to rule out an extradural haemorrhage with midline shift
  - **b** rapid resuscitation with 2 large-bore intravenous cannulae and warmed fluids
  - **c** ECG and an echocardiogram to eliminate cardiac contusion as the cause of his hypotension
  - **d** obtaining an urgent cross match
  - **e** elimination of tension pneumothorax as a cause of his symptoms/signs:

4 Which of the following is NOT considered an immediate threat to life?
  - **a** fracture of T6 with a complete spinal cord transection
  - **b** splenic injury with ongoing bleeding
  - **c** open pneumothorax
  - **d** rapidly rising intra-cranial pressures
  - **e** aspiration

46 Burns

Rodney T. Judson

Introduction

Sustaining a burn injury during one's lifetime is almost a universally shared experience. Such injuries are usually the result of minor household mishaps that occur most commonly in the kitchen and result in a small, intensely painful area of skin damage that settles spontaneously within a few days. More serious injuries with their devastating physical, emotional, social, functional and economic consequences are uncommon. The potential life-threatening nature of major burn injuries and the natural tendency for progressing deterioration in the burn wound underlie the importance of a clear understanding of the major aspects of burn injuries. Such knowledge forms the basis of rational management aimed at preventing complications, decreasing further tissue damage and securing early wound healing with minimisation of the functional and social consequences.

A burn injury most commonly results from the transfer of heat energy from a burning source to the skin. Human tissue cells are intolerant to temperature rises, and cellular damage in the form of protein coagulation commences when warming to 45°C occurs. Other agents such as chemicals, exposure to cold and external force producing friction may cause skin damage producing the clinical picture of a burn injury.

The severity of the injury is dependant on the amount of energy absorbed by the skin. The energy absorbed will be determined by the intensity of the burning or injurious agent, the length of exposure to the energy source and the degree of insulation or protection provided by clothing. The more energy absorbed by the skin the greater the degree of cellular disruption that will occur and the greater the depth to which the injury will extend. The pattern and severity of the injury can often be predicted by contemplating the circumstances of the injury. Exposure to a flash such as gas or petrol vapour explosion will produce rapid but transient heating, resulting in damage and probable death of surface cells only. A long exposure such as immersion in hot water will result in slower but greater heat absorption, producing more extensive and deeper tissue injury. The effects of the burning incident are not necessarily confined to the skin. Heat and smoke containing noxious chemicals may be inhaled, especially when a burn injury occurs in a confined space such as a house fire. The absorbed heat and smoke may affect the respiratory passages, leading to marked swelling and oedema that can cause respiratory obstruction. Inhaled smoke may irritate and damage the lung parenchyma, producing a chemical pneumonitis with impairment of gas exchange, leading to respiratory failure.

The anatomy of the skin

Skin consists of an outer layer, the epidermis, that provides a barrier to water loss and bacterial infection. This layer is derived from the constant division of the cells in the basal layer. This layer is thrown into folds, the rete pegs, that extend into the underlying dermal layer. As the basal cells divide, they push the outer cells further to the surface, during which cell death occurs. The outer layer of epidermal cells desiccate to form the stratum corneum or horny layer, which becomes very thick on the soles of the feet and palms of the hand. The epidermis is nourished, supported and strengthened by the underlying hypocellular layer known as the dermis. The dermis is rich in collagen fibres, producing its strength, and elastin, which maintains the normal contour and elasticity to the skin. The dermis is also rich in capillaries providing nutrients to the outer epidermis. The rete pegs, sweat glands and hair follicles invaginate into the underlying dermis. These structures provide a supply of epithelial cells deep within the skin, allowing

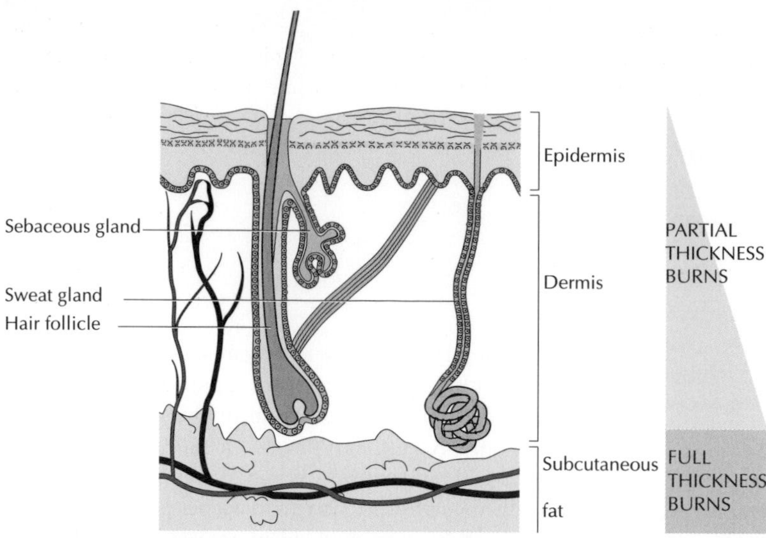

Fig. 46.1 Burn thickness in relation to skin structure.

spontaneous healing of wounds involving loss of the outer layers of the dermis (Fig. 46.1).

Epidemiology

The precise incidence of burn injury is difficult to determine as most minor burns are never reported. Less than 10% of all burn injuries will be severe enough to require hospitalisation but in approximately 10% of those hospitalised, the burn will pose a threat to the patient's life. Burns occur most commonly in the home and are the result of carelessness. Certain groups of people are significantly more prone to burn injuries as a result of physical or psychological impairment. For example, epileptics are prone to sustaining a hot water injury as a result of a seizure whilst bathing, showering or cooking. The frail and elderly may not possess the physical agility to prevent mishaps such as clothing catching alight from home heaters. Those under the influence of alcohol or other pharmacological agents may suffer burns from simple accidents such as falling onto hot stoves or open fires, and are also more likely to be victims of house fires resulting from falling asleep in bed while smoking. Burn injuries are far more common in countries with poor socioeconomic standards, where floor-level open cooking stoves are used. Children, especially toddlers, are particularly at risk from injuries such as spill scalds resulting from enquiring hands pulling cups of hot liquid or saucepans onto themselves. Industrial accidents and burns associated with motor vehicle accidents whilst often devastating are decreasing in incidence with improved work safety measures and better mechanical designs. Approximately 50% of burns to adults are the result of explosions and flame injuries and 30% from scalds. In contrast 60% of burns in children are scalds and 25% the results of flame injury. Self ignition as a suicide attempt, whilst not a common cause of burn injuries in Western society, poses a desperate situation due to the severity of the burns and the underlying psychological problems.

Pathology

The severity of the injury and the consequences to the sufferer depends upon the depth to which the burn extends and the overall size or surface area of the burn injury. The depth of the injury will determine the local consequences of the injury and the size will influence the systemic consequences.

The depth of the burn may be described in a variety of ways, but broad categorisation into superficial burns, partial-thickness burns and full-thickness burns provides a simple and clinically useful model to describe burn injuries.

Pathology of superficial burns

Rapid but transient exposure to high temperatures such as flash injuries or prolonged exposure to temperatures just above tolerable limits will produce damage or death to the surface epithelial cells only. This damage will excite an underlying inflammatory response in the tissues deep to the injury producing pain, swelling and hyperaemia, the classical triad of the inflammatory response. The surface layers of cells may peel off, leaving the sensitive deeper layers of the epidermis exposed. As the basal layer remains intact in such injuries, the epidermis will completely regenerate to normal thickness with a new outer stratum corneum. This process will usually take 7–10 days. Such a burn is described as a superficial burn.

Pathology of partial-thickness burns

If the injury occurs to a greater depth, the outer epithelium and part of the underlying dermis will be damaged. The magnitude of the underlying inflammatory response will be greater, with capillary dilatation, loss of integrity of capillary walls, leading to excessive leakage of fluid from the intravascular to the interstitial space in the area of the burn wound. This fluid consists mainly of water and electrolytes such as sodium and potassium but will contain some protein. The consequences and the clinical picture will depend on how deeply the injury extends into the dermis. If cell death occurs close to the dermal-epidermal junction, the relatively thin outer layer of dead cells may be stripped off the underlying dermis by the fluid accumulating as a result of the inflammatory response. This produces surface blisters. Beneath such blisters is a dermal layer still rich in basal cells from the retained rete pegs of the epidermis. These epidermal cells can quickly multiply and migrate to reform a confluent layer that will gradually thicken to produce a new but slightly thinner and slightly more delicate epidermis. With blistered burns this healing process, if not hampered by infection, is usually well underway by 10–14 days. Such wounds are described as a superficial partial thickness of burns.

If the line of demarcation between dead and damaged cells lies deeper within the dermis, the overlying layer of cells may either separate at the time of burning, leaving a moist, weeping, sensitive layer of exposed damaged dermis, or may remain as a blanched, waxy layer that is too thick and rigid for the fluid beneath to form a blister. The inflammatory process excited by the burn will aid autolysis of the dead cells at the line of demarcation. If the deeper layers of the dermis remain viable, scattered epithelial cells may be found within the retained sweat glands and hair follicles. These cells can multiply, forming small colonies of epithelial cells that will migrate and eventually coalesce with surrounding colonies to produce a confluent layer. This process may be slow and healing and may not be complete even beyond 6 weeks post-burn. Spontaneous healing of deep partial-thickness burns occurs with significant wound contraction and scar formation, with a very thin and friable epidermal layer. These wounds are described as deep partial-thickness burns and, although spontaneous healing may occur, the cosmetic and functional result is often unsatisfactory and inferior to that achieved with surgical wound closure.

Pathology of full-thickness burns

If cell death extends deep to the dermis, all the skin layers are lost. The burnt tissue dries, forming a thick leathery covering called an eschar. If left, this eschar gradually separates, leaving an underlying granulating deep wound that will gradually contract in size. Epithelium at the edges of this burn wound will slowly migrate into the wound in an attempt to produce wound closure. This epithelial migration is slow and spontaneous healing is only ever achieved in small full-thickness burns. The result of spontaneous healing in full-thickness burns is gross scarring and contractures.

Systemic effects of burns

With a burn injury involving less than 10% of the body surface areas, the inflammatory response leads to fluid shifts that are compensated for by normal homeostatic mechanisms such as peripheral vasoconstriction. With a burn injury to greater than 10% of the body surface area, the fluid that shifts from the intravascular to the extravascular space begins to compromise the cardiac output and overall tissue perfusion. Large burns are associated with the systemic liberation of the inflammatory mediators such as cytokines, which trigger the systemic inflammatory response syndrome, leading to generalised capillary permeability and large fluid shifts. Untreated, this process is associated with the development of hypovolaemic shock, with decreased renal perfusion resulting in renal failure and eventually multi-organ failure and death.

Infection

With burn injuries resulting in the loss of the outer protective layers of the epidermis, rapid colonisation of the wound occurs, with bacteria and fungi derived initially from the host and later from the surrounding environment. These organisms can easily invade more deeply into the exposed dermis, producing local tissue destruction, which further complicates healing and deepens the damage. If large areas of burns are infected, organisms may spread systemically leading to septicaemia. Common pathological organisms that invade and interfere with the natural healing of the burn wounds are *Staphylococcus aureus*, *Streptococcus viridans* and *Pseudomonas pyocyanea*. Meticulous wound care is necessary to prevent burn wound infection. Topical antimicrobial agents have been the preferred means of reducing burn wound infection. Systemic antibiotics are only indicated for the treatment of established or invasive burn wound infection.

Assessment and management of the burned patient

Emergency examination and treatment

Rapid assessment and treatment of major burns may be life saving. The possibility of coexisting injuries must always be considered, especially with burns associated with road traffic accidents, blast injuries and electrocution. Injuries may also occur from jumping while escaping from the heat source. The principles of initial management consist of immediate first aid, followed by primary and secondary survey with institution of simultaneous resuscitation.

First aid

Stop the burning process by smouldering flames and removing clothing to cool the burn wound.

For extensive burned areas cool water (ideal temperature 15°C) should be applied to cool the skin to normal temperatures. The patient should then be wrapped in loose dry material to prevent systemic cooling, which may lead to severe and at times fatal hypothermia. For small superficial burns, cooling will have a major analgesic effect and should be continued until the stinging sensation begins to abate.

Primary survey

The primary survey identifies and addresses immediate life-threatening conditions and consists of:

- (A) Airways maintenance with cervical spine control
- (B) Breathing and ventilation
- (C) Circulation with haemorrhage control
- (D) Disability and neurological status
- (E) Exposure and environmental control

(A) Airways maintenance with cervical spine control

Check that the airway is clear of foreign materials and, if indicated, such as in the unconscious patient, open the airway by lifting the chin or thrusting the jaw forward using pressure behind the angles of the mandible. Never hyper-flex or hyper-extend the neck during these manoeuvres as there may be an associated unstable cervical spine injury. An oropharyngeal or nasopharyngeal airway may provide a temporary airway in unconscious patients, whilst a normal speaking voice indicates a clear airway, but deterioration may occur with time if heat has been inhaled.

(B) Breathing and ventilation

Burned patients may not be ventilating adequately due to a depressed conscious state secondary to cerebral injury or hypoxia associated with the burn. Inhalation of heat and smoke, which occurs commonly in house fires, may lead to inflammation and obstruction of the airways, impairing ventilation. Smoke and chemical irritation may also irritate the lungs, leading to impaired gaseous exchange.

To assess the adequacy of breathing and ventilation, fully expose the chest and check chest expansion. If this appears adequate, supplemental oxygen should be supplied using a face mask. If there were signs of respiratory obstruction or inadequate ventilation, initial ventilation via a bag and mask should be instituted while preparing for endotracheal intubation and assisted ventilation. If there is a clinical risk of the development of airway oedema or signs of respiratory obstruction early endotracheal intubation should be performed. Delay in intubation may see the very development of gross pharyngeal oedema necessitating an emergency tracheostomy or cricothyroidotomy to secure airway.

(C) Circulation with haemorrhage control

Check the state of the circulatory system.

- Pulse and blood pressure assessment. If pulse is weak or blood pressure is low, immediate fluid resuscitation should be commenced.
- Capillary refill test. Normal return should occur within 2 seconds.
- Stop any external bleeding by applying direct pressure.

(D) Disability and neurological status

Establish and record the level of consciousness, which may be affected by direct cerebral injury or the result of hypoxia secondary to respiratory complications. A simple method of describing the disability is:

- A – alert
- V – response to verbal stimuli
- P – response to painful stimuli
- U – unresponsive.

(E) Exposure with environmental control

Remove all clothing to allow a rapid appraisal of the extent of the injury and keep the patient warm.

Secondary survey

Having stabilised any immediate life-threatening situations, a comprehensive assessment is undertaken.

History

All sources of information should be assessed including, most importantly, the information from ambulance officers or paramedics involved in the evacuation and transport of the patient (Box 46.1).

Additional salient points of the history include:

- A – allergies
- M – medication
- P – past illnesses
- L – last meal
- E – events/environment related to injury such as duration of exposure to heat, nature of the burning agent, first-aid measures applied and type of clothing worn.

Box 46.1 Key questions in taking the history of a burns patient

- When did the accident take place? What is the time delay between the accident and being seen? Long delays without treatment can be very hazardous.
- What treatment has already taken place?
- Have the appropriate measures been taken to monitor progress?
- Has resuscitation been adequate?
- How did the accident happen?
- Was flame involved?
- Explosion?
- Smoke?
- Confined space?
- Any evidence of criminal intent?
- Alcohol?
- Clothing worn at the time?

Examination

A comprehensive head-to-toe examination is necessary to fully assess the extent of the burn injury and to detect any associated injuries.

Head and neck

Assess general signs of injury. Check for corneal burns. Look for indications of possible inhalation injury, such as burns or blistering of the nose and mouth, singeing of nasal hairs, soot in the mouth or pharynx and blisters or oedema of the tongue. Carefully check for signs of cervical spine injury.

Chest

Examine the whole chest, assessing the burn injury and whether it is compromising respiration. Look for evidence of rib fractures or flail chest. Listen for breath sounds and signs that might indicate inhalation injury to the lower airways.

Abdomen

Check for signs of associated intra-abdominal injuries if burns are associated with trauma. Assess if abdominal burns are restricting respiration.

Perineum

Check for perineal burns and other injuries.

Limbs

Assess for signs of soft tissue or bony injury. Assess the burns to determine if they are full-thickness and circumferential. Such burns may lead to constriction due to skin shrinkage during the burning process. With the subsequent development of oedema following the burns, this constriction may impair the venous return from the limb, leading to further swelling and eventual cessation of arterial inflow, producing tissue ischaemia and necrosis. Impaired limb perfusion leads to pain and paresthesia, progressing to numbness, pulselessness and paralysis. When venous return from an extremity is obstructed, an escharotomy or splitting of the burned tissue must be performed rapidly to restore adequate circulation.

Assessment of the burn

As previously described, the severity of the burn injury is determined by the extent and the depth of the burn injury.

Assessment of the extent of the burn

The burn extent is described as the percentage of total body surface area (TBSA) affected. In adults this can be roughly calculated by applying the 'rule of nines' (Fig. 46.2). Each arm equals 9% body surface area, the head equals 9%, the anterior and posterior trunk equals 18% each, and each leg equals 18%. This is a simple and broadly accurate assessment tool. Estimation of small irregular burn areas may be performed using the size of the palm, which is approximately 1% of body surface area, as a measure. The use of Lund & Browder body charts is to be encouraged as they provide a permanent record of the extent of the burn injury and are more accurate as the accompanying tables taking into account the differing percentages for the limbs, trunk and head according to age.

Assessment of the depth of the burn

There is currently no accurate or readily available investigative tool for the assessment of burn wound depth

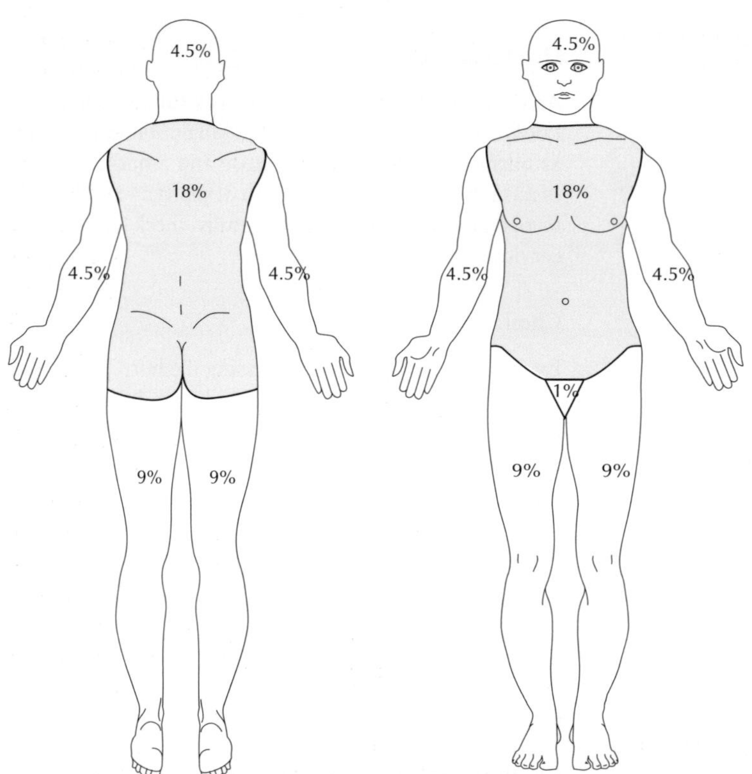

Fig. 46.2 Rule of nines.

and we must rely on the clinical characteristics. The depth, as previously described, can be broadly classified as superficial, partial-thickness or full-thickness.

Clinical features of superficial burns

Burns associated with death or damage to the outer layer of the epidermis, such as those resulting from sunburn or minor scalds, can be identified clinically by:

- erythema that blanches on pressure
- sensitivity to touch
- absence of blisters.

Clinical features of partial-thickness burns

Burns involving the outer layer of the dermis are characterised by:

- blisters suggesting superficial dermal involvement only
- a weeping moist surface suggesting deeper dermal loss
- some capillary return apparent in superficial partial-thickness burns but absent in deeper dermal burns
- sensation present and decreases the deeper the burn extends into the dermis
- the colour may vary from pale pink to blotchy red
- fresh bleeding when pricked with a needle.

Depth of full-thickness burns

Complete death of both epidermis and dermis is characterised by:

- a white waxy to a charred colour
- a firm to hard leathery texture (eschar)
- loss of sensation to pin prick
- absence of bleeding when pricked with needle.

Definitive management of the burn patient

Having fully assessed the magnitude of the clinical problem, a management plan is formulated that involves fluid resuscitation, pain management and treatment of the burn wounds.

Fluid resuscitation

Burns in adults involving greater than 10–15% TBSA and greater than 10% TBSA in children require fluid resuscitation to avoid the complications of systemic hypovolaemia.

There are a number of resuscitation formulas that have been developed to act as a guide to the volume of fluid that will be required to maintain adequate cardiac output during the early post-burn phase (first 48 hours). No resuscitation formula has been shown conclusively to have a survival advantage. The most commonly used formula is:

Adults: 3–4 mL Hartmans solution/kg bodyweight/% burn.

Children: As above plus maintenance fluids according to bodyweight using 4% glucose in one-quarter or one-fifth normal saline.

The volume commences from the time of the burn injury.

Half the calculated volume is given in the first 8 hours and the remaining half in the subsequent 16 hours. Fluid should be administered through large peripheral cannulae, preferably inserted through non-burnt tissue. Central venous access is helpful in large burns.

Monitoring adequacy of fluid resuscitation

The actual volume of fluid needed to adequately resuscitate a burn may vary considerably from the calculated volume due to the inaccuracies of burn wound assessment and the possibility of injuries such as inhalation, which will lead to a greater generalised inflammatory response. Formulas are general guides or starting points for resuscitation, which must be modified according to the clinical response. The easiest and most reliable method of assessing adequacy of fluid resuscitation is by monitoring urine output. Thus, for burns greater than 15% a urinary catheter should be inserted and urine flow of 0.5–1 mL/kg per hour for adults and of 1.0–2 mL/kg per hour for children (<30 kg) aimed for. Urine volumes greater than these levels should be avoided, as excessive resuscitation will lead to unnecessary tissue oedema and the possibility of pulmonary oedema. Red or brown discolouration of the urine indicates the presence of haemoglobin or myoglobin, suggesting muscle injury. This is commonly seen following electrocution or in the presence of a compartment syndrome. These haemochromogens, if concentrated, may become deposited in the proximal renal tubules, leading to acute renal failure. In the presence of haemochromogens, the urinary output should be maintained at a higher level, aiming for 1–2 mL/kg in adults until the urine clears. Occasionally mannitol or frusemide may be judiciously added to maintain an adequate urine flow.

Other forms of cardiovascular monitoring, such as central venous pressure or cardiac output studies, are usually only indicated for patients with premorbid cardiac disease or coexistent injuries causing blood loss.

Pain control

As in all major trauma pain, control is best achieved initially by incremental doses of intravenous narcotics, following which a continuous infusion or patient-controlled analgesia is appropriate.

Treatment of the burn wounds

The management of the burn wound is determined by the clinical assessment of the burn depth and an understanding of the pathophysiology of the burn injury.

Treatment of superficial burns

Burns not associated with significant blistering are not prone to infection and will settle rapidly if care and protection are provided. Occlusive non-adherent dressings are applied to the wound. Elevating burned limbs will minimise oedema formation. Such wounds should resolve in 7–10 days.

Treatment of partial-thickness wounds

Blistering burns and those with intact sensation should heal spontaneously in 10–14 days, providing infection does not intervene. The introduction of effective topical antiseptic agents has been one of the major breakthroughs in the management of burn wounds. While no agent exists that will effectively destroy all bacteria and fungi, silversulphadiazine, a loose chemical combination of 1% silver nitrate with the organic compound sulphonamide sulphadiazine, does cover almost the entire spectrum. This cooling, soothing cream has minimal chances of contact sensitivity or systemic toxicity and provides a highly effective surface antibacterial agent, and should be applied to the burn wound immediately and dressings changed daily. Newer biosynthetic dressings that can adhere and seal cleaned superficial burn wounds have been shown to reduce pain and accelerate spontaneous healing. Their current high costs preclude routine use for superficial burn wounds.

Treatment of deep dermal and full-thickness burns

Burns extending deeply into the dermis may slowly heal spontaneously. Such healing is associated with significant scarring and deformity and a better cosmetic result can be achieved with surgical excision and grafting. Full-thickness burns clearly require excision and grafting to achieve wound healing.

Such surgery is ideally performed as soon as practicable to minimise the risk of infection and hasten the patient's full recovery. The surgical techniques involve removal of the burned tissue down to a living vascularised layer and the application of split-thickness skin harvested from a non-burned area of the body. For partial-thickness burns, the technique of tangential excision is used, where thin layers of the burn are shaved off until a freely bleeding surface is achieved. For deep and full-thickness burns, the outer burned layer is peeled off in a single sheet usually down to the underlying investing layer of fascia. This is known as fascial excision.

Donor skin can be harvested from most sites of the body. The thighs are preferred, but with large extensive burns all unburned areas except the face may need to be used. The donor skin must contain basal epithelial cells to produce a new epidermal layer and thus skin is harvested down to the level of the rete pegs. The donor sites heal by rapid migration of the remaining keratinocytes and such donor sites may be reharvested when healing is complete. This may be in as little as 7–10 days, depending upon the thickness of the skin taken and the texture of the donor sites. To prevent blood and fluid accumulating beneath the grafted skin, which will prevent the graft from becoming vascularised, the donor skin is usually passed through a meshing machine that produces multiple slits in the graft. Depending on the length of the slits, the skin may be expanded, allowing a larger area to be covered. This technique is useful in large burns where donor sites are limited. Such widely meshed skin relies on epithelial migration to fill the gaps in the mesh.

Plastic surgery

With appropriate wound management, as detailed above, the majority of patients achieve a very satisfactory functional and cosmetic result with their primary wound healing. Severely burned patients may have damage to underlying tendons, especially on the dorsum of the hand, around the elbow or the foot, for which split-thickness grafting techniques are not appropriate. In these circumstances vascularised skin flaps may be indicated. Reconstructive surgical techniques arc also occasionally needed to correct contractures and deformities, particularly to the anterior neck and the axillary folds. Minimisation of such contractures and deformities is achieved by early wound closure and the physiotherapy and occupational therapy staff using active stretching and appropriate splinting techniques.

Nursing care of the patient

The nursing care of the burned patient is demanding both on patient and nurse. It requires a great deal of understanding and compassion from the latter and taxes the fortitude of the former, who has to put up with repeated and often painful dressing. The day-to-day care of the patient depends on good general nursing and good techniques with dressings. There is a vast array of differing techniques used for dressing the burned wounds. The basic principles to be observed are:

- keep the wound clean and protected with the appropriate antibacterial bandage or occlusive dressing
- facilitate the maximum mobility and joint function wherever possible
- minimise pain and discomfort by a combination of gentle handling and appropriate analgesics.

The techniques of continuous narcotic infusion and patient-controlled anagelsia have greatly facilitated patient comfort and wound care.

Nutrition

Energy expenditure of the extensively burned patient is high and may be several times that of the normal basal level. A rapid drop in the patient's serum proteins and significant weight loss, especially involving loss of skeletal muscle mass, may occur in major burns. Nutritional support is vital for patient survival in the setting of major burns. For moderate burns the use of food supplements and fortified drinks may be adequate. For major burns, for example those involving more than 40% TBSA, patients are usually unable to meet their metabolic demands using diet alone, and continuous nasoenteral feeding is required. This is best achieved via a nasojejunal tube, which should be placed as soon as possible, and feeding commenced early. It is possible to feed the patient enterally in the presence of gastric stasis with an appropriately placed enteral feeding tube. Parenteral nutrition is uncommonly required unless there are associated abdominal problems.

Electrical burns

Electrical injury is uncommon. Carelessness is often a factor in its occurrence. Commonly, the so-called electrical injury is the result from the discharge of electrical energy causing a fire and is thus a burn and not due to electrocution. However, if the victim does connect with an electrical circuit, death can occur due to cardiac arrhythmia or respiratory paralysis, although this is relatively unusual. Electrocution produces an entry and exit wound with variable damage to the intervening conducting tissues. If deep tissue damage is suspected, both the entry and exit points in the areas in between should be explored. Extensive limb fasciotomies and muscle debridement may be required if significant current flows through soft tissues, producing swelling and muscle necrosis. The risk of cardiac damage, especially in injuries involving conduction of current through the left arm and exiting on the right side of the body, should be remembered. Cardiac monitoring is essential if there is a history or existing evidence of a change in cardiac rhythm or elevation of cardiac enzyme. In the absence of any evidence of initial cardiac involvement, prolonged monitoring is not required. With the appropriate management of arrhythmia, recovery from a cardiac injury after electrocution is generally complete.

Chemical burns

Strong acids and alkalis used for industrial purposes are the most frequent cause of chemical injuries resulting in a burn. Immediate dowsing in water is the appropriate first aid prior to transfer to hospital. Hydrofluoric acid used in glass etching is a particularly dangerous acid as it deeply penetrates the tissues and is not quickly neutralised. Medical attention must be sought immediately. Calcium gluconate gel or 10% of calcium gluconate injected locally must be used to neutralise the effects by binding with the free fluoride radicals. Sometimes immediate surgery to excise the already damaged tissue and to prevent continuing tissue damage may be necessary.

MCQs

Select the single correct answer to each question.

1 The volume of fluid replacement required in the first 24 hours in a 70-kg adult with 30% burns is approximately:
a 2,500 mL
b 4,000 mL
c 7,500 mL
d 10 500 mL
e 12 500 mL

2 Fluid replacement in a 70-kg adult with 30% burns should maintain a urine flow of:
a 35 mL/hour
b 70 mL/hour
c 105 mL/hour
d 140 mL/hour
e 175 mL/hour

3 Mesh split skin grafts are used in burns because:
a they release haematomas
b they cause less pain
c they produce a better cosmetic result
d the donor site heals more quickly
e all of the above

4 Which of the following bacteria occur commonly in burn wound infections?
a *Klebsiella* spp.
b *Clostridium difficile*
c *Bacteroides fragilis*
d *Staphylococcus epidermidis*
e *Pseudomonas pyocyanea*

Orthopaedic Surgery

47 Fractures and dislocations

Peter Choong

Fractures

Definitions

A fracture is a loss in the normal continuity of bone following the application of a direct or indirect force to that bone. A fracture may involve a part or the entire circumference of the cortex.

Classifications of fractures

Closed

A closed fracture is one that is not associated with a breach in the overlying skin or mucous membrane.

Open

An open fracture is one where there is direct communication between the fracture and the externa through a breach in the overlying skin or mucous membrane. Open fractures are at significant risk for infection.

Types of fractures

- Transverse
- Oblique
- Spiral
- Comminuted (more than two fragments)
- Displaced
- Angulated
- Impacted
- Rotated
- Distracted
- Green stick – This occurs when only one cortex of the bone is seen to be fractured on the X-ray, and there is usually minimal deformity. This most commonly occurs in the paediatric age group.
- Intra-articular – Fractures that extend to the articular surface of a joint.
- Special fractures.
  - Pathologic fracture – fracture through an abnormal bone.
  - Stress fracture – fracture through repeated minor trauma to a normal bone (Fig. 47.1).

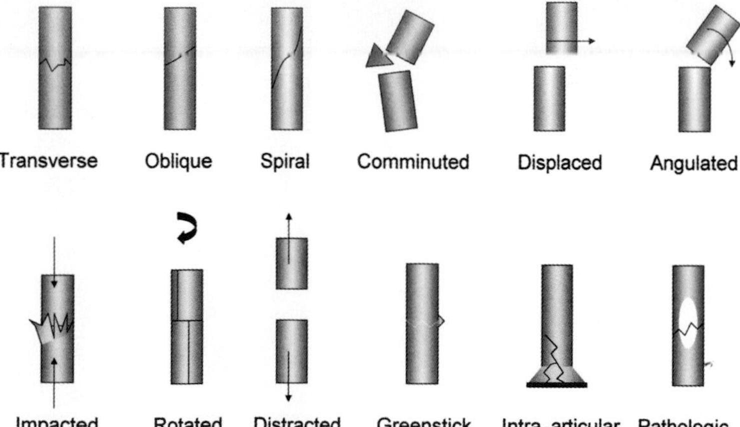

Fig. 47.1 Types of fractures.

Clinical presentation

All fractures are painful. There is normally a history of trauma except in pathological fractures where minimal trauma or no trauma is the rule. Fractures are tender, swollen, occasionally deformed, mobile at the fracture site, and associated with loss of limb function.

Investigations

Radiographs

All suspected fractures should be X-rayed in two planes (antero-posterior, lateral) (Fig. 47.2).

Bone scans

Suspected fractures, which are not obvious on plain radiographs may be identified by bone scan, which show increased isotope uptake corresponding to the site of the fracture. This maybe less apparent in the geriatric group where an osteoblastic response may be less prominent. In the elderly, a delay of one week before bone scanning is usually required to show a positive scan. Bone scans are useful for detecting femoral neck and pelvic fractures in the elderly and carpal injuries in younger patients.

Computed tomography (CT)

CT Scans are excellent for delineating cortical and trabecular bone. The plane of the CT should be

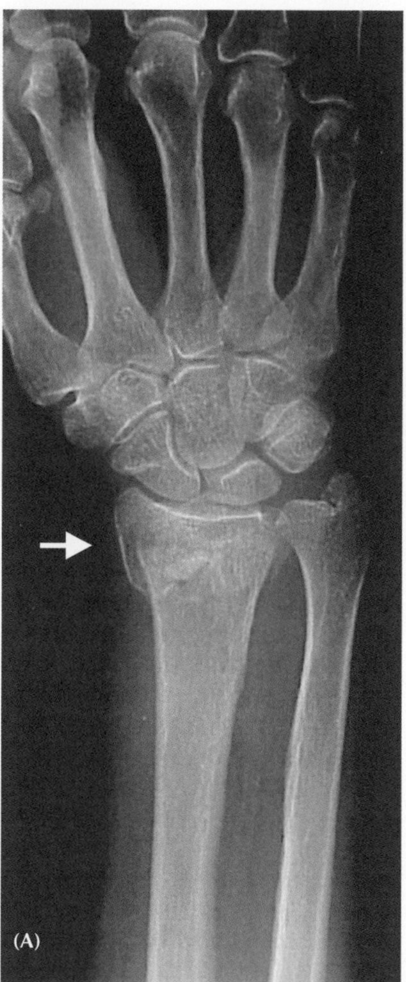

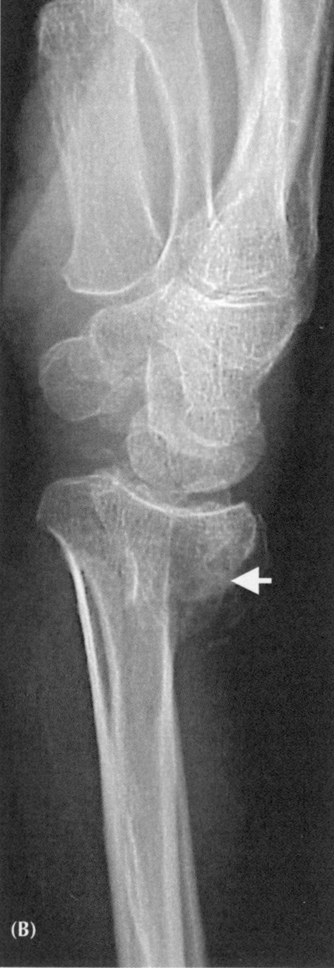

Fig. 47.2 Colles fracture.
(**A**) Antero-posterior xray of comminuted distal radial metaphyseal fracture. Note shortening and slight radial angulation of the fracture. An important sign that denotes a fracture are overlapping cortices (arrow).
(**B**) Lateral X-ray of comminuted distal radial fracture. Dorsal displacement, dorsal tilt and shortening is typical of a Colles fracture.

perpendicular or oblique to the fracture line to detect the fracture. CT is good for demonstrating periosteal new bone formation and may be valuable for diagnosing subtle stress fractures such as minimally displaced femoral neck fractures, pelvic ring fractures, and rib fractures.

Magnetic resonance imaging (MRI)

Limited MRI scans in the coronal or surgical plane are excellent for demonstrating fractures which are suspected but not readily apparent on plain X-rays. T1 weighted MRI's are able to detect the fracture immediately after injury and T2 weighted images can differentiate soft tissue inflammation from intraosseous oedema. MRI scans are excellent for early detection of undisplaced scaphoid and femoral neck fractures.

Treatment

Closed fractures

The principles of management of a closed fracture include

- correction of the deformity (reduction)
- immobilisation of the fracture
- protection until the fracture has consolidated
- rehabilitation of the muscles and joints of the affected limb.

Closed reduction

Under appropriate anaesthesia (local, regional, general) the fracture fragments should be manipulated and reduced into normal alignment. In reducing the fracture, combinations of distraction, increasing and then reducing the deformity of the fracture, and holding the reduction with 3 point fixation are employed. This technique of reduction is also used with open fractures (Fig. 47.3).

Open reduction

Open reduction is indicated when closed manipulation of bone fragments has failed to reduce the fracture into a satisfactory position, if reduction is impossible or if reduction is lost after initial closed reduction. Open reduction may be indicated to stabilise fractures securely to allow safe and effective management of the patients with multiple other bone or soft tissue injuries, or if movement of the adjacent joint is paramount.

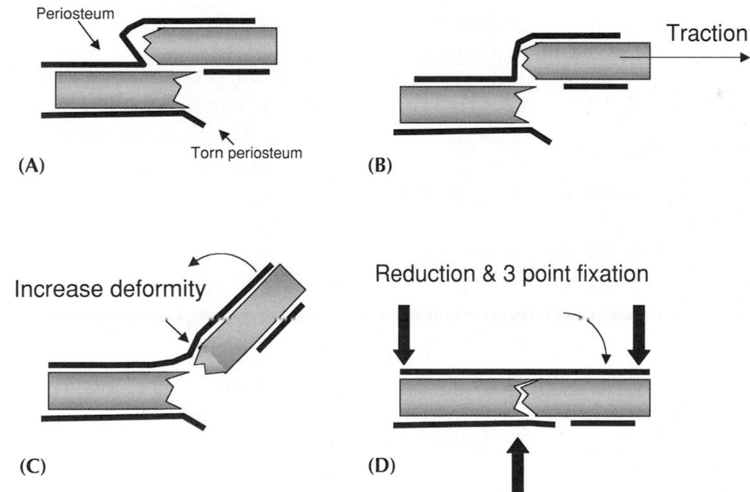

Fig. 47.3 Principles of technique of fracture reduction. (**A**) Most fractures are associated with fractures that are displaced, impacted and shortened. It is common that the periosteum on one side of the fracture is intact, while that of the other side is torn. (**B**) The first step in reducing a fracture is disimpaction where traction is applied along the axis of the bone to draw the fracture ends apart. In young patients, this may be difficult because of the very thick and resilient periosteum. (**C**) The next step is to increase the deformity so that the opposing ends of the fracture may be approximated. (**D**) The final step of reduction once the fracture ends are opposed is to correct the deformity and to apply three point fixation to hold the fracture reduction (arrows). The arrows point to areas where pressure must be applied while shaping the plaster-of-Paris cast.

Open fractures

Open fractures are at risk of developing infections (acute and chronic osteomyelitis). The principles of management include:

- Cleaning of contaminated tissue. This is usually accomplished by irrigation with copious amounts of sterile or antibiotic loaded irrigation solution. In heavily contaminated wounds, pulsatile irrigation devices are used to agitate the wound to assist in dislodging and diluting out foreign debris.
- Debridement of traumatised wound edges and tissue. This step is important to remove necrotic or ischemic tissue which may become foci for infection if colonised by infective organisms. Careful surgical handling of the tissue is mandatory to prevent extension of tissue injury.
- Stabilisation of fractures. Stability of the fracture is important to protect the surrounding soft tissue from further injury that may occur if the sharp fracture ends were allowed to move. The method of stabilisation is important and will depend on the extent of the soft tissue injury (see below).
- Closure of exposed bone by adequate soft tissue cover. On completion of wound debridement, the soft tissue defect may be closed either by direct suture or tissue grafts. Tissue grafts may be in the form of split skin grafts or tissue flaps. The decision regarding closure will depend on the degree of contamination and size of the defect.

Classification of open fractures

Open fractures are classified according to the severity of the injury and the modality of injury.

- Type 1: Puncture of overlying of skin or mucous membrane by a bony spike from within.
- Type 2: Laceration less than 1 cm overlying the fracture.
- Type 3: Laceration greater than 1 cm overlying a fracture.
- Type 3A: Raising of a soft tissue flap around the fracture.
- Type 3B: Absolute skin loss around a fracture.
- Type 3C: Deep and highly contaminated wound such as after a farm injury, gun shot injury and fractures associated with neurovascular injury.

Surgical considerations of open fractures

- Type 1 and 2 open fractures which can be thoroughly debrided, cleansed with copious amounts of fluid (6 litres) may be able to be fixed with internal fixation devices. Such injuries are also treated with prophylactic perioperative antibiotics for 48 hours: Keflin 1 gm i.v. 6 hourly.
- Type 3 open fractures are usually fixed with external fixation devices after thorough debridement, cleansing, and fracture reduction. Frequently soft tissue reconstruction is required to provide closure of the wound: Keflin 1 gm i.v. 6 hourly.
- Type 3C injuries are associated with a poor prognosis and amputation may be required in up to 60% of 3C injuries. A course of antibiotics is usually prescribed and the selection of antibiotics will depend upon the type of contamination introduced into the wound: Vancomycin 1 gm i.v. 12 hourly (adjusted to pre- and postadministration levels) and ceftriaxone 1 gm i.v. 12 hourly.

Fracture immobilisation

Splintage

Minor fractures such as those effecting the phalanges of the fingers may be treated using small metal or plastic splints.

Plaster of paris cast

Plaster of Paris cast immobilisation is a conventional method of immobilising the fracture following closed reduction. This may be either a completely encircling moulded cast or an incomplete encircling cast (plaster slab).

Traction

Some fractures, particularly those involving the lower limb, may be treated temporarily or definitively by the application of traction along the line the limb. Traction encourages normal alignment of the fracture and the increased tension of the surrounding soft tissue helps to provide internal splintage of the fracture.

External fixation

External fixation is the application of transfixing pins and bars to create a construct that lies external to the limb and acts to hold the fracture following either open or closed reduction. This method of immobilisation is selected if unstable fractures cannot be held using traditional non-operative techniques. External fixation is also indicated when an open and contaminated fracture is at risk of infection and therefore must be held immobilised by a system which does not introduce into the wound any foreign material such as metal plates and screws.

Internal fixation

Internal fixation is indicated when closed reduction has failed, when further displacement is anticipated, when closed non-operative immobilisation constitutes a risk to the patient, or when internal fixation allows earlier mobilisation, rehabilitation and earlier return to normal function. Internal fixation includes the use of transfixing wires, inter fragmentary screws, metal plates, and intra-medullary rods.

Outcome

Fracture union

Fractures treated with closed reduction are said to have united when no mobility occurs at the fracture site. Early union is normally associated with some tenderness on stressing of the fracture whilst complete union and consolidation is said to be evident when there is no tenderness of the fracture site and stressing does not reproduce symptoms of pain. Radiographic assessment of union is made by observing the development of fracture callous and the gradual disappearance of the fracture line.

Rigid and internal fixation with internal fixation devices may reduce the amount of callus formation and because of the rigidity of the fracture immobilisation may make clinical assessment of union difficult. When fractures have been openly reduced and internally fixed the union is assessed using radiographs to demonstrate the disappearance of the fracture line.

Fracture protection

All healing fractures must be protected against refracture by gradually permitting stresses along the fractured bone that is commensurate with the strength of that healing bone. In the lower limb, this may be undertaken as a combination of graduated weight bearing of the fractured limb and the use of external supports such as crutches, splints and braces after 6 to 8 weeks of non-weight bearing. In the upper limb, weighted activity may commence after 4–6 weeks.

Complications

Haemorrhage

Bleeding may occur from laceration of adjacent soft tissue, vascular structures or through fracture ends. Significant amounts of bleeding may occur into soft tissue depending upon the bone fracture, e.g. closed femoral fractures may loose up to 2 litres of blood into the thigh, and pelvic fractures up to 4 litres into the pelvic cavity.

Infection

Infection is a risk for all open injuries.

Intra-articular extension

Some fractures extend from bone into the joint. Displacement of articular fragments must be treated by anatomic reduction to reduce the risk of post-traumatic arthritis.

Vascular compromise

Excessive bleeding or swelling into the soft tissue may induce a compartment syndrome where excessive pressures within a tissue compartment prevents adequate blood flow to that compartment. Unless this is treated expediently necrosis of soft tissue and subsequent scarring may cause loss of limb function or loss of the limb itself. The signs of a compartment syndrome are dominated by pain that is not responsive to analgesia. Increasing pain following limb surgery mandates an examination to exclude a compartment syndrome. Other signs of limb ischemia include pallor, paraesthesia, paralysis, poikylothermia, and pulselessness.

Late complications

Delayed union

Delayed union occurs when a fracture has not united in a period of time that is at least 25% longer than the expected average time for fracture union at that site. The causes of delayed union include inadequate immobilisation, infection, avascular necrosis of bone, and

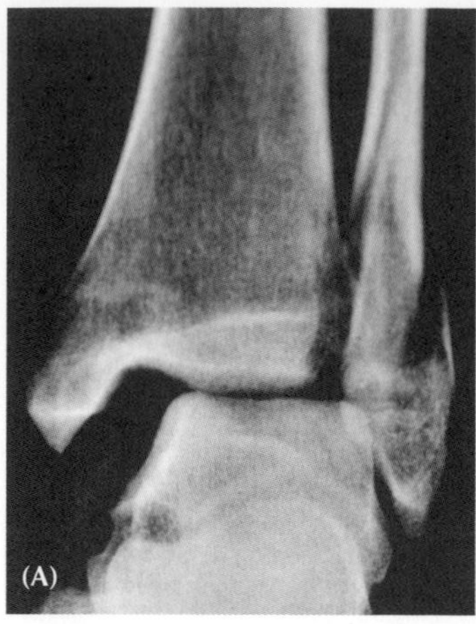

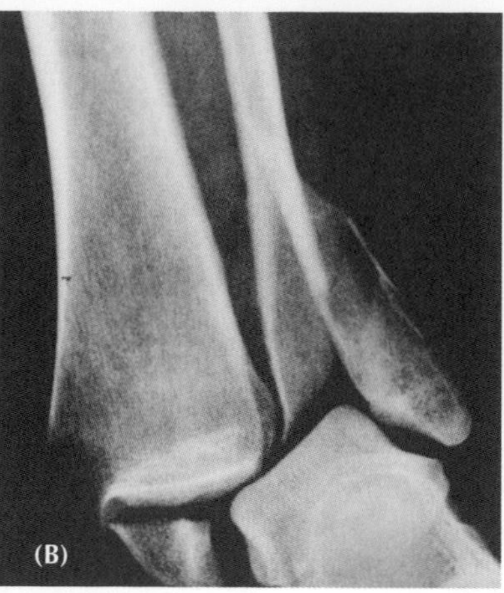

Fig. 47.4 (A) Fracture subluxation of the ankle. (B) Fracture dislocation of the ankle.

soft tissue interposition between fracture ends. Delayed union is assessed radiographically.

Non-union

Non-union is said to have occurred when no evidence of union is seen on sequential X-rays over a six-month period of time. Non-union is associated clinically with movement or pain at the fracture site. If there is copious amounts of callus formation but without bridging of the fracture a state of hypertrophic non-union is said to exist and requires rigid internal fixation for cure. If there is no evidence of callus formation, then a state of hypotrophic non-union is said to exist and bone grafting and internal fixation is required for treatment.

Mal-union

Mal-union occurs when the fracture unites with a loss of anatomical alignment. Mal-union by shortening may be acceptable but angulation and rotation of the bone following union may not be acceptable and may interfere with normal function.

Rehabilitation

On removal of a plaster cast, the joints adjacent to a fractured limb require rehabilitation to prevent or treat stiffness. This involves passive and active range of motion exercises and proprioception exercises to improve the sense of balance in the recovering joint. In addition, it is important to return the strength and endurance of the muscles in the injured limb by a regime of exercises.

Limbs treated with internal fixation may undergo earlier mobilisation because the fracture is usually more stable than those treated by plaster immobilisation.

Dislocations

Definition

Dislocation is a complete loss of contact between the articular surfaces of the bones forming a joint.

Subluxation is displacement of the joint with the loss of normal congruity but the articular surfaces remain in partial contact with each other (Fig. 47.4).

Clinical presentation

Subluxations and dislocations normally follow direct or indirect trauma. This condition may also occur voluntarily in patients with ligamentous laxity. Dislocations may also follow an epileptic seizure or electrocution, and the classic injury is a posterior shoulder dislocation. Patients complain of pain, deformity and loss of function. Examination demonstrates a loss of normal contour of the joint, marked restriction of movement and pain on attempted passive motion of the joint.

Investigations

Radiographs

Plain radiographs are sufficient to demonstrate dislocations and subluxations. Radiographs in two planes (anteroposterior and lateral) are essential for confirming the diagnosis. Occasionally associated fractures may be seen and care should be taken not to displace these fractures in an attempt to reduce the dislocation.

Treatment

The principles of treatment are to reduce the dislocation, immobilise the joint and to rehabilitate the joint.

Closed reduction of the joint under adequate anaesthesia and analgesia is undertaken with the combination of traction, rotation and angulation. At all times forceful manipulation of the joint should be avoided in order to prevent fracture of adjacent bones or neurovascular trauma.

Open reduction is undertaken when closed reduction has failed. This may occur because of the interposition of tissue or the entrapment of the dislocated bone by capsular or ligamentous attachments. Open reduction may also be undertaken if the dislocation is associated with a complex fracture or neurovascular injury that requires exploration and repair.

Chronic dislocations, that is, joints that have been dislocated for more than 1 week, are usually treated by open reduction because soft tissue scarring and fibrosis within the joint would normally prevent normal reduction.

Immobilisation

Immobilisation of the joint may be performed using a sling or splints. The purpose of immobilisation is to rest the joint to allow capsular and ligamentous healing.

Physiotherapy

Movement of the joint following reduction may be encouraged after an adequate period of time where healing of the soft tissues has occurred. Supervised movement by a physiotherapist is normally encouraged to prevent re-dislocation. The purpose of physiotherapy is to strengthen the peri-articular musculature to provide joint stability and also to improve the range of motion that is normally restricted because of capsular scarring. Strengthening exercises of the joint are only encouraged after full range of motion has been achieved.

Complications

- Neurovascular injury
- Joint stiffness
- Recurrent dislocation
- Fracture

MCQs

Select the single correct answer to each question.

1 Radiologic evidence of an acute fracture includes:
a loss of continuity in cortical bone
b osteoporosis
c sclerosis of bone
d reduced adjacent soft tissue markings
e gas in the surrounding muscle

2 In assessing the severity of an acute fracture, one must always:
a examine for subcutaneous emphysema
b examine for evidence of gangrene
c examine the status of the neurovascular system of the fractured part
d examine for a temperature and arrhythmia
e examine for evidence of a fat embolism

3 The cardinal feature of a compartment syndrome are:
a pain
b hyperthermia
c rubor
d punctate ecchymosis
e limb hyperactivity

4 When a plaster cast is applied for a fractured wrist, care must be taken to instruct the patient on symptoms of:
a pulmonary embolism
b fat embolism
c air embolism
d compartment syndrome
e Choong–Baker syndrome

5 Dislocation may be missed in the following circumstance:
a posterior dislocation of the hip
b posterior dislocation of the shoulder
c posterior dislocation of the elbow
d posterior dislocation of the sternoclavicular joint
e posterior dislocation of the knee

48 Diseases of bone and joints

Peter Choong

Infections

Acute osteomyelitis

Acute osteomyelitis is an acute bacterial infection of bone. It occurs more commonly in paediatric and geriatric patients, and in those who are immunocompromised. Infection may also follow trauma that is associated with major contamination of bone.

Organism

The commonest organism is *Staphylococcus aureus*. Other organisms include *Pneumococcus* spp., *Streptococcus* spp., *Haemophilus influenzae*, Gram-negative and mycobacteria.

Aetiology

Bacteria pass from a distant source (e.g. dental infections, open sores, urinary tract infections) via the blood stream to the metaphysis of bone (haematogenous spread). Manipulation of infected areas (e.g. tooth extractions, urethral catheterisation) may cause a bacteremia that leads to osteomyelitis. Here the entrapped organisms multiply to create firstly an acute inflammatory then suppurative lesion in metaphyseal bone. Spread of infection through the cortex may cause a subperiosteal abscess, spread into the adjacent joint may cause a suppurative arthritis and spread across the growth plate in the paediatric age group may cause growth abnormalities (Fig. 48.1).

Elevation of the periosteum by the abscess together with intra-osseous pressure caused by the metaphyseal

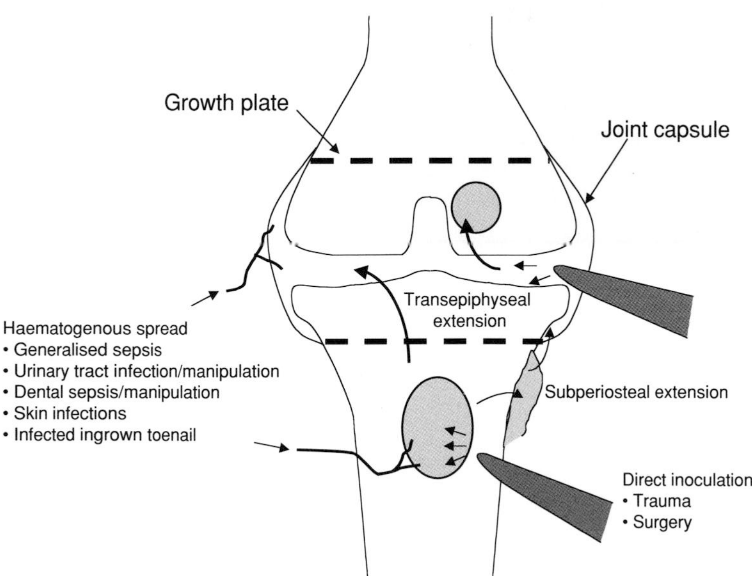

Fig. 48.1 Mechanisms of entry of infective organisms into bones and joints.

abscess may result in a vascular infarction of the involved bone. The necrotic bone is referred to as a *sequestrum*. In time, the elevated periosteum generates new bone that surrounds the sequestrum. The new tube of bone that is formed is referred to as an *involucrum*. If there is communication from the intra-medullary abscess through the skin to form a sinus this is referred to as a *cloaca*, which may discharge pus and necrotic debris. The presence of a sequestrum, involucrum and cloaca is referred to as chronic osteomyelitis.

Clinical presentation

There is often a history of minor trauma to the affected part. Trauma may give rise to a locus of decreased resistance to infection (*locus minoris resistentia*). Several days later the patient presents with a painful and swollen limb where pressure over the infected area elicits marked tenderness. Children may be reluctant to use the affected limb. With progression of infection the patient becomes constitutionally unwell (febrile, rigors, sweat, nausea, vomiting, anorexia). Fluctuance denotes the development of a subperiosteal abscess.

Investigations

BLOOD TESTS

Full blood examination – elevated white cell count, left shift, increased band forms, elevated erythrocyte sedimentation rate and C reactive protein.

BLOOD CULTURES

Blood should be taken for aerobic and anaerobic cultures on diagnosis (2 sets of cultures 1 hour apart) and at times of high fevers (>38.5°C). Blood cultures should be obtained prior to the commencement of antibiotic therapy.

RADIOGRAPHS

Radiographs early in disease commonly demonstrate soft tissue swelling or an associated joint effusion but no bone changes. After 10–14 days, radiographic changes include periosteal new bone formation, which signifies elevation or inflammation of the periosteum by oedema or infective material and osteopenia.

BONE SCANS

Infections induce a marked inflammatory response with hyperaemia of bone and increased bone turnover. Nuclear bone scans demonstrate increased (e.g. technetium-99 MDP, gallium-67) tracer uptake at the affected site (hot scan). Indium white cell scans demonstrate acute white cell collections (abscess).

MAGNETIC RESONANCE IMAGING

MRI is a very sensitive test for inflammation and bony oedema. Marked marrow and soft tissue changes on TI and T2 weighted films can be expected. The sensitivity of MRI sometimes confounds the interpretation of marked bone and soft tissue oedema, where bone oedema arising as a sympathetic response to overlying cellulitis may be interpreted as osteomyelitis.

DIFFERENTIAL DIAGNOSIS

Important differential diagnoses for a painful swollen bone include:

- Primary bone tumour, e.g. osteosarcoma, Ewing's sarcoma
- Secondary bone tumour, e.g. breast, lung, prostate
- Haematologic malignancy, e.g. lymphoma, myeloma
- Fracture, e.g. stress fracture

Treatment

ANTIBIOTIC THERAPY

Intravenous antibiotics are initiated after blood cultures have been taken (flucloxacillin 2 g i.v. 4 hourly and cephalothin 1 g i.v. 6 hourly) and continued until the organism(s) has been identified and sensitivities known. There is usually a rapid response to the initiation of antibiotics with an improvement in constitutional symptoms and signs.

IMMOBILISATION

The affected limb should be immobilised and elevated to reduce oedema and pain.

ANALGESIA

Combination of oral and intramuscular analgesia may be required.

SURGERY

Surgery is indicated if:

- There is evidence of a subperiosteal or soft tissue abscess.
- The patient's condition deteriorates despite adequate antibiotics therapy, and there is radiologic evidence of an intramedullary collection.

OUTCOME

Modern antibiotic therapy is associated with good and often complete resolution of infection. Occasionally a remnant nidus of infection will cause repeated flare-ups for which repeated courses of antibiotic therapy will be necessary. If dead bone remains in the presence of infection, a state of chronic osteomyelitis may develop.

Acute septic arthritis

This is an acute bacterial infection of a joint. It is commonly mono-articular but may occasionally affect several joints concurrently.

Organism

The commonest organism is *Staphylococcus aureus*. Other organisms include *Haemophilus* and *Meningococcus* species.

Aetiology

Septic arthritis may arise from haematogenous spread, direct inoculation, transepiphyseal spread of osteomyelitis or direct spread from a subperiosteal collection of pus (Fig. 48.1).

Clinical presentation

The patient is often febrile and toxic. Any movement of the joint causes extreme pain. In the elderly, symptoms may be less dramatic than in younger patients and the diagnosis may be missed. The joint is swollen, tender and warm. The joint need not be erythematous. An antecedent history of trauma to the limb may exist, or acute septic arthritis may follow as a complication of a local skin or bone infection.

Investigations

BLOOD TESTS

Full blood examination – elevated white cell count, left shift, increased band forms, elevated erythrocyte sedimentation rate and C reactive protein.

BLOOD CULTURES

Blood should be taken for aerobic and anaerobic cultures on diagnosis (two sets of cultures 1 hour apart) and at times of high fevers (38.5°C). Blood cultures should be obtained prior to the commencement of antibiotic therapy.

RADIOGRAPHS

Radiographs early in disease commonly demonstrate soft tissue swelling or an associated joint effusion with elevation of the extra-articular fat pad. There are usually no bone changes.

BONE SCANS

Infections induce a marked inflammatory response with hyperaemia of bone and increased bone turnover. Nuclear bone scans demonstrate increased (e.g. technetium-99 MDP, gallium-67) tracer uptake at the affected site (hot scan). Indium white cell scans demonstrate acute white cell collection (abscess).

ULTRASOUND

Joints that are difficult to palpate (e.g. shoulder, hip) may be examined with ultrasound scans.

JOINT ASPIRATION

An experienced doctor should perform a joint aspiration under sterile conditions with a large bore needle and the fluid should be submitted for microbiological examination, culture and antibiotic sensitivities. Ultrasound or CT guidance can be valuable.

Differential diagnoses

Important differential diagnoses for an acutely swollen and painful joint include:

- Gout
- Haemathrosis, e.g. post-traumatic, haemophilic, coagulopathic
- Trauma, e.g. osteochondral injury or fracture, intra-articular ligament injury
- Inflammatory arthritis
- Degenerative arthritis

Treatment

SURGERY

Arthrotomy, irrigation and drainage of the joint.

ANTIBIOTIC THERAPY

Antibiotics are instituted following blood cultures and culture of joint fluid (flucloxacillin 2 g i.v. 4 hourly and ampicillin 1 g i.v. 6 hourly) until an organism is identified and sensitivities known.

IMMOBILISATION

The limb should be immobilised in a splint and elevated until symptoms resolve.

PHYSIOTHERAPY
Gradual physiotherapy should be prescribed after symptoms resolve to regain joint motion.

Outcome

Early and adequate treatment is important to prevent cartilage destruction (chondrolysis) that may lead to stiffness and arthritis.

Chronic infective arthritis

Chronic infective arthritis is uncommon and is usually seen following Mycobacterium tuberculosis infections.

Pathology

Joint infection usually follows seeding from a distant site such as the lung or kidneys. In addition chronic tuberculosis osteomyelitis may also extend from the metaphysis or epiphysis into the articular cavity.

Clinical presentation

Pain in the joint is variable and may be extreme or slight. Typically this is most severe at night when the patient relaxes and joint movement during sleep causes severe attacks of pain (night cries). Constitutionally, the patient is unwell with fever, lassitude and loss of weight.

Affected joints are swollen with a doughy synovial thickening, effusion and gross muscle wasting. There is restriction and pain with movement but this is not as severe as acute suppurative arthritis. There may be joint sinuses and marked stiffness (fibrous or bony ankylosis).

Investigations

BLOOD TESTS
Full blood examination demonstrates an elevated lymphocyte count, elevated ESR and anemia of chronic infection.

MANTOUX TEST
Mantoux test is positive; however, in overwhelming disease there may be no reaction.

JOINT ASPIRATION AND CULTURE
Joint aspiration and culture may demonstrate acid-fast bacilli. More recent tests using polymerase chain reaction (PCR) techniques can demonstrate the characteristic DNA pattern of mycobacteria.

Treatment

- Arthrotomy irrigation and drainage of the joint if the infection is in its acute phase.
- Immobilisation of the limb until the disease is quiescent.
- Commence anti-tuberculous medication following joint and tissue culture.
- Commence physiotherapy after the disease has become quiescent.

Outcome

Anti-tuberculous therapy is usually successful in controlling or eradicating the infection. However, complications include:
- Stiffness from intra-articular fibrosis.
- Deformity from destruction of the growth plate.
- Degenerative arthritis from cartilage destruction.
- Osteomyelitis from local spread.
- Haematogenous dissemination.

Arthritides

Degenerative arthritis

Degenerative arthritis is one of the commonest conditions in orthopaedics. The commonest joints include the hip, knee, shoulder and lumbar spine. Other joints less commonly involved include the carpometacarpal joint, elbow and ankle.

Causes

- Idiopathic
- Trauma
- Infection
- Inflammation
- Metabolic, e.g. gout, pseudogout
- Avascular necrosis, e.g. steroid induced, osteochondritis dissecans

Clinical presentation

PAIN
Pain typically occurs with movement or with bearing weight (mechanical pain). This may radiate to involve

the whole limb if it is advanced. Referred pain is common, for example knee pain in severe hip arthritis.

STIFFNESS

Patients note a restricted range of motion, develop a limp and are unable to function normally, such as to run, climb stairs or twist their leg to put their shoes on.

DEFORMITY

With progressive loss of motion and the development of contractures the patient loses symmetry of his joints. This results in an abnormal gait or posture (Fig. 48.2).

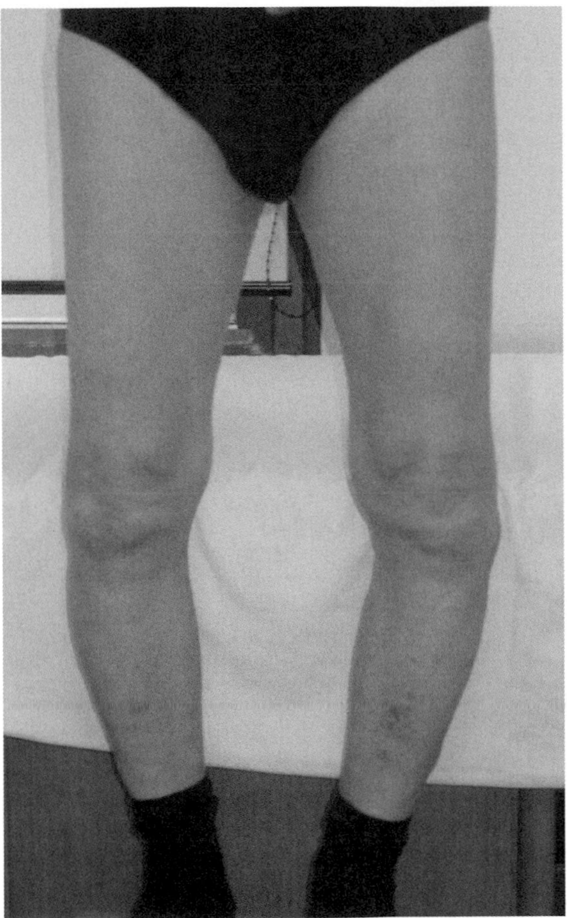

Fig. 48.2 Typical varus deformity in a patient with osteoarthritis of the knees where that part of the limb distal to the joint is deviated towards the midline. This contrasts with the knees of a patient with rheumatoid arthritis where that part of the limb distal to the joint is deviated away from the midline (valgus).

Investigations

RADIOGRAPHS

The four main radiological features of arthritis include loss of joint space, subchondral sclerosis, osteophyte formation and cyst formation (Fig. 48.3).

Treatment

NON-OPERATIVE

This usually consists of pain relief with oral analgesics and anti-inflammatory medication. The use of a walking aid such as a walking stick for lower limb arthritis and splints for upper limb arthritis may also be helpful. Physiotherapy to maintain range of motion and to prevent further loss is valuable. A mobile arthritic joint is better than a stiff arthritic joint.

OPERATIVE

- Joint replacement – This is usually recommended in the advanced stages of arthritis, particularly those involving the major proximal joint of the limbs, for example the hip, knee, shoulder and elbows. It is a very successful procedure, with the survival of joint replacements approaching 95% at 15 years from initial surgery.
- Osteotomy – Osteotomy is the division of bone and this may be used to correct the deformity of arthritis and realign the limb bio-mechanically to allow passage of forces through less-affected parts of the joints, thus reducing the pressure across the arthritic part of the joint. Osteotomy has an important role in managing knee arthritis and may provide the patient with many years of pain relief before joint replacement, which in many cases is inevitable. Osteotomy is also used with good success for the management of hallux valgus.
- Arthrodesis – Arthrodesis is the surgical fusion of a joint, which is usually undertaken in the smaller joints of the feet or hands or in very young patients. Fusion results in the permanent loss of motion but a successful fusion can also result in complete pain relief because the arthritic joint is no longer mobile.

Outcome

Arthritis is a progressive disease characterised by remissions and relapses. Non-operative treatment may slow down the rapidity of symptoms. Whilst X-rays demonstrate the extent of arthritis, symptoms may

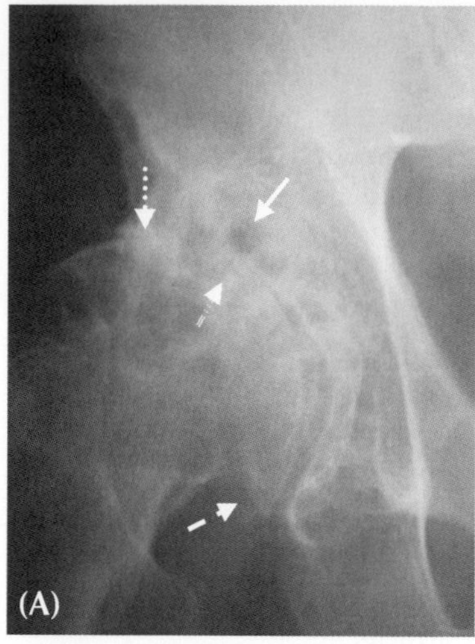

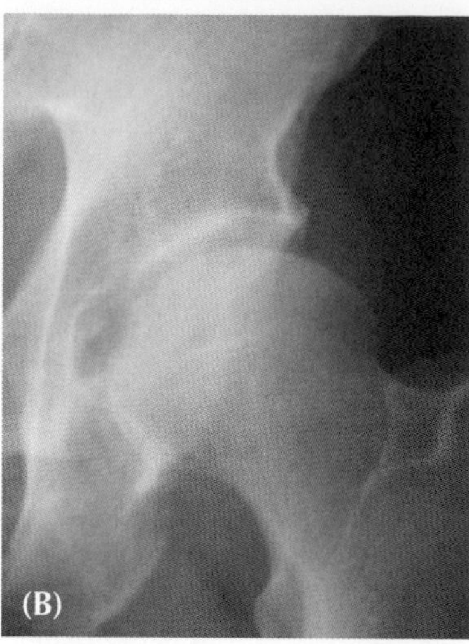

Fig. 48.3 The radiologic features of (**A**) osteoarthritis include joint space narrowing (dotted arrow), subchondral cyst formation (solid arrow), osteophyte formation (dashed arrow) and subchondral sclerosis (double body arrow). Compare this with (**B**) a normal joint.

not always correlate with the severity of radiological features.

Inflammatory arthritis

This is a spectrum of sero-positive and sero-negative arthritides characterised by acute and subacute chronic and relapsing joint inflammation. Joint involvement is part of a clinical picture that also affects bones, tendons and other organs.

Pathology

The cause of inflammatory joint disease is thought to be an autoimmune process beginning with a synovitis that causes articular cartilage destruction, disruption of the joint capsule and a proliferative synovitis.

Types

- Rheumatoid arthritis – seropositive
- Psoriatic arthritis – seropositive and seronegative varieties
- Ankylosing spondylitis – seronegative
- Reiters disease – seronegative
- Inflammatory bowel disease – seronegative
- Behcet's disease – seronegative

Presentation

Typically, patients complain of stiffness, pain and joint swelling. Characteristic exacerbations and remissions are noted, and constitutional symptoms may be present, with acute joint involvement.

Patients with rheumatoid arthritis may present with bilateral symmetric involvement of the small joints of hand, wrist and feet, and triggering of tendons. Eventually involvement of the hips, knees, shoulders and ankles are noted. Valgus deformities of the knee or a wind swept appearance with varus deformity of one knee and valgus of the other are typical. Ulnar deviation, swan neck and boutonniere deformities of the fingers are characteristic.

Patients with seronegative arthritis usually present with monoarticular arthritis involving the large joints such as the knee and hip although small joint involvement of the hand with nail changes are also seen in psoriatic arthritis. These patients also present with low-back pain. Progressive vertebral stiffness, kyphosis and sacroiliitis are typical of advancing ankylosing spondylitis. Visceral involvement of the heart, lungs, liver, spleen, bowel and eyes may occur.

Investigations

BLOOD TESTS

Full blood examination – elevated white cell count, elevated erythrocyte sedimentation rate.

SEROLOGICAL TESTS

- Rheumatoid factor
- Anti–nuclear antibody
- Anti–double-stranded DNA antibody
- HLA-B27

RADIOGRAPHS

- Seropositive disease: Radiographs demonstrate soft tissue swelling, osteopenia, joint erosions or narrowing. Symmetric, bilateral joint deformity of the hands and feet.
- Seronegative disease: Monoarticular involvement, sacroiliitis, syndesmophytes, bamboo-spine, enthesopathy, ossification of the capsular margins.

BONE SCANS

Generalised uptake around joint. Increased uptake in arterial phase demonstrating active synovitis. Bone scans are useful for identifying stress fractures from associated or steroid-induced osteoporosis.

Treatment

- Rest and immobilisation of affected joints.
- Analgesia
- Anti-inflammatory medication
- Corticosteroids
- Disease-modifying medication such as methotrexate, penicillamine, gold
- Splints or braces to prevent or correct deformities
- Surgery to correct deformities or joint destruction (osteotomy, arthrodesis, joint replacement)
- Synovectomy is the removal of inflamed synovium. This is usually indicated in early disease and may be performed by open surgery, arthroscopy or radiotherapy with intra-arterial instillation of radioisotope.

Generalised conditions of bones

Metabolic conditions

Rickets

Rickets is an uncommon condition of the immature skeleton characterised by poor mineralisation of osteoid. It is caused by a dietary lack of calcium and vitamin D or a lack of exposure to sunlight. It is usually seen in malnourished patients such as those from the Third World. Rickets may also be seen in malabsorption syndromes.

PRESENTATION

Joint tenderness, swelling and deformity. Bones typically involved include the tibia (genu varum) and ribs (rickety rosary).

X-RAYS

Gradual deformation of long bones is seen. In addition, there is expansion and loss of cortical definition of the metaphyseal region of bone. The costochondral junctions may be expanded (Rickety Rosary).

TREATMENT

- Correction of malabsorption syndromes
- Supplementation of vitamin D and calcium
- Surgical correction of long-standing bone deformity.

Osteomalacia

This is a condition of the adult skeleton characterised by inadequate bone mineralisation. The main causes of this include vitamin D deficiency, vitamin D resistance (renal failure), impaired vitamin D synthesis (liver failure, renal failure) and other metabolic disturbances.

PRESENTATION

Patients present with pathological fractures or radiological evidence of bone loss (Looser's zones), muscle aches and pains. There is no growth abnormality because osteomalacia is a condition of the mature skeleton.

INVESTIGATIONS

- Blood tests
  - Elevated serum alkaline phosphatase
  - Reduced serum calcium
  - Reduced serum vitamin D
- Radiographs
  - Looser's zones in areas of stress, e.g. pubic rami, femoral neck.
  - General osteopenia
- Bone biopsy
  - Bone biopsy shows deficient mineralisation with widened un-ossified seams of osteoid.

TREATMENT

- Correction of metabolic irregularity
- Supplement calcium and vitamin D
- Fixation of fractures if appropriate

Hormonal conditions

Hyperthyroidism (see Chapter 33)

A reduction of thyroid hormone produces growth abnormalities in infant and paediatric patients. There is stunted growth, a delay in walking and cretinism. The late appearance of secondary ossification centres suggests hypothyroidism. Early treatment with thyroid hormone supplementation is important to prevent mental retardation.

Hyperparathyroidism (see Chapter 34)

Hyperparathyroidism is an abnormality of increased secretion of parathyroid hormone. This may be caused by hypersecretion by a parathyroid adenoma or a secondary response to chronic renal failure. Increasing the secretion of parathyroid hormone raises serum calcium through bone reabsorption. Bone resorption results in a bone softening condition wherein pathological fractures are frequent.

Clinical picture

Nausea, vomiting, weight loss, abdominal pain, bone pain and muscular weakness.

Investigations

RADIOGRAPHS

There is a generalised reduction in bone density. Late in the disease bone reabsorption manifests as bone cysts. Mottling of the skull and subperiosteal erosions of the phalanges are commonly seen. Other manifestations of hypercalcaemia such as renal calculi or heterotopic calcification are seen.

BLOOD TESTS

- Elevated serum calcium
- Decreased serum phosphate
- Elevated urinary phosphate
- Elevated parathyroid hormone

TREATMENT

- Correction of metabolic irregularity.
- Surgical removal of adenoma or partial removal of the parathyroid glands.

Congenital/developmental conditions

Osteogenesis imperfecta

Osteogenesis imperfecta is an extremely rare condition characterised by bone fragility.

Pathology

This is an inherited condition, and results from an abnormality in the metabolism of Type 1 collagen. The fragility leads to bone deformity and/or fractures and soft tissue abnormalities.

Classification

Type	Inheritance	Clinical features
I	Autosomal dominant	Childhood fractures, hearing loss, blue sclera +/− opalescent teeth, commonest
II	Autosomal recessive	Lethal, multiple fractures, flattened vertebrae, blue sclera, very rare
III	Autosomal recessive	Birth fractures and progressive deformity; short stature, +/− opalescent teeth; white sclera spinal deformity and costovertebral anomalies
IV	Autosomal dominant	Skeletal fragility, no hearing loss, moderate growth failure, white sclera, may have opalescent teeth

Presentation

Patients with the severe form of osteogenesis imperfecta die at or soon after birth with multiple fractures. Patients who survive at birth may present as an abnormality of development with a typical globular shaped head, frontal bossing, stunted growth, kyphoscoliosis and hypermobility of joints. There is commonly a history of multiple fractures following minimal trauma. If presentation occurs during adolescence, normal skeletal development is seen and fracture incidence declines with increasing maturity. Fracture healing is normal but remodelling is abnormal, giving rise to bone deformities. Many survivors have blue sclera, which is due to the abnormally thin and translucent sclera highlighting the dark choroid behind it.

Radiographs

Radiographs show multiple healing or old fractures, bone deformities, ribbon shaped ribs and wormian bones in the skull and a trefoil pelvis.

Pathology

The condition is characterised by marked cortical thinning and attenuation of trabeculae. There may be persistence of hypercellular woven bone.

Treatment

Patients require protection from injury particularly when young. Treatment is aimed at correcting limb deformities by multiple osteotomies and a transfixing pin or rod. Fracture healing is excellent.

Dyschondroplasia

Also known as Ollier's disease, or multiple enchondromata, dyschondroplasia is characterised by the development during youth of multiple asymmetric intraosseous cartilage masses.

Pathology

There is an abnormality of metaphyseal bone organization. Although metaphyseal growth ceases after puberty, enchondromata may continue to grow.

Clinical presentation

Patients present with metaphyseal swelling that may be particularly severe in the fingers. This may affect joint function and the length of the bone. Limb length discrepancies are not unusual.

Investigations

RADIOGRAPHS

Radiographs show areas of lucency with central calcific stippling and endosteal scalloping. Shortening, angulation and expansion of bone can be seen.

BONE SCANS

Increased TC-99MDP uptake in the lesions implies ongoing growth and remodelling of surrounding bone. Activity in the lesions itself can be demonstrated by avidity for thallium or pentavalent dimercapto-succinic acid (DMSA).

Treatment

Troublesome lesions may be excised. Treatment is one of correcting angulation and limb length defects. The prognosis is good. Rarely, transformation to low-grade chondrosarcoma may occur. This should be suspected in lesions that show a recent increase in size and pain, and radiographs that demonstrate lysis, expansion of bone, endosteal erosion and cortical breach. Wide resection is recommended.

Outcome

A normal life expectancy is usual.

Hereditary diaphyseal aclasis

Also known as multiple cartilaginous exostoses, hereditary diaphyseal aclasis is a skeletal condition that usually presents in childhood and affects the growing ends of long bones. Occasionally, ribs, vertebrae and the pelvis may also be involved.

Pathology

There is an aberration in physeal regulation with the development of cortical exostoses at the growing end of bones. These are characterised by a cartilage cap of varying thickness. This is an autosomal dominant condition where abnormalities of chromosomes 18, 11 and 19 have been identified.

Clinical presentation

Patients present with problems of
- impingement
- deformity
- limb length discrepancy
- malignant transformation to chondrosarcoma.

Investigations

RADIOGRAPHS

Exostoses are sessile or pedunculated. Trabecular bone of the diaphysis is confluent with that of the exostosis and the cortex of the osteochondroma is continuous with that of the bone from which it arises.

BONE SCANS

Increased TC-99MDP uptake in the lesions implies ongoing growth and remodelling of surrounding bone. Activity in the lesions itself can be demonstrated by avidity for thallium or pentavalent dimercapto-succinic acid (DMSA).

COMPUTED TOMOGRAPHY

CT scans are excellent for demonstrating cortical erosion, endosteal scalloping and the large cartilage cap.

MRI

MRI scans are excellent for demonstrating the soft tissue component, intramedullary changes and the thickness of the cartilage cap (if >1 cm, suspect malignancy).

Treatment

Simple excision of the lesion at its base should suffice. Occasionally, correction of angular deformities is required. Malignant transformation is uncommon but when it occurs transformation to a low-grade chondrosarcoma is noted. Like the sarcomatous transformation noted in dyschondroplasia, removal of the tumour requires wide resection.

Outcome

A normal life expectancy is usual.

Achondroplasia

This is an autosomal dominant condition characterised by abnormalities in limb length in the presence of a normal sized trunk and an enlarged head. It is the most common skeletal dysplasia.

Pathology

It is a hereditary defect of cartilage modelling, caused by gene mutation for fibroblast growth factor receptor protein. Normal chondral calcification does not occur. Periosteal bone formation is normal. This causes thickening of bone but not lengthening of bone. Membranous bones are not affected.

Clinical presentation

The classic achondroplastic dwarf has short limbs, a normal trunk, a large head with frontal bossing and a flattened root of the nose. Patients develop the typical bow-legged appearance and an increase in the lumbar lordosis. Lumbar canal stenosis is common because of short pedicles and the increased lordosis.

Radiographs

Radiographs show short tubular bones with wide metaphyses.

Treatment

Corrective osteotomies may be required for abnormality in joint alignment, and limb-lengthening surgery may be useful for increasing height and reach. Limb bowing may lead to degenerative knee arthritis where osteotomy or joint replacement may be required. Canal stenosis may be severe enough to cause significant nerve root impingement symptoms that may require surgical decompression.

Outcome

A normal life expectancy is usual.

Bone conditions of unknown origin

Paget's disease

Paget's disease is a condition of adults in their middle age and onwards. It is a deforming condition characterised by disorganised bone formation and bone resorption. Two stages exist, an acute hyperaemic and bone-softening phase and a chronic brittle phase.

Pathology

It is thought to be of viral origin, as viral inclusion bodies have been noted within osteoclasts from affected bones.

Presentation

Patients may complain of a painless deformity of a long bone such as the femur and tibia. Alternately, patients may also complain of pain which is usually dull and constant and not related to activity. Pain may be due to Paget's disease, stress fractures or malignant change. Common bones to be involved include the skull, pelvis, femur, tibia and single vertebrae. Patients may also develop symptoms of nerve compression, pathologic/stress fractures, and high-output failure from the regional hyperaemia which may act like an arteriovenous shunt.

Investigations

- Blood tests
  Elevated serum alkaline phosphatase
- Urinary tests
  Elevated urinary calcium and hydroxyproline excretion
- Bone biopsy
  Biopsy demonstrates abundant disorganised woven bone with abnormal cement lines and abnormal-shaped lamelli, so-called crazy pavement.
- Radiographs
  Course trabeculae, thickened cortices, flame-shaped lysis, stress fractures, bone deformity, enlarged bone and malignant change.
- Bone scans
  Markedly increased uptake of radioactive tracer in active Paget's disease.

Treatment

- Pain relief – oral analgesia, non-steroidal anti-inflammatory drugs
- Anti-osteoclastic drugs – bisphosphonate, calcitonin.
- Surgery – joint replacement, correction of deformity

Outcome

Paget's may become burnt out with established deformities and hard brittle and pain-free bone. Fractures through this bone are not uncommon because of their brittle nature. Abnormality in bone architecture may predispose to arthritis. Sometimes, differentiation between the pain of Paget's disease and arthritis may be difficult. Rarely malignant transformation may occur, which carries a very poor prognosis.

Osteoporosis

Osteoporosis is an absolute loss of bone mass with an increase in fracture risk.

Pathology

There is normal mineralisation of osteoid, but the absolute amount of bone is decreased. Osteoporosis may be associated with calcium deficiency, secondary hyperparathyroidism, excess alcohol intake, immobilisation, steroid use, and malignancy.

Clinical presentation

Osteoporosis has an insidious onset characterised by a gradual loss of height with increasing age, the development of kyphoscoliosis and a predisposition to fracture after minor trauma or falls. Specific areas prone to fracture include vertebrae, the pelvis, and radius. Stress fractures of the tibia and pelvis are common.

Investigations

BLOOD TESTS

Primary osteoporosis has a normal blood profile. If associated with other causes, blood derangements may be typical of those other conditions.

RADIOGRAPHS

Lumbar vertebrae are bio-concave with herniation of the disc into and through the endplate of the vertebrae (fish shaped). There may be osteoporotic wedge fractures of the vertebrae. Stress fractures may be seen in the pubic rami, sacrum, medial tibia and sometimes the distal tibia.

BONE MINERAL DENSITY SCANS

Bone mineral density scans show low mineralised bone content. Results are compared to age- and sex-matched control data to determine the risk of fracture.

BONE BIOPSY

Bone biopsy may be required if the diagnosis and cause for apparent bone loss is unclear. Tetracycline labelling protocol is required to determine the rate and amount of bone formation within a given time.

Treatment

- Correction of metabolic deficiencies
- Correction of the underlying medical condition
- Reduction of bone resorption – bisphosphonates
- Oestrogen supplement
- Vitamin D supplementation

Fibrous dysplasia

This is a deforming condition of bone that may begin in young adulthood. It is characterised by abnormal development of cysts and fibrotic areas within bone associated with gradual deformation.

Presentation

The patient may complain of pain or the condition may be an incidental finding on X-rays.

Investigations

RADIOGRAPHS
Radiographs demonstrate thickened bone, with lytic areas containing matrix with a typical ground-glass appearance. Bone deformities include a shepherd's crook abnormality of the proximal femur, thickened corticesand expanded diaphysis.

BIOPSY
Biopsy demonstrates normal trabeculae of bone broken up into tiny islands of bone by fibrous stroma and bland cells giving a "chinese character" type appearance.

Outcome

There may be gradual deformity in a weight-bearing bone. Pathological fractures may also occur. Malignant change occurs rarely.

Conditions of joints

Charcot's disease

Charcot's disease is the consequence of conditions that result in denervation or loss of proprioceptive sense, predisposing to bone and joint destruction (neuropathic joint).

Pathology

Repeated trauma leads to fracture, poor healing and joint derangement. Predisposing causes include diabetes, alcoholism, syringomyelia, syphilis, trauma.

Presentation

Patients present with painless, deformed and swollen joints. The ankle and knee are the most commonly affected joints. Syringomyelia should be suspected with charcot's disease of the shoulder. Patients may also present with the complications of deformed joints (e.g., chronic nonhealing ulcers overlying bone prominences).

Radiographs

Typical radiographic signs include dense bone, destruction of joint, para-articular bone debris, deformity.

Treatment

BRACING
Deranged joints may be stabilised with external braces or splints. The purpose of this is to prevent further deformity rather than to correct it, which is usually permanent.

SURGERY
Surgery to correct the deformity or to arthrodese the joint is usually met by failure. Amputation is considered if the joint becomes useless and is an impediment to limb function or is complicated by persistent infection.

Gout

Gout is an abnormality of purine metabolism characterised by an excess production of uric acid or a reduction in the excretion of uric acid. Deposition of urate crystals and the subsequent inflammatory response elicits painful joint symptoms and other visceral complications.

Clinical features

Patients present with acutely painful swollen and tender joints. If severe, there may be constitutional symptoms. Joint symptoms can be mistaken for septic arthritis. Typically, the metatarsal phalangeal joint of the big toe is affected. In chronic gout deposit of urate crystals in the soft tissue (tophi) are common and this can be seen on the ear and on the phalangeal joints of the fingers and toes.

Other associated conditions include cardiac disease, hypertension and renal failure.

Investigations

RADIOGRAPHS
Radiographs may show peri-articular erosions, joint deformities and soft tissue calcifications.

BLOOD TESTS

Elevated serum uric acid. This may be normal in 30% of patients. The white cell count is elevated, in addition to elevated ESR and CRP.

JOINT ASPIRATION

Joint aspirations should be performed under sterile conditions and fluid submitted for biochemical and microbiological examination including culture. Typically, negatively birefringent needle-shaped crystals are noted.

Treatment

- Rest immobilisation and elevation of joint
- Oral and intramuscular analgesia
- Anti-inflammatory medication
- Colchicine
- Allopurinol
- Dietary control

Outcome

Patients with gout often have recurring attacks. Uncontrolled gout may lead to joint destruction and renal tubular failure.

Pigmented vilo-nodular synovitis (PVNS)

This is a rare condition characterised by a localised nodular or papillary overgrowth and inflammation of the synovium. This may cause bone erosions, subchondral cysts and large soft tissue masses. There is controversy as to whether this is an inflammatory or true neoplastic process.

Clinical presentation

Patients may present with a range of symptoms including recurrent joint swelling and pain, soft tissue masses, osteoarthritis.

Investigations

RADIOGRAPHS

Radiographs show generalised joint narrowing if the diffuse form of PVNS is present. Typically, subchondral cyst are large and situated at a distance from the joint.

MRI

MRI scans demonstrate articular soft tissue abnormalities that contain haemosiderin (chronic synovial haemorrhage). Synovitis is well demonstrated by this scan.

Treatment

- Synovectomy
- Radiation synovectomy with intra-articular isotopes
- Joint replacement

Synovial chondromatosis

This is a metaplastic condition of the synovium resulting in the formation of numerous intra-articular cartilaginous loose bodies.

Clinical presentation

These may cause painful catching, locking or osteoarthritis of the joint.

Investigation

- Radiographs
  These demonstrate intra-articular loose bodies if they are calcified. If the loose bodies remain cartilaginous they may not be detectable on radiographs.
- MRI
  MRI scans demonstrate cartilage very well and are excellent for detecting intra-articular loose bodies.

Treatment

- Synovectomy
- Removal of loose body
- Joint replacement in severe disease with associated articular degeneration

Osteochondritis dissecans

Osteochondritis dissecans is a condition of adolescence and young adulthood that is characterised by local avascular necrosis of epiphyseal bone causing fracture and/or separation of an osteoarticular fragment.

Clinical presentation

The commonest joints are the knee, elbow and ankle. It presents initially with pain on weight-bearing activity. Repeated joint effusions or clicking or locking of the joint may be noted.

Investigations

RADIOGRAPHS
Early in the condition this may be normal. Late in the condition a defect of bone may be seen and a loose fragment may be noted. Typical areas include the lateral side of the medial femoral condyle, superomedial corner of the dome of the talus, the head of the second metatarsal and the capitellar surface.

BONE SCANS
Bone scans may show increased focal activity.

CT SCANS
CT scans are excellent for demonstrating a subchondral fracture.

MRI
MRI scans are excellent for demonstrating lesions that are not visible on radiographs or CT scans. MRI can detect oedema and inflammation surrounding the area of necrosis.

Treatment

- Acute pain may be treated by rest, partial weight bearing and use of crutches.
- Arthroscopy and drilling of the fragment may assist and encourage a new blood supply and thus healing of the fragment.
- Open reduction internal fixation is indicated if the osteochondral fragment is a large fragment.
- *Ex vivo* autogenous chondrocyte culture and reimplantation is a new and exciting technique for treating this condition.

Outcome

Lesions that remain attached usually proceed to heal. Detached lesions may heal after internal fixation, but if too small may simply be discarded. The residual defect does not heal normally and may predispose to osteoarthritis if it is large and on the weight bearing surface of bone.

Orthopaedic malignancies

Malignant primary tumours

Sarcomas are primary malignancies of bone and soft tissue. The cells of origin arise from mesenchymal and neuroectodermal tissue. Two peak incidences exist (<20 years and >55 years). Males are more commonly affected. The commonest site for born sarcomas is the lower limb, particularly around the knee. The commonest site for soft tissue sarcomas is the thigh, and the majority of these tumours arise beneath the deep fascia and are larger than 5 cm.

Clinical presentation

Sarcomas present with a mass. Bone sarcomas are painful. Characteristically, the pain is constant, unremitting, nocturnal and responds poorly to oral analgesia. Soft tissue sarcomas tend to be pain-free (with the exception of synovial sarcoma and neurosarcoma). It is important to note that:

- Bone pain that is unremitting should raise suspicions of a tumour.
- All soft tissue masses larger than 5 cm and/or deep to the deep fascia should be regarded as soft tissue sarcomas until proven otherwise.

Most frequent bone sarcomas
- Osteosarcoma
- Ewing's sarcoma
- Chondrosarcoma

Most frequent soft tissue sarcomas
- Malignant fibrous histiocytoma
- Liposarcoma
- Synovial sarcoma
- Fibrosarcoma
- Neurosarcoma

Investigation

All investigations must be completed prior to biopsy because biopsy can produce imaging artefacts. Inappropriate biopsy site or procedure may jeopardise limb sparing surgery.

RADIOGRAPHS
All suspected bone tumours should be radiographed. Typical patterns are recognised for most tumours.

COMPUTED TOMOGRAPHY SCAN
Computed tomography scans provide excellent imaging of cortical and trabecular destruction. Pulmonary scans are mandatory for determining systemic spread.

MAGNETIC RESONANCE IMAGING SCAN
Magnetic resonance imaging scans provide excellent multiplanar imaging with unsurpassed soft tissue

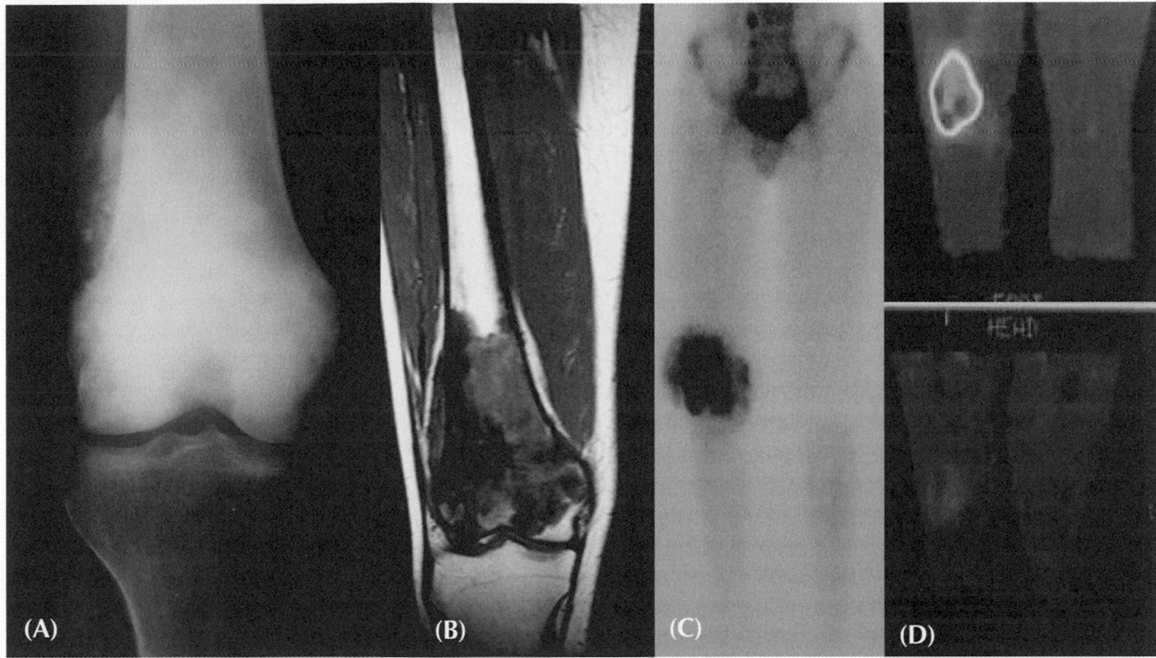

Fig. 48.4 (**A**) Radiograph of a distal femoral osteosarcoma showing typical areas of mixed lytic and blastic changes within the tumour. Note the periosteal new bone formation (arrow). (**B**) MRI clearly shows the intra- and extraosseous extension of the tumour. (**C**) Bone scanning shows the activity of new bone formation stimulated by the tumour. The changes before and after chemotherapy on bone scanning may indicate response to treatment. (**D**) Functional metabolic imaging (thallium or positron emission tomography [PET]) shows the metabolic activity of the tumour itself before chemotherapy (upper panel) and after chemotherapy (lower panel), where a good response is noted by the marked reduction in nuclear tracer activity.

contrast. Magnetic resonance images are important for determining the site, size, shape, consistency and vascularity of a tumour, and the relationship of adjacent structures. This modality is extremely important for assessing surgical margins.

NUCLEAR SCANS

^{99m}Technitium-methylenediphosphonate bone scans are excellent for demonstrating multicentric bone involvement. Such scans are also important for determining response to treatment. More recently, functional nuclear scans, e.g. thallium, PET, allow an assessment of tumour activity(Fig. 48.4).

BIOPSY

Biopsy is important for confirming the diagnosis and for determining histologic subtype. Biopsy may be performed percutaneously with fine- or wide-bore needles, or through a formal incision. More invasive methods carry a higher risk of complications and contamination of tissue planes. Each year 30% of limbs are lost through inappropriate biopsy site and technique. In principle, biopsies should be performed at a tumour centre by a specialist in tumour surgery.

Treatment

CHEMOTHERAPY

All osteosarcomas and Ewing's sarcomas are treated with protocols of pre-operative chemotherapy unless the patient's renal or cardiac function prohibits the use of chemotherapy. Chondrosarcoma is resistant to chemotherapy.

RADIOTHERAPY

Radiotherapy is indicated for soft tissue sarcomas. This may be provided pre-operatively or post-operatively. The benefit of pre-operative radiotherapy is the smaller target of irradiation. Post-operative radiotherapy requires targeting of the entire operative field. The complications of pre-operative versus post-operative radiotherapy are comparable.

SURGERY

Surgical margins may be classified as intralesional (tumour capsule is transgressed), marginal (pericapsular inflammatory zone is transgressed), wide (surrounding cuff of normal tissue) and radical (entire tumour-bearing compartment is excised). All sarcomas should be excised with at least wide margins. Intralesional and marginal margins are regarded as inadequate and are associated with the highest local recurrent rates.

Outcome

The 5-year metastasis-free survival for osteosarcoma is 75%. The 5-year metastasis-free survival for Ewing's sarcoma is 50%. The 5-year metastasis-free survival for chondrosarcoma is 80%. The 5-year metastasis-free survival for soft tissue sarcoma is 75%. All patients should follow a regular programme of surveillance with clinical examination, pulmonary CT scans and imaging of the operated area.

Secondary malignancies

Metastatic carcinomas are the commonest malignant tumours of bone. Carcinomas that commonly metastasise to bone include breast, prostate, lung, kidney and thyroid. The majority are osteolytic although prostate is unique because 95% of bone lesions are osteoblastic.

Clinical presentation

Patients present with pain, pathologic fracture, loss of limb function or as an incidental finding on other imaging. Solitary metastases are uncommon. Up to 30% of bone metastases are the initial presenting feature of carcinoma.

Investigations

RADIOGRAPHS

Radiographs of the affected limb are vital for determining the extent of disease and the likelihood of fracture.

BONE SCANS

Bone scans are important for determining multicentricity of bone disease. All 'hotspots' should be radiographed.

MRI

Magnetic resonance imaging may be important for assessing the quality and extent of bone involvement if reconstruction is being considered.

CT SCANNING

CT scanning is helpful for determining cortical destruction. Computed tomographs of the chest, abdomen, and pelvis are important for identifying the site of the primary tumour.

BLOOD TEST

Routine blood tests may indicate the extent of marrow involvement. Elevation of specific markers such as prostate-specific antigen (prostate), carcinoembryonic antigen (gastrointestinal), α-feto protein (gastrointestinal) and erythrocyte sedimentation rate (myeloma) may assist diagnosis.

Treatment

- Radiotherapy is very useful for controlling pain, lysis or growth of the tumour.
- Chemotherapy has an important role in specific carcinomas.
- Surgery is indicated for the prevention of impending pathologic fracture, or the treatment of fracture. In almost all cases, pain is a major reason for surgical intervention.

Outcome

In general, the surgical treatment of metastatic disease of bone is palliative. On occasion, resection of solitary renal or thyroid disease may affect cure.

MCQs

Select the single correct answer to each question.

1 Degenerative arthritis is a common condition characterised by:
- **a** joint pain, stiffness, contracture and deformity
- **b** recurrent haemarthroses, joint swelling and a charcot joint
- **c** high temperature, exquisite joint pain and constitutional symptoms
- **d** flitting arthralgia, skin rash and sore throat
- **e** single joint swelling, conjunctivitis and urethritis

2 The radiologic features of degenerative arthritis include:
a syndesmophytes, bamboo spine
b joint narrowing, subchondral sclerosis, osteophyte formation, cyst formation
c joint debris, density, derangement and destruction
d osteoporosis, valgus knee, marked joint synovitis

3 Crystal arthropathy may be seen in the following condition:
a hyperurecaemia
b chondrodysplasia
c haemachromatosis
d Osgood–Schlatters disease
e osteochondritis dissecans

4 Septic arthritis is associated with the following features:
a exquisite pain with attempted joint motion
b minimal constitutional symptoms
c low incidence in children
d low incidence in the elderly
e never associated with trauma

5 Septic arthritis should be managed urgently with:
a amputation
b arthrodesis
c arthrocentesis
d arthrocutaneous fistula
e arthroplasty

Neurosurgery

49 Head injuries

Andrew H. Kaye

Introduction

Trauma is the leading cause of death in youth and early middle age, and death is often associated with major head trauma. Head injury contributes significantly to the outcome in more than half of trauma-related deaths. There are approximately 2.5 deaths from head injury per 10 000 population in Australia each year and road traffic accidents are responsible for about 65% of all fatal head injuries.

Head injury may vary from mild concussion to severe brain injury resulting in death. Management of patients requires careful identification of the pathological processes that have occurred.

Pathophysiology of head injury

Most head injuries result from blunt trauma, as distinct from a penetrating wound of the skull and brain caused by missiles or sharp objects. The pathological processes involved in a head injury are:

- direct trauma
- cerebral contusion
- intracerebral shearing
- cerebral swelling (oedema)
- intracranial haemorrhage
- hydrocephalus.

In addition, it is likely that following the initial injury there is a 'secondary injury' leading to further tissue damage, involving a complex series of destructive biochemical events. These include the possible release of excitotoxic neurotransmitters, such as glutamate, and lipid peroxidation initiated by free oxygen radicals originating from the injured tissue, which leads to a cascade of oxidative damage.

Direct trauma

In penetrating injuries the direct trauma to the brain produces most of the damage, but in blunt injuries the energy from the impact has a widespread effect on the brain.

Cerebral contusion

Cerebral contusion may occur locally, under the position of the impact, but often occurs at a distance from the area of impact as a result of a 'contra-coup' injury. As the brain is mobile within the cranial cavity a sudden acceleration/deceleration force will result in the opposite 'poles' of the brain being jammed against the cranial vault. A sudden blow to the back of the head will cause the temporal and frontal lobes to slide across the skull base, causing contusion to the undersurface of the brain, and to the temporal and frontal poles of the brain as they are jammed against the sphenoid ridge and frontal bones, respectively.

Intracerebral shearing

Intracerebral shearing forces result from the differential brain movement following blunt trauma, causing petechial haemorrhages, and tearing of axons and myelin sheaths.

Cerebral swelling

Cerebral swelling occurs either focally around an intracerebral haematoma or diffusely throughout the brain. The process involves a disturbance of vasomotor tone causing vasodilatation and cerebral oedema.

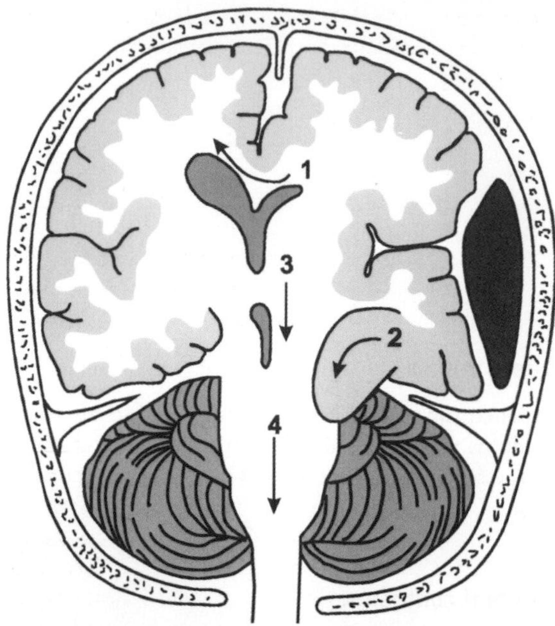

Fig. 49.1 Brain herniation. 1, subfalcine; 2, herniation of the uncus and hippocampal gyrus of the temporal lobe into the tentorial notch, causing pressure on the third nerve and mid-brain; 3, brainstem caudally; 4, cerebellar tonsils through foramen magnum. (Adapted from Kaye AH. *Essential Neurosurgery*. Oxford: Blackwell Publishing 2005. Reproduced with permission.)

Intracranial haemorrhage

Intracranial haemorrhage following trauma may be intracerebral, subdural or extradural. Intracranial haematoma or cerebral swelling may cause cerebral herniation. The medial surface of the hemisphere may be pushed under the falx (subfalcine), the uncus and parahippocampal gyrus of the temporal lobe herniate through the tentorium, causing pressure on the third nerve and mid-brain (Fig. 49.1), or there may be a caudal displacement of the brainstem and/or cerebellum herniating into the foramen magnum.

Hydrocephalus

Hydrocephalus occurs occasionally early after a head injury and may be due to obstruction of the fourth ventricle by blood or swelling in the posterior fossa, or a result of a traumatic subarachnoid haemorrhage causing a communicating hydrocephalus. This is also an uncommon but important cause of delayed neurological deterioration.

Concussion

Concussion usually involves an instantaneous loss of consciousness as a result of trauma. The term *concussion* is not strictly defined in respect to the severity of the injury. However, a minimum criterion is that the patient will have had a period of amnesia. The retrograde amnesia of most cerebral concussion is usually short-term, lasting less than 1 day. The initial retrograde amnesia may extend over a much longer period but gradually diminishes. A more reliable assessment of the severity of the head injury is the post-traumatic amnesia. The concussion is regarded as being severe if the amnesia following the head injury lasts more than 1 day.

The exact definition of concussion remains a contentious issue. The American National Football League established a Committee on Mild Traumatic Brain Injury (MTBI) who have established a much broader definition for concussion which includes an alteration of awareness or consciousness including being 'dazed', 'stunned', and with features of a 'post-concussion syndrome' that include headache, vertigo, light-headedness, loss of balance, blurred vision, drowsiness and lethargy.

Associated injuries

Cranial nerves

The cranial nerves may be injured either as a result of direct trauma by the skull fracture, cerebral swelling, brain herniation or the movement of the brain. The olfactory nerves are most commonly affected.

Eighth nerve damage is often associated with a fracture of the petrous temporal bone and deafness may be conductive, due to a haemotympanum, or sensorineural, as a result of injury to the inner ear or nerve itself.

Facial paralysis is usually associated with a fracture through the petrous temporal bone. It may be either immediate, as a result of direct compression of the nerve, or delayed, due to bleeding and/or swelling around the nerve.

The sixth cranial nerve has a long subarachnoid course and is easily damaged by torsion or herniation of the brain.

The third nerve may also be damaged by direct trauma or by brain herniation, with the herniated uncus of the temporal lobe either impinging on the mid-brain or directly stretching the nerve.

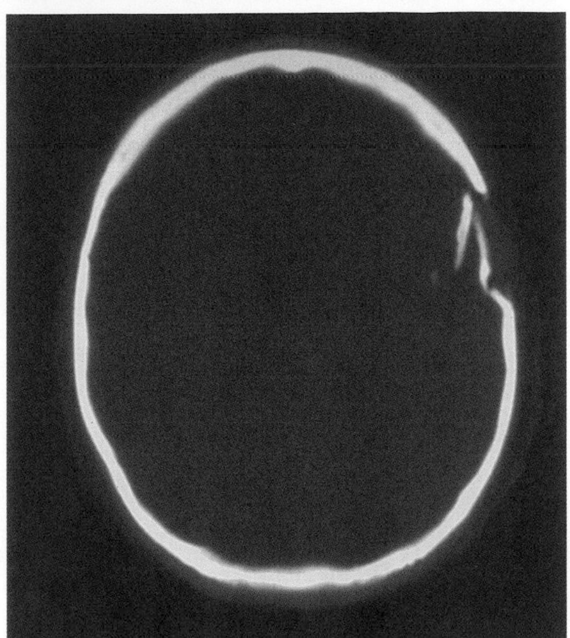

Fig. 49.2 Depressed skull fracture.

Skull fractures

Trauma may result in skull fractures that are classified as simple (a linear fracture of the skull vault), depressed (when bone fragments are depressed beneath the vault; Fig. 49.2) or compound (when there is a communication with the external environment, usually from a laceration over the fracture). A fracture of the base of the skull may have a direct connection outside the vault, via the air sinuses.

Scalp lacerations

The extent of the scalp laceration does not necessarily indicate the degree of trauma to the underlying brain.

Traumatic intracranial haematomas

Intracranial haematoma formation following head injury is the major cause of fatal injuries in which death may potentially have been avoidable. Delay in the evacuation of the haematoma may also increase morbidity in survivors.

The general classification of traumatic intracranial haematoma depends on the relationship of the haematoma to the dura and brain. They are classified as extradural, subdural or intracerebral.

Extradural haematoma

Extradural haematomas are more likely to occur in the younger age group because the dura is able to strip more readily off the underlying bone. Although an extradural haematoma may occur in the presence of a severe head injury and coexist with a severe primary brain injury, its important feature is that it may occur when the injury to the underlying brain is either trivial or negligible.

The most common sites of the extradural haematoma are the temporal region followed by the frontal area. Posterior fossa and parasagittal extradural haematomas are relatively uncommon. In most cases the haemorrhage is from a torn middle meningeal artery or its branches, but haematomas may also develop from haemorrhage from extradural veins or the venous sinuses. A fracture overlies the haematoma in nearly all (95%) adults and most (75%) children.

Clinical presentation

Frequently, extradural haematoma occurs following a head injury that has resulted in only a transient loss of consciousness, and in approximately 25% of cases there has been no initial loss of consciousness. In these patients the most important symptoms are:

- headache
- deteriorating conscious state
- focal neurological signs (dilating pupil, hemiparesis)
- change in vital signs (hypertension, bradycardia).

Headache is the main initial symptom in patients who have either not lost consciousness or who have regained consciousness. The headache is often followed by vomiting.

A deteriorating conscious state is the most important neurological sign, particularly when it develops after a 'lucid' interval. It is essential that the drowsiness that occurs in a patient following a head injury is not misinterpreted as just the patient wishing to sleep.

Focal neurological signs will depend upon the position of the haematoma. In general, a temporal haematoma will produce a progressive contralateral spastic hemiparesis and an ipsilateral dilated pupil. Further progression will result in bilateral spastic limbs in a decerebrate posture and dilated pupils related to uncal herniation. Occasionally, the hemiparesis may initially

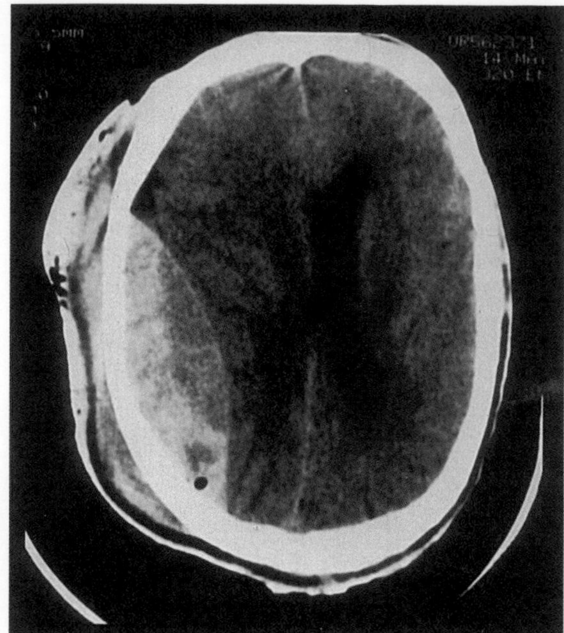

Fig. 49.3 Extradural haematoma with typical biconvex configuration.

be ipsilateral due to compression of the contralateral crus cerebri of the tentorial edge, but only rarely is the opposite pupil involved first.

A change in vital signs shows the classical Cushing response to increased intracranial pressure, that is, bradycardia accompanied by an increase in blood pressure. Disturbances in respiration will develop into a Cheyne–Stokes pattern of breathing.

Radiological investigations

A computed tomography (CT) scan will show the typical hyperdense biconvex haematoma with compression of the underlying brain and distortion of the lateral ventricle (Fig. 49.3).

Treatment

The treatment of extradural haematoma is urgent craniotomy with evacuation of the clot.

As soon as an extradural haematoma is suspected clinically, the patient should have an urgent CT scan. In some cases the rate of neurological deterioration may be so rapid that there is not sufficient time for a CT scan and the patient should be transferred immediately to the operating theatre. Infusion of mannitol (25% solution, 1 g/kg) or frusemide (20 mg i.v.) may temporarily reduce the intracranial pressure during the transfer to the operating theatre. If unconscious, the patient should be intubated and hyperventilated during the transfer. It is essential that there should be no delay in evacuating the haematoma. An extradural haematoma is a surgical emergency because the haematoma will result in death if not removed promptly.

Subdural haematoma

Subdural haematomas are classified depending on the time at which they become clinically evident following injury: acute (<3 days), subacute (4–21 days) and chronic (>21 days).

A CT scan enables a further classification depending on the density of the haematoma relative to the adjacent brain. An acute subdural haematoma is hyperdense (white) and a chronic subdural haematoma is hypodense. Between the end of the first week and the third week the subdural haematoma will be isodense with the adjacent brain.

Acute subdural haematoma

The acute subdural haematoma frequently results from severe trauma to the head and commonly arises from cortical lacerations.

An acute subdural haematoma usually presents in the context of a patient with a severe head injury whose neurological state is either failing to improve or deteriorating. The features of a deteriorating neurological state (decrease in conscious state and/or increase in lateralising signs) should raise the possibility of a subdural haematoma.

A CT scan will show the characteristic hyperdense haematoma, which is concave towards the brain with compression of the underlying brain and distortion of the lateral ventricles (Fig. 49.4). More than 80% of patients with acute subdural haematomas have a fracture of either the cranial vault or base of skull.

Chronic subdural haematoma

Chronic subdural haematoma may follow a significant and often severe head injury, but in approximately one-third of patients there is no definite history of preceding head trauma. The aetiology of the subdural haematoma in this non-traumatic group is probably related to rupture of a fragile bridging vein in a relatively atrophic 'mobile' brain. A relatively trivial injury may result in movement of the brain, like a walnut inside its shell,

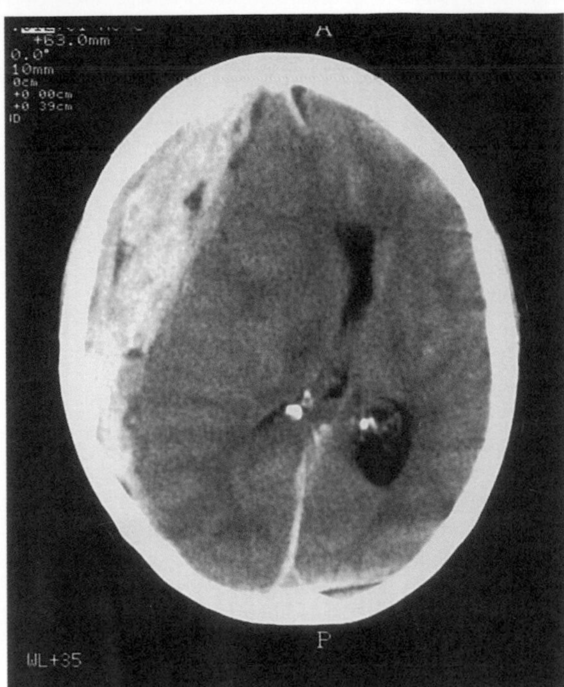

Fig. 49.4 Acute subdural haematoma with compression of ventricles.

with tearing of the bridging vein. The majority of patients in this group are more than 50 years of age.

If the patient is being treated in hospital for a head injury the presence of a chronic subdural haematoma should be considered if the neurological state deteriorates. Alternatively a patient may present without the history of a significant head injury in one of three characteristic ways:

- Raised intracranial pressure without significant localising signs. Headache, vomiting and drowsiness and the absence of focal neurological signs indicate the possible differential diagnosis of a cerebral neoplasm or chronic subdural haematoma.
- Fluctuating drowsiness.
- Progressive dementia.

Chronic subdural haematoma will be diagnosed on CT scan as a hypodense extracerebral collection causing compression of the underlying brain (Fig. 49.4). In 25% of cases the haematoma is bilateral. The chronic subdural haematoma can usually be drained through burr holes.

Intracerebral haematoma

Intracerebral haematomas occur as a result of a penetrating injury (e.g. a missile injury), a depressed skull fracture or following a severe head injury. They are frequently associated with a subdural haematoma.

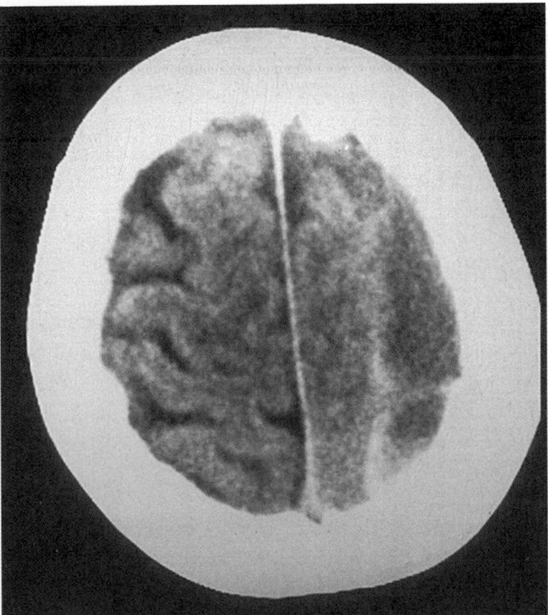

Fig. 49.5 Chronic subdural haematoma.

An intracerebral haematoma should be suspected in any patient with a severe head injury or a patient whose neurological state is deteriorating. A CT scan will show the size and position of the haematomas (Fig. 49.5).

A large intracerebral haematoma usually needs to be evacuated. Small intracerebral haematomas are not removed but should be monitored because the haematoma may expand and require evacuation.

Initial management

The key aspects in the management of patients following head injury are:

- clinical assessment of the neurological and other injuries
- determination of the pathological process involved
- recognition that a change in the neurological signs indicates a progression or change in the pathological processes.

Immediate treatment at the site of the accident involves rapid restoration of an adequate airway and ventilation, circulatory resuscitation, first-aid treatment of other injuries, and the urgent transfer of the patient to hospital. It is essential to avoid hypoxia and hypotension because both will cause further brain injury.

Clinical assessment

In the management of head injury it is essential to know the type of accident that caused the head inujury and whether the neurological condition is deteriorating. An assessment of the patient's initial neurological condition can be obtained from bystanders at the site of the accident or from the ambulance officers.

Neurological examination

Neurological examination will help to determine the type and position of the pathological process and provide a baseline for comparison with subsequent examinations. Although a full neurological examination should be undertaken special emphasis should be given to:

- the conscious state
- pupillary size and reaction
- focal neurological signs in the limbs.

An assessment should be made of the retrograde amnesia and post-traumatic amnesia, if possible.

There is a continuum of altered consciousness from the patient being alert and responding appropriately to verbal command to those who are deeply unconscious. Drowsiness is the first sign of a depressed conscious state. As the level of consciousness deteriorates, the patient will become confused. The use of the words 'coma', 'semi-coma' or 'stuporose' should be avoided because they convey different meanings to different observers. The assessment is more accurate and reproducible if the Glasgow Coma Scale (GCS) is used (Table 49.1). This scale gives a numerical value to the three most important parameters of the level of consciousness: eye opening, best verbal response and best motor response. The exact response can be shown on a chart or the level of consciousness can be given as a numerical score (the sum of the three parameters of the GCS). A score of 8 or less indicates a severe injury.

Careful evaluation of the pupil size and response to light is essential at the initial clinical assessment and during further observation. Raised intracranial pressure causing temporal lobe herniation will cause compression of the third nerve, resulting in pupillary dilatation that nearly always occurs initially on the side of the raised pressure. The pupil will initially remain reactive to light but will subsequently fail to respond at all to light. As the intracranial pressure increases, this same process commences on the opposite side.

Neurological examination of the limbs will assess the tone, power and sensation. A hemiparesis will result from an injury of the corticospinal tract at any point from the motor cortex to the spinal cord. Following a severe brain injury the limbs may adopt an abnormal 'posturing' attitude. The decerebrate posture consists of the upper limbs adducted and internally rotated against the trunk, extended at the elbow and flexed at the wrist and fingers, with the lower limbs adducted, extended at the hip and knee with the feet plantar flexed. Less frequently the upper limbs may be flexed, probably due to an injury predominantly involving the cerebral white matter and basal ganglia, corresponding to a posture of decortication.

Table 49.1 The Glasgow Coma Scale

Parameter	Response	Numerical value
Eye opening	Spontaneous	4
	To speech	3
	To pain	2
	None	1
Best verbal response	Oriented	5
	Confused	4
	Inappropriate	3
	Incomprehensible sounds	2
	None	1
Best motor response to painful stimulus	Obeys commands	6
	Localise to pain	5
	Flexion to pain (withdrawal)	4
	Flexion (abnormal)	3
	Extension to pain	2
	None	1
Total		3–15

Particular attention must be given to the patient's ventilation, blood pressure and pulse. At all times it is essential to ensure the patient's ventilation is adequate. Respiratory problems may result either as a direct manifestation of the severity of the head injury or due to an associated chest injury.

Pyrexia frequently occurs following a head injury. A raised temperature lasting more than 2 days is usually due to traumatic subarachnoid haemorrhage or may occur in patients with a severe brainstem injury.

General examination

Careful assessment must be made of any other injuries. Chest, skeletal, cardiovascular or intra-abdominal injury must be diagnosed and the appropriate management instituted. Hypotension or hypoxia may severely aggravate the brain injury.

Radiological assessment

Radiological assessment following the clinical evaluation will be essential unless the injury has been minor. A CT scan will show the macroscopic intracranial injury and should be performed if:

- the patient is persistently drowsy or has a more seriously depressed conscious state
- there are lateralising neurological signs
- there is neurological deterioration
- there is cerebrospinal fluid (CSF) rhinorrhoea
- there are associated injuries that will entail prolonged ventilation so that ongoing neurological assessment will be difficult.

The indications for a skull X-ray have diminished since the introduction of the CT scan, especially as the bony vault can be assessed by the CT scan using the bone 'windows'.

It is important to note that radiological assessment of the cervical spine is essential in all patients who have sustained a significant head injury, particularly if there are associated facial injuries.

Further management

Following the clinical and radiological assessments, subsequent management will depend on the severity of the injury and the intracranial pathology.

Minor head injury

Any patient who has suffered a head injury must be observed for at least 4 hours. The minimum criteria for obligatory admission to hospital are given in Box 49.1.

Box 49.1 Minimum criteria for obligatory admission to hospital after head injury

- Loss of consciousness (post-traumatic amnesia) for more than 10 minutes
- Persistent drowsiness
- Focal neurological deficits
- Skull fracture
- Persisting nausea or vomiting after 4 hours' observation
- Lack of adequate care at the patient's home

Further management of these patients will be by careful observation, and neurological observations should be recorded on a chart displaying the GCS scores.

Should the patient's neurological state deteriorate, an immediate CT scan is essential to re-evaluate the intracranial pathology. Further treatment will depend on the outcome of the scan.

Severe head injury

The management of a patient following a severe head injury depends on the patient's neurological state and the intracranial pathology resulting from the trauma. In general, the following applies.

The patient has a clinical assessment and CT scan as described previously. If the CT scan shows an intracranial haematoma causing shift of the underlying brain structures then this is evacuated immediately.

Following the operation, or if there is no surgical lesion, the patient should be carefully observed and the neurological observations recorded on a chart with the GCS scores. Measures to decrease brain swelling should be implemented, including management of the airway to ensure adequate oxygenation and ventilation (hypercapnia will cause cerebral vasodilatation and so exacerbate brain swelling), elevation of the head of the bed to 20 degrees, and maintenance of fluid and electrolyte balance. Normal fluid maintenance with an intake of 3000 mL per 24 hours is optimum for the average adult. Blood loss from other injuries should be replaced with colloid or blood, not with crystalloid solutions. Pyrexia may be due to hypothalamic damage or traumatic subarachnoid haemorrhage, but infection as a cause of the fever must be excluded. The temperature must be controlled because hyperthermia can elevate the intracranial pressure, will increase brain and body metabolism, and predisposes to seizure activity. Adequate nutrition must be maintained as well as routine care of the unconscious patient, including bowel and bladder care, and pressure care.

More aggressive methods to control intracranial pressure are advisable if the patient's neurological state continues to deteriorate and the CT scan shows evidence of cerebral swelling without an intracranial haematoma, there is posturing (decerebrate) response to stimuli, or the GCS score is less than 8.

An intracranial pressure monitor will also be useful in patients requiring prolonged sedation and ventilation as a result of other injuries. Measurement of the intracranial pressure will provide another useful monitoring parameter, and any sustained rise in the pressure will be an indication for careful reassessment and, if necessary, CT scan.

The techniques used to control intracranial pressure include controlled ventilation maintaining Pa_{CO2} at 33–38 mm Hg, CSF drainage from a ventricular catheter and diuretic therapy, using intermittent administration of mannitol or frusemide. Mild hypothermia, achieved by cooling the patient to 34°C is possibly of benefit. Other techniques such as barbiturate administration, to reduce cerebral metabolism and intracranial pressure, and hyperbaric oxygen have been advocated in the past but have not been shown to have any proven benefit. Steroid medication is of no proven benefit in head injury.

Management of associated conditions

Scalp injury

A large scalp laceration may result in considerable blood loss. When the patient arrives in the emergency department, 'spurting' arteries should be controlled with haemostatic clips prior to a sterile bandage being applied to the head. After initial assessment and stabilisation the wound should be closed without delay. The hair should be shaved widely around the wound, which should be meticulously cleaned and debrided. The closure should be performed in two layers if possible, with careful apposition of the galea prior to closing the skin.

If the scalp wound has resulted in loss of soft tissue the wound may need to be extended to provide an extra 'flap' of healthy tissue so that the skin edges can be approximated without tension.

Skull fractures

Simple fracture

There is no specific management for a simple skull fracture without an overlying skin injury, although it is an indication that the trauma was not trivial and it should provide a warning that a haematoma may develop beneath the fracture.

Compound fracture

A skull fracture may be compound because of an overlying scalp laceration or if it involves an air sinus. The scalp wound should be debrided and closed. A short course of prophylactic antibiotics should be administered to reduce the risk of infection.

Depressed skull fracture

If the depressed skull fracture is compound, prophylactic antibiotics and tetanus prophylaxis should be administered. Surgery, usually requiring a general anaesthetic, should be performed as soon as possible.

Cerebrospinal fluid rhinorrhoea

A fracture involving the base of the anterior cranial fossa may cause tearing of the dura, resulting in a fistula into the air sinuses. This type of fistulous connection should also be suspected if the patient suffers an episode of meningitis or if the radiological investigations show a fracture in the appropriate site. An intracranial aerocele is proof of a fistulous connection. Cerebrospinal fluid rhinorrhoea may also occur as a result of a fistula through the tegmen tympani into the cavity of the middle ear and leakage via the Eustachian tube.

Surgery should be performed if CSF leakage persists, if there is an intracranial aerocele, or if there has been an episode of meningitis in a patient with a fracture of the anterior cranial fossa.

Rehabilitation

Some form of rehabilitation is essential following any significant head injury. If the injury has been relatively minor, then the rehabilitation necessary may involve only advice and reassurance to the patient and family. Following a severe head injury, rehabilitation will also usually involve a team of paramedical personnel, including physiotherapists, occupational therapists, speech therapists and social workers.

Further readings

American Academy of Neurology. Practice parameter. The management of concussion in sports. *Neurology.* 1997; 48:581–585.

American Congress of Rehabilitation Medicine. Definition of mild traumatic brain injury. *J Head Trauma Rehabil.* 1993; 8:86–87.

Collins M, Grindal S. Relationship between concussion and neuropsychological performance in college football players. *JAMA*. 1999;282(10):964–970.
Kaye AH. *Essential Neurosurgery*. 3rd ed. Oxford: Blackwells; 2005.
Hsiang JNK, Yeung T, Yu ALM, Poon WS. High-risk mild head injury. *J. Neurosurg*. 1997;87:234–238.
Sahuquillo J, Poca M-A, Arridas M, Garnacho A, Rubio E. Interhemispheric supratentorial intracranial pressure gradients in head-injured patients: Are they clinically important? *J. Neurosurg*. 1999;90:16–26.
Zhao W, Alonso OF, Loor JY, Busto R, Ginsberg MD. Influence of early posttraumatic hypothermia therapy on local cerebral blood flow and glucose metabolism after fluid-percussion brain injury. *J. Neurosurg*. 1999;90:L510–L519.

MCQs

Select the single correct answer to each question.

1 In the treatment of head injury, the following is true:
a steroids are regularly used
b patients with a Glasgow Coma Scale score less than 8 are usually intubated and ventilated
c antibiotics are routinely used
d pyrexia is nearly always due to severe infection
e severe fluid restriction is necessary

2 The best investigation for patients with severe head injury is:
a CT Scan
b skull X-ray
c EEG
d ultrasound
e MRI

3 Traumatic *intracerebral* haematomas following blunt trauma:
a can usually be diagnosed by skull X-ray
b are usually associated with severe brain injury
c always need to be drained
d should be treated with fluid restriction
e are always associated with a skull fracture

4 An acute subdural haematoma:
a shows a characteristic hyperdense extra-cerebral mass
b is often associated with only a minor head injury
c virtually never need surgical excision
d can always be managed with diuretic therapy
e usually causes an ipsilateral hemiparesis

50 Intracranial tumours, infection and aneurysms

Andrew H. Kaye

Introduction

This chapter provides a brief overview of three important neurosurgical conditions: intracranial tumours, cerebral aneurysms and intracranial infection. A brief description of each of these pathologies will be given and the principles of treatment will be discussed.

Brain tumours

Brain tumours are responsible for approximately 2% of all cancer deaths. However, central nervous system (CNS) tumours comprise the most common group of solid tumours in young patients, accounting for 20% of all paediatric neoplasms.

The general brain tumour classification is related to cell or origin, and is shown in Box 50.1. Table 50.1 shows the approximate distribution of the more common brain tumours, some of which will be described in this chapter.

Box 50.1 General classifications of brain tumours

Neuroepithelial tumours
- Gliomas
  - Astrocytoma (including glioblastoma)
  - Oligodendrocytoma
  - Ependymoma
  - Choroid plexus tumour
- Pineal tumours
- Neuronal tumours
  - Ganglioglioma
  - Gangliocytoma
  - Neuroblastoma
- Medulloblastoma

Nerve sheath tumour – acoustic neuroma

Meningeal tumours
- Meningioma

Pituitary tumours

Germ cell tumours
- Germinoma
- Teratoma

Lymphomas

Tumour-like malformations
- Craniopharyngioma
- Epidermoid tumour
- Dermoid tumour
- Colloid cyst

Metastatic tumours

Local extensions from regional tumours
- (e.g. glomus jugular (i.e. jugulare); carcinoma of ethmoid)

Reproduced with permission from Kaye AH. *Essential Neurosurgery*. 3rd ed. Oxford: Blackwells; 2005.

Aetiology

Epidemiological studies have not indicated any particular factor, either chemical or traumatic, that causes brain tumours in humans. There is no genetic predisposition to brain tumours, but many specific chromosome abnormalities involving chromosomes 10, 13, 17 and 22 have been noted in a wide range of CNS tumours.

At present there is considerable conjecture regarding the role of trauma, electromagnetic radiation and organic solvents in the development of brain tumours, but as yet there is no convincing evidence to implicate.

Molecular biology techniques have enabled the identification of a variety of alterations in the genome of the tumour cell, including those of brain tumours. Tumour suppressor genes are normally present in the genome, and act as a 'brake' on cell transformation. Mutations in the *p53* tumour suppressor gene are the most common gene abnormality found in tumours to date, and

Table 50.1 Incidence of common cerebral tumours (%)

Tumour	%
Neuroepithelial	52
Astrocytoma (all grades including glioblastoma)	44
Ependymoma	3
Oligodendroglioma	2
Medulloblastoma	3
Metastatic	15
Meningioma	15
Pituitary	8
Acoustic neuroma	8

Reproduced with permission from Kaye AH. *Essential Neurosurgery*. 3rd ed. Oxford: Blackwells; 2005.

have been shown to occur in both astrocytomas and meningiomas.

Cerebral glioma

Gliomas comprise the majority of cerebral tumours and arise from neuroglial cells. There are four distinct types of glial cells: astrocytes, oligodendroglia, ependymal cells and neuroglial precursors. Each of these gives rise to tumours with different biological and anatomical characteristics.

Astrocytoma

The most common gliomas arise from the astrocyte cells, which comprise the majority of intraparenchymal cells of the brain. The tumours arising from the astrocytes range from the relatively benign to the highly malignant. The term *malignant* for brain tumours differs from its usage for systemic tumours, in that intrinsic brain tumours very rarely metastasise (except for medulloblastoma and ependymoma), and the term *malignant* refers to the aggressive biological characteristics and poor prognosis.

There are many classifications of brain tumours in general and gliomas in particular. The World Health Organization classification of cerebral gliomas recognises four grades. Grade 1 is assigned to the pilocytic astrocytoma, an uncommon tumour that is very slowly growing and biologically distinct from the diffuse astrocytomas, which are classified as astrocytoma (WHO grade II), anaplastic astrocytoma (WHO grade III), and glioblastoma multiforme (WHO grade IV) and comprise over 50% of the astrocytoma tumours.

PATHOLOGY

The hallmark of the pathology of cerebral gliomas is invasion of the tumour cells into the adjacent normal brain. Although in certain areas the margin of the tumour may seem to be macroscopically well defined from the brain, there are always microscopic nests of tumour cells extending well out into the brain. The histological appearance of the tumour varies with the tumour grade, with increasing cellular atypia, mitoses, endothelial and adventitial cell proliferation and necrosis with increasing grade of the tumour.

CLINICAL PRESENTATION

The presenting features of all intracranial tumours can be classified under:

- raised intracranial pressure
- focal neurological signs
- epilepsy.

The duration of the symptoms and the progression evolution of the clinical presentation will depend on the grade of the tumour (i.e. the rate of growth). A patient presenting with a low-grade astrocytoma (grade I or II) may have a history of seizures extending over many years antedating the development of progressive neurological signs and raised intracranial pressure. Patients with the more common higher grade tumour present with a shorter history, and glioblastoma multiforme is characterised by a short illness of weeks or a few months.

Raised intracranial pressure is due to the tumour mass, surrounding cerebral oedema and hydrocephalus due to blockage of cerebrospinal fluid (CSF) pathways. The main clinical features of raised intracranial pressure are headaches, nausea and vomiting, drowsiness and papilloedema.

Headache associated with increased intracranial pressure is usually worse on waking in the morning and is relieved by vomiting. Intracranial pressure increases during sleep, probably from vascular dilatation due to carbon dioxide retention.

Nausea and vomiting are usually worse in the morning.

Drowsiness is the most important clinical feature of raised intracranial pressure. It is the portent of rapid neurological deterioration.

Papilloedema is the definitive sign of raised intracranial pressure. The early features of increased pressure on the optic nerve head are those of dilatation or failure of normal pulsations of retinal veins. As the intracranial pressure rises, the nerve head becomes more swollen and the disc margins become blurred on fundoscopic examination. Flame-shaped haemorrhages develop, particularly around the disc margins and along the vessels.

Sixth nerve palsy, causing diplopia, may result in raised intracranial pressure owing to stretching of the sixth cranial nerve by cordal displacement of the brainstem. This is a so-called 'false localising sign'.

Focal neurological signs are common in patients presenting with cerebral gliomas, and the nature of the deficit will depend on the position of the tumour.

Patients presenting with tumours involving the frontal lobes frequently may have pseudo-psychiatric problems with personality change and mood disorders. Limb paresis results from interference of the pyramidal tracts, either at a cortical or subcortical level, and field defects are associated with tumours of the temporal, occipital or parietal lobes. Dysphasia, either expressive or receptive, is a particularly distressing symptom in patients involving the relevant areas of dominant hemisphere.

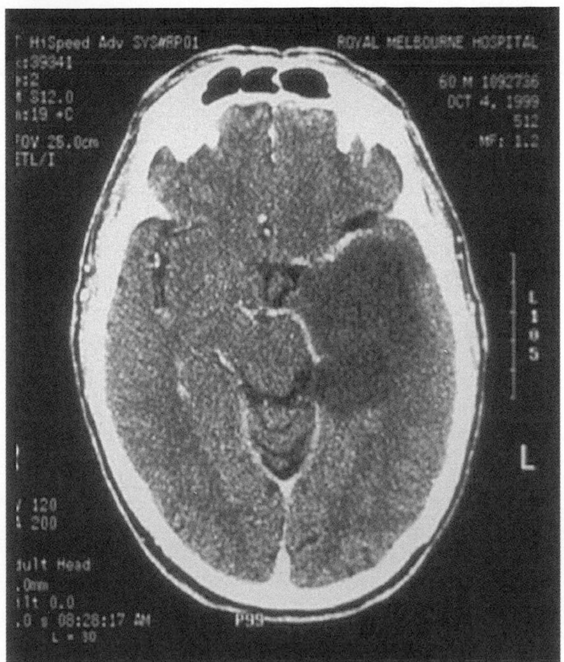

Fig. 50.1 Low-grade glioma with decreased density on T_1-weighted magnetic resonance image.

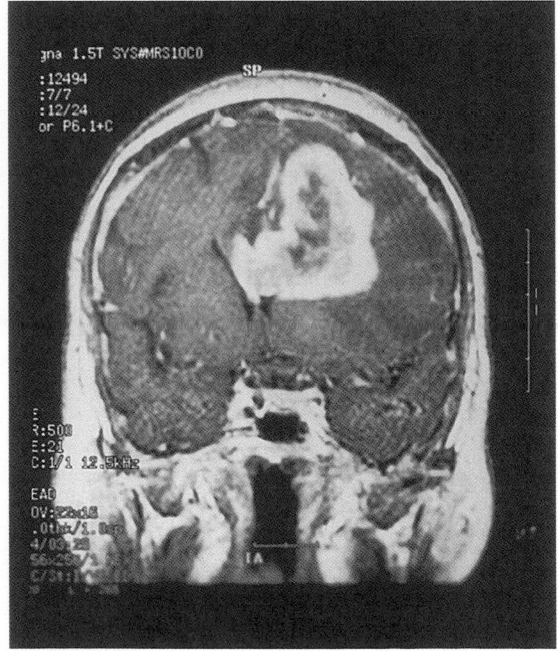

Fig. 50.2 High-grade glioma (glioblastoma multiforme) showing vivid enhancement after intravenous injection of contrast material.

INVESTIGATIONS

Computed tomographic (CT) scanning and magnetic resonance imaging (MRI) of the brain are the essential radiological investigations and an accurate diagnosis can be made in nearly all tumours.

Low-grade gliomas show decreased density on CT scanning and the T_1-weighted MRI, with minimal surrounding oedema and no enhancement with contrast (Fig. 50.1). Calcification may be present. High-grade gliomas are usually large and enhance vividly following intravenous injection of contrast material and have extensive surrounding oedema (Fig. 50.2).

Magnetic resonance imaging, particularly when used with gadolinium contrast enhancement, improves the visualisation of cerebral gliomas. Gadolinium enhancement is more likely to occur in high-grade tumours.

MANAGEMENT

Following the presumptive diagnosis of a glioma, the management involves

- surgery
- radiotherapy
- other adjuvant treatments.

Surgery: The aim of surgery is to

- make a definitive diagnosis
- reduce the tumour mass to relieve the symptoms of raised intracranial pressure
- reduce the tumour mass as a precursor to adjuvant treatments.

Radiotherapy: Post-operative radiation therapy is often used as an adjunct to surgery in the treatment of high-grade gliomas as it has been shown to double the median survival from high-grade gliomas to 37 weeks.

PROGNOSIS

At present there is no satisfactory treatment for cerebral glioma. The median survival following surgery for the high-grade glioma (glioblastoma multiforme) is approximately 17 weeks, and when radiotherapy is used as an adjunct, the median survival is approximately 37 weeks. Chemotherapy for high-grade gliomas has been disappointing and the best results for surgery, radiation therapy and chemotherapy consistently show a median survival time of less than 1 year.

Oligodendroglioma

Oligodendroglioma are much less common than the astrocytoma group, being responsible for approximately 5% of all gliomas.

Oligodendrogliomas have the same spectrum of histological appearance as astrocytomas but, as distinct from the astrocytoma series, are more likely to be slow growing. Calcium deposits are found in 90% of the tumours (Fig. 50.3).

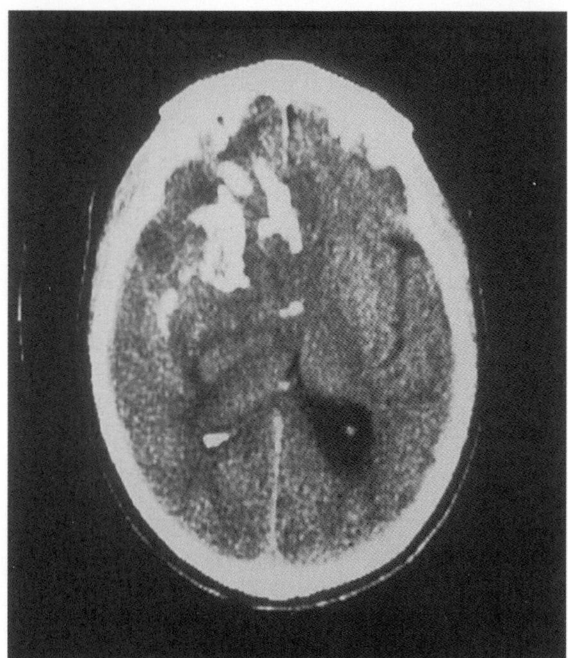

Fig. 50.3 Oligodendroglioma that is highly calcified.

The clinical presentation is essentially the same as for the astrocyte group, but as these tumours are more likely to be slow growing, epilepsy is more common.

The principles of treatment are the same as for the astrocytoma group. Surgery is necessary to make a definitive diagnosis and debulking the tumour will relieve the features of raised intracranial pressure as well as reducing the tumour burden for adjuvant therapies. Radiotherapy is probably helpful in reducing the rate of growth of any remnant tumour. Unlike the astrocytoma group, chemotherapy has been shown to be of some use in helping to control those tumours with an oligodendroglial component, especially those tumours with loss of heterozygosity on chromosome 1p or 19q.

Metastatic tumours

Metastatic tumours are responsible for 15% of brain tumours in clinical series, but up to 30% of brain tumours reported by pathologists. Approximately 30% of deaths are due to cancer and 20% of these will have intracranial metastatic deposits at autopsy. The metastatic tumours most commonly originate from

- carcinoma of the lung
- carcinoma of the breast
- metastatic melanoma
- carcinoma of the kidney
- gastrointestinal carcinoma.

In 15% of cases a primary origin is never found. Most metastatic tumours are multiple and one-third are solitary. In about half of the solitary tumours, systemic spread is not apparent. The incidence of tumours in the cerebrum relative to the cerebellum is 8 to 1. Metastatic tumours are often surrounded by intense cerebral oedema.

Clinical presentation

The interval between diagnosis of the primary cancer and cerebral metastasis varies considerably. In general, secondary tumours from carcinoma of the lung present relatively soon after the initial diagnosis, with a median interval of 5 months. Although cerebral metastases may present within a few months of the initial diagnosis of malignant melanoma or carcinoma of the breast, some patients may live many years before an intracranial tumour appears.

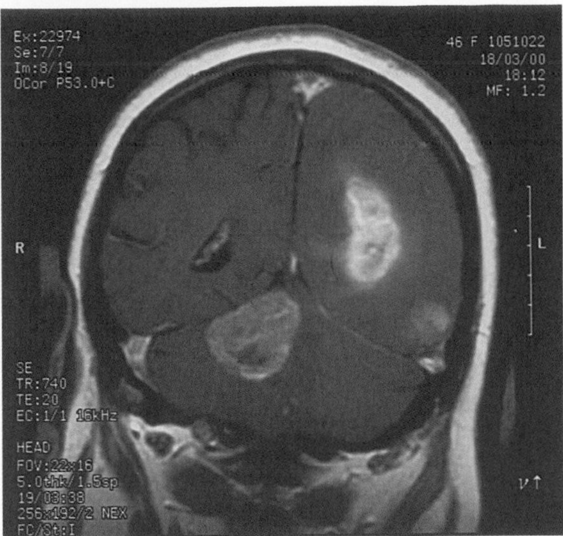

Fig. 50.4 Multiple metastatic tumours.

The presenting clinical features for cerebral metastasis are similar to those described for other tumours:

- raised intracranial pressure
- focal neurological signs
- epilepsy.

Radiological investigations

A CT scan or MRI will diagnose metastatic tumour and show whether or not the deposits are solitary or multiple. Most metastatic tumours are isodense on un-enhanced scan and they enhance vividly after intravenous contrast material. Magnetic resonance image following gadolinium contrast may demonstrate small metastatic tumours often not visible on a CT scan (Fig. 50.4).

Treatment

Steroid medication will control cerebral oedema and should be commenced immediately if there is raised intracranial pressure.

Surgery to remove the metastasis is indicated if:

- there is a solitary metastasis in a surgically accessible position
- there is no systemic spread.

Removal of a solitary secondary is preferable especially if the primary site of origin has been, or will be, controlled. Excision of a single metastasis will provide excellent symptomatic relief and consequently may be indicated even if the primary site cannot be treated satisfactorily.

Radiotherapy, together with steroid medication to control cerebral oedema is used to treat patients with multiple cerebral metastases and may be advisable following excision of a single metastasis. More recently, stereotactic radiosurgery, which uses a highly focussed beam of radiation, has been used to treat single and multiple cerebral metastases if the tumour size is less than 3 cm in diameter.

Prognosis

The 1-year median survival for patients having had a surgical excision of a solitary metastatic deposit is:

- 50% for patients with carcinoma of the breast
- 30% for patients with carcinoma of the lung
- 30% for patients with melanoma
- 50% for patients in whom the source of metastatic tumour is undetermined.

Paediatric brain tumours

Intracranial tumours are the most common form of solid tumours in childhood, with 60% of tumours occurring below the tentorium cerebelli. The most common supratentorial tumours are astrocytomas, followed by anaplastic astrocytomas and glioblastoma multiforme.

Posterior fossa paediatric tumours

Sixty per cent of paediatric brain tumours occur in the posterior fossa. The relative incidence of tumours is:

- cerebellar astrocytoma 30%
- medulloblastoma (infratentorial primary neuroectodermal tumour) 30%
- ependymoma 20%
- brainstem glioma 10%
- miscellaneous 10% (choroid plexus papilloma, haemangioblastoma, epidermoid, dermoid, chordoma).

Clinical presentation

The presenting clinical features of posterior fossa neoplasms in children are related to:

- raised intracranial pressure
- focal neurological signs.

RAISED INTRACRANIAL PRESSURE

Raised intracranial pressure is the most common presenting feature. It is due to hydrocephalus caused by obstruction of the fourth ventricle and is manifest by headaches, vomiting, diplopia and papilloedema. The raised intracranial pressure may result in a strasbismus causing diplopia due to stretching of one or both of the sixth (abducens) cranial nerves (a false localising sign).

FOCAL NEUROLOGICAL SIGNS

Focal neurological signs are due to the tumour invading or compressing the cerebellum, the brainstem and cranial nerves. Truncal and gait ataxia result particularly from midline cerebellar involvement. Horizontal gaze paretic nystagmus often occurs in tumours around the fourth ventricle. Vertical nystagmus is indicative of brainstem involvement. Disturbance of bulbar function, such as difficulty in swallowing, with nasal regurgitation of fluid, dysarthria and impaired palatal or pharyngeal reflexes result from brainstem involvement. Compression or tumour invasion of the pyramidal tracts may result in hemiparesis or sensory disturbance.

Investigations

Computed tomography scan and MRI will confirm the position of the tumour and whether there is hydrocephalus (Fig. 50.5).

Management

The treatment of posterior fossa tumours involves surgery, radiotherapy and chemotherapy.

A CSF shunt may need to be performed to control raised intracranial pressure due to hydrocephalus. The CSF diversion can be achieved with either an external drain or ventriculoperitoneal shunt. The shunt will provide immediate and controlled relief of intracranial hypertension and the subsequent posterior fossa operation can be performed as a planned elective procedure. A criticism of pre-operative ventriculoperitoneal shunt is that it may promote the metastatic spread of these tumours.

In general, the treatment of medulloblastoma and ependymoma involves surgery to excise the tumour, followed by radiation therapy, which may be to the whole neuraxis as the tumour may spread throughout the CNS, followed by chemotherapy. The 5-year survival of these tumours is approximately 40%. Many cerebellar astrocytoma tumours have a small single nodule surrounded by a large cyst. These tumours can often be cured by excision of the nodule alone, and adjuvant therapy is not necessary. In contrast, the treatment of brainstem glioma usually involves only a biopsy of the tumour to confirm the diagnosis, possibly followed by radiotherapy and/or chemotherapy. These tumours usually cause death within 24 months of diagnosis, although some patients with low-grade tumours will live longer.

(A)

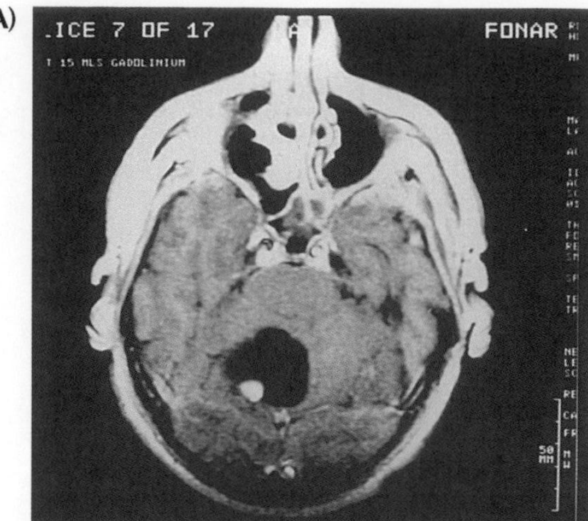

(B)

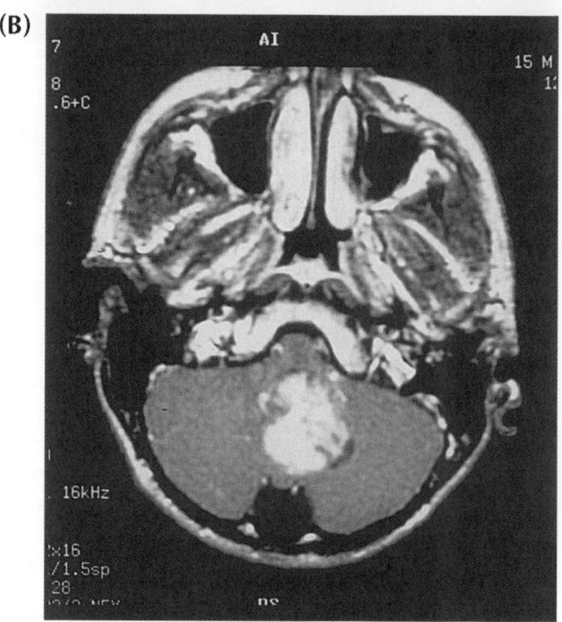

Fig. 50.5 (A) Posterior fossa cystic astrocytoma with small tumour nodule and large cyst. (B) Enhancing midline posterior fossa tumour (medulloblastoma).

Benign brain tumours

The most common benign brain tumours are:

- meningioma
- acoustic neuroma
- haemangioblastoma
- dermoid and epidermoid tumours
- colloid cysts
- pituitary tumours
- craniopharyngioma.

Meningiomas

Meningiomas are the most common of the benign brain tumours and constitute about 15% of all intracranial tumours, being about one-third the number of gliomas. Although they may occur at any age, they reach their peak incidence in middle age and are very uncommon in children.

Unlike gliomas, where the classification system is based on the histological appearance of the tumours, meningiomas are usually classified according to the position of origin rather than histology. The reason for this is that, in general, the biological activity of the tumour, the presenting features, the treatment and prognosis all relate more to the site of the tumour than the histology (Table 50.2).

CLINICAL PRESENTATION

Meningiomas present with features of:

- raised intracranial pressure
- focal neurological signs
- epilepsy.

The position of the tumour (Fig. 50.6) will determine the features of the clinical presentation. The tumours

Table 50.2 Position of intracranial meningioma (%)

Position	%
Parasagittal and falx	25
Convexity	20
Sphenoidal wing	20
Olfactory groove	12
Suprasellar	12
Posterior fossa	9
Ventricle	1.5
Optic sheath	0.5

Reproduced with permission from Kaye AH. *Essential Neurosurgery*. 3rd ed. Oxford: Blackwells; 2005.

POSITION OF MENINGIOMAS

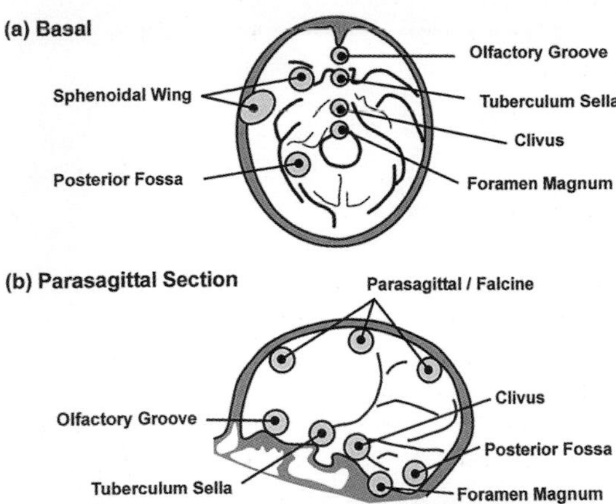

Fig. 50.6 Classical positions of meningiomas.

often grow slowly and there is frequently a long history, often of many years, of symptoms prior to diagnosis.

Parasagittal tumours often arise in the middle third of the vault, and the patient may present with focal epilepsy and paresis, usually affecting the opposite leg and foot, as the motor cortex on the medial aspect of the posterior frontal lobe is affected. Urinary incontinence is occasionally a symptom for a large frontal tumour, especially if it is bilateral.

Convexity tumours often grow around the position of the coronal suture. Patients present with raised intracranial pressure, and more posterior tumours will cause focal neurological symptoms and epilepsy.

An inner sphenoidal wing meningioma will cause compression of the adjacent optic nerve and patients may present with a history of uniocular visual failure.

Olfactory groove meningioma will cause anosmia, initially unilateral and later bilateral. The presenting features may include symptoms of raised intracranial pressure.

Suprasellar tumours arise from the tuberculum sellae and will cause visual failure with a bitemporal hemianopia.

Posterior fossa tumours may arise from the cerebellar convexity or from the cerebellopontine angle or clivus.

RADIOLOGICAL INVESTIGATIONS

Computed tomography scan and MRI show tumours that enhance vividly following intravenous contrast (Fig. 50.7). Hyperostosis of the cranial vault may occur at the site of attachment of the tumour, and these bony changes may often be seen on plain skull X-ray.

(A)

(B)

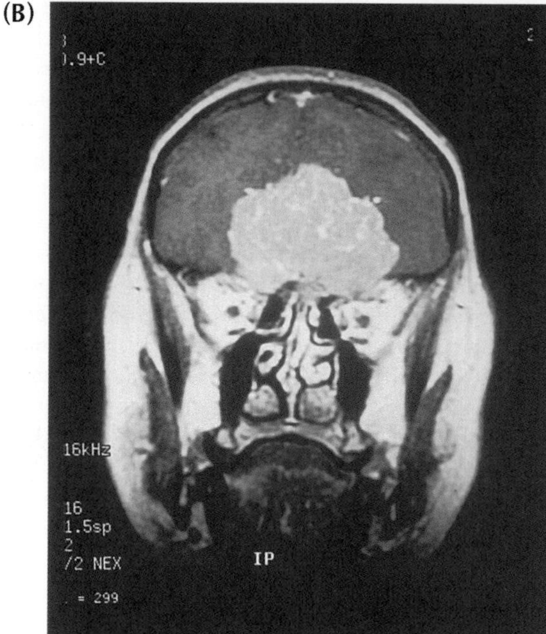

Fig. 50.7 (A) Axial magnetic resonance image (MRI) and (B) coronal MRI showing meningioma with vivid contrast enhancement arising from floor of anterior carnial fossa (olfactory groove) and growing into superior frontal lobes.

TREATMENT

The treatment of meningiomas is total surgical excision including obliteration of the dural attachment. Although this objective is often possible, there are some situations where complete excision is not possible because of the position of the tumour. Surgery may be preceded by embolisation of the main vascular supply of the tumour.

Acoustic neuroma

Acoustic schwannomas arise from the eighth cranial nerve and account for 8% of intracranial tumours. The tumours are schwannomas, with their origin from the vestibular component of the eighth cranial nerve near the internal auditory meatus.

Clinical presentation

The clinical presentation of an acoustic schwannoma will depend on the size of the tumour at the time of diagnosis. The earliest symptoms are associated with eighth nerve involvement. Tinnitus and unilateral partial or complete sensory neural hearing loss are the earliest features. With extension into the cerebellopontine angle, the tumour will compress the cerebellum, resulting in ataxia and compression of the pyramidal tracts due to a large tumour causing brainstem compression, which will cause a contralateral hemiparesis. A very large tumour will cause obstructive hydrocephalus.

Radiological investigations

Computed tomography scan or MRI will show an enhancing tumour in the cerebellopontine angle with extension into the internal auditory meatus that will be widened, indicating the tumour has arisen from the eighth cranial nerve (Fig. 50.8). Small tumours within the internal auditory meatus are best diagnosed using MRI following gadolinium enhancement.

The treatment of a large acoustic neuroma is surgical. Stereotactic radiosurgery has been advocated by some for small tumours (<2 cm diameter), although as yet its efficacy is not definitely proven in controlling the growth of the tumour and there is an increased incidence of fifth cranial nerve morbidity following radiosurgery. Intracanalicular, or very small tumours in the elderly, may be just observed and treatment advised only if there is evidence of tumour growth.

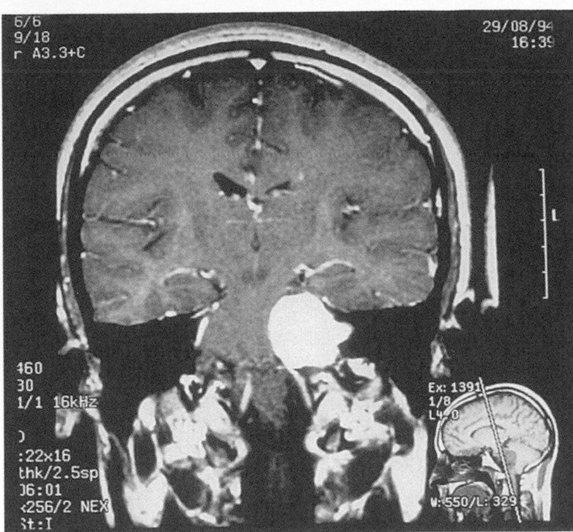

Fig. 50.8 Acoustic neuroma showing extension to tumour into internal auditory canal.

Colloid cyst of third ventricle

A colloid cyst of the third ventricle is situated in the anterior part of the ventricle and applied to the roof just behind the foramen Munro. As the cyst grows it causes bilateral obstruction to the foramena of Munro resulting in raised intracranial pressure from hydrocephalus.

Radiological investigations include MRI and CT scan, which show a round tumour in the anterior third ventricle that usually enhances following intravenous contrast (Fig. 50.9). The treatment is surgical excision.

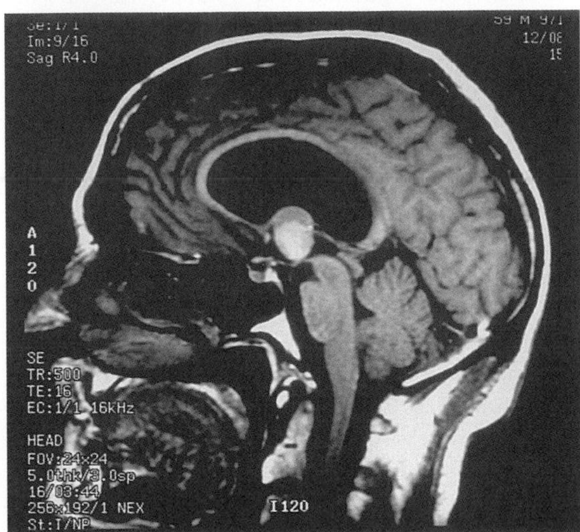

Fig. 50.9 Colloid cyst of third ventricle.

Pituitary tumours

Pituitary tumours account for 8–10% of all intracranial tumours.

Pathology

Historically, three main types of pituitary tumours were defined by their cytoplasmic staining characteristics; chromophobic, acidophilic and basophilic. The development of immunoperoxidase techniques and electron microscopy have provided a more refined classification of pituitary adenomas based on the specific hormone produced. This classification is shown in Table 50.3. The tumours can be further classified via their size with microadenomas (being tumours <1 cm diameter) and macroadenomas (>1 cm) being either confined to the sella or with extrasellar extension (Fig. 50.10).

Clinical presentation

The presenting clinical features of pituitary tumours are due to:

- the size of the tumour
- endocrine disturbance.

Headache occurs principally in patients with acromegaly and is uncommon in other types of pituitary tumours.

VISUAL FAILURE

Suprasellar extension of the pituitary tumour causes compression of the optic chiasm resulting in bitemporal hemianopia. Optic atrophy will be evident in patients with long-standing compression of the chiasm. Extension of the tumour into the cavernous sinus may

Table 50.3 Classification of pituitary adenomas

Hormone secreted	Percentage of tumours
Prolactin	40
Growth hormone	20
Null cell (no hormone)	20
ACTH	15
Prolactin and growth hormone	5
FSH/LH	1–2
TSH	1
Acidophil stem cell (no hormone)	1–2

Reproduced with permission from Kaye AH. *Essential Neurosurgery*. 3rd ed. Oxford: Blackwells; 2005.

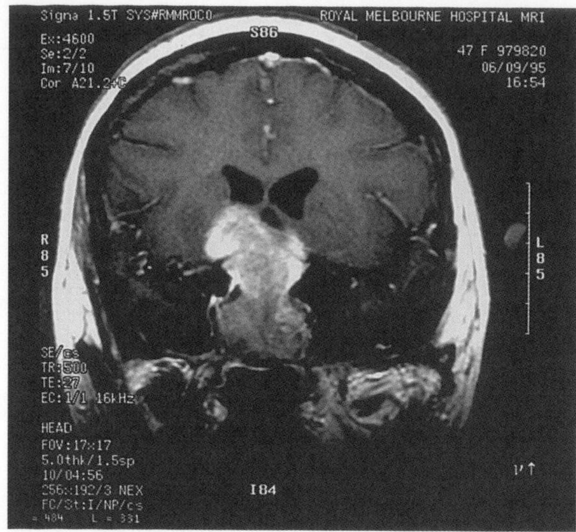

Fig. 50.10 Large pituitary tumour with marked suprasellar extension causing compression of the optic chiasma.

cause compression of the third, fourth or sixth cranial nerves.

ENDOCRINE DISTURBANCE

Endocrine disturbance is due to either hypopituitism or excess secretion of a particular pituitary hormone.

Hypopituitism results from failure of the hormone secreted by the adenohypophysis. The endocrine secretions are not equally depressed, but there is a selective failure, and the order of susceptibility is as follows: growth hormone, gonadotrophin, corticotrophin, thyroid stimulating hormone. Hypopituitarism initially results in vague symptoms including lack of energy, undue fatiguability, muscle weakness and anorexia, and when prolonged or severe will cause low blood pressure. Clinical hypothyroidism is manifest by physical and mental sluggishness and a preference for warmth. When the hypopituitarism is severe episodic confusion occurs and the patient will become drowsy.

Pituitary apoplexy results from sudden spontaneous haemorrhage into the pituitary tumour. It is characterised by sudden severe headache followed by transient and more prolonged loss of consciousness, with features of neck stiffness or vomiting and photophobia.

Prolactinoma: Prolactin-secreting tumours may be a microadenoma or a macroadenoma. The patients with microadenomas are usually women who present with infertility associated with amenorrhoea and galactorrhoea. These tumours can usually be treated with a dopamine agonist such as bromocryptine. Very large macroadenomas may occur in males who present with features of hypopituitarism and visual failure due to suprasella extension.

Acromegaly results from growth hormone-secreting pituitary adenomas. Clinical features include bone and soft tissue changes as evidenced by an enlarged supraciliary ridge, enlarged frontal sinuses and increased mandibular size, which will cause the chin to project (prognathism). The hands and feet enlarge, the skin becomes coarse and greasy and sweats profusely. The voice becomes hoarse and gruff. Systemic problems include hypertension, cardiac hypertrophy and diabetes.

Cushing's disease is due to ACTH producing pituitary adenomas. Over 80% of the tumours are microadenomas. The onset is often insidious and the disease may affect children or adults. Severe obesity occurs, the skin is tense and painful and purple striae appear around the trunk. Fat is deposited, particularly on the face (moonface), neck, cervicodorsal junction (buffalo hump) and trunk. The skin becomes a purple colour due to vasodilatation and stasis. Spontaneous bruising is common. The skin is greasy, acne is common and facial hair excessive. Osteoporosis predisposes to spontaneous fractures and there is wasting of the muscles. Glucose tolerance is impaired and hypertension occurs. Laboratory investigations are vital to confirm the diagnosis.

TREATMENT

The treatment of patients with pituitary tumours depends on whether the patient has presented with features of endocrine disturbance or problems related to compression of adjacent neural structures.

Surgical excision will be used as the primary method of treatment for:

- large tumours causing compression of adjacent neural structures, particularly the visual pathways
- growth hormone-secreting tumours causing acromegaly
- ACTH-secreting tumours causing Cushing's disease
- the occasional treatment of a prolactin-secreting adenoma when the medical treatment using bromocryptine is not tolerated.

Most tumours can be excised via the trans-sphenoidal approach to the pituitary fossa. Post-operative radiotherapy may be indicated if there has been a subtotal excision of the tumour or if the post-operative endocrine studies demonstrate residual excessive hormone secretion.

Subarachnoid haemorrhage and cerebral aneurysm

The sudden onset of a severe headache in a patient should be regarded as subarachnoid haemorrhage until proven otherwise. The most common cause of subarachnoid haemorrhage in adults is rupture of a berry aneurysm. Subarachnoid haemorrhage in children is much less common than in the adult population, and the most common paediatric cause is rupture of an arteriovenous malformation. Cerebral aneurysm as a cause of subarachnoid haemorrhage becomes more frequent than arteriovenous malformation in patients over the age of 20 years.

Subarachnoid haemorrhage

Clinical presentation

HEADACHE

The sudden onset of a severe headache of a type not previously experienced by the patient is the hallmark of subarachnoid haemorrhage. A relatively small leak from an aneurysm may result in a minor headache, sometimes referred to as a 'sentinel headache', and this may be the warning episode of a subsequent major haemorrhage from the aneurysm.

DIMINISHED CONSCIOUS STATE

Most patients have some deterioration of their conscious state following subarachnoid haemorrhage. This varies from only slight change, when the haemorrhage has been minor, to apoplectic death resulting from massive haemorrhage.

MENINGISMUS

Blood in the subarachnoid CSF will cause the features of meningismus (headache, neck stiffness, photophobia and fever or vomiting).

FOCAL NEUROLOGICAL SIGNS

Focal neurological signs may occur in subarachnoid haemorrhage due to concombinant intracerebral haemorrhage, the local pressure effects on the aneurysm (such as a third cranial nerve palsy resulting from pressure from a posterior communicating artery aneurysm) itself or cerebral vasospasm.

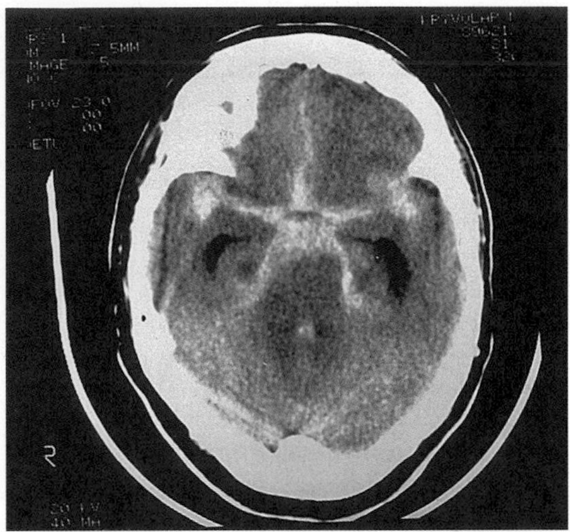

Fig. 50.11 Diffuse blood in the basal cisterns confirming the diagnosis of subarachnoid haemorrhage.

Clinical assessment

The major differential diagnosis of subarachnoid haemorrhage is meningitis, although a minor haemorrhage is often misdiagnosed as migraine. Confirmation of the clinical diagnosis of subarachnoid haemorrhage should be undertaken as soon as possible by CT scanning (Fig. 50.11). If there is any doubt that subarachnoid blood is present on the CT scan, as may occur following more minor haemorrhages, a lumbar puncture is essential. The presence of xanthochromia (yellow staining) in the CSF will confirm subarachnoid haemorrhage.

Cerebral angiography (Fig. 50.12) will confirm the cause of the subarachnoid haemorrhage and will determine the subsequent treatment.

Cerebral aneurysm

Cerebral aneurysms are the most common cause of subarachnoid haemorrhage in the adult population. The great majority of aneurysms arise at branch points of two vessels and are situated mainly on the Circle of Willis; about 85% on the anterior half of the circle and 15% in the posterior circulation (Box 50.2). Aneurysms occur in more than one position in approximately 15% of cases.

(A)

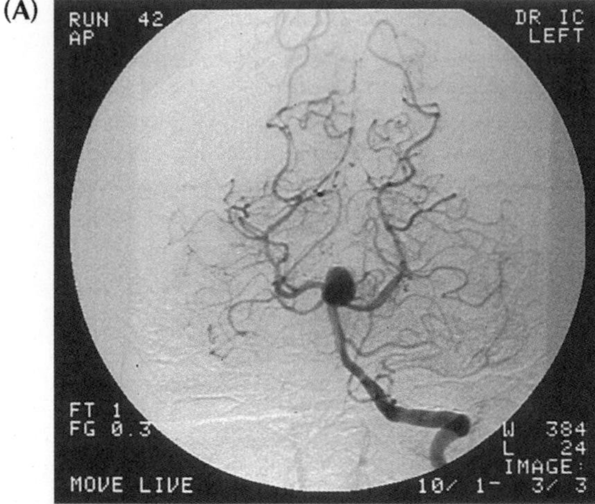

(B)

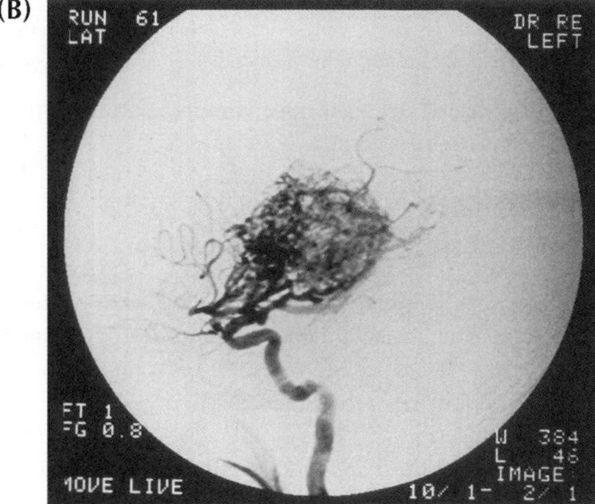

Fig. 50.12 (**A**) Cerebral aneurysm on angiogram. (**B**) Arteriovenous malformation.

Management

Management of patients following rupture of a cerebral aneurysm is determined by three factors:

- severity of the initial haemorrhage
- re-bleeding of the aneurysm
- cerebral vasospasm.

About 30% of all patients suffering a subarachnoid haemorrhage from a ruptured aneurysm either have an apoplectic death or are deeply comatose as a result of the initial haemorrhage. Re-bleeding occurs in about 50% of patients within 6 weeks and 25% of patients within 2 weeks of the initial haemorrhage. The only certain way to prevent the aneurysm re-bleeding is to occlude it from the circulation. Cerebral vasospasm occurs in 50% of patients following subarachnoid haemorrhage and in 25% it results in serious neurological complications. Clinical vasospasm is treated using hypertension and volume expansion, and consequently the treatment is most effective if the aneurysm has been occluded.

Box 50.2 Position of cerebral aneurysm

- Anterior Circle of Willis
  - Anterior communicating artery
  - Middle cerebral artery – bifurcation or trifurcation
  - Internal carotid artery
    - Posterior communicating artery
    - Terminal bifurcation
    - Anterior choroidal artery
    - Ophthalmic artery
    - Intracavernous
  - Pericallosal artery
- Posterior circulation (15%)
  - Terminal basilar artery – most common
  - Vertebrobasilar junction
  - Posterior inferior cerebellar artery
  - Anterior inferior cerebellar artery
  - Superior anterior cerebellar artery
  - Superior inferior cerebellar artery
  - Posterior cerebral artery

Reproduced with permission from Kaye AH. *Essential Neurosurgery*. 3rd ed. Oxford: Blackwells; 2005.

Surgery – endovascular occlusion

Although in the past surgery has often been delayed for fear that it might exacerbate cerebral vasospasm, the current treatment of cerebral aneurysm is immediate obliteration of the aneurysm by either surgery or an endovascular technique. Surgery is not performed on patients who are comatose or have features of decerebrate posturing unless the CT scan shows a large intracerebral haematoma resulting from the ruptured aneurysm that needs to be evacuated, or hydrocephalus as a cause of the poor neurological state. Evacuation of intracerebral haematoma or drainage of the hydrocephalus should be performed urgently, and the aneurysm occluded.

The surgical procedure involves a craniotomy with occlusion of the neck of the aneurysm. Endovascular techniques, using detachable coils, have been shown to have an increasing role in the treatment of cerebral aneurysms, particularly for posterior fossa (basilar tip) aneurysms. Most centres treating aneurysms utilise endovascular coiling in over 50% of cases.

Intracranial infection

Although infections involving the nervous system may present in many ways and involve a large variety of pathogens, the most common infections involving the neurosurgeon are acute bacterial meningitis and cerebral abscess.

Meningitis

Bacterial meningitis is a serious life-threatening infection of the meninges. Most of the common organisms that cause bacterial meningitis are related to the patient's age and to the presence and nature of any underlying predisposing disease. Table 50.4 shows the common organisms causing bacterial meningitis related to age.

The bacteria reach the meninges and CSF by three main routes:

- haematogenous spread from extracranial foci of infection
- retrograde spread via infected thrombi within emissary veins from infections adjacent to the CNS such as sinusitis, otitis or mastoiditis
- direct spread into the subarachnoid space such as from osteomyelitis of the skull and infected paranasal sinuses.

Clinical presentation

Bacterial meningitis is usually an acute illness with rapid progression of the clinical signs. The major presenting features are:

- high fever
- meningismus including headache, neck stiffness, photophobia and vomiting.

Although patients are usually alert at the commencement of the illness, they will frequently become drowsy and confused.

In infants, neonates, the elderly and the immunocompromised, the presentation of bacterial meningitis may be different. Neck stiffness and fever are often absent and the presentation includes listlessness and irritabilty in the young and confusion or obtundation in the elderly. A careful search must be made for a skin rash. Meningococcal infection frequently has a coexisting petechial rash, which occurs less frequently in other bacterial or viral infections. The original source of the infection, for example sinusitis, bacterial endocarditis, otitis media or mastoiditis may be evident and many patients have evidence of pharyngitis – bacterial meningitis sometimes follows another respiratory tract infection.

The diagnosis is made by CSF examination obtained by lumbar puncture, which should be performed immediately once the diagnosis is suspected. If the patient is drowsy, has other signs of raised intracranial pressure or if there are focal neurological signs, an urgent CT scan must be performed prior to lumbar puncture to exclude an intracranial space-occupying lesion.

The CSF features in a lumbar puncture are:

- raised cell count, predominantly a polymorphonuclear leucocytosis
- protein level greater than 0.8 g/L
- glucose level less than 2 mmol/L
- positive Gram stain in more than 70%.

Other tests that should be performed on the CSF include examination for *Cryptococcus neoformans* and for *Mycobacterium tuberculosis*. Other investigations

Table 50.4 Common organisms causing primary bacterial meningitis related to age

Age	Organism
Neonate (0–4 weeks)	Group B streptococcus, *Escherichia coli*
4–12 weeks	Group B streptococcus, *Streptococcus pneumoniae, Salmonella, Haemophilus influenzae, Listeria monocytogenes*
3 months–5 years	*Haemophilus influenzae, Streptococcus pneumoniae, Neisseria meningitidis*
Over 5 years and adults	*Streptococcus pneumoniae, Neisseria meningitidis*

Reproduced with permission from Kaye AH. *Essential Neurosurgery*. 3rd ed. Oxford: Blackwells; 2005.

should include blood cultures and radiological investigations to detect the source of the infection; chest X-ray, CT scan or skull X-ray for sinusitis.

The differential diagnoses include:

- other types of meningitis (viral, fungal, carcinomatosis)
- subdural empyema (patients are drowsy, with focal neurological signs, and usually have seizures)
- subarachnoid haemorrhage
- viral encephalitis.

Treatment

High-dose intravenous antibiotic therapy should be commenced immediately, and the selection of the antibiotic depends on the initial expectation of the most likely organism involved, taking into account the age of the patient, source of infection, CSF microbiology studies and the antibiotic that has best penetration to CSF.

There are many antibiotic regimes, but if there is no obvious site of infection initial therapy should commence immediately as follows:

- Neonates (under months) – cefotaxime or ceftriaxone plus benzoyl penicillin or amoxy/ampicillin
- Three months to 15 years – cefotaxime or ceftriaxone
- 15 years to adults – benzyl penicillin + cefotaxime/ceftriaxone
- Add vancomycin if Gram-positive streptococci are seen and there is any suspicion of intermediate and/or resistant *Streptococcus pneumoniae*.

When the organism has been identified, the most appropriate antibiotic should be used, depending on sensitivites and the ability of the antibiotic to penetrate into the CSF.

The usual specific antimicrobial therapy following identification of the organism is:

- Pneumococcus or meningococcus – Benzyl penicillin (child: 60 mg/kg up to 1.8–2.4 g intravenously 4 hourly). If the patient is sensitive to penicillin use cefotaxime (child: 15 mg/kg 6 hourly or ceftriaxone 100 mg/kg daily). About half the patients with meningococcal meningitis have petechiae or purpura. Subclinical or clinical disseminated intravascular coagulation often accompanies meningococcaemia and may progress to haemorrhage infarction of the adrenal glands, renal cortical necrosis, pulmonary vascular thrombosis, shock and death. The antibiotic therapy must be accompanied by intensive medical supportive therapy.
- *Haemophilus influenzae* – amoxy/ampicillin if organism is susceptible. If the patient is allergic or organism-resistant use cefotaxime or ceftriaxone.
- *Listeria* – benzyl penicillin or amoxy/ampicillin plus trimethoprim and sulfamethoxazole
- Hospital-acquired meningitis – vancomycin plus cefotaxime, ceftriaxone or meropenem

Complications of bacterial meningitis

Complications are more likely to occur if treatment is not commenced immediately. The major complications are:

- Cerebral oedema
- Seizures
- Hydrocephalus – communicating hydrocephalus. This may occur early in the disease or as a late manifestation
- Subdural effusion – particularly in children. Most resolve spontaneously but some may require drainage
- Subdural empyaema. A rare complication that usually requires drainage
- Brain abscess – occurs as a rare complication of meningitis.

Brain abscess

Cerebral abscess may result from:

- haematogenous spread from a known septic site or occult focus
- direct spread from an infected paranasal or mastoid sinus
- trauma causing a penetrating wound.

Metastatic brain abscesses arising from haematogenous dissemination of infection are frequently multiple and develop at the junction of white and grey matter. Most common sites of infection include skin pustules, chronic pulmonary infection (bronchiectasis), diverticulitis, osteomyelitis and bacterial endocarditis. The site of origin of haematogenous spread is unknown in approximately 25% of patients.

Direct spread from paranasal sinuses, mastoid air cells or the middle ear are the most common pathogenic mechanisms in many series. Infection from the paranasal sinuses spread either into the frontal or temporal lobe and the abscesses are usually single and located superficially. Frontal sinusitis may cause an abscess in the frontal lobe. Middle ear infection may spread into the temporal lobe and uncommonly the cerebellum.

Table 50.5 Cerebral abscess: pathogenesis and principal organisms

History	Site of infection	Predominant organism
Sinusitis – frontal	Frontal lobe	Aerobic streptococci *Streptococcus milleri* *Haemophilus* species
Mastoiditis, otitis	Temporal lobe	Mixed flora Aerobic and anaerobic streptococci Enterobacteria *Bacteroides fragilis* *Haemophilus* species
Haematogenous, cryptogenic	Brain	Aerobic streptococci Anaerobic streptococci Enterobacteria
Trauma	Brain	*Staphylococcus aureus*

Reproduced with permission from Kaye AH. *Essential Neurosurgery*. 3rd ed. Oxford: Blackwells; 2005.

Bacteriology

Table 50.5 details the pathogenesis and principal organisms in cerebral abscess. Streptococci are isolated from approximately 80% of brain abscesses. The most common single species is the alpha haemolytic carboxyphilic *Streptococcus milleri*, whose major habitat is the alimentary tract including the mouth and dental plaque. Otogenic abscesses usually yield mixed flora including Bacteroides, various Streptococci and members of the Enterobacteriaceae. *Staphylococcus aureus* is often the pathogen in abscesses resulting from trauma.

Presenting features

Presenting features include:
- an intracranial mass (raised intracranial pressure, focal neurological signs, epilepsy)
- systemic toxicity (fever and malaise in 60% of cases)
- clinical features of the underlying source of infection (sinusitis, bacterial endocarditis, diverticulitis).

Diagnosis

A CT scan and MRI (Fig. 50.13) show a ring enhancing mass often surrounded by considerable oedema.

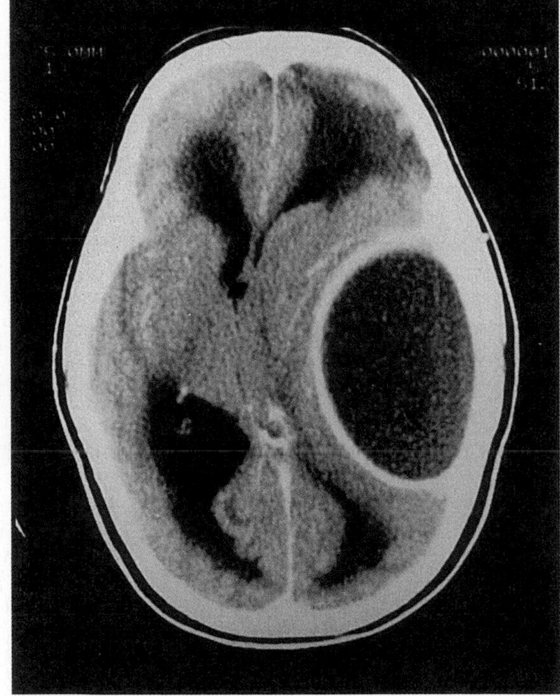

Fig. 50.13 Cerebral abscess – a ring enhancing mass. Reproduced with permission from Kaye AH. *Essential Neurosurgery*. 3rd ed. Oxford: Blackwells; 2005.

Management

The principles of treatment are:
- identify the bacterial organism
- institute antibiotic therapy
- drain or excise the abscess.

A specimen of pus is essential for accurate identification of the organism. Antibiotic therapy should be commenced as soon as the pus has been obtained. The initial choice of antibiotic, before culture results are available, will depend on the probable cause of the brain abscess and the Gram stain. The therapy will be refined once the organism is known. Anticonvulsant medication should be commenced as there is an incidence of seizures of 30–50%.

The abscess may need to be treated by either single or repeat aspiration. Surgical excision of the abscess may be necessary if there is persistent re-accumulation of the pus, or if a fibrous capsule develops that fails to collapse despite repeat aspirations. A cerebellar abscess requires excision.

Further reading

Colli BC, Carlotti CG, Machado HR, Assirati JA. Intracranial bacterial infections. *Neurosurg Quart.* 1999;9:258–284.

Dorsch NWC, King MT. A review of cerebral vasospasm in aneurysmal subarachnoid haemorrhage. *J Clin Neurosci.* 1994;1:19–26.

Kaye AH. *Essential Neurosurgery*. 3rd ed. Oxford: Blackwells; 2005.

Kaye AH, Black PMcL. *Operative Neurosurgery*. Edinburgh: Churchill Livingstone; 1999.

Kaye AH, Laws ER. *Brain Tumors*. 2nd ed. Edinburgh: Churchill Livingstone; 2001.

Stephanov S. Surgical treatment of brain abscess. *Neurosurgery.* 1988;22:724–730.

International Subarachnoid Aneurysm Trial (ISAT) of Neurosurgical Clipping vs Endovascular Coiling in 2143 patients with ruptured intracranial aneurysms: a randomised trial. *Lancet.* 2002;360:1267–1273.

Weir B. Unruptured intracranial aneurysms: a review. *J Neurosurg.* 1996;3–42.

MCQs

Select the single correct answer to each question.

1 The following is true:
- **a** meningiomas are the most common adult brain tumours
- **b** brain tumours are rare in children
- **c** high-grade cerebral gliomas are invariably fatal
- **d** metastatic cancer in the brain is uncommon
- **e** oligodendroglioma is the most common type of glioma

2 Cerebral gliomas in adults:
- **a** do not infiltrate through the brain
- **b** are best managed with chemotherapy
- **c** rarely cause raised intracranial pressure
- **d** are best visualised by MRI
- **e** most frequently occurs in the cerebellum

3 Brain tumours in children:
- **a** most commonly occur in the posterior fossa
- **b** can be cured with surgery
- **c** never metastasise
- **d** invariably have an excellent prognosis
- **e** most frequently present with epilepsy

4 Cerebral aneurysms:
- **a** usually occur on the peripheral intracranial vessels
- **b** can be definitively diagnosed by a CT scan
- **c** are the most common cause of subarachnoid haemorrhage in adults
- **d** are virtually always multiple
- **e** usually present with focal seizures

5 Subarachnoid haemorrhage:
- **a** is most commonly due to ruptured arterial venous malformation in adults
- **b** usually presents as an epileptic seizure as the initial symptom
- **c** must be evacuated as an emergency
- **d** is characterised by the onset of a sudden severe headache
- **e** is frequently due to haemorrhage from a tumour

6 In considering pituitary tumours, the following is true:
- **a** the tumour is always confined to the sellar
- **b** adults frequently present with growth retardation
- **c** prolactin-secreting tumours are best treated with surgery
- **d** ACTH-secreting tumours cause Cushing's disease
- **e** posterior pituitary function is almost always absent in patients presenting with large tumours

51 Nerve injuries, peripheral nerve entrapments and spinal cord compression

Andrew H. Kaye

Introduction

Peripheral nerves may be trapped, compressed or injured at any position along their course, although there are certain regions where they are especially vulnerable. Injury to the nerve occurs when the nerve is either relatively superficial and exposed, or lying adjacent to bone so that the jagged fractured ends of the bone may directly injure the nerve. Nerve entrapments occur particularly where the peripheral nerve passes through a tunnel formed by ligaments, bone and/or muscle.

Acute nerve injuries

Peripheral nerve anatomy

The axon projects from the cell body and is surrounded by a basement membrane and myelin sheath. The axon is covered by the endoneurium, the innermost layer of connective tissue, and a number of axons are grouped together in a bundle called a fascicle, which is invested by a further connective tissue sheath called the perineurium. The peripheral nerve consists of a group of fascicles covered by the outermost layer of connective tissue, the epineurium.

Classification of nerve injuries

There is no single classification system that can describe all the many variations of nerve injury. Most systems attempt to correlate the degree of injury with symptoms, pathology and prognosis. Seddon in 1943 introduced a classification of nerve injuries based on three main types of nerve fibre injury and whether there is continuity of the nerve (Table 51.1).

Neurotmesis

Neurotmesis is the most severe injury. The nerve is completely divided and complete distal Wallerian degeneration occurs. There is complete loss of motor, sensory and autonomic function.

Although the term *neurotmesis* implies a cutting of the nerve, the term is also used when the epineurium of the nerve is still in continuity but the axons have been destroyed and replaced by scar tissue to such a degree that spontaneous regeneration is impossible.

If the nerve has been completely divided, axonal regeneration causes a neuroma to form in the proximal stump.

Axonotmesis

Axonotmesis is characterised by complete interruption of the axons and their myelin sheaths, but with preservation of the epineurium and perineurium. Spontaneous regeneration will occur, with the intact endoneurial sheaths guiding the regenerating fibres to their distal connections. Axonotmesis is initially clinically indistinguishable from neurotmesis because there is complete and immediate loss of motor, sensory and autonomic function distal to the lesion with a similar electromyographic (EMG) picture. Regeneration occurs at a rate of 1–2 mm per day so that the time of recovery will depend on the distance between a lesion and the end organ, as well as on the age of the patient. The major types of injuries causing an axonotmesis include compression, traction, missile and ischaemia.

Neurapraxia

Neurapraxia is the most mild form of injury and is likened to a transient 'concussion' of the nerve, where

Table 51.1 Classification of nerve injuries

	Neurotmesis	Axonotmesis	Neurapraxia
Pathological			
Anatomical continuity	May be lost	Preserved	Preserved
Essential damage	Complete disorganisation, Schwann sheaths preserved	Nerve fibres interrupted	Selective demyelination of larger fibres, no degeneration of axons
Clinical			
Motor paralysis	Complete	Complete	Complete
Muscle atrophy	Progressive	Progressive	Very little
Sensory paralysis	Complete	Complete	Usually much sparing
Autonomic paralysis	Complete	Complete	Usually much sparing
Electrical phenomena			
Reaction of degeneration	Present	Present	Absent
Nerve conduction distal to the lesion	Absent	Absent	Preserved
Motor-unit action potentials	Absent	Absent	Absent
Fibrillation	Present	Present	Occasionally detectable
Recovery			
Surgical repair	Essential	Not necessary	Not necessary
Rate of recovery	1–2 mm a day after repair	1–2 mm a day	Rapid, days or weeks
March of recovery	According to order of innervation	According to order of innervation	No order
Quality	Always imperfect	Perfect	Perfect

Adapted from Seddon H. *Surgical Disorders of the Peripheral Nerves*. 3rd ed. Oxford: Blackwells; 2005. Reproduced with permission.

there is a temporary loss of function that is reversible within hours to months of the injury (with an average of 6–8 weeks). If there is initially a complete loss of function, neurapraxia cannot be distinguished from the more serious type of injury but will be recognised in retrospect when recovery of function has occurred sooner than would be possible following Wallerian degeneration.

Causes of peripheral nerve injury

The type of trauma will determine the nature of the injury to the nerve (Box 51.1).

Management of nerve injuries

The basis of management depends on a precise assessment of the damage that has been done to the nerve (Box 51.2). The types of injuries vary considerably, from an isolated single nerve lesion to a complex nerve injury in a patient with multiple trauma.

Brachial plexus injury

The mechanisms of injury are the same as for any peripheral nerve (see Box 51.1).

Birth injuries

Birth injuries include Erb's palsy due to damage to the upper trunk of the brachial plexus, Klumpke's paralysis due to damage to the lower trunk of the brachial plexus (C8 and T1; resulting from the arm being held up while traction is applied to the body during a breech delivery), and paralysis of the whole arm as a result of severe birth trauma.

Adolescents and adults

In adolescents and adults the most common cause is severe traction on the brachial plexus, resulting most frequently from a motorbike or motor vehicle accident. The trauma may result in damage to any part of the

Box 51.1 Types of trauma and the nature of nerve injury

- Lacerations cause neurotmesis, with complete or partial division of the nerve.
- Missile injuries may cause the spectrum of nerve injury from complete disruption of the nerve to a mild neurapraxia.
- Traction and stretch trauma may result in either complete disruption of the nerve or, if minor, a neurapraxia. This type of mechanism is responsible particularly for brachial plexus injuries following motorbike accidents, radial or peroneal nerve injuries. It is a common mechanism of nerve injuries associated with skeletal fractures.
- Fractures or fracture dislocation may cause nerve injuries when the adjacent nerve is either compressed by the displaced bone fragments or, less commonly, severed by the jagged edge of the bone.
- Compression ischaemia may produce a neurapraxia in mild cases or, if prolonged and severe, axonotmesis or neurotmesis. It is the cause of the pressure palsies following improper application of a tourniquet or the 'Saturday night palsy', in which the radial nerve has been compressed against the humerus.
- Injection injury results from either direct trauma by the needle or the toxic effect of the agent injected. As would be expected the sciatic and radial nerves are the most commonly affected.
- Electrical and burn injuries are uncommon causes of serious peripheral nerve damage.

Box 51.2 General guidelines for management of nerve injuries

- Determination of the exact nerve involved by (i) the clinical deficit and (ii) the position of the injury.
- Assessment of the type of nerve damaged by the mechanism of injury.
- If a neurapraxia or axonotmesis is suspected on clinical grounds, there is no specific surgical treatment for the nerve but physiotherapy should commence as soon as possible to prevent stiffness of the joints and contractures.
- Immediate or early exploration of the nerve should be undertaken: (i) if it is highly probable that the type of injury (e.g. laceration) will have caused the nerve to be severed; or (ii) if the nerve injury has been caused by a displaced fracture that needs reduction by open surgery, it is appropriate to explore the nerve at that time.
- Delayed exploration of the nerve will be indicated if the clinical and EMG findings indicate failure of regeneration of the nerve beyond the time expected; that is, the injury has resulted in a neurotmesis rather than an axonotmesis or neurapraxia.

plexus but severe traction may result in tearing of the arachnoid and dura with nerve root avulsion from the spinal cord.

Management

The management involves determination of the exact neurological injury, particularly the part of the brachial plexus involved (Fig. 51.1). A Horner's syndrome is evidence there has been avulsion of the nerve roots from the spinal cord.

A magnetic resonance imaging scan may show the pseudomeningocele, characteristic of nerve root avulsion. Electrical studies provide useful baseline studies for future comparison. It is reasonable to obtain these studies 8 weeks after the injury.

There is debate concerning the indications for surgical intervention for closed brachial plexus injuries in adults. In general there is little benefit from exploration of the plexus in closed injuries although some surgeons do advocate exploration approximately 4 months after the injury if clinical and electrical evidence shows the lesion to be complete. If the injury is improving there is no indication for surgery and management includes intensive physiotherapy and mobilisation of the joints. There is no place for surgery if there is evidence of nerve root avulsion from the cord.

Peripheral nerve entrapment

Entrapment neuropathies occur particularly when nerves pass near joints. Less common forms of entrapment neuropathies may lie at a distance from a joint. Box 51.3 shows a list of the common and less frequent entrapment neuropathies.

Carpal tunnel syndrome

This is by far the most common nerve entrapment and women are affected four times more frequently than men.

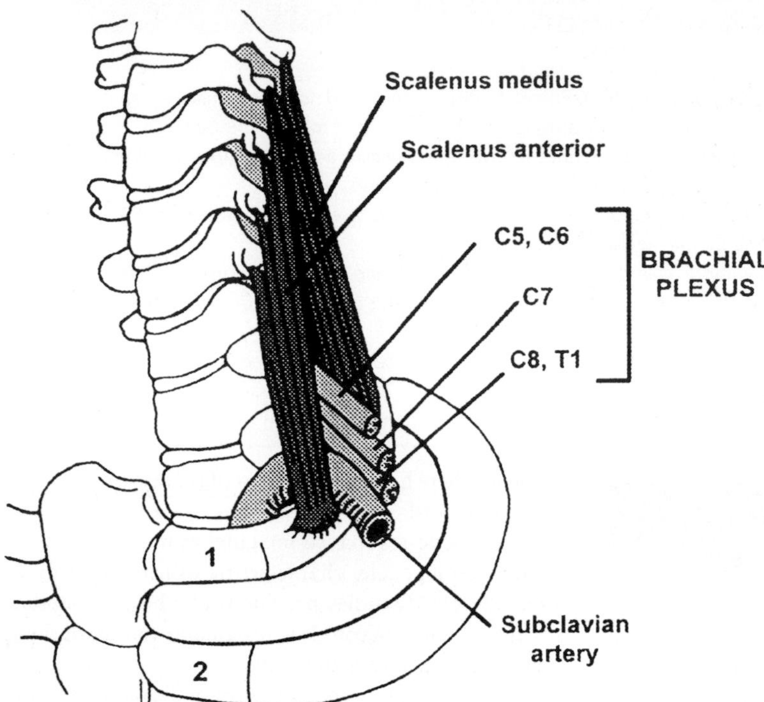

Fig. 51.1 The brachial plexus passing through the cervicobrachial junction. (Reproduced with permission from Kaye AH. *Essential Neurosurgery*. 3rd ed. Oxford: Blackwells; 2005.)

Anatomy

The carpal tunnel is a fibro-osseous tunnel on the palmar surface of the wrist (Fig. 51.2). The dorsal and lateral walls consist of the carpal bones, which form a crescentric trough. A tunnel is made by the fibrous flexor retinaculum, which is attached to the pisiform and hook of the hamate medially and the tuberosity of the scaphoid and crest of the trapezium laterally. The contents of the tunnel are the median nerve, flexor tendons of the flexor digitorum superficialis, flexor digitorum profundus and flexor pollicis longus.

Box 51.3 Entrapment neuropathies (the more common ones are shown in bold)

Median nerve
- **Carpal tunnel syndrome**
- Supracondylar entrapment
- Cubital fossa entrapment
- Anterior interosseus nerve entrapment

Ulnar nerve
- **Tardy ulnar palsy**
- Deep branch of ulnar nerve

Radial nerve (posterior interosseus nerve)
Suprascapular nerve
Meralgia paraesthetica (lateral femoral cutaneous nerve of thigh)
Sciatic nerve
Tarsal tunnel syndrome
Thoracic outlet syndrome

Aetiology

The initial symptoms occur in women during pregnancy and in both sexes when they are performing unusual strenuous work with their hands, although the features of carpal tunnel syndrome may present at any stage throughout the adult years. There are a number of systemic conditions that are associated with and that may predispose to carpal tunnel syndrome:
- pregnancy and lactation
- contraceptive pill
- rheumatoid arthritis
- myxoedema
- acromegaly.

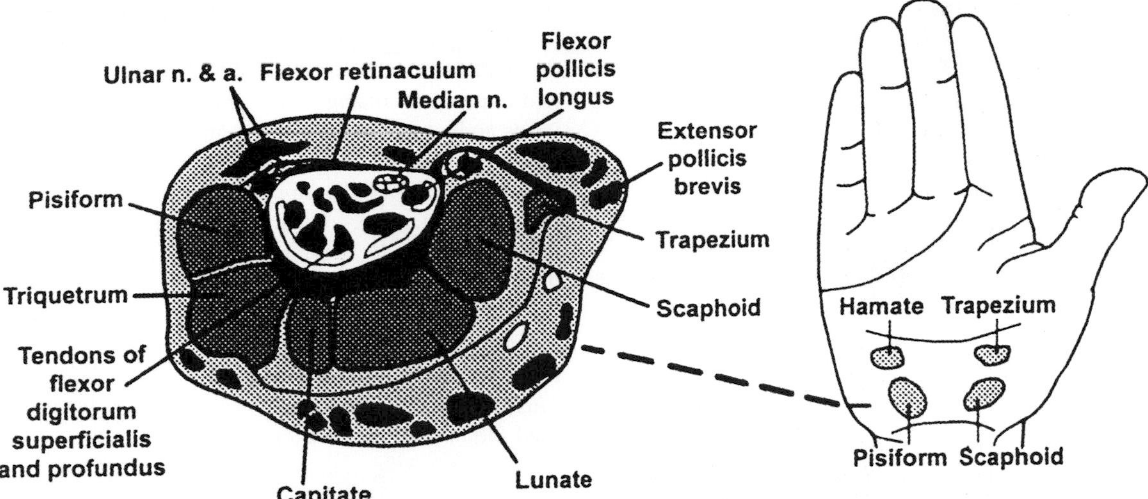

Fig. 51.2 The carpal tunnel, just distal to the wrist. (Reproduced with permission from Kaye AH. *Essential Neurosurgery*. 3rd ed. Oxford: Blackwells; 2005.)

Any local condition around the wrist joint that decreases the size of the carpal tunnel will also predispose to carpal tunnel syndrome. These include a ganglion, tenosynovitis, unreduced fractures or dislocations of the wrist or carpal bones, and any local arthritis.

Clinical features

The principal clinical features of carpal tunnel syndrome are pain, numbness and tingling.

The pain, which may be described as burning or aching, is frequently felt throughout the whole hand and not just in the lateral three digits. There is often a diffuse radiation of the pain up the forearm to the elbow and occasionally into the upper arm. The symptoms are particularly worse at night, and on awakening the patient has to shake the hand to obtain any relief.

Numbness and tingling principally occur in the lateral three and a half fingers, in the distribution of the median nerve, although the patient frequently complains of more diffuse sensory loss throughout the fingers. This symptom is also worse at night and with activity. The patient frequently complains that the hand feels 'clumsy', but with no specific weakness.

There are often only minimal signs of median nerve entrapment at the wrist. The Tinel sign (tingling in the median nerve innervated thumb, index and middle finger) may be elicited by tapping over the median nerve but its absence has little diagnostic value.

If the compression has been prolonged there may be signs of median nerve dysfunction including wasting of the thenar muscle, weakness of muscles innervated by the distal median nerve, especially abductor pollicis brevis, and diminished sensation over the distribution of the median nerve in the hand. The clinical diagnosis can be confirmed by EMG examination.

Treatment

Surgery involving division of the flexor retinaculum is a simple and effective method of relieving the compression and curing the symptoms. However, conservative treatment involving the use of a wrist splint and non-steroidal anti-inflammatory agents is appropriate if the symptoms are mild or intermittent or if there is a reversible underlying precipitating condition, such as pregnancy or oral contraceptive pill.

Ulnar nerve entrapment at the elbow

Anatomy

The ulnar nerve runs behind the medial epicondyle of the humerus and enters the forearm through a fibro-osseous tunnel formed by the aponeurotic attachment of the two heads of flexor carpi ulnaris, which span from the medial epicondyle of the humerus to the olecranon process of the ulnar forming the cubital tunnel (Fig. 51.3). During flexion of the elbow the ligament tightens, and the volume of the cubital tunnel decreases, putting increasing pressure on the underlying nerve. Compression can also be due to injuries in

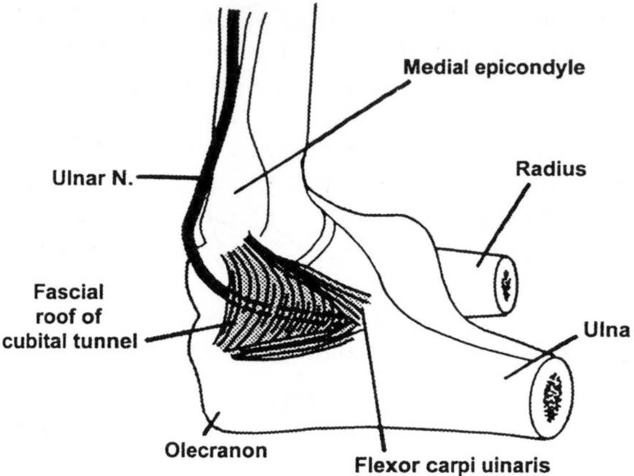

Fig. 51.3 The ulnar nerve passing behind the medial epicondyle of the humerus and through the cubital tunnel. (Reproduced with permission from Kaye AH. *Essential Neurosurgery*. 3rd ed. Oxford: Blackwells; 2005.)

the region producing deformity of the elbow, although the features of ulnar nerve entrapment do not usually appear for some years. This delay in the appearance of symptoms led to the term 'tardy ulnar palsy'.

Aetiology

In most cases there is no particular predisposing cause. In a minority there are underlying factors that predispose to nerve entrapment, including lengthy periods of bed rest from coma or major illness, and poor positioning of the upper limbs during long operations causing prolonged pressure on the nerve. Other causes include arthritis of the elbow, ganglion cysts of the elbow joint and direct trauma.

Clinical features

The clinical features include paraesthesia and numbness in the ring and little finger of the hand and the adjacent medial border of the hand, wasting of the hypothenar eminence and interossei muscles, and weakness.

In advanced cases, entrapment of the ulnar nerve will lead to weakness of the muscles of the hypothenar eminence, the interossei, the medial two lumbricals, adductor pollicis, flexor digitorum profundus (ring and little finger) and flexor carpi ulnaris. Paralysis of the small muscles of the hand causes 'claw hand', this posture being produced by the unopposed action of their antagonists. As the interossei cause flexion of the fingers at the metacarpophalangeal joints and extension at the interphalangeal joints, when these muscles are paralysed the opposite posture is maintained by the long flexors and extensors causing flexion at the interphalangeal joints and hyperextension at the metacarpophalangeal joints. This is most pronounced in the ring and little fingers as the two radial lumbricals, which are innervated by the median nerve, compensate to some degree for the impaired action of the interossei on the index and middle fingers. Froment's sign is demonstrated by asking the patient to grasp a piece of cardboard between the index finger and thumb against resistance. There will be flexion of the interphalangeal joint of the thumb because the median innervated flexor pollicis longus is used rather than the weakened adductor pollicis.

Treatment

Conservative treatment may be tried if the clinical features are minor and not progressive. The patient should avoid putting pressure on the nerve at the elbow during reading, sitting or lying and should cease heavy work with the arms.

Surgery involves decompression of the nerve and is indicated if there are progressive symptoms or signs and if there is any wasting or weakness.

Meralgia paraesthetica

Meralgia paraesthetica results from entrapment of the lateral cutaneous nerve of the thigh beneath the inguinal ligament, just medial to the anterior superior iliac spine. At this position the nerve passes between two roots of attachment of the inguinal ligament to the iliac bone and there is a sharp angulation of the nerve as it passes from the iliac fossa into the thigh.

Prolonged standing or walking and an obese pendulous anterior abdominal wall accentuates the downward pull on the inguinal ligament and may predispose to entrapment of the nerve. The syndrome is most frequently seen in middle-aged men who are overweight and in young army recruits during strenuous training.

The principal symptom is a painful dysaesthesia in the anterolateral aspect of the thigh with the patient often describing the sensation as 'burning', 'pins and needles' or 'prickling'.

The only neurological sign is diminished sensation over the anterolateral aspect of the thigh in the distribution of the lateral cutaneous nerve.

The symptoms may be only minor and the patient may be satisfied with reassurance. The unpleasant features may resolve with conservative treatment, including weight reduction in an obese patient. Surgery may be necessary if the symptoms are debilitating and the procedure involves decompression of the nerve or, if that fails, division of the nerve.

Spinal cord compression

Compression of spinal cord is a common neurosurgical problem and requires early diagnosis and urgent treatment if the disastrous consequences of disabling paralysis and sphincter disturbance are to be avoided.

Although there are a large range of possible causes of spinal cord compression in clinical practice the majority are due to:

- Extradural
  - Trauma
  - Metastatic tumour
  - Extradural abscess
- Intradural, extramedullary
  - Meningioma
- Schwannoma
- Intramedullary
  - Glioma (astrocytoma and ependymoma)
- Syrinx

Presenting features

The two major presenting features that are the hallmark of spinal cord compression are pain and neurological deficit. There is considerable variation in the manner in which these two major features present, and depend on the pathological basis, the site of the compression and the speed of the compression.

Pain

Pain is a common early feature of spinal cord compression and often precedes any neurological disturbance, sometimes by many months. The pain is due to involvement of local pain-sensitive structures, such as the bone of the vertebral column. Involvement of a spinal nerve root will cause pain radiating in the affected region. Thoracic cord compression with involvement of the thoracic nerve root will often be associated with pain radiating around the chest wall. This 'girdle' pain is an important feature associated with a lesion which may cause spinal cord compression. In addition there is also a 'central' pain due to spinal cord compression, which is described as an unpleasant diffuse dull ache with a 'burning' quality.

Flexion or extension of the neck may cause 'electric shock' or tingling sensations radiating down the body to the extremities. This is called Lhermitte's sign, and is typically associated with cervical cord involvement.

Neurological deficit

The neurological features of spinal cord compression consist of progressive weakness, sensory disturbance and sphincter disturbance.

The *motor impairment* will be manifest as a paralysis, and the level of the weakness will depend on the position of the cord compression. Thoracic cord compression will result in a progressive paraparesis of the lower limbs and if the cervical cord is involved the upper limbs will also be affected. Compression of the corticospinal pathways will result in upper motor neurone weakness with little or no wasting, increased tone, increased deep tendon reflexes and positive Babinski response. As the cord becomes more severely compressed a complete paraplegia will result. The compressing mass will also cause weakness of the nerve root segment at the involved level. In the cervical region this will result in a lower motor neurone weakness of the involved nerve roots in the upper limbs. In the lumbar region involvement of the conus medullaris may produce a mixture of lower motor neurone and upper motor neurone signs in the lower limbs. Cauda equina compression produces a lower motor neurone pattern of weakness.

Sensory disturbance

A *sensory level* is the hallmark of spinal cord compression. In the thoracic region the sensory level will be to all modalities of sensation over the body or trunk, although there may be some sparing of some modalities in the early stages of compression. A useful guide to remember is the T4 dermatome lies at the level of the nipple, the T 7 at the xiphisternum and T10 at the umbilicus.

Sphincter involvement

Sphincter disturbance often follows compression of the spinal cord, with the first symptom being difficulty in initiating micturition, which is followed by urinary retention, often relatively painless. Constipation and faecal incontinence will subsequently occur. The clinical signs include an enlarged, palpable bladder, diminished perianal sensation and decreased anal tone.

In summary the clinical features of spinal cord compression are:

- Pain – local and radicular.
- Progressive weakness of the limbs.
- Sensory disturbance – often a sensory level.
- Sphincter disturbance.

Management

Spinal cord compression is a *neurosurgical emergency*. Investigation and treatment must be undertaken as a matter of urgency once the diagnosis is suspected.

The radiological studies undertaken to confirm the diagnosis of spinal cord compression include:

- Plain spinal X-rays
- MRI
- CT scan (with intrathecal contrast).

The MRI is of considerable value in diagnosing the cause and position of spinal cord compression and is by far the best investigation, as it will clearly show the pathological changes in the vertebral body, spinal canal, spinal cord and paravertebral region, thereby aiding with planning the treatment. Plain X-rays and CT scan will help show the focal bony destruction.

Treatment

The standard treatment for spinal cord compression is urgent surgery, except in some cases of compression due to malignant tumour, in which treatment with high-dose glucocorticosteroids and radiotherapy may be indicated.

Common causes of spinal cord compression

Malignant spinal cord compression

By far the most common cause of spinal cord compression, this results from extradural compression by malignant tumours. The most common tumours are:

- Carcinoma of the lung
- Carcinoma of the breast
- Carcinoma of the prostate
- Carcinoma of the kidney
- Lymphoma
- Myeloma.

Surgical management for malignant spinal cord compression utilises either:

- Decompressive laminectomy (posterior approach)
- Vertebrectomy and fusion (anterior approach).

Urgent radiotherapy, combined with high-dose glucocorticosteroids may be effective in controlling the tumour causing spinal cord compression and is sometimes advisable if the patient has a known primary tumour that is radiosensitive and if there is a partial incomplete neurological lesion that is only slowly progressive.

Schwannoma (neurofibroma)

Schwannomas are the most common of the intrathecal tumours and may occur at any position. They arise invariably from the posterior nerve roots and grow slowly to compress the adjacent neural structures. Occasionally the tumour extends through the intervertebral foramen to form a 'dumbell' tumour, which may rarely present as a mass in the thorax, neck or posterior abdominal wall.

The presenting features are those of a slowly growing tumour causing cord compression. There is frequently some degree of a Brown–Séquard syndrome due to the lateral position of the tumour. The treatment is surgical excision.

Spinal meningioma

Spinal meningiomas occur particularly in middle-aged or elderly patients and there is a marked female predominance. The tumour grows extremely slowly and there is usually a long history of ill-defined back pain, often nocturnal, and a slowly progressive paralysis prior to diagnosis.

Intramedullary tumours

Ependymoma and astrocytoma of the spinal cord are uncommon, with the presenting features depending on the level of cord involvement. Ependymomas not infrequently arise in the filum terminale and will cause features of cauda equina compression. There is often a history of low back and leg pain, progressive weakness in the legs (often with radicular features) sensory loss over the saddle area and eventually sphincter disturbance.

Intervertebral disc prolapse

Intervertebral disc herniation is a common cause of nerve root compression, but occasionally the disc may prolapse directly posteriorly (centrally), causing compression of the spinal cord in the cervical or thoracic region and of the cauda equina in the lumbar region.

Urgent surgery is essential to relieve the compression.

Spinal abscess

Spinal abscess is an uncommon condition requiring urgent treatment. The spinal cord compression is due to both inflammatory swelling and pus, and presenting features include severe local spinal pain with rapidly progressive neurological features of spinal cord compression. There are frequently constitutional features of infections such as high fever, sweating and tachycardia. The MRI is the preferred investigation and treatment consists of urgent surgery with appropriate antibiotic medication.

Cervical myelopathy

Cervical myelopathy results from cervical cord compression due to a narrow cervical vertebral canal. The constriction of the canal enclosing the cervical cord is due to a combination of congenital narrowing, and cervical spondylosis involving hypertrophy of the facet joints and osteophyte formation, hypertrophy of the ligamenta flava and bulging of the cervical disc. The myelopathy results from both the direct pressure on the spinal cord and ischaemia of the cord due to compression and obstruction of the small vessels within the cord or to compression of the feeding radicular arteries within the intervertebral foramen.

There is frequently a history of slowly progressive disability, although it is not unusual for the neurological disability to deteriorate rapidly, particularly following what might be even a minor or trivial injury.

Muscular weakness manifest by clumsiness involving the hands and fingers, impairment in fine-skilled movements and dragging or shuffling of the feet is the most common initial symptom. *Sensory symptoms* are frequent, and occur as diffuse numbness and paraesthesia in the hands and fingers.

The MRI will confirm the severity of the cord compression and show the exact pathological basis for the compression. An additional benefit of MRI is that it may show myelomalacia (high signal within the cord) indicating the severity of the compression and a poorer prognosis following surgery.

Surgery is indicated for clinically progressive or moderate or severe myelopathy. The operation may involve either a posterior decompression laminectomy or, if the compression is predominantly anterior to the cord, an anterior approach with excision of the compressive lesion and fusion is preferred.

Spinal injuries

Trauma to the spinal column occurs at an incidence of approximately 2–5 per 100 000 population. Adolescents and young adults are the most commonly affected, with most serious spinal cord injuries being a consequence of road traffic accidents and water sports (especially diving into shallow water), skiing and horse riding accidents.

MECHANISM OF INJURY

Although severe disruption of the vertebral column usually causes serious neurological damage it is not always possible to correlate the degree of bone damage with spinal cord injury. Minor vertebral column disruption does not usually cause neurological deficit, but occasionally may be associated with severe neurological injury. The mechanism of the injury will determine the type of vertebral injury and neurological damage.

Trauma may damage the spinal cord by direct compression by bone, ligament or disc, haematoma, interruption of the vascular supply and/or traction.

CERVICAL SPINE

Flexion and flexion–rotation injuries are the most common type of injury to the cervical spine, with the C5/6 level being the most common site. There is often extensive posterior ligamentous damage and these injuries are usually unstable. Compression injuries also most frequently occur at the C5/6 level. The wedge fracture injuries are often stable because the posterior bony elements and longitudinal ligaments are often intact. However, those with a significant retropulsed fragment are likely to have disruption of the associated ligaments and are considered unstable. When combined with a rotation force in flexion, a 'tear drop' fracture may occur, with separation of a small anterior-inferior fragment from the vertebral body, and these should also be considered unstable.

Hyperextension injuries are most common in the older age group and in patients with degenerative spinal canal stenosis. The bone injury is often not demonstrated and the major damage is to the anterior longitudinal ligament secondary to hyperextension.

THORACOLUMBAR SPINE

Flexion-rotation injuries most commonly occur at the T12/L1 level and result in anterior dislocation of T12 on the L1 vertebral body.

Compression injuries are common with the vertebral body being decreased in height. These injuries are usually stable and neurological damage is uncommon.

Open injuries may result from stab or gunshot wounds that result in damage to the spinal cord.

Neurological impairment

There is a state of diminished excitability of the spinal cord immediately after a severe spinal cord injury, which is referred to as 'spinal shock'. There is an areflexic flaccid paralysis. The duration of spinal shock varies, with minimal reflex activity appearing within a period of 3–4 days or being delayed up to some weeks.

COMPLETE LESIONS

The most severe consequence of spinal trauma is a complete transverse myelopathy in which all neurological function is absent below the level of the lesion, causing either a paraplegia or quadriplegia (depending on the level), impairment of autonomic function including bowel or bladder function, and sensory loss.

INCOMPLETE LESIONS

There are numerous variations of neurological deficit manifest in incomplete lesions but with some specific syndromes:

- *Anterior cervical cord syndrome* – due to compression of the anterior aspect of the cord resulting in damage to the corticospinal and spinothalamic tracts with motor paralysis below the level of the lesion and loss of pain, temperature and touch sensation but relative preservation of light touch, proprioception and position sense, which are carried by the posterior columns.
- *Central cord syndrome* – due to hyperextension of the cervical spine with damage located centrally causing the most severe injury to the more centrally located cervical tracts, which supply the upper limbs. There is a disproportionate weakness in the upper limbs compared with the extremities. Sensory loss is usually minimal.
- *Brown–Séquard syndrome* – from hemisection of the cord resulting in ipsilateral paralysis below the level of the lesion with loss of pain, temperature and touch on the opposite side.

Management of spinal injuries

As little can be done to repair the damage caused by the initial injury, major efforts are directed towards prevention of further spinal cord injury and complications resulting from the neurological damage. The general principles of management are:

- Prevention of further injury to the spinal cord
- Reduction and stabilisation of bony injuries
- Prevention of complications resulting from spinal cord injury
- Rehabilitation.

The initial first-aid management of patients with injuries to the spinal column and spinal cord require the utmost caution in turning and lifting the patient. The spine must be handled with great care to avoid inflicting additional damage. Sufficient help should be available before moving the patient to provide horizontal stability and longitudinal traction. Spinal flexion must be avoided. A temporary collar should be applied if the injury is to the cervical spine. Hypotension and hypoventilation immediately follow an acute traumatic spinal cord injury and this may not only be life-threatening but also may increase the extent of neurological impairment. Respiratory insufficiency may require oxygen therapy and ventilatory assistance. Loss of sympathetic tone may result in peripheral vasodilatation with vascular pooling and hypotension. Treatment will include the use of intravascular volume expanders, alpha-adrenergic stimulators and intravenous atropine. Careful attention should be paid to the body temperature as the spinal patient is poikilothermic and will assume the temperature of the environment. A nasogastric tube should be passed to avoid problems associated with vomiting due to gastric stasis and paralytic ileus and a urinary catheter is necessary. Prophylaxis for deep vein thrombosis and subsequent pulmonary embolus should be commenced as soon as possible.

Radiological investigations will include plain X-rays, computer tomography and MRI.

High-dose dexamethasone is usually administered as soon as possible for patients with spinal cord compression but there is no conclusive proof of its effectiveness.

Spinal reduction and stabilisation

Skeletal traction for restoration and/or maintenance of normal alignment of the spinal column is an effective treatment with a variety of cervical traction devices available. The traction must be commenced under X-ray or fluoroscopic control and great care should be taken to avoid distraction at the fracture site, as traction on the underlying cord will worsen the neurological injury. Reduction of facet dislocations may involve either manipulation under fluoroscopic control with the patient under general anaesthesia or may require open surgery. This management must only be undertaken in specialised neurosurgical or spinal injury departments. Following reduction the position is usually maintained with either skeletal traction or halo immobilisation.

Injuries of the thoracolumbar spine can usually be managed conservatively by postural reduction in bed.

There has been considerable controversy over surgical intervention with spinal cord injuries. The damage to the spinal cord occurs principally at the time of the injury and there has been no evidence to show improved neurological function from acute operative decompression of the spine. The following are the general indications for surgical intervention:

- Progression of neurological deficit is an absolute indication
- Patients with a partial neurological injury who fail to improve, with radiological evidence of persisting compression of the spinal cord
- An open injury from a gunshot or stab wound
- Stabilisation of the spine if there is gross instability or if it has not been possible to reduce locked facets by closed reduction.

Further management

Following reduction and immobilisation of fractures, the principles of continuing care involve avoidance of potential complications in patients who are paraplegic or quadriplegic and early rehabilitation, which commences as soon as the injury has stabilised.

Further reading

Kaye AH. *Essential Neurosurgery.* 3rd ed. Oxford: Blackwells; 2005.

Kline DG, Judice DJ. Operative management of selected brachial plexus lesions. *J Neurosurg.* 1983;58:631–649.

Pang D, Wessel HB. Thoracic outlet syndrome. *Neurosurgery.* 1988;22:105–121.

MCQs

Select the single correct answer to each question.

1 Carpal tunnel syndrome:
- **a** most frequently occurs in men
- **b** is due to the compression of the ulnar nerve at the wrist
- **c** usually causes severe weakness in the hand
- **d** is especially associated with pregnancy and lactation
- **e** causes decreased sensation on the dorsum of the hand

2 In considering spinal cord compression, the following is true:
- **a** the most common cause is an intramedullary spinal cord tumour
- **b** the management of compression by a malignant metastatic tumour is best undertaken utilizing chemotherapy
- **c** the usual treatment for spinal cord compression due to malignant tumours is urgent surgery or radiotherapy
- **d** spinal pain is a late feature of spinal cord compression
- **e** metastatic tumours are rarely a cause of spinal cord compression

3 In considering nerve injuries, the following is true:
- **a** a neurapraxia almost never recovers
- **b** neurotmesis is a mild form of injury, likely to be transient
- **c** an Erb's palsy is due to damage of the upper trunk of the brachial plexus
- **d** Horner's syndrome in association with a brachial plexus injury is indicative of an excellent prognosis
- **e** injury to the radial nerve in the upper arm causes weakness of finger flexion

4 Considering peripheral nerve entrapments, the following is true:

a the ulnar nerve is frequently trapped at the elbow in front of the medial epicondyle

b carpal tunnel syndrome is due to entrapment of the radial nerve at the wrist

c meralgia paraesthetica is due to entrapment of the lateral cutaneous nerve of the thigh

d the principal symptom of meralgia paraesthetica is weakness of the leg

e the early features of ulnar nerve entrapment at the elbow is numbness involving the thumb and index finger

Vascular Surgery

52 Disorders of the arterial system

John Harris

Introduction

The clinical approach to peripheral vascular disease should be based on knowledge of the natural history of the particular disorder, options for non-operative management, particularly risk factor modification and the likely outcome of any proposed intervention.

Epidemiology

Patients with peripheral arterial disease usually die from co-existent coronary or cerebrovascular disease. Heart, stroke and vascular disease combined caused 37.6% of all deaths in Australia in 2002, more than any other disease group. The prevalence of diabetes has doubled over the last 20 years and now affects 8% of the adult population.

Atherosclerosis

In 90% of adults with peripheral arterial disease, the cause is atherosclerosis. The other 10% of less common causes include peripheral thromboembolism either from the heart or an aneurysm, trauma, fibromuscular disease and rare inflammatory conditions.

The pathogenesis of atherosclerosis is complex and can begin in the second decade of life, with implications for the timing of preventative measures. It may take many years for atherosclerotic plaque to enlarge enough to narrow an artery. Peripheral vascular disease may therefore remain asymptomatic for many years.

The earliest detectable pathological feature of atherosclerosis is fatty streaking, which later evolves into the fibrous plaque. More complex lesions occur with intra-plaque haemorrhage, calcification or disruption of the overlying fibrous cap.

Once the diameter of an artery is reduced beyond 60%, the stenosis becomes critical, reducing blood flow. To compensate, a collateral circulation forms. The clinical outcome of arterial occlusion depends on the adequacy of the arterial collateral. If there is little collateral present then ischaemia can be extreme. With well-developed collateral, arterial occlusion may even be asymptomatic.

Aneurysms

An aneurysm is defined as a permanent, localised dilation of an artery that has at least a 50% increase (1.5 times) in diameter as compared with the expected normal diameter of that artery. When an artery dilates it may rupture causing internal bleeding (typical of large abdominal aortic aneurysms) or form laminated thrombus in the aneurysm sac that can embolise or thrombose (typical of popliteal aneurysms) resulting in limb loss.

Patterns of arterial aneurysmal disease

The aetiology of abdominal aortic aneurysms is multifactorial. There is a 10% familial association in first-order siblings and an association with genetic disorders such as Marfan's or Ehlers–Danlos syndrome.

A patient with an abdominal aortic aneurysms is likely to have other aneurysms involving the iliac arteries in 40% and popliteal in 15%. Conversely, aortic aneurysms are present in about 30% of patients with bilateral popliteal aneurysms. An aneurysm in one anatomic location should therefore prompt a search for aneurysms elsewhere.

Epidemiology

The prevalence of abdominal aortic aneurysm increases with age from 4.8% in men aged 65–69 years to 10.8% for men aged 80–83 years and is higher in men, those with hypertension, smokers and in Caucasians. The mortality from a ruptured abdominal aortic aneurysm is over 75%, with most patients dying before they can reach hospital. Even with surgery there is a 50% mortality rate. Every effort therefore must be made to identify and treat abdominal aortic aneurysm before rupture occurs.

Once an aneurysm reaches a diameter greater than 5 cm, the risk of rupture increases exponentially with further expansion. At a diameter of 5–6 cm, the 5-year risk of rupture is 25%, from 6–7 cm 35% and over 7 cm it is 75%.

Clinical presentation

Most abdominal aortic aneurysms are asymptomatic unless rupture is impending, in which case, the presentation can be dramatic, with hypotension and abdominal pain radiating through to the back. More usually, an abdominal aortic aneurysm is an unexpected finding, either on astute routine physical examination or on incidental ultrasound or CT scanning.

Evaluation

The diagnosis of a suspected abdominal aortic aneurysm is best initially confirmed by ultrasound examination, although calcification of the aortic wall can be seen in plain X-rays. Three-dimensional computed tomographic (CT) reconstruction can show the morphology of an aortic aneurysm in exquisite detail. Ultrasound examination is also the best modality for population screening or to follow patients with small abdominal aortic aneurysms to check for expansion and the easiest way to confirm the diagnosis of a suspected popliteal aneurysm.

Treatment

Small abdominal aortic aneurysms can be observed for expansion by regular ultrasound examination. There is general agreement that once the diameter of an abdominal aortic aneurysm exceeds 5 cm, the risk of rupture is sufficient to justify intervention.

Endoluminal repair of aneurysms

The endovascular method of treating an abdominal aortic aneurysm involves the insertion of an aortic graft through the common femoral artery via a catheter, avoiding the morbid open abdominal incision.

Not all patients are suitable to treat by the endoluminal method. In order to anchor the aortic endograft, enough normal aorta (>2.5 cm) is needed below the renal arteries to securely fix the device in place. Secure fixation may be impossible if this segment of aorta is too dilated. Narrow, calcified and tortuous iliac and femoral arteries also pose technical challenges. Many of these anatomic limitations may be overcome with further technical advances in endograft design and delivery systems.

The same concept can be extended to treat other peripheral aneurysms, for example in the thoracic aorta or popliteal artery.

Open surgical repair of aneurysms

The open method of treating an abdominal aortic aneurysm has been used for more than 50 years, and late graft failure and rupture is rare. Conventional repair of an abdominal aortic aneurysm involves a laparotomy, clamping of the aorta and sewing in a prosthetic arterial graft to replace the aneurysmal aorta. This can be done in a straight or bifurcated configuration.

In other settings, the aneurysm can be ligated and circulation maintained by a bypass procedure. This is the commonest form of treatment for popliteal aneurysms.

Complications

Randomised trials have confirmed a short-term advantage with endovascular repair with a lower perioperative mortality of 1.2% compared to 4.6% for open repair. General complications, particularly cardio-respiratory, are more common with open repair, but there is a higher incidence of local vascular or implant related complications after endovascular repair. It is not yet known if the immediate advantage of endovascular repair will be sustained in the longer term because of late problems that can develop with endografts, including device failure or migration causing endoleak (blood flow communicating with the aneurysm sac), leading to ongoing aneurysm expansion and possible late rupture.

Ruptured aneurysms or more extensive aneurysms involving the thoracoabdominal aorta are generally not suitable to treat by the endoluminal method, although this is now being investigated, and the complication rate is higher. Serious complications include renal dysfunction, paraplegia and ischemic colitis. Late prosthetic graft infection is rare but can occur after open or endovascular repair and lead to graft-enteric fistula years after surgery.

Chronic limb ischaemia

Chronic limb ischaemia is the commonest clinical problem occurring in patients with peripheral vascular disease (Box 52.1).

Clinical presentation

Patients may present with intermittent claudication, a characteristic muscle pain induced by exercise, relieved by rest and recurring on walking the same distance again. Similar pain occurs less commonly on a neurogenic basis from spinal cord or nerve root compression but can be distinguished from arterial claudication by physical examination and exercise testing.

The risk of limb loss is low, with less than 10% chance of amputation in 10 years. A mortality of 5% per year can be expected from associated medical co-morbidities, with coronary events the usual cause of death. The outlook is worse in claudicants with diabetes who continue to smoke.

With more severe ischaemia, pain can affect the limb at rest and is usually worse at night. The next stage is the onset of ischaemic ulceration or gangrene. In either situation, the risk of limb loss is high. Without restoration of adequate blood supply, the chance of amputation is about 30% within 3 months. A mortality rate of 10% per year can be expected, with the higher mortality reflecting the more severe, generalised disease in such patients.

Box 52.1 Patterns of disease affecting the lower limb

Superficial femoral artery (approximately 60%)
The most common site for atherosclerotic occlusion or stenosis is at the lower end of the superficial femoral artery where it passes through the hiatus in the adductor magnus muscle into the popliteal fossa.

Aorto-iliac disease (approximately 30%)
Common patterns include disease of the lower aorta involving the common iliac arteries and disease of the external iliac artery extending into the common femoral and profunda femoris arteries. Severe aortoiliac disease can result in Lé Riche syndrome involving buttock and thigh claudication with impotence.

Combined disease (approximately 10%)
These patients have significant disease of both systems. Other recognised patterns include disease of the common femoral or profunda femoris artery and disease of the tibial arteries associated with diabetes.

Clinical evaluation

The aorta and femoral pulses should be palpated in every routine physical examination. The femoral pulse is generally easy to feel and therefore a good site to check cardiac rate and rhythm. The degree of arterial calcification can be estimated by the rigidity of the pulse.

Palpation of the popliteal artery is more difficult. Whenever the popliteal pulse is prominent and easy to feel, a popliteal aneurysm should be suspected.

Investigations

As atherosclerosis is a generalised disease, investigations should be carried out to assess risk factors and the involvement of other arterial beds, thinking particularly of the coronary and carotid arteries.

Measurement of ankle pressure

The Ankle Brachial Index (ABI) can be derived by dividing the highest ankle systolic pressure by the arm systolic blood pressure. This measurement adds a degree of objectivity to the detection and grading of any arterial occlusive disease present.

Normal range >0.95
Intermittent claudication 0.9–0.4
Rest pain 0.4–0.15
Gangrene <0.15

In patients with diabetes or chronic renal failure their arterial walls may be calcified and not compressible by a blood pressure cuff, resulting in falsely elevated ABI determination.

Duplex ultrasound imaging

Ultrasound can also be used to image blood vessels, with the anatomic display of the artery complementing the physiological information derived from ankle systolic pressure measurement. This is the simplest and most cost-effective way to confirm the diagnosis and anatomic location of suspected peripheral arterial disease.

Angiography

Angiography is regarded as the diagnostic 'gold-standard'. The complication rate is low, related to arterial injury or adverse reaction to the contrast agent used. Ultrasound has replaced angiography for many applications because these risks are avoided. Angiography is now more selectively used on an 'intention to treat' basis after duplex imaging.

Management

Non-operative management (Fig. 52.1)

Conservative treatment should be offered as the initial treatment for patients with intermittent claudication, summarised in the advice 'Stop smoking, lose weight and exercise.'

Intervention should be considered if intermittent claudication affects essential daily activity or threatens employment.

Endovascular procedures

Arterial stenoses or occlusion may be dilated or stented by minimally invasive catheter technology. Balloon angioplasty enlarges the lumen by a controlled dissection. The risk of serious complications is about 2%. In the iliac arteries an initial success rate of about 90% is well maintained over a period of 5 years. In the superficial femoral artery the results are less satisfactory. Metallic stents may be deployed to maintain the lumen after angioplasty, improving durability of arterial dilatation but adding to the cost of intervention. Many of the local complications of balloon angioplasty can be controlled by stent placement.

Operative management

Surgical bypass is done by anastomosing a conduit to carry blood around an occluded arterial segment, even down to the tibial arteries in the foot. A prosthetic graft may be needed if autogenous vein, the preferred graft material, is unavailable.

Femoropopliteal bypass has an operative mortality of 1–2% and a 5-year patency of 50–70%, with the best results achieved when autogenous vein can be used as graft material. Aortofemoral bypass has an operative mortality of 2–5% and a 5-year patency of 80%. This operation is now infrequently performed because of the comparable results and lower morbidity of endovascular methods such as iliac arterial dilatation and stenting.

Surveillance

Whether the patient has been treated by endovascular means or by bypass surgery, regular surveillance is required to detect and correct late structural problems. Re-stenosis is usually due to neointimal hyperplasia, which occurs most frequently in the first 18 months after intervention and can be detected by ABI measurement and ultrasound scanning.

The diabetic foot

Patients with long-standing diabetes mellitus are predisposed to foot complications on the basis of arterial occlusive disease, neuropathy and infection. Co-existent arterial disease, with calcification of the tibial arteries, is most likely in diabetics who smoke.

Diabetic neuropathy may affect motor, sensory and autonomic nerves. Sensory neuropathy results in loss of pain sensation. Motor neuropathy results in paralysis and atrophy of the small muscles of the foot. This produces clawing of the toes, with neuropathic ulceration forming under the metatarsal heads, maximum area of load bearing. Diabetics are also susceptible to infection.

Clinical presentation

The foot lesion may be the presenting feature of maturity-onset non–insulin-dependent diabetes mellitus (NIDDM). The patient may present with a 'punched out' ulcer or area of localised gangrene, or acutely with a major infection in the foot.

Assessment is directed at determining the extent of local tissue damage and the adequacy of the blood supply. Plain X-rays of the foot will reveal any underlying orthopaedic abnormality such as metatarsal phalangeal dislocation or show evidence of osteomyelitis.

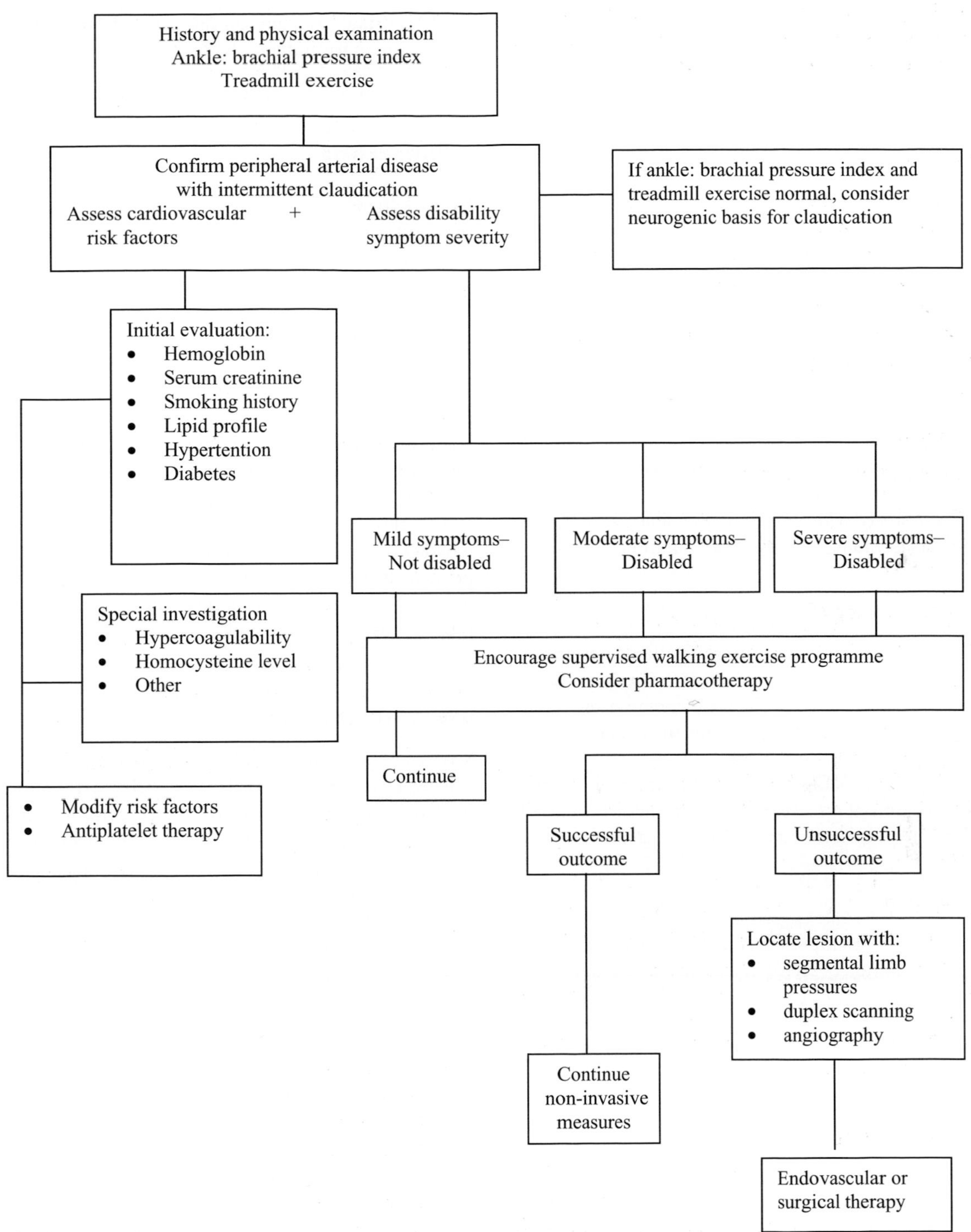

Fig. 52.1 Suggested management algorithm for intermittent claudication. Modified from ACS Working group. Management of peripheral arterial disease (PAD). *J Vascular Surgery* 31, Part 2, January 2000.

Management

Prevention is a major goal by careful control of the diabetes and foot care, to removing callus that can precede ulceration. Surgery has an important role, requiring inter-disciplinary co-operation. Vascular surgeons are involved in improving lower extremity blood supply and orthopaedic surgeons in correcting local bone or soft tissue complications of diabetes. The outlook is worst for patients with diabetic foot ulceration due to peripheral arterial disease who continue to smoke.

Acute limb ischaemia

Acute arterial ischaemia can be caused by trauma (see the section "Vascular Trauma") or by non-traumatic conditions, notably arterial embolism or thrombosis of a pre-existing diseased arterial segment. Unless blood flow is restored within hours, irreversible tissue damage will occur, leading to possible amputation.

Pathophysiology

The common causes of non-traumatic acute limb ischaemia are embolus, thrombosis or graft occlusion following prior surgery. The most common site of origin of an embolus is the heart, due to atrial fibrillation or after myocardial infarction.

Arterial thrombosis can be precipitated by pre-existing arterial disease, resulting in sudden occlusion at the site of an atheromatous arterial stenosis.

Evaluation

Features such as rapid onset of ischaemia, presence of atrial fibrillation or recent myocardial infarction, or absence of a history of claudication are more common in patients with embolus. The ABI will indicate the severity of the ischaemia. In almost all cases angiography is necessary to define the site and extent of obstruction.

Treatment

The survival of the limb is threatened if there is loss of sensation and muscle tenderness or weakness. The aim is to restore arterial inflow, which may done by thrombolytic therapy to dissolve the occluding thrombus, which is successful in 30% of cases, decreasing the need for surgical thrombectomy or bypass.

The mortality remains on the order of 10% and the rate of amputation about 20%.

Upper extremity

Upper extremity ischaemia occurs far less commonly than lower extremity ischaemia and is usually due to non-atherosclerotic causes.

Thoracic outlet syndrome

The subclavian artery, vein and T1 nerve root pass over the first rib to enter the arm. These structures can be compressed in the presence of cervical ribs or with the hypertrophic musculature that follows hard work or in athletes.

The clinical presentation will vary, depending on whether the artery, vein or nerve is predominantly compressed. In selected patients, removal of the first rib, usually by a transaxillary approach, will relieve arterial, venous or neural compression.

Vasospastic disorders

Raynaud's syndrome describes the changes which result from intermittent vasospasm of the arterioles in the hands or feet which occurs after exposure to cold. There is a classic sequence of colour change from pallor to cyanosis to redness as the arterioles first spasm, then slowly recover.

This can be secondary to an underlying connective-tissue disorder such as scleroderma or rheumatoid arthritis.

Management is directed towards treating the underlying condition but with severe digital ischaemia causing tissue loss, vasodilator therapy or occasionally endoscopic surgical sympathectomy is indicated to dilate the digital arteries and improve cutaneous circulation.

Vascular trauma

Vascular injury may be blunt or penetrating. Most arterial injury in Australia is due to blunt trauma sustained in motor vehicle accidents, but there is an increasing incidence of penetrating trauma related to urban violence.

Patterns of arterial injury

Arterial transection

This will present with haemorrhage and evidence of distal ischaemia. The severity of the ischaemia depends on the collateral circulation. With complete transection, arterial spasm and contraction occurs so that bleeding may spontaneously stop as the distal end of the artery thromboses. With partial transection, arterial contraction cannot occur so bleeding can be profuse while the distal pulses remain present.

Arteriovenous fistula

If a penetrating injury involves the adjacent artery and vein, a fistula between the two may develop, with shunting of blood from artery to vein. External bleeding may therefore be minimal.

Closed injury/intimal dissection

This type of injury is most commonly encountered with blunt injury and is dangerous because there may be no external haemorrhage and therefore the possibility of arterial injury overlooked. The artery wall usually remains intact but may weaken, producing a false aneurysm classically seen with traumatic dissection of the thoracic aorta.

Certain orthopaedic injuries such as supracondylar fracture of the humerus or dislocation of the knee are associated with concomitant arterial injury.

Clinical presentation

Vascular injury should be suspected when there is pulsatile bleeding, signs of distal ischemia, an expanding haematoma or a thrill or bruit overlying a site of suspected arterial injury.

Diagnosis

Regular clinical review with a high index of suspicion is essential in detecting arterial injury. Prompt assessment in an operating theatre, ideally equipped for intra-operative angiography, is required for arterial injury associated with ongoing haemorrhage or acute ischaemia. Less obvious arterial injury will usually be detected with measurement of the ABI, duplex scanning and diagnostic angiography. Arterial spasm should not be assumed as an explanation for limb ischaemia after injury unless intimal disruption has been excluded by angiography or surgical exploration.

Treatment

Arterial inflow must be restored within 4–6 hours of acute injury to prevent permanent muscle damage and limb loss.

The technique of arterial repair depends on the pathology of the injury. In some cases of lacerated wounds direct repair can be performed. If a segment of artery has been damaged an interposition graft may be necessary to bridge the defect. Covered stents are also used in selected cases.

Reperfusion syndrome can occur when blood supply is restored to muscle damaged by ischaemia, so that the breakdown products from ischaemic muscle necrosis are washed into the general circulation. Systemic features of reperfusion syndrome include hyperkalaemia and myoglobinuria that can cause sudden death, adult respiratory distress syndrome and cardiac or renal failure.

If muscle swelling is anticipated following restoration of blood flow, a fasciotomy will relieve high intracompartmental pressure.

MCQs

Select the single correct answer to each question.

1 Which of the following is true about a pulsatile mass in the abdomen?
- **a** it must be an aortic aneurysm
- **b** an ultrasound would be the best initial investigation
- **c** no imaging is needed if the mass is not tender
- **d** immediate surgery is indicated
- **e** immediate angiography is indicated

2 Which of the following suggest that acute arterial ischaemia is due to embolus in a 70-year-old woman?
- **a** she is in atrial fibrillation
- **b** her symptoms developed slowly over a month
- **c** she has had long-standing intermittent claudication
- **d** she smokes
- **e** she is an insulin-dependent diabetic

3 Which of the following is true about arterial trauma?
- **a** all arterial injury is associated with pulsatile bleeding
- **b** the commonest cause in Australia is penetrating injury
- **c** the distal pulses will be absent
- **d** there is no relationship to major joint dislocations
- **e** bleeding is more likely with partial than with complete arterial transection

4 Which of the following is true about the diabetic foot complications?
- **a** the neuropathy is only sensory
- **b** there is no relation to ongoing smoking
- **c** the metatarsal phalangeal joints do not dislocate
- **d** the prognosis is worse with arterial disease and ongoing smoking
- **e** there is no place for surgical management

53 Extracranial vascular disease

John Harris

Introduction

The term stroke encapsulates the potentially devastating consequences when blood supply to the brain is disrupted. There are two main types of stroke:

- Ischaemic stroke due to inadequate blood supply, usually by embolisation from or occlusion of an artery that supplies the brain.
- Haemorrhagic stroke due to bleeding from a ruptured cerebral blood vessel in the brain.

More than 40,000 Australians each year experience a stroke, nearly a third of which are fatal. Another third of patients who suffer a stroke will be left with significant neurological deficit, making up almost one in four of Australia's chronic disabled population. The already considerable economic impact of stroke is likely to rise with Australia's ageing population.

Unlike cellular recovery after liver injury, dead neurons in the brain cannot regenerate. There is therefore an increasing emphasis on the emergency nature of impending stroke so that intervention can be undertaken before irreversible cerebral damage occurs. Like 'heart attack' the concept of 'brain attack' has arisen.

The four major arteries that supply the brain are the vertebral arteries originating from the subclavian arteries forming the basilar artery and supplying the posterior cerebral circulation and the internal carotid arteries. These arise from the carotid bifurcation in the neck and lead onto the middle cerebral arteries, the most important branches in the anterior cerebral circulation. The Circle of Willis provides potential communication between the anterior and posterior cerebral circulations but may be inadequate to fully compensate for an occluded internal carotid artery in about 20% of individuals.

Incidence

Although the death rate from stroke has more than halved since 1980 in common with other forms of cardiovascular disease, cerebrovascular disease remains the third commonest cause of death after heart disease and cancer, accounting for 10% of all mortality in the Australian community. Predominantly middle-aged males are affected but the incidence of stroke increases exponentially with age, with 50% of all strokes occurring in patients over 75 years of age.

Risk factors for stroke

Stroke arising from extra-cranial arterial disease is most likely to occur when there is a high grade (>70%) stenosis of the internal carotid artery, particularly if there have been recent transient ischaemic attacks (TIAs).

Risk factors for stroke include high blood pressure, tobacco smoking, heavy alcohol consumption, high cholesterol, obesity, diabetes and insufficient physical activity. Hypertension is associated with both ischaemic and haemorrhagic stroke. Improved medical management of high blood pressure has contributed to the decreasing incidence of stroke (Box 53.1). Carotid stenosis occurs more frequently in patients who have co-existent coronary artery disease or lower extremity peripheral arterial disease.

Embolic stroke is most likely in patients with atrial fibrillation or after an acute myocardial infarction.

Pathogenesis

Overall, 70% of strokes are ischaemic and 15% haemorrhagic, either from primary intracranial

Box 53.1 Management algorithm presentation

Asymptomatic bruit
- Check for co-existent coronary artery disease
- Carotid duplex scan
  - >60% internal carotid stenosis, consider carotid endarterectomy

Symptomatic
- TIAs
  - Carotid duplex scan
    - >60% internal carotid stensois
      - If patient fit
        - carotid endarterectomy
      - If patient unfit
        - Consider carotid stenting
      - Correction of underlying risk factors
  - Evolving stroke
    - CT scan/MRI
      - Intracranial haemorrhage
      - Ischaemic stroke
        - Heparinise
        - Investigate for cardiac embolic source
          - ECG
          - Cardiac echography
        - Investigate for extra-cranial arterial disease
          - Carotid duplex scan
          - MRI
          - CT angiography

hemorrhage (11%) or subarachnoid hemorrhage (4%). Haemorrhagic stroke can be readily differentiated from ischaemic stroke by computed tomography (CT) or magnetic resonance imaging (MRI) and will not be considered further.

Ischaemic stroke results in cerebral infarction, due to atherosclerosis affecting the large arteries in 75%, from cardiac embolism in 15% or from small vessel occlusion, usually related to hypertension, causing lacunar infarction in 10%.

Atherosclerosis affecting the extracranial circulation most commonly occurs at the carotid bifurcation, particularly at the origin of the internal carotid artery, where there is a region of turbulent flow as the common carotid artery divides into the high-resistance external carotid artery and low-resistance internal carotid artery.

There are two main theories of how disease at the carotid bifurcation may cause transient ischaemic attacks and stroke.

Embolic theory: Embolisation of atherosclerotic material or thrombus can arise from the carotid bifurcation. This is more likely to occur, with complicated atherosclerotic plaques forming a tight (>70%) stenosis.

Haemodynamic theory: Blood flow to the brain may be reduced by a tight stenosis or occlusion of the carotid arteries. The effect of such lesions will depend on the extent of intracranial collateral circulation. This is the mechanism of stroke after profound hypotension from any cause.

The theories are not mutually exclusive, as the likelihood of embolisation from carotid plaque and occlusion of the internal carotid artery increases with the degree of stenosis.

Extracranial arterial pathology

Atherosclerosis is the pathological basis of extracranial arterial disease in about 90% of cases, with less common conditions occurring in 10%, including fibromuscular disease, dissection, aneurysm, arteritis such as Takayasu's disease and carotid body tumours. Recurrent stenosis of the carotid artery due to neointimal hyperplasia can occur after surgery or carotid stenting.

Fibromuscular dysplasia occurs mainly in young females and causes irregular webs and dilatations, causing a 'string of beads' sign on angiography in the internal carotid artery or even dissection or aneurysm formation. Takayasu's disease is a non-specific arteritis that can occlude the major branches of the thoracic or abdominal aorta (hence the term *pulseless disease*). Carotid body tumours are rare, arise from the chemoreceptors, and are therefore highly vascular and occasionally malignant. They present as a pulsatile mass in the neck that can be moved from side to side and should not be biopsied.

Subclavian steal

Another mechanism of haemodynamic cerebral hypoperfusion occurs on basis of 'subclavian steal'. If the left subclavian artery or more rarely the innominate artery is stenosed or occluded, then the vertebral artery becomes an important collateral pathway to sustain blood flow to the arm. When the arm is exercised, vertebral arterial flow reverses resulting in cerebral hypoperfusion. This is usually asymptomatic unless there is co-existent internal carotid stenosis.

Clinical presentation

Extracranial cerebrovascular disease may be either symptomatic or clinically silent. This will depend on whether the carotid plaque is affecting blood flow or embolising and on the sensitivity of the affected part of the brain. Symptoms will depend on whether the anterior (carotid) or posterior (vertebrobasilar) circulations are involved. The left hemisphere, largely supplied by the anterior circulation, is usually dominant in a right-handed person, so emboli to the left cerebral hemisphere are more likely to result in disabling symptoms.

Asymptomatic

A bruit in the neck may indicate asymptomatic extracranial arterial disease. It is important to distinguish between bruits arising from the heart or great vessels and bruits due to turbulence at the carotid bifurcation, which are loudest in the neck. A carotid bruit is a poor marker of internal carotid stenosis and is probably a better guide to the presence of general atherosclerosis, particularly coronary artery disease. Only about a third of patients with a carotid bruit will have a significant stenosis of their internal carotid artery and a bruit is rarely present with the most severe stenosis (>90%) because of reduced blood flow.

An asymptomatic internal carotid stenosis is an occasional incidental finding on duplex ultrasound scanning.

Symptomatic

All the major clinical trials have confirmed that the likelihood of symptoms and stroke is directly related to the severity of internal carotid stenosis. Microemboli from carotid plaque induce a transient cerebral ischaemia in either the carotid (anterior) or vertebrobasilar (posterior) circulation. Symptoms may occur as an isolated event or may recur or progress to a major stroke.

Transient ischaemic attacks

A TIA is a reversible neurological deficit that resolves in 24 hours, but is usually briefer, lasting for less than 15 minutes and resolving without a persistent neurological deficit. Classical carotid (anterior circulation) TIAs involve ipsilateral retinal ischaemia manifest as amaurosis fugax (fleeting blindness) described as a curtain coming down over the eye. Cholesterol emboli (Hollenhorst plaques) and fibrin–platelet emboli (Fisher plugs) can be seen on fundoscopy in the retinal arteries, and both are strongly indicative of ulcerative atheromatous disease of the carotid arteries, particularly at the carotid bifurcation in the neck.

Motor and sensory symptoms involve the contralateral limbs because of the crossover of the major motor and sensory neural pathways. The symptoms and signs are focal and may be motor, with weakness, paralysis, poor function, or clumsiness in one or both extremities. There may be sensory symptoms, with numbness or paraesthesiae affecting one or both extremities on the same side. Dysphasia with speech disturbance is common, particularly when the dominant hemisphere is affected (usually the left in a right-handed individual).

When the vertebrobasilar system is involved, the symptoms are less specific but may affect both sides of the body, with bilateral visual disturbance. Symptoms such as ataxia, imbalance, unsteadiness and vertigo can also be caused by middle ear disorders or bradycardia causing the patient to collapse (Stokes Adams attacks).

Headache more commonly occurs with intracranial hemorrhage, migraine or a space-occupying neoplasm.

Clinical examination will often fail to reveal any neurological deficit but there may be a bruit in the neck. This condition is one diagnosed on history and should prompt further investigation to define the state of the extracranial blood vessels.

Stroke in evolution/complete stroke

If the neurological deficit fluctuates and a progressive motor or sensory deficit is evident, then a stroke-in-evolution, potentially leading to a complete stroke, should be suspected. This is a medical emergency, requiring prompt neurological evaluation.

Investigations

In a patient who presents with focal neurological symptoms investigations are needed to determine the cause, particularly whether cerebral infarction or haemorrhage has occurred and if there is correctible extra-cranial arterial disease responsible.

With the advent of CT and carotid duplex scanning it has become easier to define those patients who are likely to have hemispheric neurological symptoms on a potentially correctible basis of thromboembolic phenomenon arising from the carotid bifurcation.

General medical evaluation includes cardiovascular evaluation with blood pressure measurement to detect hypertension and electrocardiography to assess any cardiac rhythm disturbance like atrial fibrillation or evidence of co-existent coronary artery disease. Haematological disorders such as polycythaemia, leukaemia or coagulopathies can cause stroke and should be sought. Similarly, renal function, lipid and glucose levels are measured to exclude renal failure, hyperlipidaemia and diabetes respectively.

CT scanning or MRI will identify intracranial blood if a haemorrhagic stroke has occurred and will demonstrate cerebral infarction or space-occupying lesions such as a brain tumour. Although sophisticated 3-D reconstruction of the extracranial vasculature can be done with both MRI and CT, these are usually not the first-line investigations to assess the carotid arteries.

Duplex ultrasound is used in most centres as the initial diagnostic test to evaluate the carotid arteries and used as the definitive investigation by many vascular surgeons in planning carotid endarterectomy. Duplex ultrasound is operator-dependent but in good hands can show the morphology of the carotid bifurcation and accurately identify the degree of stenosis present (Figure 53.1).

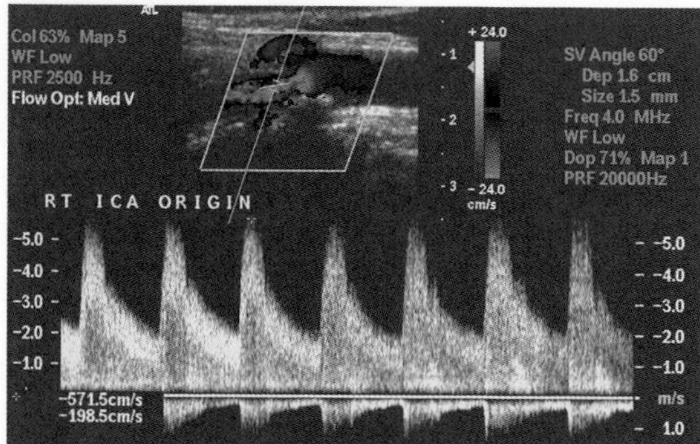

Fig. 53.1 Carotid duplex scan showing turbulent flow at the origin of the internal carotid artery with a peak systolic velocity of 571.5 cm/s and an endiastoic velocity of 198.5 cm/s indicating more than 80% stenosis of the artery.

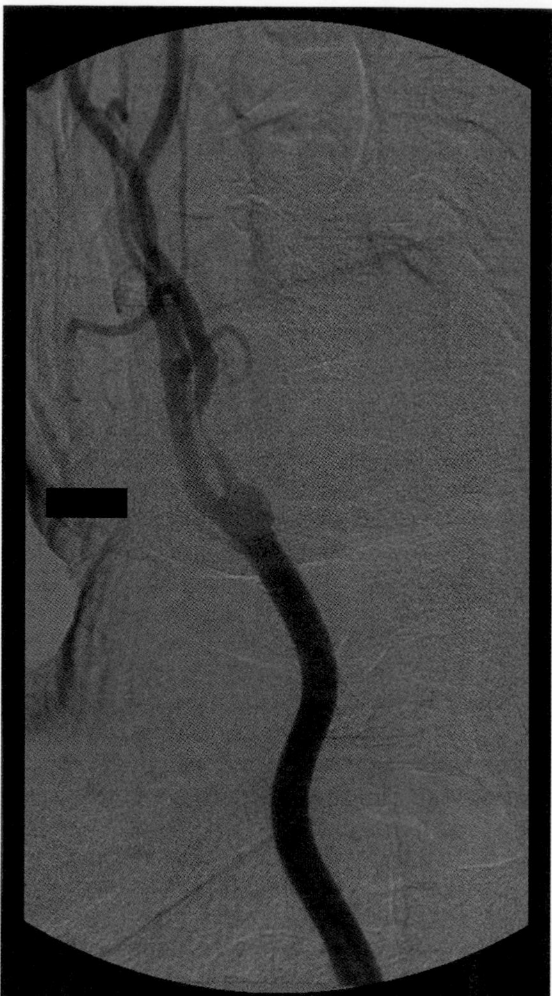

Fig. 53.2 Carotid angiogram showing more than 80% stenosis at the origin of the internal carotid artery.

Carotid angiography, considered the diagnostic gold standard, is now used more selectively, particularly if the ultrasound findings are uncertain, or if the major aortic arch branches need to be imaged in planning carotid stenting (Figure 53.2).

Treatment

Optimal medical control of risk factors, in particular hypertension and smoking, have significantly reduced the risk of stroke and remains the most important part of overall management. Anti-platelet aggregate

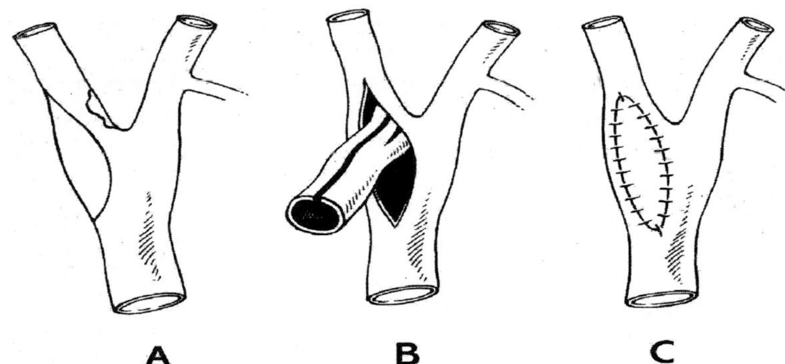

Fig. 53.3 After the carotid arteries are clamped, the plaque (A) is removed (B) and the arteriotomy closed either primarily or with a patch (C).

therapy, usually with aspirin, will help prevent recurrent TIAs but does not reduce the risk of stroke.

There are defined sub-groups of patients who will benefit from surgery or endovascular intervention to remove an identified embolic source or improve cerebral blood flow. Age should not preclude treatment that would otherwise be indicated.

Fortuitously, the carotid bifurcation is the commonest site for extra-cranial stenotic disease, as it is surgically accessible unlike the aortic arch branches or vertebral arteries that pose more complex treatment problems.

Symptomatic carotid disease

Two major clinical trials have confirmed the clear advantage of surgery over best medical management for patients with recent TIAs associated with a high-grade (>70% angiographic diameter reducing) stenosis of the relevant internal carotid artery.

Asymptomatic carotid disease

Although the benefit of carotid endarterectomy is not as great for asymptomatic patients as it is for symptomatic patients with an equivalent stenosis, guidelines prepared by the American Heart Association recommend prophylactic carotid endarterectomy for asymptomatic patients with higher than 60% stenosis of the internal carotid artery, if the surgical risk is estimated at less than 3% and life expectancy is at least 5 years. Surgery is generally not recommended if the surgical risk is higher or with limited life expectancy. There is a tendency in the Australian setting to consider surgery only for more severe (>80%) asymptomatic stenoses.

Carotid endarterectomy

The carotid bifurcation is exposed in the neck and, after heparinisation, the carotid arteries are clamped so that artery can be opened to core out the atherosclerotic plaque (Figure 53.3). There is a plane between the diseased portion of the carotid artery and the outer media so that a smooth surface can be restored to the artery. A patch is often used to close the artery to ensure a widely patent lumen and to decrease the risk of re-stenosis. A shunt is occasionally used during carotid surgery to maintain cerebral blood flow if the cerebral collateral circulation is judged inadequate.

Occasionally a bypass procedure is needed to restore cerebral perfusion; for example an occluded common carotid artery can be treated by a bypass from the subclavian artery to the internal carotid artery.

Carotid stenting

Carotid stenting is a more recent technical advance and remains a controversial aspect of carotid therapy. Carotid angioplasty has for some time been the therapy of choice for symptomatic fibromuscular dysplasia, a relatively rare condition occurring in less than 3% of patients with symptomatic carotid arterial disease. There has been continuing improvement in the reported results of balloon dilatation and stenting for atherosclerotic carotid arterial disease. The proposed benefit of carotid artery stenting is that an anaesthetic can be avoided as can the neck incision and risk of cranial nerve injury. However, there have been concerns about a higher risk of peri-procedural cerebral embolisation and stroke and late recurrent stenosis. The risk of peri-procedural stroke has been reduced with cerebral protection devices, designed to catch embolic material before it can pass into the brain.

Controlled clinical trials should resolve the relative merits of carotid stenting and endarterectomy. Until that time, carotid endarterectomy is the established intervention for high-risk patients with high-grade symptomatic internal carotid stenosis.

Angioplasty and stenting is usually indicated to treat subclavian artery stenosis or occlusion causing subclavian steal.

Peri-operative management

Close monitoring is essential after any form of cerebrovascular intervention to observe for neurological deficit, to guide blood pressure control and to decrease the risk of adverse cardiovascular events. Patients are usually started on Aspirin therapy soon after surgery to decrease the risk of thrombosis at the endarterectomy site.

The incidence of carotid re-stenosis due to neointimal hyperplasia after surgery can be reduced by use of a patch to close the artery. Re-stenosis is more common after stenting. Post-operative surveillance using ultrasound is commonly done to monitor the operated or stented carotid artery.

Procedural complications

There is a 2–3% risk of ipsilateral stroke after carotid endarterectomy or stenting related to embolisation from the carotid during the manipulation of intervention or to the interruption of cerebral blood flow. Labile blood pressure is common and hypertension is related to the risk of post-operative intracerebral hemorrhage. Co-existent coronary artery disease is an important cause of post-operative myocardial infarction and death. Important local complications after surgery are neck haematomas and cranial nerve injuries, which can include the hypoglossal and recurrent laryngeal nerves. Sensory loss in the distribution of the greater auricular nerve is commonly observed. Neck haematomas are an occasional problem and, if severe, can obstruct respiration, requiring prompt return to the operating theatre.

Prognosis and results of surgery

The North American Symptomatic Carotid Endarterectomy Trial (NASCET) showed that the risk of stroke in symptomatic patients with greater than 70% stenosis of the relevant internal carotid could be reduced at two years from 26% to 9% with carotid endarterectomy, provided that the surgery is done with an acceptably low morbidity and mortality. A recent audit of carotid surgery in New South Wales confirmed that in an Australian setting, carotid endarterectomy is being performed with less than 2–3% combined stroke/death rate, in keeping with NASCET recommendations.

The overall benefit is not as great for asymptomatic carotid stenosis. However, the Asymptomatic Carotid Atherosclerosis Study did confirm an advantage for surgery for asymptomatic patients with more than 60% internal carotid stenosis. The surgical group in this study incurred a 2.3% peri-operative risk of stroke or death, and had a 5.1% cumulative 5-year risk of ipsilateral stroke, peri-operative stroke or death. The medical group had an 11% cumulative risk of the same late endpoints. Surgery reduced the absolute risk by 5.9% and relative risk by 53% at 5 years. Although there was therapeutic benefit at 1 year, the benefit was greater at 5 years. The benefit appeared greater for men than women.

Future developments

Carotid endarterectomy is the most frequently performed peripheral vascular surgical operation, with its efficacy confirmed by Level 1 evidence. Carotid stenting is evolving as a less invasive alternative and is being subjected to rigourous evaluation through controlled trials.

There is an increased focus on preventing stroke by risk factor modification and by identification of subgroups at high risk of stroke who will benefit from prophylactic intervention.

MCQs

Select the single correct answer to each question.

1 Which of the following is not true about the anatomy of extracranial arterial disease?

- **a** the left subclavian artery arises directly from the aortic arch
- **b** the vertebral artery is a branch of the subclavian carotid artery
- **c** the vertebral arteries form the basilar artery
- **d** there is no communication between the anterior and posterior cerebral circulations
- **e** there is a low-resistance flow pattern in the internal carotid artery

2 An 80-year-old woman presents with transient right hemiparesis, lasting 15 minutes and resolving completely. She is otherwise healthy and independent. Her carotid duplex scan shows >80% stenosis of her left internal carotid artery. Despite aspirin therapy, she has a further episode. Which of the following statements is true?
- **a** she is best managed on warfarin therapy
- **b** left carotid endarterectomy is indicated
- **c** carotid stenting is a preferred option to surgery
- **d** she is facing a cumulative 5% stroke within the next 3 years
- **e** lowering her blood cholesterol level will reduce her immediate risk of stroke

3 Which of the following is true about the pathology of extracranial arterial disease?
- **a** atherosclerosis is the commonest cause of internal carotid stenosis
- **b** recurrent stenosis occurs in >50% of patients after carotid endarterectomy
- **c** carotid body tumours arise from the vertebral arteries
- **d** fibromuscular disease is commonest in young men
- **e** Takayasu's disease is commonly known as 'pulsing disease'

4 Which if the following is true about carotid endarterectomy?
- **a** it is associated with a high (>5%) risk of peri-operative stroke
- **b** closure with a patch decreases the risk of recurrent stenosis
- **c** there is a plane between the atheromatous plaque and the intima
- **d** it is the procedure of choice for fibromuscular disease
- **e** it precludes the use of a carotid stent for recurrent stenosis

5 A 65-year-old man presents with angina, and a left neck bruit is heard. Which of the following statements is correct?
- **a** the first priority is investigation of the bruit
- **b** the bruit may be arising from the aortic valve
- **c** a carotid angiogram in indicated
- **d** there is no relationship between angina and a carotid bruit
- **e** the left internal carotid artery must be occluded

54 Venous and lymphatic diseases of the limbs

M. Grigg and C. Miles

Varicose veins

Introduction

Varicose veins are a common condition occurring in 20% of adults. The characteristics of varicose veins are that they are

- visible
- dilated
- elongated
- tortuous

Varicose veins result from incompetent valves in the venous system.

Anatomy of the venous system

The veins of the lower limb can be classified into three groups: superficial, deep and perforating.

Superficial veins

The superficial veins are collected in two major systems. These are the tributaries and main trunks of the long and short saphenous veins.

The long saphenous system begins on the dorsum of the foot and runs anterior to the medial malleolus, along the medial aspect of the calf and thigh and ends at the saphenofemoral junction, where it joins the common femoral vein. This junction is 2–3 cm below and lateral to the pubic tubercle. A major tributary, the posterior arch vein, joins the long saphenous vein just below the knee. This drains blood from much of the medial side of the calf and communicates with the deep venous plexus of the calf by way of several perforating veins – so named because they 'perforate' the deep fascia. In the thigh, there are large medial and lateral tributaries and thigh perforating veins. A number of tributaries join the long saphenous vein close to its termination. These are important in the surgery for saphenofemoral incompetence since failure to deal with these will result in recurrence of the varicose veins.

The short saphenous system begins behind the lateral malleolus of the ankle and then runs along the lateral and then the posterior aspect of the calf to penetrate the deep fascia in the upper calf. It terminates in the popliteal fossa by joining the popliteal vein in the vicinity of the knee crease. The exact level of the junction is variable and may be either a few centimetres above or below the knee crease.

Deep veins

The deep veins run as venae comitantes of the major arteries in the foot and calf, where they receive tributaries from the muscles of the calf, including the venous sinusoids in the calf muscles. The venous sinusoids within the calf muscles are important as part of the venous pump mechanism. They are a frequent site of origin for venous thrombosis. The deep system also receives the perforating veins from the superficial system. At about the level of the knee joint a single popliteal vein is formed in most cases. This runs proximally in company with the main artery to become the femoral vein and then the external iliac vein as it passes beneath the inguinal ligament.

Perforating veins

The perforating veins join the superficial and deep systems. They contain valves which direct blood flow from the superficial to the deep system. Perforating veins are variable in number and position, but usual sites are the medial side of the lower third of the calf between the posterior arch vein and the posterior tibial veins and at about the junction of the middle and lower thirds of the thigh between the long saphenous vein and the femoral vein. Other perforating veins join the anterior tibial veins, the peroneal veins and the superficial veins. The inconstancy of these veins makes precise localisation difficult and is an important reason for the development of recurrent varicose veins following treatment.

Physiology

The superficial veins collect blood from the superficial tissues. During the relaxation phase of the calf muscle cycle, the pressure in the superficial veins is greater than the pressure in the deep veins thus blood flows from superficial to deep. Each contraction of the calf muscles results in high pressure (approximately 250 mm Hg) being generated in the calf compartments. This empties the veins in the muscles and transmits a pulse of blood proximally.

Retrograde flow, or reflux, due to gravity is prevented by valves. If the valves in the veins directing venous return proximally or if the perforating veins are incompetent the venous return from the leg is less efficient. This results in higher pressures in the superficial system and progressive dilatation occurs, causing more valves to become incompetent. This is accompanied by elongation of the superficial veins, which results in tortuosity. The high pressure in the superficial veins, particularly in the most gravitationally dependent part of the leg around the ankle, may be sufficient to impair the nutrition of the subcutaneous tissue and dermis and contribute to ulcer formation.

Varicose veins are a disorder of the superficial and perforating veins. In most cases the disorder is inborn although the mode of inheritance is uncertain. Varicose veins often first appear in young adults. Females are affected more commonly and the veins are more prominent during pregnancy due to the combined effects of the muscle-relaxing effects of hormonal (especially progesterone) changes and the pressure effects of the pregnant uterus, which also acts as an arteriovenous fistula in the pelvis. Partial regression occurs following delivery but there is a progression of the varicosities with succeeding pregnancies. Tributaries of the internal iliac vein and even the ovarian vein may be involved, producing posterior thigh and vulval varices.

Clinical presentation

Patients with varicose veins most commonly present for cosmetic reasons. Some patients present with tiny veins – telangiectasia or venous flares. Others present with huge veins that may have been present for 10–20 years or longer.

Symptoms

Symptoms result from fluid congestion of gravitationally dependent superficial tissues due to inadequate venous return and increased venous pressure. Patients may complain of tiredness and aching of the lower legs at the end of the day. This is relieved by rest and elevation of the legs. They may develop mild ankle swelling, particularly in warmer weather. Leg pain is a common complaint and the presence of varicose veins may be coincidental.

Complications

Thrombophlebitis

Thrombosis in a segment of varicose vein is common. The patient presents with signs of inflammation spreading from a hard lump, which is the thrombosed vein. The redness, pain and heat falsely suggest the presence of infection. The condition usually resolves over a period of days provided the thrombosis does not extend into the deep venous system, when pulmonary embolus becomes a risk. Hence thrombus extending from the long saphenous vein into the common femoral vein can be very dangerous. The thrombus often extends 15 cm or more proximal to the clinical signs of inflammation, and a duplex scan will readily demonstrate the true level of the clot. Urgent operative ligation of the saphenofemoral junction or full anticoagulation needs to be considered for thrombophlebitis extending above the level of the knee joint.

Haemorrhage

The subcutaneous varices of the lower calf and around the ankle may rupture through the skin causing profuse bleeding. This bleeding will continue unabated whilst the limb remains dependent, even to the point of exsanguination. The patient should lie down immediately and elevate the limb. Pressure should be applied over the bleeding point. This pressure can be reinforced by a firm bandage. A tourniquet must not be used. The rise in venous pressure produced by a tourniquet may worsen the bleeding.

Ulceration

Prior to the advent of duplex scanning, which enabled noninvasive evaluation of the venous system, it was mistakenly believed that superficial varicose veins rarely caused venous ulceration. It is now realised that severe, long-standing varicose veins are a common cause of leg ulcers. Before the development of frank ulceration, secondary venous tissue changes occur. These tissue changes include pigmentation due to haemosiderin deposition, lipodermatosclerosis, and atrophe blanche.

Other complications

Rare presentations occur in children and are associated with major congenital abnormalities of the venous system, often associated with arteriovenous malformations.

Examination

The examination is directed at identifying the sites of incompetent valves that allow reflux of blood from the deep to the superficial veins. The patterns of disease are:

- long saphenous incompetence
- short saphenous incompetence
- incompetence of thigh or calf communicating veins
- combinations of the above

The patient is examined standing. The size and distribution of varicose veins are examined. If the veins are predominantly medial and if they involve the thigh, it is likely that the long saphenous vein is involved. If they are posterior and lateral in the calf, it is likely that the short saphenous vein is involved. Remember that there are many communications between the two systems so that, for example, incompetence in the long saphenous system may fill varices on the posterior and lateral aspects of the calf. The presence of any secondary venous tissue changes is noted. If long saphenous incompetence is suspected a cough impulse over any prominent vein confirms the diagnosis of saphenofemoral incompetence.

The examiner should also be aware of findings which signify that the patient does not have 'straightforward' varicose vein problem. For example:

- varices of the medial aspect of the upper thigh may indicate pelvic venous insufficiency
- the presence of significant leg oedema is unlikely to be due to varicose veins alone
- prominent superficial veins extending above the level of the inguinal ligament in the suprapubic area suggests that these veins are dilated collaterals which have formed in response to deep venous obstruction
- ulcers sited proximal to the mid-calf level are unlikely to have a venous aetiology.

A tourniquet test is performed to systematically search for the sites of incompetence. The findings on inspection will indicate where these are likely to be. The patient lies on an examination couch. The leg to be examined is elevated to drain the blood from the superficial venous system. It is convenient to rest the patient's heel on the examiner's shoulder. A narrow tourniquet is placed around the thigh as high as possible. A narrow tourniquet is used because it occludes the superficial veins but does not affect the deep veins. A length of rubber tubing makes a good tourniquet. With the tourniquet in place, the patient is asked to stand. The leg is inspected to see if the veins that had been seen previously are full or empty. The veins will fill slowly (30–60 seconds) because of arterial inflow or rapidly because of venous reflux. If the veins remain empty during the first 30 seconds it means that there are no incompetent valves allowing reflux into the superficial veins below the level of the tourniquet. The most likely cause of the patient's varicose veins is incompetence at the saphenofemoral junction. The tourniquet is released and rapid refilling of the superficial veins can be seen.

If the veins are not controlled by this manoeuvre, the examination is repeated with the tourniquet placed above the patella. This tests for the middle lower third of thigh perforator. If the veins are not controlled, the tourniquet is placed below the knee to test the short saphenous system. If no measure controls the filling of the veins, the site of incompetence is below the tourniquet and therefore involves the calf communicating veins.

This examination is sufficient in many cases of untreated varicose veins. More elaborate clinical tests, usually described with the name of their originator, may be used. The accuracy of these clinical tests have been called into question when compared with the results of ultrasound examination as detailed below.

Investigations

Doppler ultrasound probe

A hand-held Doppler ultrasound probe may assist in identifying incompetence of the long and short saphenous systems. With the patient standing and the muscles of the leg relaxed, the probe is placed over the upper end of the vein. The limb is compressed distally by squeezing the calf with the hand in the case of the short saphenous system. This produces a sharp augmentation of the flow of blood in the vein. The compression is relaxed and if the valves in the vein are competent blood flow stops. If the valves are incompetent, the flow signal continues indicating reflux of blood in the vein.

Duplex ultrasound

More information is provided by duplex ultrasound, which provides both an image and information about the blood flow velocity. Many surgeons recommend routine duplex scanning prior to any varicose vein surgery, but there are four major indications for this investigation:

- if there is clinical doubt about incompetence involving either of the major saphenous systems
- for identification of the level at which the short saphenous vein enters the popliteal vein (this level may be variable and performance of the operation is much easier with precise information about the level of the junction)
- for locating incompetent perforating veins (duplex ultrasound is the best method because the veins can be seen and the direction of blood flow in them identified)
- for patients with recurrent varicose veins as information about the sites of recurrence is critical to planning treatment.

There are three major causes of recurrence. First, recurrence in a system not previously treated (e.g. short saphenous incompetence that has developed later or was not initially detected). Second, recurrence in the groin following saphenofemoral ligation. This may be due to inadequate surgery where a major tributary in the groin has been missed or sometimes due to 'neovascularisation' where the recurrence is due to the development of multiple tiny channels between the deep and superficial systems through scar tissue at the site of the saphenofemoral ligation. Finally, recurrence due to incompetence of perforating veins (e.g. at the junction of the middle and lower thirds of the thigh).

Venography

Venography is an obsolete investigation for these patients and should be avoided because of the poor risk-to-benefit ratio.

Treatment

There are few serious sequelae of untreated varicose veins (see 'Complications') so treatment is not essential, except in those patients with pre-ulcerative secondary venous tissue changes in the lower calf or with complications (see 'Symptoms').

Elastic stockings

Elastic stockings will not cure varicose veins but will provide relief from symptoms of swelling and tiredness in the legs and prevent complications. They are particularly helpful for the pregnant patient with varices. A range of stockings are available – low-, medium- and high-grade compression and below- and above-knee lengths. For patients with varicose veins, a below knee stocking of moderate compression (Grade 2, 20–30 mm Hg pressure) will suffice. If there is doubt that the veins are the cause of the symptoms in a particular patient, relief of symptoms while wearing stockings supports the diagnosis of varicose veins and, conversely, failure of stockings to relieve symptoms suggests that other causes should be sought. Graduated compression stockings should be prescribed with caution for patients in whom pedal pulses are not palpable.

Injection–compression therapy

Injection therapy should not be considered while there are major uncontrolled sites of deep to superficial incompetence. When these sites have been controlled by surgery, injections may be used to control small veins that may remain. An important part of injection therapy is compression, which keeps together the surfaces irritated by the sclerosant. This facilitates fibrous organisation and inhibits re-canalisation of the vein. Recently, techniques have been introduced for injecting very small cutaneous veins. These often cause cosmetic disability because they are prominent blue or red lines in the skin that are hard to disguise. Injections of small amounts of hypertonic saline will result in sclerosis of these veins.

Operation

Operation is the most appropriate method of control for major sites of incompetence. The aims of operation are to obliterate the major sites of deep to superficial incompetence and to remove the larger varicose veins. The presence of varicose veins predisposes to the development of post-operative deep vein thrombosis so appropriate prophylaxis should be undertaken.

Saphenofemoral ligation

Saphenofemoral ligation is the procedure performed most commonly. The saphenofemoral junction is exposed through a skin crease incision about 3 cm long placed below and lateral to the pubic tubercle and 1 cm above the groin crease. The long saphenous vein and its tributaries are dissected. All tributaries are ligated and divided. Once the junction between the long saphenous and femoral veins has been clearly identified, the long saphenous vein is divided and ligated flush with the femoral vein. The femoral vein is explored for 2 cm proximal and distal to the junction to ensure that there are no more tributaries entering the vein. Any that are found are ligated and divided.

Saphenopopliteal ligation

Saphenopopliteal ligation is carried out in a manner analogous to saphenofemoral ligation. The dissection may be difficult because of the fat in the popliteal fossa and is greatly facilitated by precise knowledge from duplex ultrasound scanning of the exact level of the saphenopopliteal junction. Care is necessary to avoid inadvertent injury to the sural nerve which runs with the short saphenous vein.

Stripping

Stripping of the long saphenous vein from the groin to the knee removes a large dilated vein which, if left, may be the site of thrombophlebitis or recurrence. A varicose long saphenous vein is not useful for later coronary or leg artery bypasses. Stripping the long saphenous vein between the ankle and the knee should not be performed since it is unnecessary and may result in troublesome neuritis of the saphenous nerve.

Multiple extractions

Most of the obvious varicosities are removed through multiple small incisions. The veins are then grasped either by small artery forceps or specially designed hooks. As much as possible of the dilated vein is removed. The next incision is made 2–4 cm away and the process repeated until all the major varices have been removed.

Ligation of incompetent perforating veins

This usually involves an incision over the perforating vein as it passes through the deep fascia. Pre-operative duplex scan provides accurate localisation. Endoscopic techniques have been developed particularly for patients with multiple incompetent perforating veins. The vein is ligated and divided beneath the deep fascia. Ligation of perforating veins is usually reserved for patients undergoing operation for recurrent veins or patients who have significant secondary venous tissue changes or ulceration. It is not a cosmetic procedure.

Post-operative care

The leg is firmly bandaged to promote haemostasis from the extraction sites. Early and continued mobility is encouraged to reduce the risk of DVT. Patients having bilateral operations or operation for major recurrences usually stay in hospital overnight. The outer bandages are removed 24–48 hours after operation and elastic stockings are applied. These are worn for about 2 weeks while there is a tendency for the leg to swell.

Prognosis and results of surgery

The result of surgery that has been carefully planned and carried out should be good. The immediate cosmetic result should satisfy the patient. With well-performed surgery the recurrence rate is 15–20% at 5 years. Injection therapy may be used to obliterate telangiectatic vessels that it is not possible to remove surgically.

Further reading

Houghton AD, Panayiotopoulos Y, Taylor PR. Practical management of primary varicose veins. *Br J Clin Pract.* 1996; 50:103–105.

Rutherford R, ed. *Vascular Surgery*. 5th ed. Philadelphia: WB Saunders;2000:1907–2093.

Lymphoedema

Introduction

Lymphoedema is the consequence of abnormal amounts of fluid and protein in the interstitial spaces of the skin and subcutaneous tissues particularly with respect to the limbs. The high protein content of the fluid distinguishes this type of swelling, or brawny oedema, from that seen occurring as a result of filtration oedema of heart and kidney failure, venous obstruction and hypoproteinaemia (pitting oedema).

Incidence

This is an unusual cause of limb swelling. There are two principal types:

i) a congenital abnormality of the lymphatic channels (primary lymphoedema)
ii) secondary lymphatic obstruction resulting from infection, trauma (including surgery and radiotherapy), secondary metastatic tumours and, occasionally, primary tumours such as lymphoma.

Physiology

The brain and the spinal cord are the only body tissues that do not have significant lymphatic vessels. For all other structures, lymphatic vessels function to collect lymph – tissue fluid including protein that leaks from the capillary bed – and then convey this to the regional lymph nodes, to the major lymphatic trunks and ultimately into the thoracic duct, which terminates by joining the junction of the subclavian and internal jugular vein in the left side of the neck.

The lymphatic capillaries are thin-walled endothelial tubes, the endothelium being supported on collagen with occasional smooth muscle cells. The onward progression of the lymph in these channels is maintained by the presence of valves and the compression applied by neighbouring structures, such as the contraction of muscles and the varying pressure and movement of the gut in the abdominal cavity. The onward flow is also enhanced by the changes in the intrathoracic pressure generated by respiration. The composition of the lymph will vary with the drainage site. If this is the intestine, it will contain chylomicrons. In all cases there is a high concentration of albumin. The lymph flow in the thoracic duct varies from 1 to 4 L per day and the proportions of its final composition will depend on the relative flow from the various sites of the body and the food intake at the time.

Pathogenesis and pathology

The pathogenesis of lymphoedema is invariably a consequence of inadequate lymphatic flow, either because the lymph vessels are congenitally abnormal or deficient, or because of obstruction to the vessels or the draining lymph nodes. Less frequently, temporary lymphoedema can occur in a limb on account of muscle inactivity, as occurs with prolonged sitting, but resolves swiftly with muscle activity.

Primary lymphoedema

Primary or idiopathic lymphoedema refers to swelling due to intrinsic abnormalities of the lymphatic vessels. This can be a familial abnormality and is often bilateral and symmetrical. The lymphatic vessels are aplastic in 15% and hypoplastic in 65% of patients, being fewer and smaller in calibre than is normal. They may be varicose, dilated and incompetent in 20% due to fibrosis in the draining lymph nodes. In this group with an intrinsic abnormality present at birth, lymph may reflux into the skin, leak through the skin (especially between the toes), into the peritoneum as chyloperitoneum, into the thorax as chylothorax and into the urine as chyluria.

Acquired lymphoedema

Acquired lymphoedema often affects only one limb, except when the obstructing lesion is due to an infective agent such as the filarial nematode *Wuchereria bancrofti*. This is a mosquito-borne parasite of tropical regions. The other infective agents that cause secondary lymphoedema are lymphogranuloma inguinale, tuberculosis and recurrent non-specific infection.

Tumour-induced secondary lymphoedema is most commonly associated with metastatic tumour of the breast causing upper limb lymphoedema and pelvic tumours of the cervix, ovary and uterus in the female, and of the prostate in males giving rise to lower limb lymphoedema.

Iatrogenic or trauma-induced lymphoedema occurs most frequently as a result of block dissections of either the axilla or groin, or in association with radiation of the same region.

The pathological complications of lymphoedema include recurrent infection such as cellulitis and chronic thickening of the skin with hyperkeratosis. In the very long term, lymphangiosarcoma may develop (see Chapter 56).

Clinical presentation

Primary lymphoedema

Primary or idiopathic lymphoedema can manifest clinically at various ages. Congenital lymphoedema is apparent at, or within a few weeks of, birth, often in association with some other congenital abnormality.

Lymphoedema praecox refers to lymphoedema not present at birth but which appears before the age of 35 years. It usually affects adolescent women.

Lymphoedema tarda becomes evident after the age of 35 years. This group of patients, usually females, may have uni- or bilateral limb swelling which can affect the upper or lower limbs. There may be a temporal relationship with a minor injury or surgery on the limb that preceeds the onset of the swelling. Initially the swelling is soft and pitting but with time the tissues become more indurated and fibrous. This change is hastened and accentuated by attacks of cellulitis.

Lymphoedema tends to affect the foot and the toes. In the later stages, the skin becomes thickened and hyperkeratotic with wart-like excrescences. In the severe and chronic stage, the limb has a tree trunk–like appearance and can be distinguished from venous oedema by the absence of prominent pigmentation and the chronic venous ulceration commonly seen in severe venous insufficiency oedema.

Secondary lymphoedema

The swelling of secondary lymphoedema develops more rapidly, often in an older age group and may be associated with dragging discomfort. This form of lymphoedema is frequently secondary to an obstructing lesion; thus there may be changes at the site of obstruction such as scarring, swelling and local erythema. As with primary lymphoedema, these patients are prone to episodes of cellulitis and lymphangitis.

Investigation

It is important to distinguish lymphoedema from venous oedema or if the swelling involves the lower limbs, or there is compression in the popliteal fossa. The clinical presentation, history and examination will usually suggest either of these conditions but each can be readily excluded by the use of duplex scanning of the lower limb venous system. If the scan does not demonstrate venous obstruction or venous valvular incompetence, the swelling is more likely to be lymphatic in origin. It is important to ensure that the iliac venous system has been sonographically interrogated before a venous cause is excluded.

Oedema associated with generalised problems, such as hypoproteinaemia, nephrotic syndrome or cardiac failure, will be excluded on clinical examination, biochemical tests (e.g. liver function tests, serum protein levels, urea, creatinine and electrolytes) and an examination of the urine for protein.

Specific investigations for lymphoedema are not usually employed as they rarely impact on management. They include lymphoscintography. Radioactive labelled colloids can be injected into the interdigital spaces and should appear within 30 minutes in the regional nodes if the lymphatic vessels are normal. Reduced uptake implies hypoplastic or obliterated lymphatic vessels. In obstructive secondary lymphoedema the radionucleotide uptake in the regional nodes is often normal. It may be slow in the more proximal nodes, indicating an obstruction at that level.

Computed tomography scanning of the regional node area will give an assessment of nodal enlargement if these are obstructive. In primary lymphoedema the number and size of nodes may be diminished.

Lymphangiography is now seldom used because it may accentuate the obliterative process of primary lymphoedema and give rise to infection or an inflammatory process that may relate to the contrast medium used. It will give information about the type and site of lymphatic obstruction and valvular incompetence in the lymph vessels in particular cases.

Hence the diagnosis of lymphoedema, particularly in primary lymphoedema, tends to be a diagnosis of exclusion.

The extent and severity of lymphoedema should be determined and recorded as baseline information to gauge subsequent treatment. The minimum is precise measurements of limb circumference with reference to defined bony points, for example 2 cm above the medial malleolus.

The major aim of investigating a patient with lymphoedema is to determine whether or not underlying pathology exists.

Treatment

The treatment of lymphoedema is essentially conservative.

Conservative treatment aims to preserve the quality of the skin, prevent lymphangitis and reduce limb size. Skin quality can be maintained by careful avoidance of trauma and regularly applying a water-based skin lotion. Non–skin drying soaps should be used to minimise the loss of oil from the skin.

Patients with lymphoedema are predisposed to cellulitis and spreading lymphangitis. The problem is that infection will further damage the lymphatic system. Patients should be warned to avoid trauma and to seek early and aggressive management of skin sepsis. Streptococci are the most common organisms causing cellulitis. Early treatment with systemically administered penicillin is indicated if any form of skin sepsis develops. The most common portal of entry is via associated interdigital fungal infection with tinea pedis. If a patient has recurrent attacks of cellulitis, long-term daily prophylaxis with 250 mg of pencillin twice daily is appropriate. For those allergic to penicillin, erythromycin may be given as treatment for acute infections. Any interdigital fungal infection should be treated regularly with an anti-fungal powder, and if there is an established infection, oral griseofulvin can be taken. If the infection fails to respond to standard treatment, alternative antibiotics can be considered.

Limb swelling is best managed with graded compression stockings. The patient should sleep with the foot of the bed elevated on the equivalent of two house bricks and graded compression stockings fitted before the patient gets out of bed. The stockings may range from 30 to 50 mm Hg in their compression depending on the tolerance of the patient. For those with whole limb swelling, the pantyhose or thigh stocking should be used. Similar stockings can be used for those with arm oedema.

Intermittent pneumatic compression may help to reduce limb swelling. The pneumatic compression is applied as a multi-cell unit arranged concentrically. The multi-cell unit inflates successively from peripheral to proximal and thus has a 'milking' action driving fluid from the periphery to the centre. The outcome for the use of compression stockings and the intermittent use of external pneumatic compression devices will achieve very satisfactory limb size control in the majority of patients.

Surgical treatment is rarely performed, being reserved for the few patients who cannot have their swelling controlled by compression, have repeated bouts of sepsis or in whom skin changes and the persisting swelling might suggest there is a risk of a neoplasm. Surgery may either involve excision of subcutaneous tissue (Charles operation) or attempts at lymphatic bypass – the latter being still experimental.

Prognosis and results of treatment

The majority of patients can control their leg swelling with compression stockings during the day and nocturnal elevation. The ability to achieve this goal is largely dependent upon the determination and compliance of the patient. This can be facilitated by putting the patient in touch with the local lymphoedema society (see 'Further reading').

Further reading

Davies D, Rogers M. Morphology of lymphatic malformations: a pictorial review. *Australas J Dermatol.* 2000; 41: 1–5.

Gloviczki P. Principles of surgical treatment of chronic lymphoedema. *Int Angiol.* 1999;18:42–46.

Szuba A, Rockson SG. Lymphoedema: Classification, diagnosis and therapy. *Vasc Med.* 1998;3:145–156.

www.lymphoedema.org.au

MCQs

Select the single correct answer to each question.

1 With regards to varicose veins, which of the following is *incorrect*?
  - **a** varicose veins are dilated, tortuous and visible when the patient is standing
  - **b** valvular incompetence is an integral component of the pathogenesis of varicose veins
  - **c** the principal superficial venous systems of the lower limbs are the long and the short saphenous systems
  - **d** the principal route of venous drainage from the lower limb is via the superficial venous system
  - **e** the principal driver of venous drainage from the legs in the erect position is the calf pump

2 Which of the following is incorrect? Patients with varicose veins may present to their doctor because of:
  - **a** calf pain after walking 200 m that is relieved by resting for 5 minutes
  - **b** a superficial ulcer on the ankle
  - **c** aching discomfort in the calf after prolonged standing
  - **d** superficial thrombophlebitis
  - **e** spontaneous bleeding from a varix

3 Which ONE of the following is correct?
  - **a** venography is an accurate method for investigating varicose veins
  - **b** duplex scanning has little to add to the pre-operative investigation of varicose veins
  - **c** the most frequent cause of recurrent varicose veins is neovascularisation
  - **d** due to frequent, serious late complications, all patients with varicose veins should be advised to have surgery
  - **e** patients with varicose veins and who have haemosiderin deposits and liposclerosis at the ankle should be treated

4 Which of the following is NOT true in the management of patients with varicose veins?
  - **a** below-knee-length elastic stockings may be definitive treatment in the patient in whom surgery is contraindicated because of co-morbidities
  - **b** injection with a sclerosing agent followed by elastic compression for 4–6 weeks can be beneficial
  - **c** using a below-knee elastic stocking may help decide if calf symptoms are due to varices
  - **d** surgical trials have demonstrated that it is not necessary to remove the long saphenous vein in the thigh
  - **e** endoscopic techniques to divide incompetent perforating veins have been developed

5 Primary lymphoedema:
  - **a** should be differentiated from oedema due to varicose veins with a duplex scan
  - **b** should be investigated with lymphoscintography before deciding on treatment
  - **c** is more common in women
  - **d** usually responds to nocturnal elevation and elastic compression during the day
  - **e** the response to therapy is monitored by serial measurement of limb circumference

Urology

55 Genitourinary tract

R. Gardiner

Anatomy and development

The kidney develops through three phases to form the metanephros, which migrates proximally as the tissue differentiates into the nephron and tubules, the calyces and the renal pelvis. At the same time, the urogenital sinus differentiates into the bladder and urethra and the ureteric bud, which communicates with the upper ureter arising from the metanephros. The prostate develops as an outgrowth of the urethral epithelium.

The kidneys lie retroperitoneally at the level of L1–2 and normally are supplied by single arteries, although up to 30% of people may have multiple arteries. The renal vein is again normally single on each side, draining into the inferior vena cava. Renal lymphatics drain to the para-aortic nodes.

The adult ureter is approximately 25 cm in length in adult life and runs retroperitoneally before swinging medially at the level of the ischial spine to pass through the bladder wall. The bladder lies within the pelvis but can expand upwards into the abdominal cavity. Arterial supply to the bladder and the lower ureters is via the internal iliac artery, and lymphatic drainage parallels venous drainage to the internal iliac nodes.

The male urethra passes through the prostate and is joined by the ejaculatory ducts. The prostate itself is a fibromuscular gland that drains into the urethra and, in terms of structure, is divided into peripheral, transitional and central zones (see Fig. 55.1). The arterial supply to the urethra and prostate is through the inferior vesical artery, and venous drainage is through the periprostatic plexus to the internal iliac veins. Lymphatic drainage is to the obturator and internal iliac nodes.

Clinical conditions

Disorders of the male external genitalia will be considered in a separate chapter (Chapter 56). Specific disorders of the genitourinary tract will be considered under the headings of urinary tract calculi, urinary tract infection, prostatitis, urethral stricture, benign prostatic hyperplasia, prostatic cancer, renal cell carcinoma and urothelial cancer.

Urinary tract calculi

Urinary calculi are defined as insoluble substances formed from the constituents of urine. They consist of crystalloids deposited on an organic matrix. In developed countries most stones are in the upper tract and present in about 2% of the population.

Aetiology

Urinary tract calculi are divided into infective and metabolic stones. Infective stones are caused by bacteria, mostly *Proteus* species containing the enzyme urease, which splits urea to form an insoluble complex of magnesium-ammonium-calcium phosphate. Bacteria become embedded in these stones, which form cast or staghorn calculi in renal pelves to produce a combination of obstruction and infection with eventual destruction of the kidney.

Most metabolic stones contain calcium (in combination with oxalate and/or phosphate) and, unlike most gallstones, are radio-opaque on plain X-ray. There is often a familial susceptibility. Although the aetiology is multifactorial, defined predisposing conditions such as primary hyperparathyroidism, Paget's disease

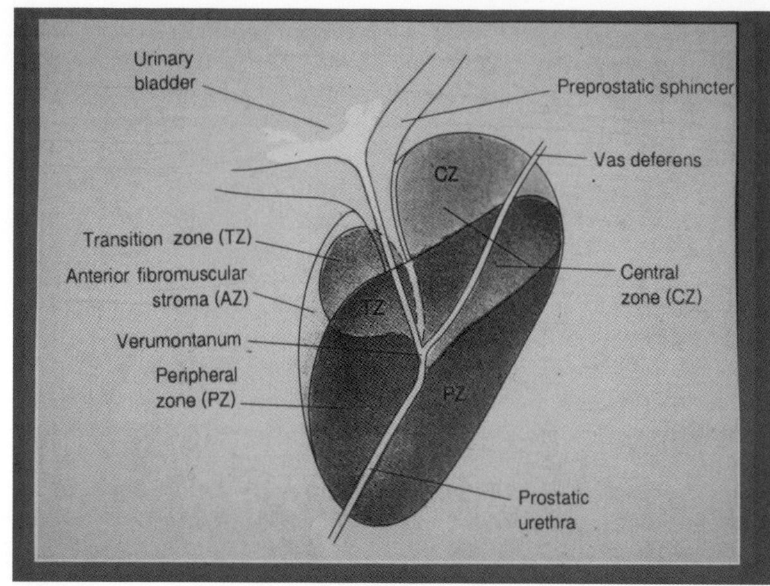

Fig. 55.1 Anatomy of the prostate.

and other bone demineralisation conditions, hyperthyroidism, sarcoidosis, impaired ileal function, renal tubular acidosis and medullary sponge kidneys are identifiable in a minority of patients.

Uric acid stones are radiolucent. Patients with gout and clinical states characterised by rapid protein catabolism are at risk of urate stone formation. Urate stones form in patients whose urinary pH is invariably lower than 6.5. Pure cystine stones also form in acid urine. Cystine stones (about 3% of calculi) are faintly identifiable on plain radiographs. This disorder is inherited in autosomal recessive fashion.

The principles of stone formation in the majority of patients, who do not have defined clinically predisposing conditions, can be considered in terms of hypersecretion and hyperconcentration of solutes, anatomical factors including a foreign body serving as a nidus, the role of inhibitory substances, and the part played by macro-molecules and matrix in crystal precipitation and aggregation.

Clinical presentation

Infective stones will be discussed in the section on urinary tract infection (UTI). Metabolic stones usually present with pain called renal, or more correctly, ureteric colic. This is an extremely severe pain that, classically, occurs without warning. The patient cannot find a comfortable position and rolls around or paces about in agony. He (patients are more often male) may notice pain radiating to the groin and the genital region and, generally, the lower the pain, the lower the stone. Pain in the loin suggests arrest at the pelviureteric junction, pain in the flank or groin suggests arrest at the pelvic brim, and pain in the genitalia suggests arrest at the ureterovesical junction. Vomiting is not a dominating feature although it is not uncommon for the patient to have vomited once. Some tenderness in the loin and along the line of the ureter is often present.

The differential diagnosis is that of an acute abdomen so the patient should be assessed as for an acute abdomen. Microscopic blood is usually present in the urine (routinely detected by dip-stick). Macroscopic blood is uncommon with ureteric colic from stone disease. The absence of blood on ward-testing does not exclude a diagnosis of ureteric colic and, conversely, a positive result may occur with other conditions.

Stones in the lowermost ureter may cause frequency and burning attributed to inflammation of distal ureteric smooth muscle, which extends into superficial trigone and urethra. A UTI may need to be excluded.

Diagnosis

The diagnosis is confirmed by intravenous urography (IVU; see Fig. 55.2) or, alternatively, especially if another cause for the pain is entertained, a spiral CT scan

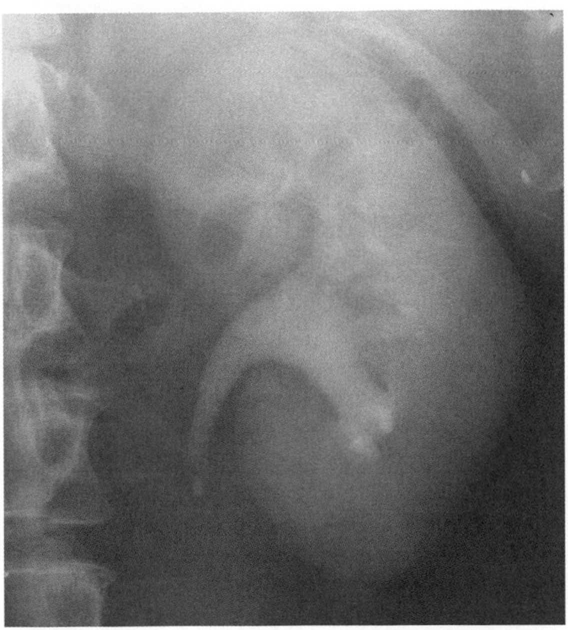

Fig. 55.2 Intravenous urogram showing a distended pelvicaliceal system with contrast tracking down to an obstructing stone in the upper ureter.

(which permits visualisation of the whole of both upper tracts). A plain radiograph by itself is insufficient, because phleboliths (calcified veins), calcified lymph nodes and, less commonly, radiolucent calculi may mislead. Unilateral partial obstruction is common at the time of acute presentation. Delay in excretion with dilatation of the collecting system above the obstruction is usually seen. Consequently delayed films may be required and, because excreted contrast medium is heavier than urine, patients should be in prone or erect positions for a little time before and during the taking of delayed radiographs so that contrast tracks to the level of obstruction.

Radiolucent stones cause filling defects. Ultrasound has little, if any, place diagnostically, because definition below the uppermost ureter is usually not provided. Furthermore, dilatation does not equal obstruction. Uncommonly, obstruction does occur without dilatation so that a functional study such as an IVU is much more informative.

Management

A definitive diagnosis by IVU or spiral CT scan is essential soon after presentation. Narcotic analgesia is recommended initially. Subsequent analgesia may be provided by indomethacin suppositories (± paracetamol) rather than repeated doses of narcotic analgesia. Intravenous fluids should only be given to replenish fluids if the patient is too nauseated to drink normally or is dehydrated. A diuresis is to be avoided at this stage, because this may exacerbate obstruction and worsen pain. It is not the hydrostatic pressure from a distended ureter that causes advancement of the stone, but rather coaptation of the ureteric walls above the stone advancing it distally.

Approximately 80% of upper tract stones pass spontaneously. Calculi of 4 mm diameter almost always pass without intervention, but most stones greater than 6 mm will not. Indications for surgical intervention include a stone too large to pass, complete obstruction (a rare occurrence), obstruction and infection, as well as the very relative indication of persisting pain without any progress in stone movement.

Chemolysis is often effective in causing dissolution of urate stones. A dilute urine with a pH higher than 7 is advised (usually induced by sodium bicarbonate). Allopurinol is also prescribed to minimise further uric acid formation.

Large renal stones are usually treated primarily by percutaneous nephrolithotomy with stone disintegration by extracorporeal shock wave lithotripsy (ESWL) used for calculi that are less than 2 cm in diameter; ESWL involves focusing a shock wave, generated outside the body, onto a stone localised by X-rays or ultrasound. Open renal surgery is now practised infrequently, its main role being stone removal *en passant* at the time of corrective surgery for predisposing anatomical abnormalities such as pelviureteric junction obstruction.

Stone basketry has been used for many years. With distal ureteric calculi, basketry may be performed through a cystoscope without ureteroscopy. However, basketry without ureteroscopic guidance is not recommended for stones above the distal few centimetres of ureter because of the risk of ureteric intussusception. Disintegration of ureteric stones may be effected by intracorporeal targeting with a ureteroscope (using laser, ultrasound, shock wave and physical energy sources) as well as ESWL (most effective in the upper ureter). An internal ureteric stent may facilitate passage of a stone by relieving obstruction (urine flowing mainly around the stent) and serving as a 'slide' for the calculus. The stent needs to be removed soon after it has served its purpose, as it may serve as a nidus for stone formation.

Apart from a chest X-ray and routine biochemical profile to exclude predisposing and correctable underlying medical conditions, together with chemical analysis of the calculus, other investigations are reserved for recurrent stone formers. All patients should be induced to drink sufficient fluid so that their urine is visibly dilute at all times.

Urinary tract infection

Introduction

Urinary tract infections (UTIs) are extremely common in females, with most women experiencing at least one in a lifetime.

Causative organisms are *Escherichia coli* (approximately 80% of UTI in the community and about 50% in hospitals), *Proteus* species (the presence of which should always alert to the possibility of an infective stone), *Pseudomonas*, *Klebsiella* and *Enterobacter*, as well as the Gram-positive cocci *Streptococcus faecalis* and, occasionally, *Staphylococcus aureus*.

Pathogenesis

Both bacterial and host factors are relevant. Bacteria from the bowel or external genitalia colonise the urethral meatus then migrate in a retrograde fashion into the bladder. Other forms of access to the urinary tract (such as haematogenous, lymphatic and innocula introduced with instrumentation) are less common. Variation in bacterial virulence factors (such as adhesin expression and phase variation) and host-cell receptivity to bacteria (due to intrinsic and extrinsic factors) dynamically affect the host–bacteria relationship.

Clinical presentation

The most common site of bacterial infection in the male is the prostate. A diagnosis of UTI is based on a combination of symptoms and bacteriological findings. Patients complain of burning and frequency, with a feeling of wanting to void continually. Lower abdominal discomfort is common. If haematuria is present this requires thorough investigation subsequently.

A significant proportion of female patients with these symptoms do not have a UTI. The differential diagnosis includes detrusor instability, vaginitis, abacterial cystourethritis and, rarely, carcinoma *in situ*. Consequently, urinary bacteriology is essential to make an accurate diagnosis. Normal urine is abacteriuric. By convention, more than 10^5 organisms per millilitre from a freshly voided midstream specimen is regarded as infection, as this figure indicates a higher than 90% probability of UTI rather than contamination.

Increased numbers of leucocytes are to be expected in a UTI. Increased numbers of epithelial cells strongly suggest contamination.

Acute pyelonephritis is diagnosed on the basis of loin pain and tenderness in association with fevers in a constitutionally unwell patient. Persisting pyuria may be due to resolving UTI, stone, foreign body, sloughed papilla and, uncommonly in Australasia, tuberculosis (TB). Schistosomiasis due to *Schistosoma haematobium* contracted in Africa or the Middle East may also cause pyuria although non-specific UTIs do occur as with genito-urinary TB.

Treatment

Patients presenting acutely with symptoms of UTIs need to be treated as having a UTI until an alternative diagnosis is proven. After providing a specimen for urine microscopy and bacteriology, patients are advised to take a single dose (200 mg nitrofurantoin or 600 mg trimethoprim) or a 3–5-day course of combination amoxycillin/clavulinic acid, trimethoprim or nitrofurantoin.

A further micro-urine examination is required following treatment of an uncomplicated UTI to confirm eradication of the offending organism. If there is a recurrence of symptoms, further microscopy and bacteriology are required to determine whether this is another UTI and, if so, whether this is due to a different organism (recurrent infection) or a recrudescence of a prior, partially treated UTI (relapse). Approximately 90% of subsequent UTI episodes are due to different organisms (i.e. recurrent infections).

For relapsing UTI a reason for failure of eradication needs to be sought. This may be due to not taking the medication, a large residual urine in the bladder, a stone or foreign body or renal scarring as a consequence of childhood vesico-ureteric reflux.

Patients with acute pyelonephritis require intravenous fluids together with gentamicin and amoxycillin during the acute phase followed by maintenance trimethoprim, or oroquinolones for 2–4 weeks. An IVU during the period of hospitalisation will identify those patients who have a complicating stone.

As a principle, before prescribing any medications for women or adolescent females, enquire regarding the patient's current pregnancy status and, if in doubt, prescribe a medication approved for use in pregnancy.

Investigations

All men with UTIs and women with complicated UTIs (which include relapsing and upper tract infections) require investigation. An IVU may provide information regarding renal scarring and stone formation with suspected incomplete bladder emptying confirmed by catheter or trans-abdominal ultrasound estimation of residual urine. Occasionally a technetium-99m dimercapto-succinic acid (^{99m}Tc DMSA) renal scan will be required to demonstrate scarring.

Special considerations

Infective stones

A *Proteus* UTI should always raise the possibility of an infective stone. Cast or staghorn calculi form with bacteria entrapped so that a combination of obstruction and infection ensues, with destruction of renal parenchyma as the end result. Antibacterial therapy alone is ineffective. Stone clearance is required.

Perinephric abscess

If untreated, a pyonephrosis may develop from an infective stone to extend to form a perinephric abscess. This may become large, inducing chronic ill health and anaemia. Perinephric abscesses can also develop from renal carbuncles that are metastatic infections to the renal cortex, the bacteria in these cases most often being staphylococci. Perinephric abscesses require drainage followed by treatment of underlying predisposing causes. Abdominal ultrasound is valuable in diagnosis and in instituting drainage.

Asymptomatic bacteriuria

Asymptomatic bacteriuria in healthy women seldom needs treatment because it is self-limiting and usually transitory. Similarly, asymptomatic patients with indwelling catheters and bacteriuria should not be prescribed antibacterial drugs because, apart from the untoward risks and costs associated with drug therapy, resistant organisms are likely to emerge. However, treatment of asymptomatic bacteriuria is advised in girls and pregnant women because of the considerable likelihood of symptomatic UTI developing.

Genitourinary tuberculosis

Genitourinary TB, always secondary to TB elsewhere (usually in the lung), may present as a non-specific UTI. If suspected a chest X-ray and three early morning urine specimens for culture for acid-fast bacilli are indicated. Microscopy alone is not sufficient, because acid-fast contaminants may cause a misdiagnosis. Long-term monitoring is imperative. Treatment is undertaken with standard anti-tuberculous drugs.

Urinary tract infections in children

Children need to be regarded differently because of the higher likelihood of underlying congenital abnormalities. In the neonatal period girls and boys are afflicted in comparable numbers, but girls predominate subsequently. Urinary tract infections are diagnosed in approximately 5% of schoolgirls, highlighting the frequency of such infections.

Haematogenous spread of infection to the kidney is common in neonates, while the ascending route via the urethra predominates in older children. *Escherichia coli* is the offending organism in 80% of cases.

Before the age of 2 years children often present looking ill with fevers and non-specific symptoms of vomiting and diarrhoea with dehydration. In older children, burning, frequency and back pain may be present, although some have symptoms not referable to the urinary tract.

Abdominal ultrasound examination is routine. If the child is less than 2 years old or an abnormality is detected, a micturating cystourethrogram is ordered. The underlying conditions of particular importance that are sought are vesico-ureteric reflux, and urethral valves in boys. Vesico-ureteric reflux in the presence of a UTI and intrarenal reflux (of the compound calices at the upper and lower poles) result in scarring. Long-term sequelae are chronic pyelonephritis and hypertension.

Ideally, management of vesico-ureteric reflux is orchestrated by liaison between a paediatric urologist or a paediatric surgeon and a paediatric nephrologist. Most children require long-term maintenance antibacterial prophylaxis, with only the most severe cases needing surgical intervention. The presence of urethral valves is an indication for prompt intervention.

Prostatitides

The conditions previously constituting the prostatitides were reclassified in 1997. New National Institute of Health categories of chronic pelvic pain syndromes (CPPS) are acute and chronic bacterial prostatitis (CPPS I & II), chronic abacterial prostatitis (CPPS IIIa) and prostatodynia (CPPS IIIb). Category CPPS IV consists of asymptomatic inflammatory prostatitis, with the diagnosis made incidentally by prostatic biopsy or by white cells in expressed prostatic secretions or semen, identified during evaluation of other disorders.

CPPS I, II and IIIa are those in which white cells are detected in prostatic secretions, post-prostatic massage urine or semen from symptomatic men, with accompanying bacteria for both CPPS I and II, but not CPPS IIIa. With the exception of acute prostatitis (CPPS I), which is a distinct clinical entity, CPPS II (chronic bacterial prostatitis) and both CPPS III sub-category patients have clinically indistinguishable chronic pelvic pain.

Acute bacterial prostatitis

This is a potentially life-threatening affliction characterised by high fever, chills, rigors, lower urinary tract symptoms and the presence of a tender, often hot, swollen prostate on digital rectal examination (DRE). To minimise any risk of septic emboli, DRE should be performed gently. Gram-negative bacteria are present in urine samples.

Treatment, after obtaining urine and blood samples for bacteriology, consists of parenteral gentamicin and amoxycillin with intravenous fluids initially. A minimum of 8 weeks of trimethoprim or one of the new oroquinolones, after the patient is no longer toxic, is recommended. If urinary retention develops, a stab suprapubic catheter is advocated in preference to a urethral catheter.

Chronic prostatitides (CPPS II, IIIa and IIIb)

Patients are young adult to middle-aged, complaining of urethral burning, perineal pain, suprapubic discomfort and frequency. The prostate is not abnormal on DRE. Differentiation between the three clinical conditions is provided by microscopy and bacteriological culture of an initial voided (urethral) specimen, followed by a midstream urine (bladder) analysis, prostatic fluid expressed by prostatic massage and a urethral massage (post-void urine).

Chronic bacterial prostatitis (CPPSII)

Patients have episodes of urinary infection with intermittent asymptomatic periods of days to months. Prostatic fluid contains increased numbers of white cells and Gram-negative bacilli (most often *E. coli*). Absolute bacterial counts and white cell numbers are less important than their presence.

Treatment options are limited by the small number of antibacterial drugs able to concentrate in adequate levels in the prostate. Trimethoprim and the new oroquinolones, in particular ciprofloxacin, are effective, with protracted treatment required for resistant cases.

Abacterial prostatitis (CPPS IIIa)

The aetiology remains unknown. A 4–8-week course of tetracycline or erythromycin may benefit some, although these men often return with further symptoms. Non-traditional dietary supplements are sometimes beneficial, with quercin recently shown to demonstrate clinically significant relief in a double-blind, placebo trial.

Non-inflammatory chronic pelvic pain syndrome (CPPSIIIb)

Non-inflammatory pelvic pain syndrome patients may have a non-prostatic cause for their symptoms and the differential diagnosis includes interstitial cystitis (IC), drug effects, such as the non-steroidal anti-inflammatory drugs tiaprofenic acid and diflunisal and DO. After voided urinary cytology, cystoscopy and urodynamic studies may reveal a cause.

Urethral stricture

Strictures represent a pathological narrowing of the urethral lumen, causing both anatomical and functional obstruction.

Aetiology and classification

Strictures may be congenital or acquired, or due to inflammation or trauma (from both internal and severe external trauma), although often the cause remains unknown (idiopathic). Submeatal and bulbomembranous regions are the most common sites.

Presentation and diagnosis

The classical presentation is with a narrowed or weak flow. By the time the stream is noticeably thin, the luminal diameter is reduced considerably.

An ascending urethrogram is the most useful diagnostic investigation. For a urethrogram to be considered normal, dye should outline an anterior urethra of regular calibre and needs to be seen entering the bladder without having extravasated.

Treatment

Dilatation by either rigid or flexible dilators remains the most common form of management. Flexible dilators may be introduced under direct urethroscopic vision or blindly. Patients may keep their urethral lumina patent by self-catheterisation once or twice a week. Catheters are passed completely into the bladder to ensure that the whole of the urethra is traversed.

Urethrotomy under vision is unlikely to be successful if there is full-thickness bulbo-spongio-fibrosis but may be of value in partial-thickness strictures. Excision and re-anastomosis is suitable for some short strictures, with substitution (buccal mucosa or skin) urethroplasty employed in others.

Complications

Restricturing is common after dilatation or urethrotomy. Bacteraemia may occur during treatment (particularly dilatation). Prophylactic pre-procedural gentamicin and amoxycillin are administered routinely to these patients in order to avoid this problem.

Benign prostatic hyperplasia

Introduction

If they live long enough nearly all men will develop microscopic benign prostatic hyperplasia (BPH). About half of these men will develop macroscopic enlargement of the gland, with only one half again developing symptomatic BPH.

Pathogenesis and pathology

BPH is a result of hyperplasia of both epithelial and stromal elements of the transition zone (see Fig. 55.1) with stromal elements (mostly smooth muscle and connective tissue) predominating.

Clinical presentation

BPH may cause bladder outflow obstruction (BOO), which is a functional obstruction with catheters and instruments able to be passed in an antegrade fashion, usually without difficulty. Prostatic size bears no relationship to whether or not BOO is present.

Symptoms attributed to BPH are predominantly those of bladder dysfunction, with only hesitancy and slow stream reported to correlate with BOO. What is perceived as poor flow may be due to small volumes voided. The irritable symptoms of urgency, urgency incontinence and frequency are non-specific.

Frequency, excluding polyuria, is due to a functionally small (rarely an anatomically small) bladder. The functionally reduced bladder capacity may be due to sensory or motor causes (or both).

DO due to inappropriate bladder muscle contractions with generation of raised intravesical pressures, occurs in most patients with significant BOO. Once BOO is relieved, DO usually disappears, but may persist if the cause is neuropathic or idiopathic. (An idiopathic aetiology is increasingly common with ageing, for both genders).

Incomplete bladder emptying does not equal obstruction and there is a group of patients with poorly contracting detrusors who do not have BOO and for whom prostatic resistance lowering strategies are unlikely to be helpful. Chronic urinary retention is considered when residual urine is less than 300 mL. Patients with high-pressure chronic retention classically present with nocturnal enuresis and few, if any, urinary symptoms. These men may also have bilateral hydronephrosis and impaired renal function due to back-pressure.

Acute urinary retention (painful bladder distension) is more common. It may be precipitated by a diuresis (with or without alcohol), alpha-stimulant drugs or anticholinergic medication, a rectum loaded with faeces, acute prostatitis or prostatic infarction. The possibility of a neuropathic cause should always be considered.

Diagnosis

The severity of symptoms should be assessed. The significance to the patient may be semi-quantified by symptom scores (e.g. the International Prostate Symptom Score [IPSS]) completed independently by the patient.

Nocturia, the most disruptive symptom, should be considered in context with length of slumber and whether or not the patient's bladder wakens him. Fluid and drug (including alcohol) taking patterns and a voiding time-volume chart (recording every volume voided with the time of micturition over several representative 24 hour periods) are pertinent. Nocturnal polyuria may result from nocturnal diuresis after evening alcohol ingestion, fluid redistribution in cardiac failure or abnormal anti-diuretic hormone (ADH) production from sleep apnoea or tumours. Following abdominal and limited neurological examination, DRE is essential.

Investigations

A micro-urine examination and urine culture are essential to exclude infection. Transabdominal ultrasound examination of the upper tracts with a plain X-ray of the abdomen and pelvis (rather than IVU) is recommended. Ultrasound of the lower tracts also permits estimation of residual urine.

As an accurate diagnosis of BOO from BPH cannot be made on symptoms alone, a voided urinary flow rate and urodynamic studies, with bladder pressure/voided urine flow recordings, may be used to provide objective evidence of BOO. However, sustained symptomatic relief following effective lowering of bladder outflow resistance does not correlate accurately with the presence or absence of demonstrable obstruction prior to treatment.

Treatment

Apart from acute urinary retention in the presence of preceding symptoms supportive of BOO and chronic retention with upper tract dilatation and bladder calculi, indications for treatment are relative. In the short term, symptoms due to BOO fluctuate, although with time they gradually worsen. Treatment strategies available for BOO include pharmacological and procedural approaches.

Pharmacological approaches

There is evidence that the "natural product" saw palmetto (*Serenoa repens*) can be effective in reducing lower urinary tract symptoms.

5α-reductase inhibitor drugs competitively inhibit conversion of testosterone to dihydrotestosterone, causing a reduction in prostatic size due to an effect on epithelial cells with an associated decrease in prostate-specific antigen (PSA) levels by approximately 50%. Patients with larger prostates are more likely to experience symptomatic relief, after 3 to 6 months, and a reduced likelihood of acute urinary retention. Several placebo-controlled trials confirm the durability of 5α-reductase inhibitor drugs in the management of BOO which, unlike α-1 blocking agents, are better tolerated in the longer term. α-1 blocking agents reduce urethral and prostatic smooth muscle tone, producing a symptomatic effect within weeks. There is comparable efficacy for all members of this family of drugs, with postural hypotension the main untoward effect. Although a selective α-1_A subtype antagonist is available, dizziness remains problematical as an unwanted effect.

Surgical procedures

The operative procedure of transurethral resection of prostate (TURP) is the standard operation for relieving BOO due to BPH. Open enucleative prostatectomy is now reserved for large, vascular glands and selected patients with narrowed or strictured urethras.

There is an erroneous view that TURP is a simple 're-bore' of the prostate able to be performed almost mechanically on any patient. It requires regional or general anaesthesia and is associated with peri-operative and post-operative morbidity and mortality (albeit low). Retrograde emission is to be expected following TURP because the bladder neck is resected. Potency difficulties are not commonly a problem. Dribbling and urgency incontinence may occur post-operatively, with strictures and chronic urinary infections as the possible long-term sequelae.

A less invasive procedure, better suited to small prostates, is bladder neck incision (BNI), which involves making one or two incisions completely through the region of the bladder neck extending to just above the distal sphincter. This enables the prostatic urethra to open and funnel during voiding, thus relieving BOO. Retrograde emission is less likely, because the bladder neck is incised rather than resected. Consequently, the bladder neck should continue to remain closed during ejaculation (when the distal sphincter relaxes), only opening with detrusor contractions.

Of a number of other procedures introduced over the recent past, those which have established a niche as being less invasive than TURP yet effective and durable include transurethral microwave thermotherapy and radio-frequency-needle ablation thermotherapy. Laser techniques have evolved over the past few years such that laser prostatectomy is now comparably effective with TURP as well as providing the advantages of minimal peri-operative blood loss and shorter inpatient times.

Prostatic cancer

Introduction

This is the most common cancer diagnosed clinically in men and the second most common cause of male cancer deaths in Australasia. The lowest rates are in Asia and the highest rates in Scandinavia and the United States, particularly in African Americans.

The significance of prostate cancer as a major health issue is underestimated. The oft-quoted line that 'more men die with prostate cancer than from it' misleads, falsely implying an innocuous nature. Importantly, age has no significant prognostic effect in contemporary series. The morbidity that prostate cancer exacts from middle-aged and elderly men, both from the disease itself and its various treatments is considerable, the magnitude of unwanted effects (and costs) escalating with advancing stage of disease.

Aetiology and pathology

Prostate cancer is rare before 40 years, with prevalence increasing with age. Family susceptibility is regarded as comparable with that of breast cancer, with the risk of developing prostate cancer increasing with the number of genetic relatives diagnosed with this disease.

The large majority of tumours are adenocarcinomas. Because of their heterogeneous nature histologically, the Gleason scoring system has become accepted as most useful clinically. Most prostate cancers progress slowly so that, with contemporary earlier diagnosis, the overall 10-year survival expectancy is comparable with men without prostate cancer but at 15 years, there is a considerable difference. However, for patients with higher Gleason scores the average life expectancy is approximately 5–10 years.

Diagnosis

Clinically, prostatic cancer presents late either with BOO or with symptoms from metastases. There are no early symptoms of this disease. Approximately 10–15% of patients who have TURP for what is clinically BPH have carcinoma diagnosed in the resected fragments: 25% of prostatic cancers arise in the same (transition) zone as BPH, with 70% in the peripheral zone and 5% in the central zone. About 50% of solitary nodules felt by DRE will be malignant. A histological diagnosis of prostatic cancer is required before any form of treatment is contemplated.

Prostatic cancers also present as sciatica, anaemia, weight loss or with bony pain.

Investigations

Prostate specific antigen

Raised serum PSA levels occur with BPH, bacterial prostatitis (CPPS I & II), prostate cancer and following instrumentation. A normal DRE is unlikely to cause elevation. PSA is a labile enzyme, fluctuating diurnally. Raised PSA levels are found in 90% or more of patients diagnosed with prostatic cancer. However PSA is not a test for cancer because it is neither sensitive nor specific enough, and should be employed together with DRE.

Adaptations to improve the discriminatory ability of PSA include PSA velocity (rate of increase in PSA with time) and age-related PSA changes. Assays vary so PSA velocity assessments need to be made using the same assay. The ratio of free to total PSA is also useful with a lower free component present in patients with prostate cancer. However, ejaculation may result in a temporary surge of free PSA in the serum.

Although serum PSA is definitely not a specific screening or diagnostic test for prostatic cancer, once a tumour has been diagnosed, it usually serves as a very sensitive indicator of progress of disease and response to treatment.

Transrectal ultrasound

Transrectal ultrasound (TRUS) permits definition of prostatic anatomy, but not prostatic cancer. Its main value is for spatial positioning of spring-loaded needles for transrectal prostatic biopsies. These biopsies are uncomfortable procedures with a small but definite risk of septicaemia despite routine pre-procedural enema and antibacterial prophylaxis. Haematospermia, blood on faeces and haematuria with difficulty voiding are not unexpected short-term sequelae.

Staging

Prostate cancer spreads by local extension to periprostatic tissues, lymphatic spread to obturator, internal iliac and presacral nodes, and venous spread to involve the axial skeleton, predominantly with osteosclerotic metastases.

Prostate cancer is only curable when localized to the prostate. Lymph node involvement indicates systemic disease. Currently, radionuclide bone scanning is the standard method for detecting bony metastases. However, even when the cancer is thought to be localised clinically, up to 25% of patients have occult metastases.

Treatment

Management options include a role for 'watchful waiting', with radiotherapy and total (radical) prostatectomy remaining the only potential curative therapies for tumours confined to the prostate. Androgen suppression affords palliation for most patients with metastatic disease. There is no established place for chemotherapy in routine treatment.

Localised prostatic cancers usually progress slowly with an estimated doubling time of 2 years. As all interventional strategies are associated with unwanted effects and co-morbidity is common in the elderly, a place for a watch and wait (close surveillance) policy remains appropriate, especially if life expectancy is less than 10 years. Most men die with, rather than from, their prostate cancers. However, because of its proclivity to metastasise to the axial skeleton, men dying of prostate cancer have the potential to die badly.

Total (radical) prostatectomy

Radical prostatectomy is generally regarded as the reference treatment, with a 90% 10-year disease-specific survival for organ-confined tumours. The incontinence rate is approximately 7% at 12 months and the impotence rate is at least 30%. Other significant complications are urethral stricture, lymphocele, and deep venous thrombosis. Morbidity is greater in elderly patients and there is a definite, albeit low, peri-operative mortality of less than 0.5%.

Radiotherapy

The other potentially curative form of treatment is radiotherapy. Supervoltage radiotherapy is probably comparably effective as radical prostatectomy with lower mortality and incontinence rates. Impotence following supervoltage radiotherapy for prostate cancer is not uncommon, with varying degrees of proctitis; rectal bleeding and faecal soiling remain incapacitating for a minority well beyond the end of therapy – sometimes requiring definitive surgical treatment subsequently. The routine use of many months of peri-procedural androgen suppression therapy adjunctively, shown to improve survival in the intermediate term, adds a further dimension to the unwanted effect profile with contemporary supervoltage treatment.

Over the past few years, a resurgence of interest has developed regarding local radiotherapy (brachytherapy) alone or in combination with supervoltage radiotherapy. Improved imaging and isotope placement techniques have resulted in excellent cancer control in the medium to long term in selected patients. Brachytherapy is attractive because of its minimal invasiveness and perceived lack of side effects. While irritative voiding and minor proctitis problems are common in the short term, long-term unwanted effects are less of a problem. Patients with severe preceding urinary symptoms and those who have previously had a TURP are most at risk to have continence problems subsequently: potency difficulties are not uncommon following brachytherapy.

Androgen suppression

Androgen suppression is the mainstay of treatment for non-localised disease. Approximately 80% of patients demonstrate a durable response, with a median duration response of 24–36 months. The faster the PSA returns to the normal range, the better the response and prognosis. Methods currently used for androgen suppression include bilateral orchidectomy (the reference treatment), depot injections of long-acting luteinising hormone-releasing hormone (LHRH) analogues and anti-androgens.

There is no clear evidence that commencing androgen suppression early improves survival. An initial testosterone surge ("flare effect"), loss of muscle mass, osteoporosis, anaemia, hot flushes and adverse cognitive changes accompany LHRH analogue administration; liver dysfunction, depression, drowsiness and gynaecomastia result from anti-androgen therapy. Loss of sexual desire and impotence have been identified as the most important factors adversely affecting the quality of life of these men. Unfortunately, not all unwanted effects are reversible, negating the benefit of intermittent androgen blockade (IAB) compared with a delay in commencing androgen suppression initially. The use of maximal androgen blockade (MAB) to also address adrenal androgens affords little if any benefit in terms of tumour control but certainly increases the likelihood and magnitude of unwanted effects.

Renal cell carcinoma

Renal cell cancer (RCC) constitutes approximately 2–3% of malignancies. Approximately 60% of RCCs are diagnosed in men, with the incidence increasing from the mid-fifties.

Aetiology and pathology

The aetiology remains unknown, but RCC arise more commonly in patients afflicted by Von Hippel–Lindau (VHL) disease. A VHL gene mutation rate of 33–70% has been reported in sporadic RCCs. RCCs usually develop *de novo* as solid, parenchymal lesions but may arise in the wall of complex, septated cysts.

Clear cell (75–85%), chromophilic (papillary) (15%), chromophobic (5%), oncocytic (uncommon) and collecting duct (rare) tumours constitute the 5 subtypes of RCC. The best prognostic projection from histology is afforded by the nuclear grading system of Fuhrman. Descriptions of other mass lesions are given in Box 55.1. Direct spread, with a predilection for venous propagation and metastases and lymphatic spread to hilar and retroperitoneal lymph nodes are features of this neoplasm.

Clinical presentation

In the past RCC presented late, being clinically quiescent until quite large with haematuria, the most common presenting symptom. Increasingly, RCC is being diagnosed as an incidental finding on abdominal imaging studies.

Local effects

Pathological kidneys are prone to injury with even trivial trauma. Pain occurs from local extension and clot colic. A varicocele that develops after early adulthood raises the possibility of a left testicular vein obstruction from a propagated renal tumour thrombus (see Chapter 56).

Toxic effects

A pyrexia of unknown origin as a mode of presentation occurs in only a small percentage of patients, although fever is said to occur in approximately 20% of patients during their clinical course. Anaemia may result from bone marrow metastases, but also from toxic effects, as can a hepatopathy with abnormal lactate dehydrogenase and serum alkaline phosphatase levels as well as impaired prothrombin production. These effects are reversible with removal of the tumour.

Box 55.1 Other mass lesions of the kidney

- Angiomyolipomas are chorostomas containing considerable amounts of fat readily evident in CT scans. They are more common in women, who may present following intra-lesional haemorrhage, especially if the lesion is less than 4 cm diameter. A proportion have stigmata of tuberous sclerosis.
- Complex renal cysts
- Phaechromocytoma
- Sarcomas form rarely in the connective tissues of and surrounding the kidney. Fibrosarcomas and leiomyosarcomas, in particular, pursue aggressive clinical courses with rapid growth and vascular spread.
- Polycystic kidney may present as a renal mass, although usually bilateral and with a strong family history. Adult polycystic kidney disease has an autosomal dominant inheritance pattern. Cysts may be present in liver and pancreas.
- Wilms' tumour (nephroblastoma) is the most common abdonimal neoplasm in children, and is uncommon in adults. A mass detected by palpation or imaging is the usual mode of presentation. CT scanning of abdomen and chest, because of possible lung metastases, is routine. Treatment consists of nephrectomy with radiotherapy and chemotherapy.

Endocrine effects

Renal cell carcinomas are able to produce many hormones. Erythrocytosis is the most common manifestation. Ectopic renin and other tumour products causing hypertension may contribute to the development of heart failure, and high-output cardiac failure may develop as a result of shunting through large pathological vascular channels.

Investigations

A CT scan with radiocontrast (see Fig. 55.3) is the next investigation following ultrasound of a space-occupying lesion (SOL) not demonstrating the classical

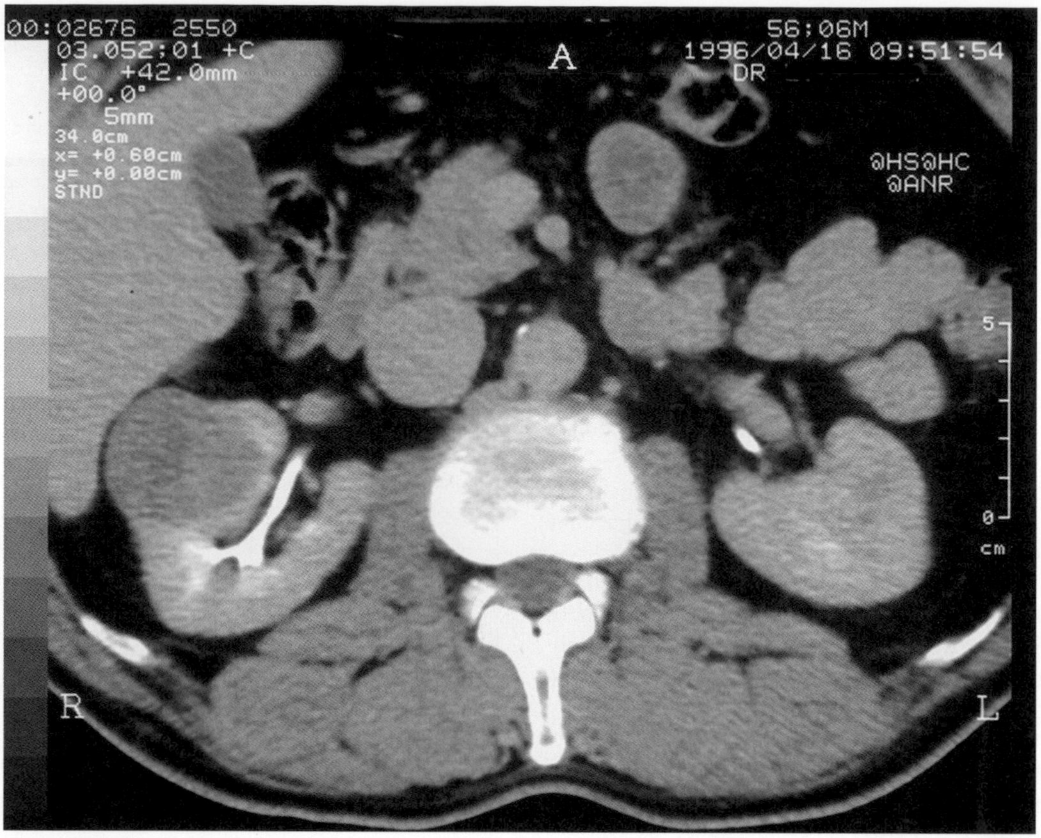

Fig. 55.3 Computed tomography scan through both kidneys following intravenous contrast injection. There is a slightly enhancing space-occupying lesion in the right kidney protruding beyond the kidney.

features of a simple cyst (viz. anechoic with posterior wall accentuation). Classically, RCCs protrude from and replace renal parenchyma and/or distort the pelvicaliceal arrangement. They 'contrast enhance' in the post-injection phase in most instances by virtue of their vascularity. If an upper pole tumour is suspected, the adrenal gland must be identified, as adrenal tumours (especially phaeochromocytomas) may be difficult to distinguish. The possibility of tumour thrombus should be sought, with ultrasound often useful in this regard. Identifiable hilar, paracaval and para-aortic lymph nodes may be due to follicular hyperplasia or secondary deposits. The contralateral kidney, liver, lung fields and vertebrae should be examined thoroughly in the search for possible metastases.

Radioisotope bone scanning using a labelled phosphate compound that concentrates in sites of increased phosphate metabolism in bone remains the standard for detecting metastatic osseous deposits. Reference plain X-rays may be required to exclude false-positive 'hot spots' from non-metastatic lesions such as Paget's disease, and healing fractures.

Treatment

Radical nephrectomy with a surrounding envelope of fat and fascia, which remains the only effective form of treatment, has little place for patients with secondary tumours unless performed to relieve local symptoms. With few exceptions, if lymphatic metastases are present, the patient has systemic disease, with less than 35% chance of surviving 5 years. Where the tumour is confined to the kidney or within Gerota's fascia, 5-year survival rates of around 60% can be expected.

Propagation of tumour thrombus into the venous system, seemingly in preference to direct and lymphatic spread in some patients, involves the IVC in 5–10% of cases and may extend into the right atrium. Tumour thrombus in the IVC does not cause the tumour to be inoperable, because prognosis relates to the presence or absence of lymphatic and other metastases. However, in general terms, the higher the tumour thrombus the worse the prognosis because of the increasing likelihood of coexisting metastases.

Urothelial cancer

Introduction

The urothelium is the epithelial lining of the urinary tract extending from the collecting tubules to the urethral meatus.

Although urothelial cancers can involve any part of the urothelium, most arise in the bladder. In the upper tract, renal pelvis and lower ureter are the most common sites. Upper tract to lower tract rate is approximately 1 : 30. The incidence of bladder cancer has increased by 50% in the past 35 years and this tumour now forms approximately 3% of all new cancers. The male to female ratio is 7 : 3.

Aetiology

Cigarette smoking is considered responsible for approximately 40% of bladder cancers, with 25% attributed to occupational exposure. Occupations considered to be 'at risk' include those associated with handling of chemicals, especially naphthylamine, magenta, auramine and benzidine.

Phenacetin has been incriminated as the carcinogenic agent in compound headache powders containing aspirin, phenacetin and caffeine (APC) that were ingested habitually in Australia in the past. These patients also developed papillary necrosis and renal failure, although these manifestations are now less common with legislation that bans the sale of such compound powders. Bilharziasis from *Schistosoma haematobium*, a common condition in Egypt and East Africa, predisposes to bladder cancer, particularly squamous cell carcinoma.

Pathology

These are largely transitional cell carcinomas (90–95%), with squamous cell carcinoma and occasional adenocarcinomas constituting the remainder. Adenocarcinoma of the bladder is a rarity and is a secondary tumour (mostly from bowel) until proven otherwise.

Superficial tumours are limited to the mucosa and lamina propria (70–75%), invasive tumours involve the muscularis propria and beyond (20–25%), with the remainder being widespread flat carcinoma *in situ* (CIS). In the bladder, CIS is a malignancy rather than a premalignant condition.

Clinical presentation

The presenting symptom in the vast majority of patients is haematuria, with day- and night-time frequency (often without haematuria) the dominant symptom for CIS. A history of haematuria, even if fleeting, must never be ignored, with prompt exclusion of a urothelial cancer of paramount importance.

Investigations

Voided urine cytology is the most useful adjunctive, non-invasive test but, by itself, is insufficiently sensitive to replace the definitive investigations below. Cytology is particularly valuable for detecting the presence of CIS.

Upper tract urothelial tumours produce filling defects or obstruction on IVU or helical CT scan with radiocontrast. The status of the upper tracts should be determined before cysto-urethroscopy to permit the option of retrograde studies, mostly retrograde pyelograms and saline lavaging to disaggregate tumour cells for cytology, at the time of endoscopic examination. Alternatively ureteroscopy (± biopsy) may also be performed.

The non-contrast phase of CT scans distinguishes radiolucent calculi from other causes of a filling defect on IVU. Tumours, blood clots and sloughed papillae are of tissue density. In addition, a CT scan of the pelvic region may aid in determining extravesical extension, although early tumour extension into the bladder wall is not reliably demonstrable radiographically.

Cysto-urethroscopy forms the basis for the diagnosis of bladder and urethral cancers, initial inspections being performed increasingly by flexible instruments. Tumours are biopsied through the working element of the cystoscope and adequate biopsy will allow the depth of invasion of the bladder wall (stage) to be determined and the degree of anaplasia (grade) to be assessed.

Treatment

Tumours of the upper and lower tracts require different forms of treatment.

Ureteric and renal pelvic urothelial cancers

Treatment for ureteric and renal pelvic urothelial cancers is by nephro-ureterectomy, together with excision of a cuff of bladder. Periodic check cystoscopies are performed because further tumours are likely to develop subsequently.

Superficial bladder cancer

Superficial and submucosally invasive tumours of the bladder are treated by endoscopic transurethral resection of the bladder (TURB), using a resectoscope with cutting and coagulating diathermy. The tumour base is resected separately to facilitate histopathological staging. There is a high risk of recurrence after treatment of the initial lesion, with at least 50% of tumours recurring, with up to 25% of those recurrences progressing to invasive cancer, with a worsening of prognosis. In order to reduce this tendency to recur, it is now common practice to instill mitomycin C into the bladder in the immediate post-operative period.

Cystoscopy, in conjunction with voided urinary cytology, remains routine for monitoring and diagnosing tumour recurrences. In general, with the exception of a small group of patients whose superficial tumours are recognisably aggressive so that treatment as for invasive disease is indicated, current practice is to commence with an examination every 3 months, extending these progressively to 12-month intervals if findings remain negative. These patients are prone to further tumour formation indefinitely and must be followed for life.

Fulguration is used extensively for recurrent small tumours without obvious invasion, although biopsy of at least some lesions is essential to record stage and grade.

Intravesical chemotherapy with epirubicin and mitomycin C, and immunotherapy with Bacillus Calmette–Guérin (BCG) are effective in reducing the likelihood of recurrences. Although BCG is the most effective agent, it is also potentially more toxic. Viability of the bacilli may be jeopardised by antibacterial drugs which, in addition to anticoagulant and anti-inflammatory agents which impair fibronectin attachment, should be avoided during the periods of intravesical therapy. If haematuria is present or traumatic catheterisation occurs, BCG should not be introduced into the bladder as there is an increased risk of systemic infection from this organism.

Invasive bladder cancer

Approximately 50% of patients with invasive bladder cancer have micrometastases at the time of presentation, so local therapy alone is very unlikely to effect cure in these patients. Radical cystoprostatectomy (± urethrectomy) is generally regarded as superior to radical radiotherapy with and without concurrent use of radiosensitising cytotoxic drugs. Salvage cystectomy for persisting cancer post-radiotherapy is associated with increased rates of morbidity and mortality. Chemotherapeutic regimens for metastatic disease remain toxic and add, at best, little to overall survival.

MCQs

Select the single correct question to each question.

1 Which of the following is *not correct* with respect to upper tract urinary calculi?
- **a** approximately 80% of upper tract stones pass spontaneously
- **b** calcium oxalate is the commonest component of these stones
- **c** diuresis at the time of an episode of ureteric colic facilitates spontaneous passage of the stone
- **d** urate calculi may be dissolved with alkalinisation of urine
- **e** infection stones are most commonly associated with *Proteus* species of bacteria, which contain urease

2 Which of the following is *correct* with respect to prostate cancer?
- **a** compared with men under the age of 65 years, prostate cancer in the elderly is very rarely an aggressive cancer
- **b** most patients diagnosed with prostate cancer present with lower urinary tract symptoms
- **c** 80% of men presenting with an elevated serum prostate specific antigen (PSA) have prostate cancer
- **d** approximately 95% of prostate cancer patients have a durable response (>36 months) to androgen suppression therapy
- **e** the obturator, internal iliac and presacral lymph nodes are commonly involved in prostate cancer metastases

3 Which of the following is *correct*?
- **a** 'obstructive symptoms' of hesitancy, a reduced flow and terminal dribbling indicate bladder outflow

obstruction (BOO) in more than 90% of men 50 years and over

b benign prostatic hyperplasia (BPH) is predominantly a stromal hyperplasia

c a residual of more than 100 mL on three consecutive occasions is diagnostic of BOO

d the size of the prostate on digital rectal examination (DRE) is a reliable indicator of the presence or absence of BOO

e all men with chronic urinary retention benefit clinically from transurethral resection of the prostate

4 Which of the following is *not correct*?

a a mid-stream specimen of urine (m/s/u) submitted for microscopy, culture and sensitivities (m/c/s) remains the standard approach for diagnosing a urinary tract infection

b vesico-ureteric reflux of infected urine in infancy causes reflux nephropathy

c patients with reflux nephropathy are at risk for developing chronic pyelonephritis, hypertension and renal failure

d *E. coli* is the bacterium responsible for most urinary tract infections

e first-line management of a 20-year-old woman with her first episode of lower urinary tract symptoms of acute onset involves obtaining an m/s/u for m/c/s and prescribing a 10-day course of one of the new quinolone drugs (ciprafloxacin or norfloxacin)

5 Your recommendation for a 45-year-old man with a history of suspected haematuria 2 weeks earlier, who is currently asymptomatic, is:

a an m/s/u submitted for m/c/s, voided urinary cytology and ultrasound examination of both upper and lower tracts

b an m/s/u submitted for m/c/s, voided urinary cytology, intravenous urography and cystourethroscopy

c reassurance with advice to return if and when the bleeding recurs for investigation at that time

d an m/s/u submitted for m/c/s and voided urinary cytology

e an m/s/u submitted for m/c/s, voided urinary cytology and CT scan of the urinary tract

56 External genitalia in the male

Anthony Costello

Introduction

The external genitalia of the male consist of the penis and the scrotum and its contents. These parts are involved in the processes of urination, intercourse and reproduction.

Penis

The penis protrudes from the anterior aspect of the male pelvis. It has two functions, that of facilitation of urination, and the process of erection and ejaculation.

Anatomy

The penis is made up of three cylinder-like arrangements of erectile tissue, the two corpora cavernosa and the corpus spongiosum. The penile urethra travels invested in the corpus spongiosum, which also constitutes the glans penis. The corpora are filled with sinusoidal tissue which becomes engorged with blood during erection. The distal end of the penis is occupied by the glans penis, which is a continuation of the corpus spongiosum which lies between and beneath the two corpora cavernosa. The penis is invested with penile skin which is continued from the skin of the anterior abdominal wall, and is doubled back on itself at its distal end over the glans, forming the foreskin.

The penis is richly supplied by arteries which are all branches of the internal pudendal artery. The penis is drained through a complex of veins, both superficial and deep, which drain to the periprostatic plexus.

The lymph drainage of the skin of the penis, the corporal tissue and glans penis is to the superficial and deep inguinal nodes.

The penis is richly supplied by the dorsal nerves, which follow the course of the dorsal arteries, and are especially prevalent in the glans. The cavernous nerves ramify in the erectile tissue, providing sympathetic and parasympathetic supply to the erectile tissue.

Penile lesions

Phimosis

The presence of a tight foreskin which cannot be retracted behind the glans is known as phimosis. This can lead to the overgrowth of smegma bacillus under the foreskin due to inability to cleanse the area. Alternatively the glans and foreskin may undergo scarring and fibrosis secondary to balanitis xerotica obliterans, giving rise to phimosis. This situation can be resolved by circumcision.

Paraphimosis

If the retracted foreskin becomes stuck behind the coronal sulcus and cannot be replaced over the glans, this gives rise to the painful condition of paraphimosis, with swelling of the glans distal to the constricting band of tissue, which may result in necrosis of the glans unless the condition is relieved. Treatment is by compression and manual reduction; if this is unsuccessful, urgent surgery in the form of a dorsal slit to release the constricting band is performed, with later circumcision.

Priapism

Prolonged persistence of erection is known as priapism and nowadays is often related to the injection of medications for the treatment of erectile dysfunction. Other causes include trauma, which leads to high-flow priapism, often through the formation of an arteriovenous fistula, or recreational drug use, leading to the more dangerous low-flow priapism, where the penis is engorged with deoxygenated blood, which can lead to penile necrosis and tissue loss. Treatment is by drainage of the blood from the penis, which if unsuccessful, necessitates the formation of a shunt between corporal and cavernosal tissue or directly from the cavernosal tissue to a large vein, such as the transposed saphenous vein.

Peyronie's disease

Abnormal curvature to the penis is often the result of the formation of a plaque of fibrotic tissue in the tunica albugina causing limited expansion and thus curvature in the opposite direction during erection. This may follow trauma but if the process is stable and interfering with intercourse, surgical correction can be undertaken.

Penile cancer

Penile cancer is an uncommon disease that usually occurs in the older patient and is almost exclusively found in the uncircumcised male. Risk factors include smoking and exposure to the human papilloma virus. It is usually a squamous cell carcinoma and can present in the form of carcinoma *in situ*. Treatment is penectomy, either total or partial, if a sufficient disease-free margin can be attained. If a total penectomy is undertaken, the urethra is rerouted through the perineum as a perineal urethrostomy to allow for voiding. Typically, the inguinal lymph nodes on one or both sides are found to be clinically enlarged. This is often secondary to superinfection of the cancer, so 6 weeks of treatment with antibiotics is often used before reassessing these clinically. If still enlarged, the patient may require staged lymphadenectomy with possible subsequent radiotherapy.

Scrotum and testes

Anatomy

The scrotum is the bag-like structure which hangs below the penis and contains the male reproductive units, the testes and other associated structures. The scrotum is divided into two spaces by a fibro-muscular septum in the form of the median raphe. The normal adult testes are ovoid in shape, 2–3 cm in transverse and antero-posterior diameter and 3–5 cm in length. They are approximately 30 mL in volume.

The scrotum is covered by hair-bearing skin, thrown up into multiple rugae. Under the skin lies the dartos muscle layer. The testes descend from an intra-abdominal position and takes coverings from the layers that it passes through as it transverses the abdominal wall via the inguinal canal. Thus the external oblique muscle continues as the external spermatic fascia, and the internal oblique muscle continues as the cremasteric muscle. The internal spermatic fascia is a continuation of the tranversalis fascia and the tunica vaginalis is a continuation of the peritoneal layer. These layers constitute the spermatic cord, which also contains the vas deferens, testicular artery and vein and lymphatics. The testes themselves are surrounded by the tunica vaginalis, which has two layers – a visceral and a parietal layer. This is a potential space that can normally contain 2–3 mL of fluid. Deep to the tunica vaginalis lies the extremely tough tunica albugina, the dense fibrous capsule of the testes. The seminiferous tubules leading from the lobules of the testes coalesce and enter into the rete testis, which passes into the epididymis. This communicates with the vas deferens, travelling upwards via the spermatic cord.

The blood supply of the scrotum is derived from the external pudendal arteries anteriorly and the perineal arteries posteriorly. These vessels do not cross the median raphe, allowing for a relatively bloodless incision. The testis draws its own blood supply with it from the abdomen, and thus the testicular artery which travels in the spermatic cord originates from the aorta. Further arterial supply to the testis and vas deferens comes from the artery to the vas, and a large area of anastamosis occurs at the epididymis with the cremasteric, vasal and testicular arterial branches, allowing for a rich blood supply to the testis.

Venous drainage of the scrotum is via the external pudendal veins at the front and the posterior scrotal branches of the perineal vessels at the back. The testis is drained by many veins forming the pampiniform plexus. These may anastomose extensively with the cremasteric, vasal and external pudenal veins, and are usually in two to three branches in the inguinal canal. The testicular veins drain into the inferior vena cava on the left and the renal vein on the right.

The delineation of scrotal lymph drainage from that of the testes is of vital importance in the surgical treatment of testis cancer. The skin of the scrotum is drained by the superficial inguinal lymph nodes of the ipsilateral side. The testis drains via the spermatic cord to the para-aortic nodes on the same side. This implies that scrotal integrity should not be breached when performing an orchidectomy for testis cancer, as this will ensure that two areas of lymphatic drainage are now involved (see below).

The scrotal skin is innervated by the genital branch of the genitofemoral nerve, with a further input from the perineal branch of the posterior femoral cutaneous nerve. The testes are supplied by nerves from the renal and aortic plexuses, as well as by contributions from the pelvic plexuses accompanying the vas deferens.

Testicular torsion

Torsion involves rotation of the testis and usually occurs in teenage (postpuberty) or early adult life. The condition is due to high reflection of the tunica vaginalis, incomplete fixation or an excessively long mesorchium. The patient presents with sudden onset of pain and swelling, commonly after exertion or intercourse; epigastric pain may be present. The testis is extremely tender and often elevated due to cremasteric spasm but the spermatic cord is not tender. The differential diagnosis is acute epididymitis (see below). Doppler ultrasonography usually shows ischaemia of the testis, although false negative results also occur. The treatment is early surgical exploration since ischaemic necrosis of the testis will result if the torsion is not released as a matter of urgency. Following release of the torsion, the testis is fixed to the scrotum to avoid recurrence.

Scrotal masses

Hydrocoele

Primary hydrocoele represents a collection of fluid within the tunic vaginalis which obscures palpation of the underlying testis and is readily transilluminable. It is treated initially by aspiration; if recurrent, subtotal excision of the parietal tunica is performed.

Secondary hydrocoele is usually a response to underlying pathology in the testis or epididymis, so that treatment is directed to the underlying pathology.

Spermatoceles/Epididymal cysts

These fluid collections occur in relation to the head of the epididymis. They are of no importance unless they become large and uncomfortable, when they can be excised surgically.

Varicocoele

This presents as a dilatation of the pampiniform plexus, visible and palpable only in the erect position. It usually occurs only on the left side and is believed to be due to a deficiency in the valves in the left spermatic vein, which drain directly into the left renal vein.

No specific treatment is required, although when varicocoele is found during the investigation of infertility, it is common to suggest correction by high ligation of the spermatic vein. Sudden onset of varicocoele on the left side may suggest occlusion of the left renal vein due to renal tumour, and the rare right-sided varicocoele suggests situs inversus or, more rarely, vena caval occlusion.

Epididymitis

Clinical presentation

Acute epididymitis is a disease of young men, resulting from unprotected intercourse, commonly due to Chlamydia organisms, or of elderly men with bacterial urinary tract infection, when the organism is commonly *Escherichia coli*.

The presenting symptom is scrotal pain, usually gradual in onset (as distinguished from the sudden onset in testicular torsion). On examination, there is marked swelling and tenderness of the posterior part of the scrotal contents and the spermatic cord, and commonly a small secondary hydrocoele. There is usually a moderate pyrexia and accompanying leucocytosis.

Investigations

Urine culture is required, although it is common for there to be no positive findings in the young. Doppler ultrasound shows a high blood flow in contrast to the ischaemia of torsion.

Treatment

Bedrest, scrotal support, analgesia and antibiotics are required. If there is no positive urine culture, young men are treated with tetracycline and the elderly with trimethoprim. In the elderly, follow-up should include determination of the source of infection, usually stasis due to prostatic enlargement.

Testicular cancer

Testicular cancer is uncommon, but is the most common solid organ cancer of young males. It most commonly occurs between the ages of 20 and 35 years and usually presents with a painless testicular mass, which must be differentiated from an extra-testicular mass. Up to 50% of patients may present with metastatic disease.

Aetiology

The tumour is markedly more common in those with a history of undescended testes, especially if the testis is ectopic, i.e. found lying outside the normal path of testicular descent from the abdomen. In approximately 5%, a second tumour develops in the contralateral testis.

Pathology

Testicular cancer is most commonly (95%) originates from the germ cell, that is, it arises in the reproductive cells, although Leydig cell tumours and other tumours such as lymphomas can occur. The cancer types are broken down into two types, those which are seminomas and those which are not. These are known as non-seminomatous germ cell tumours (NSGCTs). These are a mixed group of tumours which may have a single cell type or be mixed in composition and are much more aggressive than pure seminomas. They consist of embryonal cancers, choriocarcinoma, teratomas, yolk sac tumours and mixed tumours. NSGCTs may express characteristics of trophoblastic or synctiotrophoblastic cells, and thus can produce proteins related to these, which can be used in diagnosis and monitoring of treatment outcome. The relevant proteins are alphafetoprotein (AFP), beta human chorionic gonadotropin (βHCG) and lactate dehydrogenase (LDH). Eighty to 90% of patients with NSCGTs will have a rise in one or both of AFP or βHCG, whilst a rise in βHCG will be seen in less than 10% of patients with seminoma, and rise in AFP is almost never seen. This rise may be due to an undetected element of NSGCT in the tumour or production by synctiotrophoblasts. LDH reflects bulk of tumour and is very useful in follow-up of metastatic disease.

Box 56.1 Staging of testicular tumours

Stage I	Lesion in testis only
Stage II	Metastases to lymph nodes below diaphragm
	a. <2 cm diameter
	b. 2–5 cm diameter
	c. >5 cm diameter
Stage III	Metastases to lymph nodes above diaphragm
Stage IV	Pulmonary or hepatic metastases

Clinical presentation

The first sign is a lump in the scrotum noticed while bathing or by a sexual partner. Pain is an unusual feature but one not to be ignored.

Examination demonstrates a hard, heavy testis or a localised nodule, and there may be a secondary hydrocoele.

Investigations

Serum samples are taken for αFP, βHCG and LDH. Staging (see Box 56.1) involves computed tomography (CT) scanning of the abdomen and chest initially.

Treatment

Treatment is initially by inguinal (not scrotal) orchidectomy, so as not to violate the scrotal lymphatic drainage area, and classically the vasculature is occluded prior to tumour manipulation to avoid potential seeding of metastatic disease. Seminomas confined to the testis are treated with low-dose radiotherapy to the abdominal nodes. NSGCTs confined to the testis with low or negative marker levels and favourable histology may be followed intensively with regular tumour markers, chest X-rays and CT scans. Alternatively, they may be offered a primary retroperitoneal lymph node dissection (RPLND). Patients with retroperitoneal nodal disease and/or more distant metastatic disease will be given platinum-based chemotherapy, and RPLND will be offered to those patients with residual masses post-chemotherapy. Follow-up requires regular review of the tumour markers and CT scan as indicated.

Outcome

Testicular cancer represents one of the best examples of the immune benefits of multi-modality treatment of cancer, with a cure rate of less than 50% prior to 1970 rising to 95% at the present time.

MCQs

Select the single correct answer to each question.

1 Penile cancer has the following characteristics except:
- **a** almost exclusively found in the uncircumcised male
- **b** commonly associated with the human papilloma virus
- **c** usually a squamous cell carcinoma
- **d** commonly involves the inguinal lymph nodes
- **e** is most commonly treated with radiotherapy

2 Which of the following features is true of testicular cancer?
- **a** is most common in elderly men
- **b** arises most commonly from germ cells
- **c** commonly metastasises to the inguinal nodes
- **d** is insensitive to radiation therapy
- **e** has a 75% cure rate

Cardiothoracic Surgery

57 Principles and practice of cardiac surgery

James Tatoulis and Julian A. Smith

Introduction

Cardiac surgery is a modern surgical specialty. The development of the heart–lung machine in 1953 provided total circulatory support and oxygenation while intracardiac procedures were performed on the empty, and preferably still (asystolic), heart. Other milestones were the successful introduction of cardiac valve replacement in 1960, and coronary artery bypass surgery in 1968.

Cardiopulmonary bypass: heart–lung machine

Cardiopulmonary bypass (CPB) had revolutionised cardiac surgery, allowing precise intracardiac repair while vital-organ perfusion, oxygenation and function were maintained. The essential components of the CPB circuit are described in Box 57.1.

The duration of CPB for most operations is between 1 and 2 hours. Complex operations may require 3–4 hours of CPB and occasionally several days or weeks (see 'Circulatory Support'). Major shortcomings are blood cell destruction (roller pump) leading to haemoglobinuria and thrombocytopenia, coagulation factor consumption and systemic inflammatory response (due to contact with silastic tubing), as well as neurologic, renal, and hepatic dysfunction. All these problems are time-related, becoming noticeable after 2 hours of CPB.

Hypothermia (30–34°C) is used to help protect vital organ function against brief periods of possible hypotension. Haemodilution (haematocrit 25–30%) is used to help reduce blood product use, reduce red cell loss during surgery, and improve small vessel blood flow in hypothermic conditions. For complex thoracic aortic arch aneurysm surgery, CPB is used to cool the patient to 18°C (profound hypothermia), blood is drained into the CPB reservoir, and the circulation arrested for up to 60 minutes, allowing excellent, rapid, asanguineous access to major vessels, yet maintaining cerebral and renal protection. At the completion of the vascular procedure the patient is rewarmed to 37°C over 30–40 minutes.

Myocardial protection

In some conditions it is possible to perform an excellent cardiac operation using CPB but with the heart normally perfused and beating (e.g. closure of an atrial

Box 57.1 Cardiopulmonary bypass circuit

Venous cannula(e)	Drains blood from right atrium or both venae cavae
Suckers	Return shed blood from operative field back to the reservoir
Reservoir	Drainage sump for venous and shed blood to be collected, and then oxygenated
Oxygenator	Venous blood oxygenated across a membrane
Heat exchanger	Cool and rewarm blood (and thereby the patient)
Roller or centripetal pump	Performs function of left ventricle, flow rates of 4–6 L/min.
Arterial cannula	Return oxygenated blood back to the distal ascending thoracic aorta or other major artery

septal defect [ASD]). However, precise coronary artery anastomoses and complex valvular procedures are best performed in a still flaccid heart.

Ideally, this state is achieved by clamping the distal ascending thoracic aorta and infusing 'cardioplegia solution' (oxygenated blood with additional potassium, magnesium, lignocaine and amino acid substrates) at 10–20°C to arrest the heart, to reduce its metabolic requirements and provide appropriate substrates, thus protecting the heart while being operated upon and being deprived of its normal coronary blood flow. There are many formulae of cardioplegic solutions, and methods of administration, although the principles remain the same. The usual cardiac arrest times are 30–90 minutes, although up to 180 minutes is possible with preservation of cardiac function. Sinus rhythm is usually restored, within 1–2 minutes of re-establishing coronary blood flow.

Closed cardiac surgery

Many procedures do not require CPB. The early operations were performed with the heart beating. Such operations are possible where they are remote from the heart (e.g. closure of patent ductus arteriosus [PDA]), or where disruption of cardiac function is transient and can be well tolerated (mitral valvotomy). Coronary surgery can also be performed on the beating heart without CPB (see 'Off-Pump Coronary Surgery'). Operations commonly performed without CPB are listed in Box 57.2. The vast majority (>90%) of cardiac operations worldwide are performed using CPB.

Coronary artery surgery

Coronary atherosclerosis is a major disease process in Western countries, and is rapidly increasing in incidence in developing countries. Coronary angiography (by retrograde cannulation of the coronary ostia via the femoral or brachial artery under local anaesthetic) was introduced in 1962. Coronary bypass surgery became established in 1968, and coronary angioplasty in 1977.

Box 57.2 Cardiac surgery without CPB

PDA closure
Coarctation of aorta repair
Mitral valvotomy (for mitral stenosis)
Pericardiectomy
Coronary bypass (selected cases)

Pathology

Atherosclerotic, stenotic lesions develop proximally at the origins of main coronary branches or at major branching points. The coronary vessels are usually free of disease distally. A stenosis of more than 50% diameter loss is considered significant. Atheromatous plaques may disrupt, occlude, or suffer from intraplaque haemorrhage, causing acute spasm, occlusion and possible thrombosis. Gradual progressive chronic stenosis causes angina. Acute spasm results in ischaemic chest pain at rest, and thrombotic occlusion results in acute myocardial infarction.

Risk factors for coronary artery disease include family history, male gender, diabetes, hypertension, smoking, hypercholesterolaemia and obesity.

Symptoms

Angina pectoris on exertion is the most common symptom. Ischaemic chest pain occurring spontaneously at rest (unstable angina) also occurs and is associated with spasm in the vicinity of the stenotic plaque, and/or transient coronary artery occlusion. Myocardial infarction occurs with prolonged or permanent coronary occlusion resulting in severe chest pain lasting several hours. Diabetic patients may not experience chest pain because of neuropathy.

Investigations

Chest X-ray may indicate cardiomegaly or left ventricular aneurysm as a result of prior myocardial infarction.

Electrocardiogram may show ST segment elevation or depression with acute chest pain, or 'Q' waves due to old myocardial infarction.

Stress test (treadmill or bicycle with electrocardiograph (ECG) monitoring), where positive, will result in chest pain, ST segment depression on the ECG and a fall in blood pressure.

Thallium, sestamibi, and positron emission tomography (PET) scans may indicate areas of hypoperfusion, ischaemia, viability and reversibility of left ventricle (LV) function.

Coronary angiography is the definitive investigation, objectively outlining the number, location and severity of the stenotic lesions, and the size and quality of the vessels beyond.

Medical management

Low-dose aspirin, nitrates (sublingual, spray or topical), beta-blockers (metoprolol, atenolol), calcium antagonists (nifedipine, amlodipine, felodipine) and cholesterol-lowering agents (simvastatin, privastatin) are used.

Coronary angioplasty

Discrete, appropriately located, stenotic plaques in one or two arteries may be treated by percutaneous transluminal coronary angioplasty (PTCA) to dilate the plaque to its normal lumen size (2–2.5 mm), and the plaque held open by placement of a stent. However, re-stenosis rates of between 5% and 10% at 1 year are reported.

Coronary artery bypass graft surgery

Multiple severe coronary artery stenoses associated with chronic uncontrolled angina, or unstable angina, are best treated surgically. Coronary artery bypass graft (CABG) comprises 75% of all adult cardiac operations. There are many variations of surgical techniques but the general principles are as follows.

Sternotomy is performed. The left internal thoracic artery (LITA) is harvested and is usually anastomosed to the left anterior descending artery (LAD), which is considered to be the most important artery. In younger patients (<60 years) the right internal thoracic artery (RITA) is harvested and anastomosed to the second most important affected coronary vessel. Other coronary vessels are grafted using either the saphenous vein or radial artery (Fig. 57.1).

Cardiopulmonary bypass is used with the patient at 30–34°C. The heart is arrested while performing the distal anastomoses. The proximal graft anastomoses may be performed to the ascending thoracic aorta while the heart is arrested, or using a specially designed clamp. Alternatively the proximal inflow may be from the subclavian artery or the construction of pedicled grafts off the internal thoracic artery (ITA). A typical operation takes 3–4 hours, including cardiac arrest for 30–60 minutes, and bypass times of 60–90 minutes, depending on the number of bypasses performed (average of three to four bypasses). The pericardium is usually closed, drain tubes placed behind the sternum and into the pleural cavities if they have been entered, and the sternum is re-wired so that it is extremely stable.

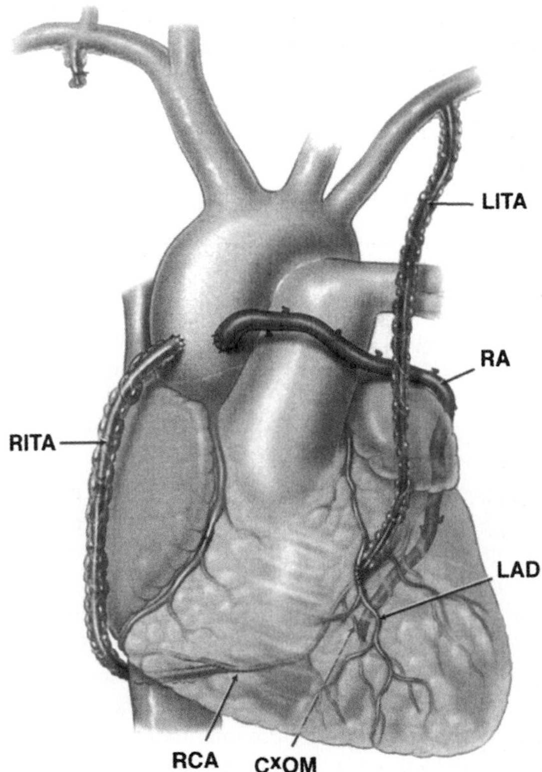

Fig. 57.1 Typical coronary artery revascularisation of the anterior, lateral and inferior walls of the heart. LITA, RITA, left and right internal thoracic artery; RA, radial artery; LAD, left anterior descending artery; RCA, right coronary artery; C^XOM, circumflex (obtuse) marginal artery.

The patient spends 24–48 hours in the intensive care unit, where blood pressure, right atrial pressure, pulmonary artery pressure, left atrial pressure, and cardiac and urine outputs are measured and interventions performed as appropriate.

The patient is mobilised on the first or second postoperative day, and aspirin and calcium antagonists recommenced. Most patients are discharged 5–7 days post-operatively. Recovery is rapid with most returning to work in 4 weeks, and to full activity within 3 months.

Results of coronary artery bypass graft

The operative mortality is 1% (although higher in reoperations or where LV function is poor). The main

Table 57.1 Coronary bypass graft patency

Conduit	5-year	10-year
Left internal thoracic artery	96%	95%
Right internal thoracic artery	93%	90%
Radial artery	90%	80%
Saphenous vein	75%	50%

morbidity relates to peri-operative stroke (1%), myocardial infarction (2%), sternal and mediastinal infections (1%), and haemorrhage (2%) (see 'Complications of Cardiac Surgery').

Graft patency is best for the left ITA and worst for the saphenous vein (Table 57.1).

Long-term freedom from recurrent angina pectoris is 85% at 5 years and 70% at 10 years (recurrence rate of approximately 3% per annum).

Long-term survival is excellent; 90–95% at 5 years and 80–85% at 10 years. Survival is significantly influenced by age at surgery (current mean age 68 years), presence of diabetes, extent of left ventricular dysfunction, and control of risk factors post-surgery. The presence of one or more internal thoracic artery grafts enhances survival and long-term freedom from angina, and it is hoped that coronary revascularisation using artery grafts only will produce further benefits, although this is not yet proven.

Coronary surgery confers prognostic benefits (over medical management), to patients that have stenosis of the left main coronary artery, those with high-grade proximal left anterior descending stenoses, those with triple vessel coronary disease (left anterior descending [LAD] artery, right and circumflex coronary arteries) and where there is left ventricular dysfunction. These groups account for approximately 85% of patients undergoing coronary surgery.

Surgery for complications of myocardial infarction

Complications of coronary artery disease, especially myocardial infarction, may require treatment in conjunction with the coronary artery bypass grafting. Myocardial infarction involving the left ventricular wall, including papillary muscles of the mitral valve, in combination with left ventricular dilatation may result in severe ischaemic mitral regurgitation (MR). This would need correction by mitral valve repair or replacement (operative mortality approximately 10%). Left ventricular aneurysms, particularly in relation to occlusion of the LAD, may require excision and repair (operative mortality 3%).

Extensive infarction may result in left ventricular free wall rupture into the pericardium (tamponade) or rupture of the interventricular septum (acute cardiogenic shock). These complications are almost universally fatal. Surgical repair using appropriate techniques (patches and biological glues) is essential, although operative mortality is high (25%), relating predominantly to the precarious pre-operative state of the patients.

New concepts in coronary artery bypass graft

Total arterial coronary revascularisation may produce even better long-term results and possibly avoid the need for re-operation.

Endoscopic harvesting techniques for saphenous vein are being developed that minimise incisions, discomfort and infection.

Performance of coronary surgery on the beating heart without use of CPB is also evolving.

Cardiac valve surgery

The initial valve operations were performed on the beating heart (mitral valvotomy). The first successful aortic and mitral valve replacements were performed in 1960. Valve pathology is still a significant factor in clinical cardiac disease. A high incidence of rheumatic valve disease persists in developing countries (India, China, Indonesia, South America). In Western countries the most common valve problems are due to degenerative processes and ageing, which have increased in incidence, while rheumatic pathology has declined.

Pathology

The two most common valve pathologies in Western countries are calcific aortic stenosis, and degenerative myxomatous mitral regurgitation. Aortic stenosis results from dystrophic calcification of either a bicuspid aortic valve, or as part of the degenerative ageing process, and is more commonly seen in older patients (a result of improved living standards and longevity). There is progressive narrowing of the aortic valve orifice with resultant left ventricular hypertrophy, and left ventricular failure in advanced cases. Aortic valve distortion may also result in aortic regurgitation with additional deleterious effects.

Myxomatous degeneration predominantly affects the mitral valve (collagen and elastin abnormalities, and increased mucopolysaccharide production). It results in varying degrees of annulus dilatation, chordae tendineae elongation, leaflet redundancy and prolapse and, in extreme cases, rupture of chordae tendineae and mitral leaflet flail, resulting in massive mitral regurgitation. Sequelae are left ventricular and left atrial dilatation and eventually left heart failure, atrial fibrillation and pulmonary hypertension. Myxomatous degeneration affecting the aortic valve results in progressive aortic regurgitation.

The chronic affects of rheumatic fever are cardiac valve leaflet thickening and retraction. In the aortic valve this results in a combined lesion of aortic stenosis and regurgitation. In the mitral valve, stenosis is the predominant effect of leaflet thickening, fusion at commissures, and shortening of chordae tendineae. Regurgitation occurs with severe leaflet fibrosis, retraction, and failure of leaflet coaptation.

Symptoms

The key symptom is dyspnoea, although this occurs late in the course of valve disease as each of the valve pathologies is generally well tolerated because of left ventricular reserve, and the initial compliance of the left atrium. Dyspnoea requires immediate investigation and aggressive intervention because it indicates exhaustion of the cardiac compensatory mechanism and a poor prognosis and rapid demise for the patient if left untreated.

Angina and syncope may be additional symptoms in aortic stenosis due to pressure loss across an extremely stenotic aortic valve and resultant poor coronary and cerebral perfusion.

Cerebral emboli or endocarditis may occur if the valve lesions are complicated by valvular or left atrial thrombus, infections or vegetations.

Investigations

Chest X-ray may show cardiomegally, calcification in the aortic or mitral valves, and pulmonary congestion.

Electrocardiogram may show left ventricular hypertrophy, a wide bifid P wave in severe mitral stenosis, or atrial fibrillation.

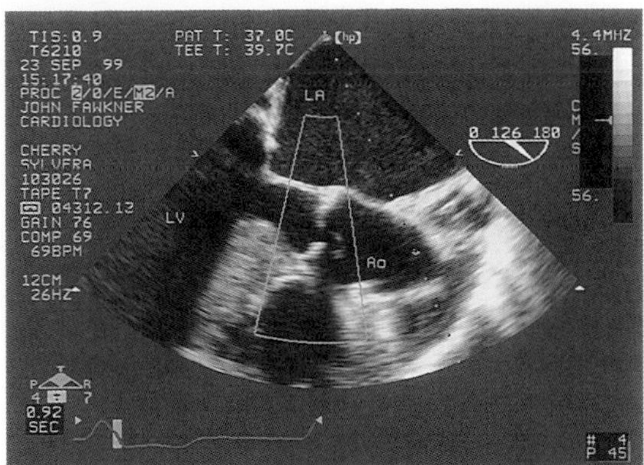

Fig. 57.2 Transoesophageal echocardiogram to evaluate the aortic valve (centre of image). LA, left atrium posteriorly; LV, left ventricle; Ao, ascending thoracic aorta. Dots represent 1-cm markings.

Echocardiography is the key investigation in valvular heart disease. Accurate measurements can be made of the cardiac chambers, pulmonary artery pressure and the valvular orifices. Calcification, degree of stenosis or regurgitation, leaflet excursion, flow, valve area, gradient and annular size can be precisely measured and compared to prior or future measurements. Transthoracic echocardiography (TTE) is an excellent screening tool. Transoesophageal echocardiography (TOE) gives greater anatomic detail of valves and their pathologies and is particularly useful in the intraoperative setting (Fig. 57.2).

Coronary angiography is performed in patients older than 40 to screen for coexistent coronary artery disease. Thirty per cent of patients undergoing cardiac valve surgery require concomitant coronary artery bypass surgery.

Medical management

Where patients are asymptomatic, and echo shows normal function and cardiac chamber size and normal pulmonary artery pressures, conservative management is indicated. Peripheral vasodilating medications such as calcium antagonists (nifedipine, amlodipine), or angiotensin-converting enzyme (ACE) inhibitors (captopril, enalapril, etc.), are useful in aortic regurgitation and mitral regurgitation to reduce the afterload for left ventricular ejection. Diuretics (fruse-mide) are required for pulmonary congestion. Warfarin anticoagulation and digoxin may be required if there is atrial fibrillation.

Aortic valve surgery

A mean gradient of more than 40 mm Hg in aortic stenosis or a left ventricular end-diastolic diameter of more than 60 mm in aortic regurgitation are indications for surgery. The mean age for aortic valve replacement (AVR) is 69 years. Sternotomy and CPB are required. The aorta is opened transversely 2–3 cm above the aortic valve. Rarely the valve can be repaired. The valve is excised, all calcium removed from the annulus, and an aortic valve prosthesis is placed using non-absorbable sutures. The aortotomy is then closed, and air is evacuated from the heart prior to reestablishment of circulation through the heart. Carbon dioxide in the operative field (heavier and more soluble than oxygen and nitrogen) is used to minimise potential air embolism. The ascending aorta is usually occluded for 60 minutes, CPB time 80 minutes, and total operative time approximately 3 hours.

Mitral valve surgery

Rheumatic mitral stenosis may be treated by percutaneous balloon valvuloplasty. The procedure is carried out by catheterisation of the femoral vein, passing superiorly into the right atrium, across the interatrial septum into the left atrium and eventually dilatation of the mitral valve.

Alternatively, closed mitral valvotomy via a left thoracotomy and trans-left atrial or trans-left ventricular dilatation of the mitral valve is performed. These procedures are performed under TOE guidance, and are best when the valve leaflets are pliable and there is no valve calcification, nor thrombus in the left atrium.

Valve leaflet thickening, calcification, fused chordae and left atrial thrombus are all indications for open operation (via sternotomy and CPB), which may include commissurotomy to free the fused commissures between the anterior and posterior mitral leaflets, debridement of calcification, and fenestration or resection of portions of thickened chordae. A severely distorted valve, especially if additionally regurgitant, will require replacement. Myxomatous degenerative mitral valve regurgitation is most commonly due to elongated and ruptured chordae, leading to prolapse and flail, of the central scallop of the posterior mitral valve leaflet, usually in combination with mitral annular dilatation. If the gross changes are localised to a specific part of the valve (e.g. central scallop of the posterior leaflet), mitral valve repair is possible. If the changes are widespread with multiple areas of prolapse, flail and lack of leaflet coaptation, then valve replacement is indicated.

Mitral valve repair is performed via a sternotomy, CPB and direct left atriotomy. Many techniques are used and include quadrangular resection of the flail or prolapsed segment, annulus and leaflet repair, placement of an annuloplasty ring to reinforce the annulus repair, correct annular dilatation and valve geometry. Leaflet prolapse can also be corrected by shortening or replacing elongated or ruptured chordae and relocating the heads of the papillary muscle. Retention of the native mitral valve avoids the need for warfarin anticoagulation in the long term (if the patient is in sinus rhythm), and maintains the geometry and function of the left ventricle.

Mitral valve replacement (MVR) is performed if the valvular pathology is too extensive. However, as much of the subvalvular mechanism (including leaflet tissue, chordae and papillary muscles) is retained to maintain left ventricular geometry and function, hence resulting in a low operative mortality, and improved long-term left ventricular function and patient survival. Low-profile mechanical valves are used in patients less than 70 years (see below). Warfarin anticoagulation is always required when a mitral valve prosthesis has been placed.

Cardiac valve prosthesis

There are two categories of valve prosthesis available for implantation: mechanical and tissue.

Mechanical valves are made of pyrolytic carbon with a Dacron sewing cuff, are low-profile, inert, and commonly have two semicircular leaflets (St Jude, CarboMedics, ATS). Mechanical valves always require warfarin anticoagulation maintaining International Normalised Ratio (INR) values between 2.5 and 3.5.

Tissue valves (bioprostheses) are derived from humans (allograft–human cadaver aortic valve) pulmonary valve autografts (discussed later) or xenografts (specially treated porcine or bovine valves). Additionally, tissue valves may be mounted on a stent for ease of implantation, or may be stentless to enhance haemodynamics, allowing a larger valve and orifice into any anatomic situation.

Advantages and disadvantages of each type of valve are indicated in Table 57.2.

In the mitral position mechanical valves are used in patients younger than 70 years, or if the patient is to be on long-term warfarin (AF). Xenograft tissue valves

Table 57.2 Cardiac valve prosthesis

Valve type	Advantages	Disadvantages
Mechanical	Durable	Warfarin anticoagulation Higher bleeding and thromboembolic rates
Tissue	No anticoagulation	15-year durability (Ca^{++}, dehiscence), re-operation
	Better haemodynamics (stentless valves)	

may be used in older patients, often with lesser degrees of warfarin anticoagulation. However, xenografts fail rapidly in young patients.

In the aortic position there are a number of choices determined by age and patient lifestyle. In patients older than 70, a xenograft tissue valve is generally used. Only low-dose aspirin is required long-term if the patient is in sinus rhythm.

In patients younger than 70, generally a mechanical valve together with warfarin anticoagulation is used. A human cadaver allograft is used if warfarin is to be avoided (e.g. patient lives in a remote area, patient participates in contact sports) or when there is endocarditis affecting the aortic valve annulus. However, allografts are relatively difficult to procure and are in short supply.

Some younger patients (15–50 years) have a pulmonary autograft (Ross) procedure in which the diseased aortic valve is replaced with the patient's own pulmonary valve, which in turn is replaced with a human cadaver pulmonary valve allograft. This is an extensive procedure, but well tolerated in young patients. Anticoagulation is avoided. However, long-term results beyond 5 years are not established.

Unfortunately, all tissue valves are subject to wear and tear and gradual degeneration. Inevitably, if any type of bioprosthesis is used in patients younger than 60, there is a very high probability that re-operation will be required, although this is uncommon within 10 years.

Post-operative management

Peri-operative prophylactic antibiotics are given to protect against endocarditis (prior to anaesthesia, and for 48 hours post-operatively) and meticulous care taken to avoid any sepsis. Warfarin anticoagulation (if appropriate) is commenced 24 hours post-operatively, and a therapeutic INR of 2.5–3.5 achieved by day 7. Warfarin is continued indefinitely (except in mitral repair or where aortic tissue valves have been used). Diuretics and ACE inhibitors are usually required for several weeks or months. General post-operative management and progress is similar to that of patients undergoing coronary artery surgery.

Other valve conditions

Severe endocarditis affecting either the aortic or mitral valve is usually caused by *Staphylococcus aureus* and results in fever, aortic or mitral regurgitation and eventual renal and hepatic dysfunction. It is best managed aggressively with appropriate antibiotic loading and early surgery to eradicate the infection and either replace or repair (uncommon but possible) the affected valve. Tricuspid valve surgery is uncommon. Tricuspid regurgitation may be the end product of chronic aortic or mitral valve disease, left heart failure and pulmonary hypertension. The mechanism is that of right ventricular and tricuspid valve annular dilatation and loss of central leaflet coaptation. The leaflets and chordae are otherwise normal. Tricuspid valve annuloplasty to correct the tricuspid annulus size and shape to normal is performed at the time of aortic or mitral surgery. Organic tricuspid valve stenosis or regurgitation due to rheumatic disease is rare, and is managed following the principles of mitral valve surgery.

Results

Operative mortality varies from 1% (AVR, MVR) to 3% (MVR). Operative mortality for combined CABG and valve surgery is 3–5%, and for re-operation is 10%. Long-term results are excellent. Survival following mitral valve repair, or AVR, is 90% at 5 years, and 80% at 10 years. Survival following MVR is a little less than this due to late referral and excision of the subvalvar apparatus in the previous era.

Morbidity of valve replacement surgery

Unfortunately each valve prosthesis has a group of long-term problems associated with its use:

- anticoagulant-related haemorrhage, which may be extremely serious (cerebral, gastrointestinal)

- thromboembolism from small thrombi that form around the annulus or within the prosthetic valve
- endocarditis from an infection on the valve prosthesis
- peri-valvular leaks, or structural deterioration of tissue valve which, when severe enough, would require re-operation.

Each of the above complications occur with an annual incidence of approximately 0.5–1.0%, and hence the potential for a patient to be totally free from any one of these complications over the course of 10 years is only of the order of 70%.

Congenital cardiac surgery

Cardiac anomalies occur in 8 per 1000 live births. The range of anomalies is extensive. Only the common ones are discussed below. Congenital cardiac abnormalities are best corrected as early as possible after birth (preferably in the first 3 months). Some, such as a large, persistent PDA, which creates a huge shunt from the aorta to the pulmonary artery, or severe coarctation of the aorta, which places a large afterload on the left ventricle, need urgent correction at birth.

Patent ductus arteriosus

A PDA allows blood flow from the pulmonary artery trunk to the aorta when the lungs and pulmonary circulation are not functioning *in utero*. The PDA usually closes at birth. A persistent, small PDA is vulnerable to endocarditis. Persistent, large PDAs allow shunting of blood from the aorta back into the pulmonary circulation, overloading it as well as the right heart, eventually leading to pulmonary hypertension and right heart failure. Closure of the PDA is essential and this can be achieved either by percutaneous catheter closure, or by direct suture ligation or division and oversewing by thoracoscopy, or a small left thoracotomy.

Coarctation of the aorta

The most common site is just distal to the left subclavian artery, the lumen of the aorta often narrowed to 1–2 mm. Left untreated, upper body hypertension, left ventricular hypertrophy and left ventricular failure develop. Correction is by either percutaneous retrograde (from the femoral artery) catheter balloon dilatation, or surgical resection and repair via a small left thoracotomy.

Atrial septal defect

Atrial septal defects occur as a result of failure of development of the interatrial septum and can be high (sinus venosus), mid (ostium secundum) or low (ostium primum) defects. A significant ASD is more than 1 cm in diameter and if left uncorrected results in a persistent left atrium to right atrium shunt, eventually leading to right atrial and ventricular enlargement, atrial fibrillation, and pulmonary hypertension. Life expectancy may be reduced by 10–30 years (depending on the size of the ASD and shunt).

Echocardiography gives excellent depiction of the anatomic location, size of the ASD and the flow through it, as well as the size of the cardiac chambers and pressure in the right ventricle and pulmonary artery.

Atrial septal defect closure is indicated if the pulmonary circulation flow is more than 1.5 times the systemic circulatory flow. Surgical repair is readily performed (using CPB) by either direct suture or a patch of autologous pericardium with an extremely low mortality (1 : 400). Percutaneous ASD closure via the femoral vein with a catheter-mounted baffle-type device has been developed and is applicable where the ASD is well circumscribed with a defined rim circumferentially. Early experience has been promising.

Ventricular septal defect

Ventricular septal defects (VSDs) occur when ventricular septal development is incomplete and may be single or multiple and placed either just below the tricuspid valve and the origin of the great vessels, or more inferiorly in the body of the muscular septum. Most commonly they occur in isolation, but may also be present as part of a more complex cardiac anomaly (e.g. Tetralogy of Fallot). Small VSDs, particularly in the central muscle septum, may close spontaneously with cardiac growth. Larger VSDs associated with pulmonary-to-systemic flow ratios of more than 1.5 : 1 are repaired to avoid endocarditis, and also the sequelae of pulmonary and right heart overload (see above). Surgical closure is by using CPB, and by direct suture or patch. The main specific complication is heart block as the conducting bundle passes near the inferior rim of the VSD, and care is taken not to damage the conducting bundle with sutures at VSD closure.

Other congenital abnormalities

Some other congenital abnormalities that may be surgically corrected with excellent long-term results include pulmonary valve stenosis, Tetralogy of Fallot, transposition of the great vessels and endocardial cushion defects (aortic valve canal). However, there are numerous rarer, more complex conditions (e.g. hypoplastic left heart syndrome, single ventricle, tricuspid atresia) where surgery is also possible, but often multiple procedures are required, with suboptimal results. (The reader is directed to texts of paediatric cardiology and cardiac surgery).

Surgery of the thoracic aorta

Aneurysms of the thoracic aorta, especially the transverse arch, are challenging. The most common pathology is myxomatous degeneration of the aortic wall media, leading to aneurysmal dilatation and eventually rupture or dissection. Marfan's syndrome is one entity that is part of the spectrum of myxomatous degeneration of connective tissues. Hypertension and atherosclerosis are now better controlled in the population and are less common contributing factors to thoracic aneurysms. Dilatation of the thoracic aorta to a diameter of more than 5 cm is associated with a marked increase in the possibility of rupture or dissection and so elective repair/replacement is advised.

The patients are usually asymptomatic. The aneurysm is often noted on routine chest X-ray. Rupture or dissection is associated with severe chest and interscapular pain, possibly collapse, hypotension (due to blood loss into the mediastinum, pleural cavity or pericardium) and unequal pulses (due to dissection around the origins of the large artery). The ECG is usually normal.

Transoesophageal echocardiography is the most important diagnostic test, and should be performed urgently. It will show the size and location of the aneurysm, any dissection flaps, the site of the aortic wall tear, extent of dissection, and the function of the aortic valve, which may partly dehisce from the outer aortic wall and become regurgitant.

Elective repair is indicated when the aneurysm is more than 5 cm in diameter. This may involve replacement of the aneurysm with a Dacron tube graft, but may also require AVR, re-implantation of the coronary artery ostia, or even replacement of the transverse arch with re-implantation of the great vessels. Results of elective surgery are excellent, with operative mortality generally less than 5%.

If rupture or dissection has occurred, emergency surgery is indicated with the TOE as the sole investigation (which can be performed in the operating room prior to anaesthesia induction). Similar operative techniques are used preserving the aortic valve if possible. Biological glues are used to glue together and stiffen the fragile myxomatous layers of the aorta at the site of anastomoses and repair. This complex surgery is usually facilitated by use of deep hypothermia (18°C) and total circulatory arrest (see 'Cardiopulmonary Bypass: Heart–Lung Machine'). Major morbidity may result from these urgent, difficult operations and includes post-operative haemorrhage, stroke and renal dysfunction. The operative mortality is between 10% and 30%.

Vigilant long-term follow-up with control of hypertension, and serial computed tomography (CT) scans or echocardiograms, are required because other parts of the aorta (descending thoracic or abdominal) may dilate over time.

Pacemaker and dysrhythmia surgery

Degenerative fibrosis associated with age can affect the cardiac conducting mechanism to produce heart block. The heart rate may fall to 30 beats per minute (ventricular escape rhythm) and result in dizziness or syncope. This is a common clinical problem in older patients. Occasionally, heart block may result from trauma to the conducting bundle at cardiac surgery, or from some anti-arrhythmic medications (verapamil, sotolol).

Treatment is relatively simple and achieved by implantation of a pacing lead into the right ventricle via the cephalic or subclavian vein below the clavicle and implantation of a lithium-powered, low-profile pacemaker generator, all performed under local anaesthesia. The pacing rate is adjusted to 70–80 beats per minute as required. An atrial lead can also be inserted to allow sequential atrial/ventricular pacing, which is more efficient. The pacemaker may be programmed to allow spontaneous increase of pacing rates according to patient activity.

Programmed sequential biventricular pacing may be beneficial in patients with left ventricular dilatation, severe dysfunction and cardiac failure.

Rapid atrial arrhythmias (atrial fibrillation, atrial flutter, junctional tachycardia) that remain uncontrolled on medication (digoxin, sotolol, amiodarone) and are significantly symptomatic, can be treated either surgically or more commonly by percutaneous catheter radiofrequency ablation.

Life-threatening rapid ventricular arrhythmias (ventricular tachycardia, ventricular fibrillation) may also be treated by implantable cardioverter defibrillators (ICD) with minimal operative mortality and morbidity, and excellent long-term results.

Circulatory support

Circulatory support may be required to allow time for cardiac recovery after a temporary but reversible insult, or permanently.

Afterload-reducing agents

Nitroprusside and nitroglycerine infusions allow rapid peripheral, arterial and venous dilatation.

Calcium antagonists (nifedipine, amlodipine) and ACE inhibitors (captopril, enalapril) are oral medications that cause peripheral vasodilatation and reduce cardiac afterload, allowing myocardial contraction and ejection of stroke volume against a lower systemic vascular resistance.

Inotropic agents

Inotropic agents are usually given as infusions for short-term use (hours or days) and include dopamine, dobutamine, adrenaline, isoprenaline, milrinone and calcium. All have varying properties and effects, but the underlying mechanism is an enhanced inotropic effect on the myocardium.

Intra-aortic balloon pump

Intra-aortic balloon pump (IABP) is indicated when hypotension and poor cardiac output persist despite appropriate inotropic support. A catheter with a 34- or 40-mL balloon is introduced into the descending thoracic aorta usually percutaneously by the femoral artery. The balloon inflates (helium) and deflates in sequence with the ECG. It inflates in diastole, suddenly increasing diastolic pressure, mean blood pressure and organ perfusion, especially coronary blood flow and myocardial perfusion. The balloon rapidly deflates just prior to cardiac systole, dramatically reducing the afterload for the left ventricle. The usual duration of IABP support is between 1 and 5 days, but use up to 21 days has been reported.

Potential problems include leg ischaemia, systemic infection and mechanical blood cell destruction leading to anaemia and thrombocytopenia.

Ventricular assist devices

Ventricular assist devices (VADs) provide additional mechanical support (when inotropes and IABP are insufficient). Typically, cannulae are placed on the inlet side (left atrium) and into the outlet side (aorta) with a mechanical device in between, effectively performing the work of the left ventricle. (A similar circuit can be constructed for the right side of the heart.) Numerous devices are available (Biopump, Thoratec, Novacor, Heartmate, Abio-Med) with varying characteristics relating to size, implantability, portability, ease of use and expense. Ventricular assist devices may be *in situ* from 3 to more than 100 days.

Extracorporeal membrane oxygenation (ECMO)

Where support of both the circulation and also oxygenation is required (e.g. virulent but reversible pulmonary infection or asthma, where oxygenation cannot be maintained with mechanical ventilation, 100% O_2, and maximum positive end-expiratory pressure), extracorporeal membrane oxygenation (ECMO) can be used. Extracorporeal membrane oxygenation is identical to regular CPB but with special cannula and circuit modifications for long-term use. The management is extremely demanding as the patient requires anticoagulation and constant supervision.

Cardiac transplantation

The first human cardiac transplant was performed in 1967 by Dr C. Barnard in South Africa. This was preceded by extensive laboratory work by Dr N. Shumway and coworkers at Stanford University, USA. The initial results were suboptimal because of difficulties with rejection and fulminating infections.

Cyclosporine, which was introduced in 1980, dramatically reduced the severity of the rejection and infection episodes to readily manageable levels, promoting renewed interest. Other advances included superior donor heart preservation, better tissue typing, myocardial biopsy surveillance, and more efficient anti-rejection regimens.

Indications for cardiac transplantation include permanent severe heart damage and failure from myocarditis, cardiomyopathy and multiple myocardial infarctions. Donor hearts are usually procured following brain death from motor vehicle trauma or cerebral trauma. Recipients are usually less than 65 years of age with no other significant coexisting medical or psychological problems.

The results or cardiac transplantation are very good with an operative mortality of 2–3%, 1-year survival of 90% and 5-year survival of 80%. Approximately 100 cardiac transplants are performed in Australia each year and almost 3000 are performed annually worldwide; however, numbers are limited by donor shortages. In response to this, much development is centred on implantable 'artificial hearts'.

Complications of cardiac surgery

Operative mortality

Most cardiac operations have an operative mortality of approximately 1% (including the first 30 days post-operation). Mortality rates are increased in reoperations (5%), multiple procedures (5%) and with increasing age (>80 years, 10%), age being a marker for multiple associated co-morbidities.

Stroke

The incidence of major neurologic events in the perioperative period is 1–2%. Causes include primary cerebrovascular disease in older patients, atheroembolism from the ascending thoracic aorta, hypoperfusion during CPB, and air or particulate embolism during valve surgery. Fortunately there is usually a significant recovery. In addition, subtle neuropsychologic dysfunction can occur, with abnormalities lasting up to 6 months.

Sternal and mediastinal infection

Sternal and mediastinal infection is a devastating complication, with an incidence of 1–2%. Risk factors include diabetes, obesity, bilateral ITA grafting, prolonged pre-operative hospitalisation and multiple instrumentations. Prophylactic antibiotics are used in all cardiac surgery. Protection against mediastinitis is afforded by closure of the thymus and pericardium behind the sternum. Common bacteria are *S. aureus* (including methicillin-resistant *S. aureus*).

Clinical features are fever, increased sternal discomfort, redness and movement of a previously stable sternum. Early diagnosis is essential, as established mediastinitis has a mortality of 30%.

Treatment depends on the extent of pathology, from intravenous antibiotics, to local debridement and sternal rewiring, to extensive debridement and use of omental and myocutaneous flaps.

Post-operative haemorrhage

Post-operative haemorrhage occurs with an incidence of 2–5%. Specific causes include bleeding from sutures lines, branches of grafts, and the ITA bed. However, in the majority no specific bleeding point is found but reoperation is useful to remove retained blood and clots from the pericardium, mediastinum and pleurae, and establish haemostasis from the oozing areas. Aspirin and other anti-platelet drugs within 7 days of cardiac surgery may be contributing factors.

Numerous other complications may also develop and include atrial fibrillation, pulmonary atelectasis, pneumothorax, and fluid retention. These are all readily treatable and reversible.

Minimally invasive cardiac surgery

Over the past 5 years there has been much interest in less invasive surgery, in minimising trauma, improving cosmesis and, where possible, avoiding the deleterious effects of CPB.

Small incisions

Shorter upper sternal and right parasternal incisions have been used for aortic valve surgery. Right submammary and short lower sternal incisions have been used for ASD repair and for mitral valve surgery (especially in young females). Left submammary incisions are used for isolated coronary bypass to the LAD. Occasionally, groin cannulation of the femoral artery and vein are used in conjunction with small thoracic incisions.

The value of these approaches is not established. Limited exposure may compromise safety and lengthen the duration of the procedure. Additionally, femoral vessel cannulation has been complicated by aortic dissection, leg ischaemia and venous thrombosis. These incisions are of great value when cosmesis is important.

Off-pump coronary surgery

Devices and techniques have been developed that allow excellent stabilisation of the coronary arteries, making it possible to perform precise coronary anastomoses, especially to the LAD and diagonal arteries (antero-lateral aspects of the heart), while the heart is beating and maintaining circulation. Similarly, but to a lesser extent, the circumflex and right coronary arteries may be grafted.

Potential advantages are avoidance of CPB and manipulation of the aorta (by cannulae and clamps), which may be an important factor in older patients or where the aorta is atheromatous or calcified, thereby reducing the possibility of bleeding or stroke.

There are potential economic gains through avoidance of CPB: consumables, personnel and potential to reduce intensive care and hospital stays; however, these have not been proved thus far.

There are also potential disadvantages, with greater operative difficulty, possible coronary artery damage, and episodes of hypotension with excessive displacement and manipulation of the heart. The role of off-pump coronary surgery (OPCAB), beating heart coronary surgery is still being evaluated.

The future of cardiac surgery

The number of cardiac operations performed worldwide per annum continues to increase. Interventional cardiology techniques such as angioplasty have changed the spectrum of cardiac surgery to more complex and re-do operations, and the mean age of patients is older. Robotics, in relation to cardiac surgery, are being developed, which promises to assist minimally invasive techniques. Substantial endeavour continues in improving prosthetic cardiac valve and artificial heart technology.

Further reading

Buxton BF, Frazier OH, Westaby S. *Ischaemic Heart Disease: Surgical Management*. Mosby International Ltd, UK;1999.

Cohn LM, Edmunds LH Jr. *Cardiac Surgery in the Adult*. 2nd ed. New York: McGraw Hill; 2003. Also at www.ctsnet.org

Topol EJ, Califf RM, Isner J et al. *Textbook of Cardiovascular Medicine*. 2nd ed. Philadelphia: Lippincott Williams & Wilkins;2002.

Townsend CM, Beauchamp RD, Evers BM, Mattox KL. *Sabiston Textbook of Surgery. The Biological Basis of Modern Surgical Practice*. 16th ed. Philadelphia: WB Saunders; 2001.

MCQs

Select the single correct answer to each question.

1 The coronary artery bypass graft conduit with the highest patency after 5 and 10 years is:
- **a** left internal thoracic artery
- **b** right internal thoracic artery
- **c** left radial artery
- **d** right radial artery
- **e** left or right long saphenous vein

2 Regarding the results of coronary artery bypass grafting:
- **a** an operative mortality of over 10% is common
- **b** patients with poor left ventricular function have a higher operative mortality
- **c** older patients have less post-operative morbidity
- **d** diabetes has no influence on post-operative morbidity
- **e** the use of an internal mammary artery improves survival but does not provide long-term freedom from angina

3 Regarding cardiac valve prosthesis:
- **a** mechanical valves require no long-term anticoagulation
- **b** tissue valves are highly durable
- **c** mechanical valves have lower bleeding and thromboembolic rates
- **d** tissue valves are generally preferred in the mitral position
- **e** structural failure is extremely rare in mechanical valves

4 Complications of cardiac valve replacement surgery include:
- **a** anticoagulant (warfarin) related haemorrhage
- **b** cerebral thromboembolism
- **c** prosthetic valve endocarditis
- **d** structural deterioration of tissue valves after 10 to 15 years
- **e** all of the above

58 Common topics in thoracic surgery

Julian A. Smith

Introduction

Thoracic surgical topics discussed in this chapter are related to disorders of the chest wall, pleural space, lungs and mediastinum. Other conditions managed by general thoracic surgeons include diseases of the oesophagus and chest trauma. Both of these topics are presented in Chapters 10, 11 and 45.

Presentation of thoracic disorders

Symptoms

Common thoracic symptoms include cough, chest pain, shortness of breath (on exertion or at rest), excessive or abnormal sputum production, haemoptysis, wheeze or stridor. Many conditions (especially neoplasms) are asymptomatic and are first detected on chest X-ray.

Examination findings

On examination, the patient may appear quite normal or severely short of breath (e.g. from a spontaneous pneumothorax). Clues to intrathoracic problems may be found in the other parts of the body such as clubbing of the finger nails, peripheral cyanosis and lymphadenopathy. The jugular venous pressure may be elevated (e.g. from neoplastic superior vena caval obstruction or tension pneumothorax) and the trachea may be deviated from the midline. Signs found in the chest in some common thoracic conditions are given in Table 58.1. Again, in some conditions, the findings on examining the chest can be completely normal.

Non-invasive diagnostic investigations

Chest X-ray

All patients with a suspected thoracic problem should have an erect postero-anterior and lateral chest X-ray. This will help define the location and extent of the problem.

Pulmonary function testing and arterial blood gases

Pulmonary function tests (PFTs) help to define the degree of respiratory impairment on presentation, the amount of functional reserve, and hence the ability of the patient to tolerate lung surgery and, at follow-up, the response to therapy. There are two major types of PFT:

- those that assess the movement of air in and out of the lungs (e.g. forced expiratory volume in 1 second, forced vital capacity, peak flow, total lung capacity, residual volume)
- those that measure the ability to transfer gas across the alveolar–capillary membrane (e.g. tests of carbon monoxide diffusing capacity).

When considering surgical therapy for a given patient, it may be evident that the patient has insufficient ventilatory capacity to withstand a chest wall incision or a major pulmonary resection, and alternative therapies will need to be offered.

Arterial blood gas analysis is an important investigation in patients with acute and chronic thoracic conditions. Parameters measured include Pa_{O2}, Pa_{CO2}, pH, bicarbonate level and arterial oxygen saturation.

Computed tomography

High-resolution images of the chest wall, pleural space, lungs and mediastinum are provided in cross-section.

Table 58.1 Physical signs in thoracic disease

	Chest wall movement	Mediastinum and trachea	Tactile voca fremitus	Percussion note	Breath sounds
Large pleural effusion above	Reduced on affected side	Shift to opposite side	Absent	Stony dull	Absent. May be bronchial, fluid level
Large pneumothorax	Reduced on affected side	Shift to opposite side	Decreased	Increased	Decreased
Massive lung collapse	Reduced on affected side	Shift to affected side	Absent	Dull	Decreased
Pneumonic consolidation	Reduced on affected side	Central	Increased	Dull	Bronchial
Advanced emphysema	Reduced on both sides 'barrel chest'	Central	Decreased	Increased	Decreased

Tissue density is quantified and a fairly accurate map of pathological lesions throughout the chest is obtained. Serial computed tomography (CT) scanning is helpful in following up suspicious lesions. Percutaneous needle biopsy of pulmonary or pleural lesions is frequently performed under CT guidance. The upper abdomen should also be scanned in patients with known or suspected pulmonary malignancy to assess the liver and adrenal glands, which are common sites for secondary deposits. Magnetic resonance imaging (MRI) is also used in centres where it is available.

Invasive and operative investigations

Bronchoscopy

Diagnostic bronchoscopy, using a flexible or rigid instrument, provides direct visualisation of airway lesions for biopsy. Lesions of the lung parenchyma or lymph nodes in the subcarinal space may be biopsied using a transbronchial technique. Most commonly, diagnostic bronchoscopy is performed by respiratory physicians with the flexible bronchoscope. This is performed using a combination of topical anaesthesia and intravenous sedation. More difficult and potentially complicated situations are handled by thoracic surgeons in the operating room. Occasionally, therapeutic rigid bronchoscopy is required to control massive haemoptysis, to remove aspirated foreign bodies, or to clear retained inspissated sputum leading to post-operative lung or lobar collapse.

Mediastinoscopy

The mediastinoscope is a lighted cylindrical instrument used to biopsy paratracheal and subcarinal lymph nodes, most commonly in the work-up to stage a patient with known or suspected lung cancer. This investigation usually precedes any major pulmonary resection for lung cancer. It is also used in the investigation of mediastinal masses. The instrument is introduced via a transverse suprasternal incision and passed caudally in a plane deep to the pretracheal fascia. The mediastinoscope passes close to the superior vena cava (to its right), the innominate artery and arch of aorta (in front) and the recurrent laryngeal nerves (to the left and right posterolaterally). Care should be taken to avoid biopsying vascular structures such as the superior vena cava, azygos vein and pulmonary artery. Access is obtained to the upper middle and posterior mediastinum except for the subaortic area below the aortic arch, which is best approached via an anterior mediastinotomy.

Anterior mediastinotomy

Anterior mediastinotomy is a left parasternal, intercostal incision employed to access tissue from the anterior mediastinum (e.g. thymic lesions). A short

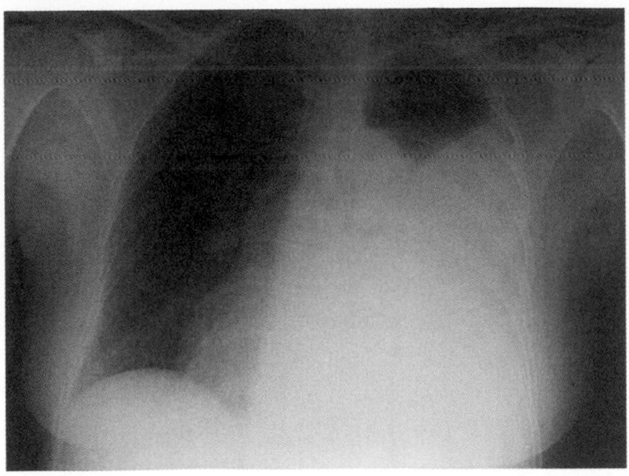

Fig. 58.1 Chest X-ray showing a large left-sided pleural effusion.

horizontal or vertical incision may be made either in the second or third intercostal space or by resecting a costal cartilage. A left anterior mediastinotomy allows excellent access to the subaortic lymph nodes, the primary site of spread for tumours in the left upper lobe.

Pleural aspiration and biopsy

When a pleural effusion is present (Fig. 58.1), pleural fluid may be aspirated (thoracocentesis) using a needle and syringe. Cytological, microbiological and biochemical analyses may provide a clue as to the cause of the pleural effusion. Pleural biopsy can be performed at the same time using an Abram's needle.

Percutaneous biopsy

Many chest wall, pleural, pulmonary or mediastinal masses can be biopsied under CT control. This allows a tissue diagnosis to be made prior to any surgical intervention. It must be noted that a negative biopsy result does not exclude malignancy.

Video-assisted thoracoscopy

Thoracoscopy, the thoracic equivalent of laparoscopy, uses cameras, telescopes and television monitors to inspect the pleural space, lung and mediastinum. Biopsy material may be taken from lesions in all these areas. The most common application is for lung and pleural biopsy. Three ports made by 2-cm incisions in the chest wall are used in the hemithorax, one for the telescope with the camera and light source and two for the instruments. Some therapeutic procedures, especially the management of recurrent spontaneous pneumothorax and thoracodorsal sympathectomy, are carried out using video-assisted thoracoscopy (VATS) techniques.

Thoracotomy

Rarely, a diagnostic thoracotomy is required when less invasive procedures are inappropriate or have failed to provide a diagnosis. Access is obtained to the mediastinal lymph node groups, the great vessels, oesophagus, lung and pericardium for tissue sampling. Frozen section analysis usually provides an immediate diagnosis and this result will determine what further intraoperative measures, if any, are required.

Basic thoracic surgical techniques

Pleural aspiration

Pleural aspiration may be used in diagnosis, as the primary treatment of a pleural collection or as a preliminary measure prior to the insertion of a chest tube for the drainage of a pleural effusion. The presence of fluid should be confirmed on physical examination and chest X-ray (Fig. 58.1) prior to commencement. With the patient in a comfortable position sitting up, the chest is widely prepared and the puncture site chosen. Local anaesthetic is infiltrated liberally down to the pleura. The aspiration needle is inserted at the upper edge of the rib and up to 1 L can safely be removed at a given sitting. Upon completion, the needle is removed and a small dressing applied. A chest X-ray is then performed to exclude a pneumothorax.

Chest tube insertion and management

Common indications for chest tube insertion include spontaneous pneumothorax, tension pneumothorax, a large pleural effusion or empyema and post-traumatic haemothorax. Chest tubes are placed routinely at the completion of intrathoracic operations. In all situations, it is mandatory that an experienced operator insert the tube, because a badly performed placement is extremely dangerous.

The usual site for insertion is the fourth or fifth intercostal space in the mid-axillary line, but for the drainage of specific air, fluid or blood collections, the appropriate location on the chest wall should be chosen. The patient should be in a comfortable and relaxed position, and adequate local analgesia is essential. Following antiseptic skin preparation and infiltration of local anaesthetic into the skin, muscle layers and pleura, a skin incision is made over the middle of the chosen intercostal space. The incision is deepened using blunt dissection (with artery forceps) down to and through the pleural layer. Final dissection into the pleural space is made with a finger, and the point of entry can be widened by opening the artery forceps widely in two directions at 90° to each other. If a tension pneumothorax is present this manoeuvre will result in a rush of air and immediate relief for the patient. The chest drain is inserted through the chest wall and firmly retained in position with strong non-absorbable sutures. The drain tube is then connected to an underwater drainage system. In almost all situations the drain should be connected to wall suction, usually high flow and low pressure (e.g. 20 cm of water). A chest X-ray must always be performed following chest tube insertion to confirm tube position and to exclude a large pneumothorax.

A chest drain should be removed only when all air leak and fluid drainage has ceased. The lung should be fully expanded on chest X-ray. A chest tube must never be 'clamped' prior to removal. The patient is asked to breathe in maximally while the tube is briskly removed and an occlusive dressing placed over the wound.

Tracheostomy

Tracheostomy is the making of a surgical opening in the trachea. Recent modifications have included percutaneous tracheostomy and minitracheostomy.

Indications for tracheostomy

The common indications for tracheostomy are listed in Box 58.1. The benefits of a tracheostomy are that it overcomes respiratory tract obstruction, allows control of secretions, reduces respiratory dead space and allows mechanical ventilation other than via an endotracheal tube.

Box 58.1 Indications for tracheostomy

Respiratory tract obstruction
Tracheobronchial toilet/retained secretions
Prolonged mechanical ventilation
Elimination of respiratory dead space
Radical laryngeal surgery

Method

An elective surgical tracheostomy is performed in the operating room usually under general anaesthesia. Alternative settings include the intensive care unit (percutaneous tracheostomy) or the bedside (minitracheostomy). Via a midline lower cervical incision, a stoma is created at the level of the second and third tracheal rings through which a cuffed tracheostomy tube is placed. The lower airway is suctioned with a fine catheter and, after the tube is secured in position and the cuff inflated, ventilation can commence.

Complications

The complications of tracheostomy are listed in Box 58.2.

Thoracotomy

Posterolateral thoracotomy

Posterolateral thoracotomy is the standard approach for major pulmonary resections. The incision is located below the inferior angle of the scapula, the latissimus dorsi is divided and the pleural space is entered along the superior surface of the fifth or sixth rib.

Lateral thoracotomy

Lateral thoracotomy is used when only limited access is required, such as in the operative treatment of recurrent

Box 58.2 Complications of tracheostomy

Operative

- Haemorrhage
- Pneumothorax
- Tube malposition

Post-operative

- Tube obstruction or dislodgement
- Haemorrhage
- Tracheal stenosis
- Dysphagia
- Tracheo-oesophageal fistula
- Tracheo-innominate fistula

pneumothorax. The incision is made between the anterior and posterior axillary lines.

Anterior thoracotomy

Anterior thoracotomy is used for open lung biopsy. An incision is made beneath the male nipple or female breast. There is a low incidence of post-thoracotomy neuralgia using this approach.

Median sternotomy

Median sternotomy or 'sternal split' gives excellent access to the anterior mediastinum, pericardium, heart and great vessels. Anterior mediastinal tumours (e.g. thymomas) and apices of each lung (in lung volume reduction operations) can be removed via this approach.

Common thoracic disorders

Chest wall

A classification of common chest wall conditions is given in Box 58.3. Chest injuries are presented in Chapter 45. Soft tissue tumours and primary bone tumours will not be discussed further (see Chapters 42 and 48).

Pectus excavatum

In pectus excavatum or 'funnel chest', there is a variable amount of depression of the sternum, lower costal cartilages and ribs. Frequently asymmetric, the deformity may displace the heart into the left chest. Heart and respiratory function are seldom impaired. Surgery, when indicated, is entirely cosmetic to correct the deformity.

Box 58.3 Classification of chest wall conditions

Congenital anomalies: pectus excavatum, pectus carinatum
Chest injuries
Soft tissue tumours: lipomas, neurofibromas, fibrosarcomas, liposarcomas
Primary bone tumours: chondromas, fibrous dysplasia, osteosarcomas, Ewing's tumour, myeloma
Secondary chest wall tumours
Chest wall infections
Thoracic outlet syndrome

Pectus carinatum

In pectus carinatum or 'pigeon chest', the opposite deformity exists, where the sternum protrudes forward like the keel of a boat. Again, surgical correction is possible if the deformity is cosmetically unacceptable.

Secondary chest wall tumours

Involvement of the ribs and sternum by secondary tumours far exceeds that by primary bone tumours. Direct extension to the chest wall may occur in breast or lung carcinomas. Chest wall mestatases are often multiple and commonly originate in the lung, prostate, kidney, thyroid, stomach, uterus or colon. Tumours with multiple chest wall secondary deposits usually have a very poor prognosis.

Chest wall infections

De novo infections of the chest wall are extremely rare, and currently infection is most associated with a recent sternotomy or thoracotomy wound. Risk factors for post-operative wound infection include diabetes and morbid obesity. Abscesses can occur within the soft tissue planes and very rarely an empyema thoracis can 'point' through the chest wall ('empyema necessitans').

Pleural effusion

The pleural space is a potential cavity that normally contains negligible amounts of fluid due to equilibrium between its production and absorption. The accumulation of fluid within this space may be a manifestation of local or systemic disease.

Classification and aetiology

There are two types of pleural effusion: a transudate or exudate. The common causes of each are given in Box 58.4.

Pathophysiology

A transudate (specific gravity <1.016 and a protein content <3 g/dL) results from the altered production or absorption of pleural fluid. There is elevated systemic or pulmonary capillary pressures, lowered plasma oncotic pressure or lowered intrapleural pressure. There is no disorder of the pleural surfaces. An exudate (specific gravity >1.016 and a protein content >3 g/dL) is

Box 58.4 Causes of pleural effusion

Transudate
- Congestive heart failure
- Cirrhosis
- Nephrotic syndrome
- Hypoalbuminaemia

Exudate
- Infective (post-pneumonic)
- Malignancy
- Chylothorax

found in the presence of diseased pleural surfaces or lymphatics where there is increased capillary permeability or lymphatic obstruction.

Surgical pathology

Pneumonia of any cause may be complicated by the formation of a pleural effusion. Should pus form within the pleural space, the collection is known as an empyema thoracis. Currently, the most common cause of a post-pneumonic pleural effusion and empyema is bacterial infection.

Malignant pleural effusions can result from secondary pleural deposits, extension of the primary (lung) tumour to the pleural surface or lymphatic obstruction. Metastatic lung or breast carcinoma is the most common cause of malignant pleural effusions, but other common primary sites include the ovary, colon and kidney. There are frequently associated pulmonary metastases, but in some instances the intrathoracic metastatic lesion may be confined to the pleural space. The effusions are often blood stained (serosanguineous), with positive cytology in up to 70% and a positive pleural biopsy in 80% of malignant effusions.

Chylothorax refers to the accumulation of chyle within the pleural space due to disruption of the thoracic duct. Very rarely a congenital anomaly of the thoracic duct and seldom from tumour involvement, chylothorax is usually the result of surgical trauma to the duct somewhere along its course.

Clinical features

Common symptoms of a pleural effusion include pleuritic chest pain, shortness of breath, cough and haemoptysis (malignant effusion). The physical signs of a large pleural effusion are shown in Table 58.1.

Box 58.5 Investigations of pleural effusion

Chest X-ray
Computed tomography scan of chest
Diagnostic pleural aspiration
Pleural biopsy (needle, video-assisted thoracoscopy or thoracotomy)
Bronchoscopy

Investigations

Investigations are listed in Box 58.5. Chest X-ray (Fig. 58.1) will determine the extent of the effusion and may demonstrate underlying lung disease. Computed tomography scanning will also reveal significant intrathoracic disease. Diagnostic pleural aspiration will reveal the type of effusion based on appearance and cytological, microbiological and biochemical analysis. Pleural biopsy should be performed if the diagnostic pleural aspiration is unsuccessful or non-diagnostic. Should the effusion prove to be the result of a malignant process, it is important to adequately stage the disease prior to the commencement of therapy.

Management

Therapy should be directed to any underlying cause such as pneumonia (antibiotics), congestive heart failure (diuretics), or malignancy (chemotherapy or radiotherapy).

The prognosis in patients with a malignant pleural effusion is poor; an average survival of 6 months follows diagnosis. Treatment of the effusion is therefore, at best, palliative. Closed chest tube drainage will provide short-term symptomatic relief, but the effusion usually re-accumulates upon tube removal. An attempt should be made to obliterate the pleural space (pleurodesis) to prevent the effusion reaccumulating. This may be achieved by introducing a sclerosing agent (e.g. talc) into the pleural space via a chest tube or at operation (VATS or thoracotomy) following drainage of the effusion.

Chylothorax usually responds to non-operative therapy; that is, chest tube drainage of the collection and measures to reduce chyle flow (no-fat diet, parenteral nutrition). Should the effusion persist or reaccumulate, operative intervention (thoracic duct ligation and/or pleurodesis) is indicated.

Box 58.6 Types of pneumothorax

Primary spontaneous pneumothorax
Secondary spontaneous pneumothorax
Tension pneumothorax
Traumatic pneumothorax

Empyema is managed in its early stages with dependent chest tube drainage. The pleural space may be irrigated with antiseptic solution. In chronic cases, a thick fibrous wall or cortex forms around the pus-filled pleural space. Treatment options include prolonged closed chest tube drainage, open chest tube drainage after resection of a segment of rib and open surgical decortication to remove the entire abscess wall. This releases the restricted chest wall and diaphragm and allows the lung to re-expand.

Pneumothorax

Pneumothorax refers to the presence of air within the pleural space. The air usually originates from the lung itself, but it may come from outside (after penetrating trauma) or from the oesophagus (after endoscopic perforation). The common types of pneumothorax are listed in Box 58.6. Traumatic pneumothorax is discussed in the chapter on chest injuries (see Chapter 45).

Primary spontaneous pneumothorax

Primary spontaneous pneumothorax is the most common type of pneumothorax and usually results from the rupture of a tiny bleb or bulla at the lung apex. Occurring in tall, thin, young adults of either sex, it presents with acute chest pain and shortness of breath. Physical findings are given in Table 58.1. Chest X-ray reveals an absence of peripheral lung markings and often a poorly defined line marking the border between lung and air (Fig. 58.2). The lung may be completely collapsed at the hilum.

If the pneumothorax is small, it may need no therapy other than observation and a repeat chest X-ray to confirm lung re-expansion or it may be aspirated with a needle. If the pneumothorax is large or under tension (discussed later), or if there is an associated pleural effusion, a formal chest tube should be inserted. As air is evacuated from the pleural space, the lung expands and presses against the chest wall, thereby sealing the site of the air leak. Once the tube stops bubbling it can be removed.

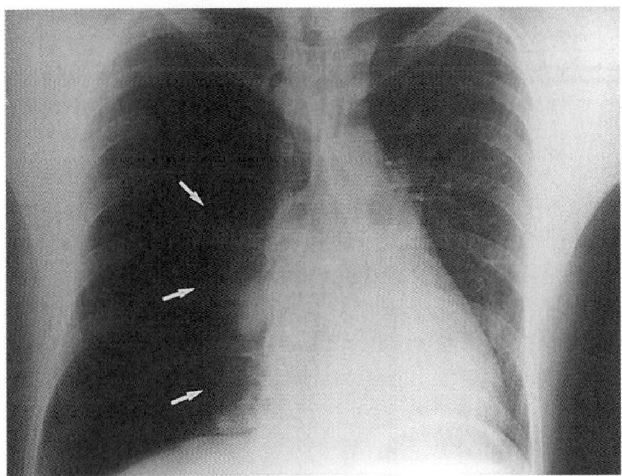

Fig. 58.2 Chest X-ray showing a large right-sided spontaneous pneumothorax. Arrows show the collapsed lung edge.

Secondary spontaneous pneumothorax

Secondary spontaneous pneumothorax occurs in the presence of significant underlying lung or pleural disorders such as primary or secondary malignancy, chronic airway disease (especially bullous emphysema) and pulmonary infections (bronchiectasis and lung abscess). The clinical features reflect the underlying disorder, and the presentation and initial management of the pneumothorax is as above.

Tension pneumothorax

A tension pneumothorax is present when the site of air leak in the lung acts as a one-way valve such that air enters the pleural space during inspiration and coughing but prevents its escape during expiration, thus raising the pressure within the pleural space. Such pressure or tension compresses the lung and shifts the mediastinum towards the other side. This compresses the normal lung and may also kink and distort the superior vena cava. The diagnosis should be suspected when signs of a large pneumothorax are associated with mediastinal shift and an elevated jugular venous pressure. This constitutes a medical emergency. A large-bore needle should be inserted to the affected side and if the diagnosis is correct will be met by the hiss of escaping air and a relief of the immediate problem. A formal chest tube should then be inserted.

Recurrent spontaneous pneumothorax

Approximately 30% of primary spontaneous pneumothoraces will recur and after a second episode this figure rises to 70%. If the same side has been affected twice or more, and especially if tension has occurred, a definitive procedure should be considered. Approaches via VATS or a limited thoracotomy include stapling of apical bullae to prevent further air leakage, and pleurodesis (either abrasive or chemical) or pleurectomy, which allows the visceral pleura to adhere to the parietal pleura or the bare chest wall.

Carcinoma of the lung

Carcinoma of the lung is the most common cause of cancer deaths in males and the second most common cause of cancer deaths after breast cancer in females. Usually occurring in patients older than 50, the overall incidence in both sexes continues to rise.

Aetiology

Cigarette smoking is the single most common predisposing factor. Environmental or occupational exposure to asbestos, arsenic, nickel, chromium and hydrocarbons also play a role. The highest geographical incidence is in parts of Scotland, suggesting a possible genetic influence.

Surgical pathology

The pathological types of lung carcinoma are listed in Box 58.7.

Squamous cell carcinoma accounts for about 35% of all lung carcinomas. Most often centrally located, these tumours arise from metaplasia of the normal bronchial mucosa. Varying degrees of differentiation are seen depending on the presence of keratin, epithelial pearls, prickle cells, basal pallisading, cell size and mitotic activity.

Box 58.7 Pathological types of lung carcinoma

Non–small-cell lung cancer
- Squamous cell carcinoma
- Adenocarcinoma
- Large-cell carcinoma
- Mixed (adenosquamous)

Small-cell carcinoma

Adenocarcinoma represents about 45% of lung carcinomas. More often found in women and located peripherally in the lung, the histopathology reveals acinar or papillary glandular elements. The tumour may form in long-standing scars (e.g. post-tuberculosis) and spreads via the bloodstream. Alveolar cell carcinoma is a highly differentiated form of adenocarcinoma. Tall columnar epithelial cells proliferate and spread along the alveolar walls. The tumour may be solitary, multinodular or diffuse (pneumonic). It may be indistinguishable from metastatic adenocarcinoma to the lung.

Large cell carcinoma comprises another 15% of malignant lung tumours. Peripherally located, there is abundant cell cytoplasm with a cellular pattern that is predominantly anaplastic.

Adenosquamous carcinoma is the most common of the mixed non–small-cell types of lung carcinoma. Tending to be peripheral in location, their behaviour is based upon the most prominent cell type.

Small cell carcinomas make up about 10% of malignant lung tumours. Mostly centrally located, they are the most malignant and carry the worst prognosis. The cells are small, round or oval in appearance ('oat cell'). Ectopic formation of the hormones adrenocorticotrophic hormone (ACTH) or antidiuretic hormone (ADH) may occur. Lymphatic and pleural invasion is common. Seventy per cent of tumours have extrathoracic involvement at presentation.

Clinical features

Approximately 10–20% of lung cancers are asymptomatic and present as a chance finding on routine chest X-rays. Symptoms may be thoracic or extra-thoracic.

Thoracic symptoms include cough, haemoptysis, shortness of breath, chest pain (pleuritic or retrosternal), hoarseness of voice (involvement of recurrent laryngeal nerve), arm pain and weakness (Pancoast's syndrome; apical tumour involving brachial plexus).

Extra-thoracic symptoms include those of metastases (e.g. bone, central nervous system, liver, adrenals) and those of non-metastatic paraneoplastic syndromes. These include the production of ectopic ACTH, ADH and parathyroid hormone. Wrist and ankle pain due to hypertrophic osteoarthropathy and a variety of myopathies are also found.

Physical findings include hypertrophic pulmonary osteoarthropathy, fingernail clubbing, supraclavicular and cervical lymphadenopathy, signs of brachial plexus

Box 58.8 Investigations for lung carcinoma

Chest X-ray
Sputum cytology
Computed tomography scan of chest and upper abdomen
Needle biopsy under computed tomography control
Bronchoscopy and biopsy
Mediastinoscopy or anterior mediastinotomy
Video-assisted thoracoscopic biopsy
Positron emission tomography scan

involvement, Horner's syndrome (ptosis, miosis, anhidrosis, enophthalmos from involvement of the cervical sympathetic ganglia), elevated jugular venous pressure and facial oedema (superior vena caval obstruction). In the chest there may be signs of a pleural effusion or lung collapse (Table 58.1).

Investigations

Investigations are listed in Box 58.8 and will provide a tissue diagnosis and aid in determining the extent of intrathoracic disease. Figures 58.3A and B show typical findings on chest X-ray and CT scan, respectively. If metastatic disease is suspected in sites such as bone or the brain, additional scans of these areas should be included so as to accurately stage the disease and to avoid unnecessary surgical intervention. Positron emission tomography (PET) scanning is showing promise in the evaluation of regional lymph nodes and also distant metastases. Radioactive tracers detect differences in metabolism between normal and malignant tissue. Metastatic disease has been found in up to 15% of lung cancers thought to have resectable disease. The number of these investigations required by a given patient is determined by the ease with which a tissue diagnosis and accurate staging is reached.

Staging of lung cancer

Staging of non–small-cell lung cancer is clinical and is based upon descriptors for the size and location of the primary tumour (T), the spread to lymph nodes within the thorax (N) and to the presence or absence of distant metastases (M). TNM subsets are grouped together into stages 0 through IV and these stages provide information about prognosis, allow a comparison of outcomes from different clinical series and also guide therapy.

(A)

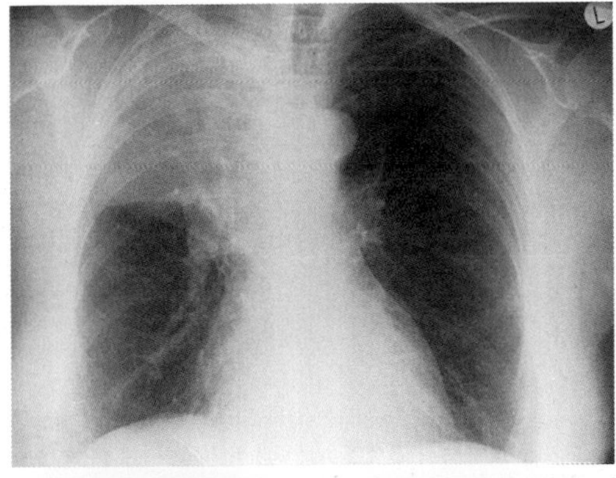

(B)

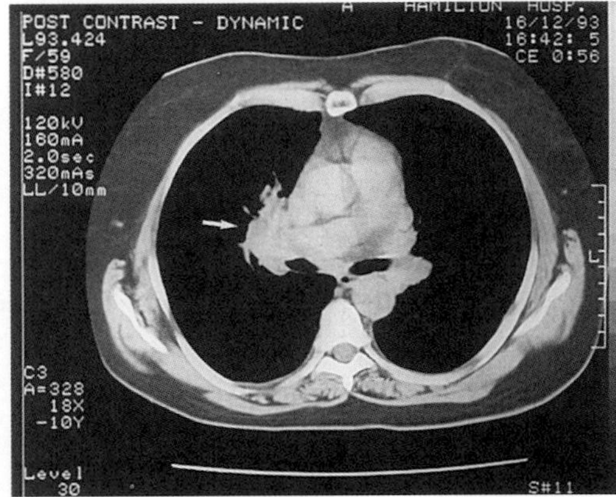

Fig. 58.3 (A) Chest X-ray showing a right hilar lung cancer with collapse and consolidation of the right upper lobe. (B) Computed tomography scan showing the right hilar lung cancer.

Differential diagnosis

Carcinoma of the bronchus presenting as a solitary pulmonary nodule ('coin lesion') in the lung periphery should be differentiated from the following:

- secondary tumours
- benign lung tumours (bronchial adenoma)
- non-specific granuloma
- tuberculous granuloma.

Management

Unfortunately, two-thirds of patients are incurable at presentation owing to spread evidenced by one or more of the following:

- distant metastases
- a malignant pleural effusion

• involved cervical lymph nodes
• superior vena caval obstruction
• recurrent laryngeal nerve palsy.

If the patient has an otherwise resectable tumour and adequate respiratory reserve, surgical resection offers the only hope of long-term survival.

Surgical treatment consists of a thoracotomy with removal of the entire lung or lobe along with regional lymph nodes and contiguous structures. Where possible, lobectomy is the procedure of choice. Pneumonectomy is used if the tumour involves the main bronchus, extends across a fissure or is located such that wide excision is required. Survival following 'curative' resection is approximately 30% at 5 years and 15% at 10 years. The best results are found in squamous cell carcinoma followed by large-cell carcinoma and the adenocarcinoma. There are very few survivors of small-cell carcinoma beyond 2 years.

Radiotherapy may be 'curative' in patients with early stage disease unfit for surgical resection. However, the usual role for radiotherapy is in the palliation of pain from bone secondaries, superior vena caval obstruction or haemoptysis. Combinations of radiotherapy and platinum-based chemotherapy provide the best palliation for patients with good performance status and non-resectable disease.

Multi-agent chemotherapy is indicated for small cell carcinoma. There is a small survival benefit from palliative combination chemotherapy in non–small-cell lung cancer. Trials are currently underway to determine whether there is a role for induction chemotherapy in patients with locally advanced non–small-cell lung cancer. Responders, if downstaged, can be offered surgical resection with a view to long-term survival. This management strategy remains controversial and should currently only be offered in the context of a properly conducted randomised clinical trial.

Mediastinal tumours

The mediastinum is a midline space between the pleural cavities. It is divided into the superior, anterior, middle and posterior compartments. Mediastinal tumours may be primary or secondary in origin. Secondary neoplasms most often result from lymphatic spread to mediastinal lymph nodes. Common primary sites are lung, oesophagus, larynx, thyroid and stomach. A classification of primary mediastinal tumours is given in Box 58.9.

Box 58.9 Classification of primary mediastinal tumours

Anterosuperior masses
• Germ cell tumours
• Thymoma
• Lymphadenopathy
• Retrosternal thyroid
• Aneurysm of the aortic arch

Middle mediastinal masses
• Lymphadenopathy
• Mediastinal cysts
• Aneurysm of ascending aorta

Posterior mediastinal masses
• Neurogenic tumours (benign and malignant)
• Peripheral intercostal nerves: neuro-fibroma, neurilemmoma
• Sympathetic ganglia: ganglioneuroma, neuro-blastoma
• Paraganglia: phaeochromocytoma, paraganglioma
• Oesophageal: duplication, tumours, diverticulae
• Hiatus hernia
• Bronchogenic cyst

Clinical presentation

Approximately half are asymptomatic and have no abnormal findings on examination. They are discovered by chance on a plain chest X-ray. Lesions in the young and those with symptoms are more likely to be malignant.

Thoracic symptoms result from compression of adjacent structures and include pain (back or chest), shortness of breath, cough or dysphagia. Systemic symptoms may be fever, malaise, weight loss and night sweats. Local findings include cervical lymphadenopathy, facial and/or arm swelling and tracheal shift. General findings may be testicular masses, hepatosplenomegaly and muscle weakness.

Surgical pathology

Neurogenic tumours are the most common mediastinal tumours and are found almost exclusively in the posterior mediastinum. About 10% are malignant and this feature is more frequent in children. All nerve types may be affected (Box 58.9).

Germ cell tumours are the most common anterior mediastinal tumours and are more common in the young. Types include teratoma, seminoma and non-seminomatous. Tumour markers may be elevated in non-seminomatous types and can be used to monitor the response to therapy.

Mediastinal lymphoma is usually associated with widespread disease and is seldom the only site (5%). Ninety per cent are either lymphoblastic (Hodgkin's) or diffuse large cell (non-Hodgkin's) in type.

Thymoma is more common in adults than children. About 30% of patients have myasthenia gravis and about 15% of patients with myasthenia gravis develop thymoma. The differentiation between benign (encapsulated) and malignant (invasive) thymoma can be difficult.

Investigations

Investigations are summarised in Box 58.10. In some instances, the combination of clinical features and findings on imaging allow a precise diagnosis. A patient with myasthenia gravis and an anterior mediastinal mass will most likely have a thymoma. The site of the lesion will determine the type of biopsy required.

Box 58.10 Investigation of mediastinal tumours

Imaging
- Chest X-ray
- Computed tomography scan with contrast
- Magnetic resonance image (neurogenic or vascular)
- Angiography (vascular)
- Barium swallow (posterior mediastinum)
- Radionucleide (thyroid or parathyroid; gallium for lymphoma)

Biochemistry
- Lactate dehydrogenase (elevated in lymphomas, seminomas)
- Beta human chorionic gonadotrophin (may be elevated in seminomas)
- Alpha fetoprotein (non-seminomatous germ cell tumours)

Tissue diagnosis
- Fine-needle aspiration biopsy
- Mediastinoscopy
- Video-assisted thoracoscopy
- Thoracotomy

Box 58.11 Management of common mediastinal tumours

Asymptomatic cysts	
• Pericardial	Aspirate
• Bronchogenic	Observe
Symptomatic cysts	Surgical resection
Neurogenic tumours	
• Benign, asymptomatic	May observe
• Symptomatic	Surgical resection
• Malignant	Surgical resection
Thymoma	
• Benign	Surgical resection
• Malignant	Surgical resection and chemotherapy
Lymphoma	Chemotherapy, radiotherapy (rarely surgical resection)
Germ cell tumours	Chemotherapy, radiotherapy, surgical resection

Management

Options in management include simple observation and follow-up, aspiration, surgical resection, radiotherapy, chemotherapy and combinations of surgical resection, radiotherapy and chemotherapy. A summary of the approach to management of the common primary mediastinal tumours is given in Box 58.11.

Further reading

Kaiser L, Singhal S. *Surgical Foundations: Essential of Thoracic Surgery*. CV Mosby;2004.

Shields T W, LoCicero J, Ponn R B, Rusch V W. *General Thoracic Surgery*. 6th ed. Vols 1 and 2. Lippincott Williams & Wilkins;2004.

MCQs

Select the single correct answer to each question.

1 Which of the following clinical signs is NOT present in a patient with a tension pneumothorax?

a tachypnoea
b hypotension
c elevated jugular venous pressure

d tracheal deviation towards the side of the pneumothorax
e hyper-resonant percussion note on the side of the pneumothorax

2 Immediate insertion of a chest tube may be lifesaving in which condition?
a carcinoma of the lung
b pulmonary embolism
c tension pneumothorax
d pleural effusion
e lung abscess

3 The pathological type of carcinoma of the lung with the worst prognosis is:
a small-cell carcinoma
b large-cell carcinoma
c adenocarcinoma
d squamous cell carcinoma
e adenosquamous cell carcinoma

4 The greatest chance of long-term survival in a patient with a localised carcinoma of the lung is provided by:
a chemotherapy
b radiotherapy
c combined chemotherapy and radiotherapy
d surgical excision
e immunotherapy

Problem Solving

59 Chronic constipation

Yik-Hong Ho

Introduction

Constipation is one of the most common presenting symptoms. Chronic constipation occurs when symptoms persist for more than 6 weeks. These symptoms may be (a) less than 3 bowel movements a week, (b) straining during defecation for more than 25% of the time or (c) frequent inability to evacuate the rectum completely. Chronic constipation by itself is not a life-threatening disorder; although dangerous disorders such as colorectal cancer should be excluded by colonoscopy as appropriate. It should only be treated if it causes complications which interfere significantly with quality of life. Such complicatons include abdominal distension, stercoral ulcers and anorectal problems. It should be remembered that chronic constipation is a symptom and not a disease. Management involves diagnosing the underlying cause and treating it. An understanding of colorectal motility physiology is required for this.

Physiology and physiologic testing

A solid meal passes from the mouth to enter the caecum in 4 hours. Residue in this meal reaches the rectosigmoid by 24 hours. Colonic motility causes the bowel contents to be retained and mixed, to facilitate absorption; it takes 3–4 days for the meal residue to be finally evacuated in the stools. The frequency of bowel movement in most normal humans ranges from 3 per week to 3 per day. About 70% of stool consistency is water, and inadequate water intake may result in harder stools that are difficult to evacuate.

The motility of the colon has 3 patterns: (a) *retrograde peristalsis*, which occurs mainly in the right colon (b) *segmentation*, which results in minimal transit over the colon and occurs mainly in the left colon and (c) *mass movement*, which results in propelling contents over long distances but occurs only a few times daily. Motility is likely controlled by a pacemaker in the transverse colon, which also acts as the main region of storage. Colonic motility is under enteric nervous and endocrine control. It can be significantly affected by physical activity, dietary fibre and emotional states. The transit which results from colonic motility can be assessed by imaging studies. Transit marker studies involve ingesting non-absorbed radio-opaque markers. Colonic transit is estimated by taking plain X-rays after standardized time intervals. The proportion and distribution of any retained markers are then assessed. Alternatively, some hospitals are using radio-isotope scintigraphy techniques.

The rectum is usually empty until faeces arrives periodically from the colon. Distension of the rectal or pelvic muscle walls causes an urge to defecaete. Initially, this can be suppressed by contraction of the anal sphincters and pelvic floor muscles. Further arrival of faeces will eventually make defecation unavoidable. At defecation, expulsion is aided by raised intra-abdominal pressure and colonic contraction. The pelvic floor muscles and the anal sphincters relax so the faeces can be discharged through the anus. Afterwards, the pelvic floor muscles and the anal sphincters resume their tone, in order to maintain bowel continence. Disorders of evacuation can be assessed by defecating proctography. The rectum is filled with radiological contrast and the patient attempts defecation on a radiolucent toilet seat. The progress of the instilled contrast is assessed by flouroscopy. The integrity of the intrinsic innervation of the rectum and anus is tested at anorectal manometry. The rectosphincteric inhibitory reflex is tested by inflating a rectal balloon looking for a transient drop in the anal pressures. This reflex is classically absent in Hirschsprung's disease.

Aetiology of constipation

The causes of chronic constipation can be worked out from an understanding of the physiology. A classification of the more common causes is given in Box 59.1

Box 59.1 Aetiology of constipation

Dietary
- Poor fibre intake
- Poor fluid intake

Functional
- Irritable bowel syndrome
- Immobility
- Pregnancy
- Psychiatric and psychological causes (e.g. depression, confusion)

Medications
- Neurological – e.g. anticonvulsants, anti-Parkinsonian drugs
- Psychiatric – e.g. antidepressants, antipsychotics
- Narcotics and opiates
- Calcium channel blockers
- Antacids
- Barium sulphate
- Iron tablets
- Fibre supplements with inadequate fluids

Metabolic, endocrine and collagen-vascular diseases
- Diabetes mellitus, hypopituitarism, hypothyroidism, hyperparathyroidism
- Hypercalcaemia, hypokalaemia
- Scleroderma
- Chronic renal failure

Neuromuscular
- Cerebral – e.g. cerebrovascular accidents, Parkinsonism, tumours
- Spinal – e.g. cauda equina tumour, multiple sclerosis, paraplegia
- Peripheral
  - Hirschsprung's disease
  - Autonomic neuropathy
  - Chagas' disease

Physiologic disorders
- Slow-transit constipation (colonic inertia)
- Intestinal pseudo-obstruction (Ogilvie's syndrome)
- Outlet obstruction
  - Anismus/puborectalis paradoxus
  - Rectocele, rectal intussusception, sigmoidocele

Evaluation of the patient with chronic constipation

The evaluation of chronic constipation can be worked out from an understanding of the more common causes (see Figure 59.1).

History

A detailed medical and dietary history must be taken of the patient history as well as bowel habit. First, it must be ascertained that the severity and chronicity of the symptoms described qualifies to be evaluated as chronic intractible constipation. Sporadic episodes of acute constipation respond readily to laxatives and do not justify subjecting the patient to extensive investigations. In addition, chronic constipation must be differentiated from recent change in bowel habits, especially with rectal bleeding. Obviously, a colonic neoplasm must be exluded in the latter case. In chronic constipation there is unhindered passage of flatus, but in colonic obstruction there is obstipation. However, chronic constipation with faecal impaction can cause intestinal obstruction, but this is usually only in the elderly nursing home or spinal cord injury patients. Sometimes, chronic constipation with faecal impaction can present paradoxically as overflow diarrhoea or faecal incontinence.

Second, the impact of the symptoms upon the patient's quality of life should be assessed by the amount of laxatives needed, complications of chronic constipation and interference with the patient's happiness. Sometimes patients may even need anal or vaginal digitation to help evacuate the stool. Third, appropriate associated questions related to the common causes may clinch the diagnosis.

Physical examination

Although the physical examination will concentrate on the abdomen and anorectum, careful systemic examination is important to exclude systemic causes of constipation (Box 59.1). Physical examination in patients with chronic constipation is usually unremarkable or may reveal abdominal distension with a colon full of faeces.

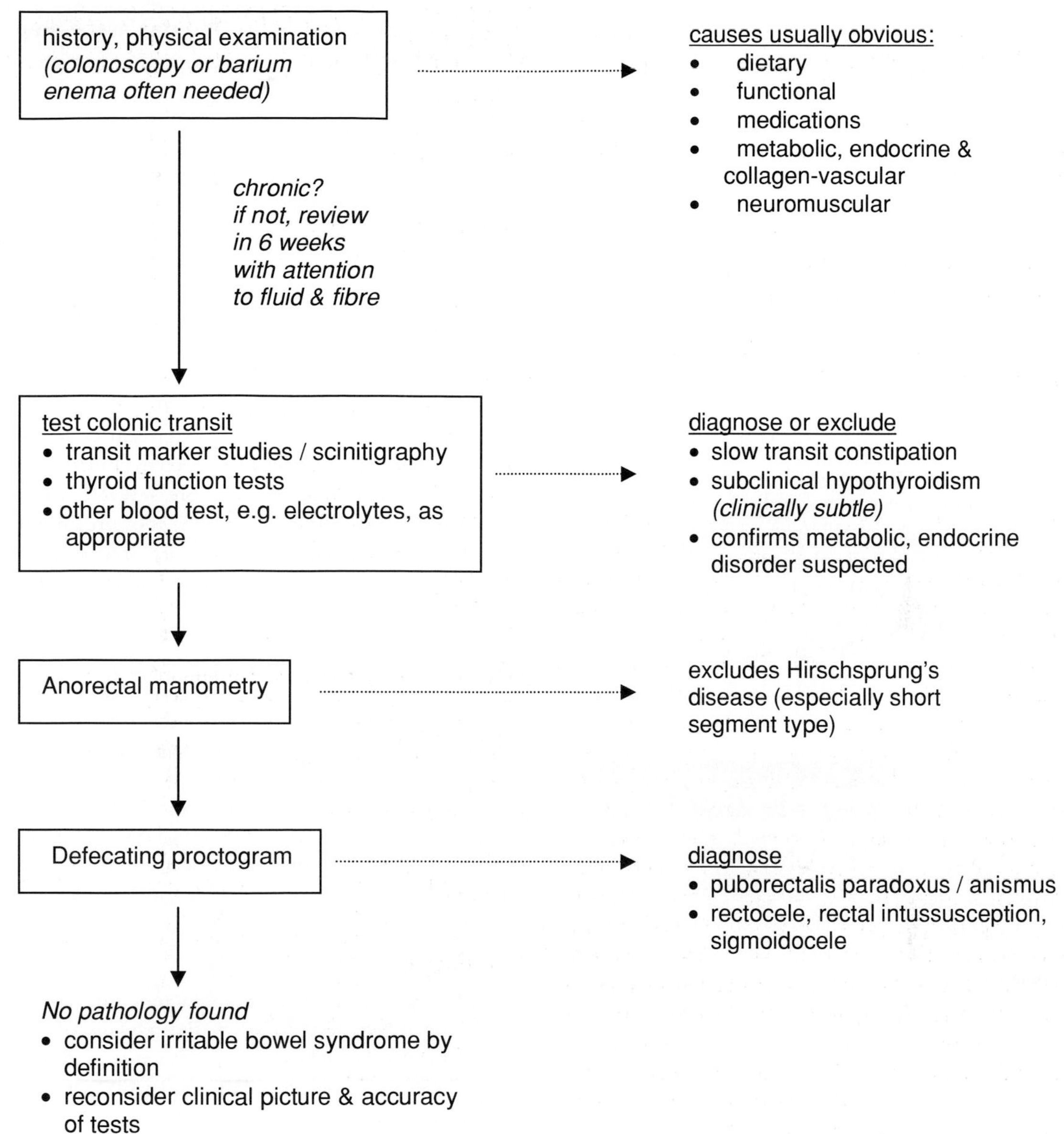

Fig. 59.1 Diagnostic algorithm for chronic constipation.

Diagnostic investigations

A colonoscopy or double-contrast barium enema is very often needed to exclude dangerous organic pathology such as neoplasm. In chronic constipation, a barium enema is preferable because the colon can be dilated and tortuous, especially with megacolon. This would make colonoscopic intubation difficult. The tests commonly used to help identify surgically treatable causes of constipation are transit marker studies, anorectal manometry and defecating proctogram. Their nature (see 'Physiology and Physiologic Testing') and application (see Figure 59.1) have already been described above. In some specialist colorectal units, personality testing is also used in assessing the patient for surgery because chronic constipation is commonly associated with pschological problems.

Management

Management is directed towards the primary cause of the constipation (see Box 59.1). The student is referred to standard textbooks of internal medicine for the management of the various systemic causes of constipation. When the primary pathology does not lend itself to treatment or when no pathology is identifed, management is symptomatic. This consists of dietary advice, improving bowel habits, encouraging exercise and the use of laxatives, enemas or suppositories. At least 30 g of dietary fibre together with sufficient fluids are needed to have an adequately bulky but soft stool each day. Other simple measures like developing regular bowel habits and not ignoring the need to pass stool may be all that is required to correct simple constipation. Regular exercise also improves bowel function. Faecal impaction should be digitally cleared to enable the other measures to work properly. A classification of the commonly used laxatives is given in Box 59.2. No evidence is available as to which laxative or laxative regime is superior.

Box 59.2 Laxatives

Bulking agents (dietary fibre/bulk laxatives)
- Ispaghula husk
- Methylcellulose
- *Sterculia*

Stimulants
- Bisacodyl
- Senna
- Sodium picosulphate

Faecal softeners
- Liquid paraffin
- Agarol

Osmotic laxatives
- Lactulose
- Fleet phosphosoda
- Magnesium sulphate

Rectal preparations
- Suppositories
- Enemas

Management of specific conditions associated with constipation

Irritable bowel syndrome

Irritable bowel syndrome is the most common gastrointestinal disease, occuring in 15% of adults in Western societies. It is a characterized by altered bowel habits, abdominal pain and absence of detectable organic pathology. Diagnosis includes a history of at least 3 months and there are 3 types of clinical presentation: (a) abdominal pain and constipation, (b) alternating constipation and diarrhoea, or (c) chronic painless diarrhoea.

The majority of patients with milder symptoms will be satisfied with the reassurance that dangerous diseases like colorectal cancer have been excluded for example by colonoscopy. Those more severely affected may require counselling to avoid stress or precipitating factors, dietary advice, drugs for symptomatic relief of pain and bowel frequency problems, and rarely formal psychological management.

Slow-transit constipation (colonic inertia)

Slow-transit constipation is likely a disorder of colonic innervation, but this is still poorly understood. Women in the second or third decades of life are most commonly affected. Transit marker studies typically show retention of more that 20% markers 5 days after ingestion, in a diffuse pattern. Total colectomy with ileorectal anastomosis is recommended for intractible cases.

Puborectalis paradox (anismus)

The puborectalis and anal sphincters normally relax during defecation, to allow the passage of stool. Puborectalis paradoxus occurs with inadequate relaxation, resulting in pelvic outlet obstruction. It is possible that a rectal motility problem also exists. The diagnosis is made at anorectal manometry and defecating proctography. Recommended treatment is anorectal biofeedback, to supposedly re-train the puborectalis muscle to relax properly during rectal evacuation.

Rectocele

Rectocele is a weakness of the anterior rectal wall, the rectovaginal septum and the posterior vaginal wall. At defecation, the weakness allows faeces to be diverted into a pouch in the vagina. Patients often have to reduce this pouch with a finger, in order to initiate defecation. Where a rectocele specifically causes constipation symptoms, surgical management is best directed at the rectal side where there is a high pressure zone. A transanal rectocele repair is recommended.

Other causes

The specific conditions like rectal intussusception, sigmoidocele, Hirchsprung's disease (especially short-segment disease in adults) and Chaga's disease are relatively rare. The interested student is directed to standard textbooks on colorectal surgery.

Further reading

Lembo A, Camilleri M. Current concepts; chronic constipation. *N Eng J Med.* 2003;349:1360–1368.

Tjandra JJ, Ooi BS, Tang CL, Dwyer P, Carey U. Transanal repair of rectocele corrects obstructed defecation if it is not associated with anismus. *Dis Colon Rectum.* 1999;42:1544–1550.

MCQs

Select the single correct answer to each question.

1 The most common cause of constipation is:
- **a** slow-transit constipation
- **b** inadequate dietary fibre and fluids
- **c** obstruction from colorectal cancer
- **d** hypothyroidism
- **e** rectocele

2 A 31-year-old lady lawyer has chronic constipation not responding to laxatives. She has 80% of transit markers retained in the ascending colon 5 days after ingestion. Thyroid function tests, defecating proctogram and anorectal physiologic tests were otherwise normal. The most appropriate management is:
- **a** use a combination of laxatives, enemas and rectal washout
- **b** right hemicolectomy
- **c** total colectomy and ileorectal anastomosis
- **d** electro-colonic stimulation
- **e** aerobic dancing (high-impact type)

3 A 24-year-old female secretary has constipation for 3 weeks after starting a new job. There are no other abdominal symptoms and no family history of colorectal cancer. The most appropriate management is:
- **a** try taking enough dietary fibre and fluids
- **b** colonoscopy and anorectal physiology tests
- **c** anorectal biofeedback therapy
- **d** teach self digital extraction of faeces from rectum
- **e** repeat thyroid function tests at least 3 times

4 A 43-year-old mother of two children complains of difficulty in initiating rectal evacuation. She feels there is a lump in the perineum which requires vaginal reduction prior to effective evacuation. The most appropriate management is:
- **a** teach good hygienic practices
- **b** avoid excessive sexual relationships
- **c** transit marker studies
- **d** defecating proctogram
- **e** anorectal biofeedback

5 After a previous hysterectomy, a 55-year-old mother of 3 children complains of constipation. Defecating proctogram showed lack of relaxation of the puborectalis paradoxus at defecation. The most appropriate management is:
- **a** yoga taught by genuine Indian guru
- **b** regular use of St. Mark's anal dilator prior to defecation
- **c** anorectal biofeedback therapy
- **d** mandatory use of squatting posture at defecation
- **e** avoid laxatives but teach rectal washout instead

60 Faecal incontinence

Joe J. Tjandra

Introduction

Faecal incontinence is defined as the inability to defer passage of faeces until an appropriate time. The maintenance of normal faecal continence is achieved by the interplay of functional anal sphincters, rectal compliance, anorectal sensation, and the composition of the faeces. The internal anal sphincter, a smooth muscle, is responsible for 80% of resting anal tone. It relaxes in response to rectal distension (rectoanal inhibitory reflex). The striated external anal sphincter is innervated by the pudendal nerve (S2, S3, S4). The external anal sphincter encircles the internal sphincter and continues cephaled as the puborectalis muscle (Fig. 60.1). Together, they function as a sphincter that exerts voluntary contraction when the intra-abdominal pressure is raised, such as in coughing or straining or when one wishes to defer defecation.

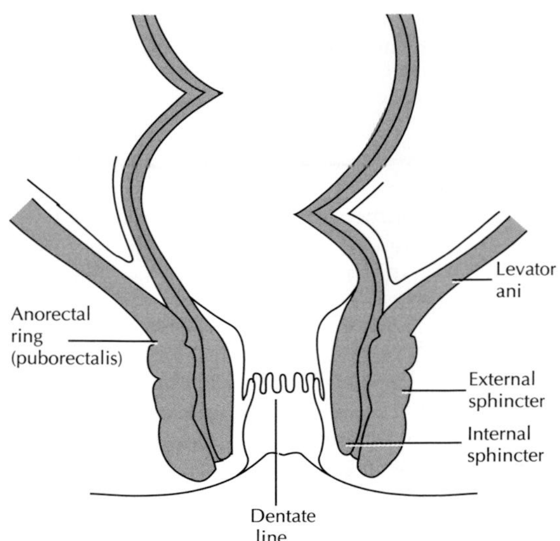

Fig. 60.1 Anal canal and rectum.

Box 60.1 Causes of faecal incontinence

Incontinence with abnormal sphincters
- Sphincter defect: obstetric, previous anorectal surgery, perineal trauma
- Neuropathic sphincters: lower motor neurone lesions (e.g. stretch pudendal neuropathy, diabetes, demyelination), upper motor neurone lesions (e.g. stroke, cerebral tumours, demyelination)
- Rectal prolapse
- Anorectal/pelvic cancer
- Congenital anorectal abnormalities

Incontinence with normal sphincters
- Faecal impaction
- Severe diarrhoea
- Dementia or mental retardation

The anal canal has a rich sensory network to provide anorectal sampling to discriminate between gas, liquids and solids. Mechanoreceptors lie within the rectal wall and pelvic floor to detect rectal fullness. With reduction in rectal compliance as in Crohn's disease or radiation proctitis, diarrhoea may cause urgency at stool and further threaten continence, even if the sphincter mechanism is intact.

The causes of faecal incontinence are given in Box 60.1.

Clinical assessment

Careful history with regard to the severity and nature of faecal incontinence is essential. Many patients are incontinent as a result of diarrhoea and urgency at stool. Neurological symptoms or any possible causative factors should be documented.

Careful examination of the perineum, anus and rectum should be performed, noting any scars, evidence of soiling, a patulous anus, perianal fistula or a rectal or uterine prolapse with straining. Digital rectal examination will provide a good assessment of the anal sphincters at rest and on voluntary contraction. Proctosigmoidoscopy is performed to exclude inflammatory bowel disease, neoplasia, mucosal prolapse and haemorrhoids.

Investigations

Endo-anal ultrasound

Endo-anal ultrasound is an outpatient procedure using a rotating hand-held ultrasound probe inserted transanally. No special bowel preparation or sedation is necessary. This procedure is operator-dependent and its use is best restricted to major specialist colorectal centres.

Endo-anal ultrasound provides high resolution images of both the internal and external anal sphincters. Defects in the anal sphincters are clearly defined (Fig. 60.2) and may then be amenable to surgical repair.

Anorectal manometry

This is performed using a balloon-tipped or microtransducer-tipped catheter inserted into the anal canal. The pressures produced by the internal sphincter (resting pressure) and the external sphincter (voluntary contraction pressure) are measured along the length of the anal canal. The length of the high pressure zone of the anal canal can then be defined.

Rectal sensation is measured by gradually distending a balloon in the rectum and recording when distension is first perceived. Compliance of the rectum and integrity of the rectoanal inhibitory reflex can also be documented.

While anorectal manometry provides interesting measurements for surgical research, it has not made a major impact on surgical management. It is generally restricted to use in specialist colorectal research and to aid in the management in complex cases.

(A)

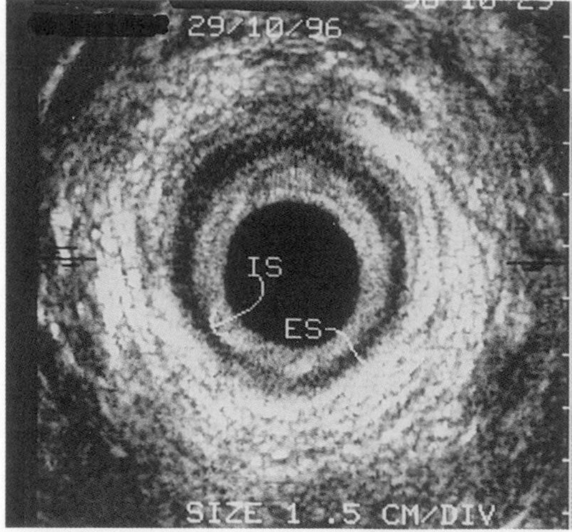

(B)

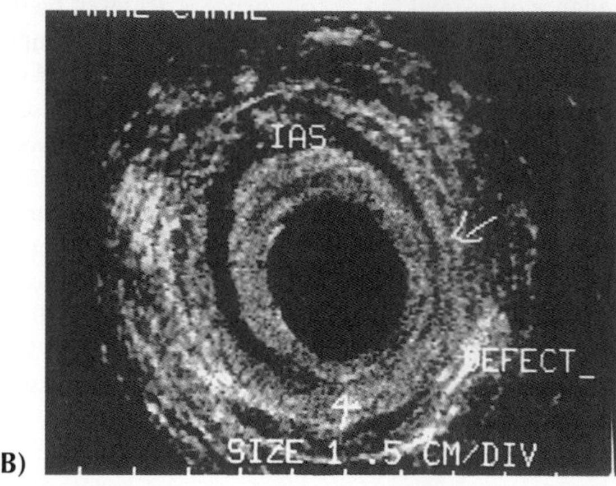

Fig. 60.2 Endo-anal ultrasound showing **(A)** normal and intact anal sphincters (IS, internal sphincter; ES, external sphincter) and **(B)** internal anal sphincter defect.

Treatment

Underlying pathology such as inflammatory bowel disease, cancer or rectal prolapse must be treated. Conservative treatment aims at producing a solid bulky stool. A low-fibre diet and codeine phosphate or loperamide are helpful. Daily phosphate enema may further reduce the risk of accidental soiling.

Pelvic floor exercises and biofeedback conditioning are used to strengthen the anal sphincters. These techniques are time-consuming and have not been proven to have a long-term benefit.

Surgery is undertaken when conservative treatment has failed or if there are identifiable sphincter defects clinically or on endo-anal ultrasound.

Surgical approaches

Sphincter repair

This is a direct repair of a defect of the anal sphincters. A perianal incision is made and both ends of the divided anal sphincters are then repaired either directly or in an overlapping fashion. About 85% of patients will derive some functional improvement after sphincter repair, if the pudendal nerve function is intact.

Injectable silicone biomaterial

This is a newly developed treatment by the Melbourne group for internal sphincter dysfunction. The silicone biomaterial is injected under guidance of endoanal ultrasound into the internal anal sphincter and the inter-sphincteric space. The injected silicone biomaterial (PTQTM) forms a template to allow ingrowth of collagen tissues, thereby increasing the bulk of the internal sphincter. Clinically it would take 6 to 8 weeks before any improvement in passive incontinence. Clinical improvement will continue up to 12 months after injection. The procedure is simple and can be performed under local anaesthesia with a mild sedative.

Sacral nerve stimulation

The innervation that controls defecation is mediated by S2, S3 and S4 nerve roots. Stimulation and modulation of the sacral nerves may increase the anal canal pressures through recruitment of the anal sphincter muscles. Melbourne is one of the pioneering centres to evaluate this particular approach and has reported outstanding success in patients with severe end-stage faecal incontinence. An electrode is inserted under fluoroscopic guidance to the S3 nerve root. Having established the optimal position of the electrode by eliciting the appropriate motor and sensory responses for S3, the electrode is connected to the stimulator. A screening phase for about 1 week is usually performed to establish the clinical benefits of sacral nerve stimulation, before a permanent neurostimulator is connected and implanted. The permanent neurostimulator is about the size of a cigarette lighter and is implanted subcutaneously in the buttock or lower abdominal wall. The procedure is safe and simple to perform.

Artificial bowel sphincter

Artificial bowel sphincter is a prosthesis using a fluid-filled, solid silicone device that is implanted around the anal canal with an occlusive cuff. A control pump is placed in the scrotum or labium to transfer fluid between the occlusive cuff and the presure-regulating balloon placed in the subcutaneous tissue of the abdominal wall. While artificial bowel sphincter can be successful in end-stage faecal incontinence, sepsis requiring removal of the prosthesis occurs in over one-third of patients. As a result, this is unlikely to be a popular treatment for faecal incontinence.

Diverting stoma with a colostomy or ileostomy

In patients with severe faecal incontinence and in whom sphincter repair or reconstruction is unsuitable or has failed, a good stoma will greatly improve the quality of life and should be considered (see Chapter 30).

MCQs

Select the single correct answer to each question.

1 Which of the following is CORRECT with faecal incontinence?
- **a** none of the treatments for faecal incontinence is satisfactory
- **b** faecal incontinence should only be managed by a specialist
- **c** sphincteroplasty is performed only if there is an intact sphincter
- **d** specialised testing with endoanal ultrasond and anorectal physiology could be helpful in managing severe faecal incontinence
- **e** specialised treatment such as sacral nerve stimulation is not available in Australia

2 Faecal incontinence:
- **a** is more common in men than in women
- **b** is more common than urinary incontinence
- **c** is often improved by pelvic floor exercises
- **d** is usually managed by surgery
- **e** is usually due to complications of anorectal surgery

61 Rectal bleeding

Joe J. Tjandra

Chronic rectal bleeding

Rectal bleeding is alarming although most causes are benign. Bleeding may be overt when noticed by the patient or occult when invisible blood loss is detectable by faecal occult blood test only. Management of rectal bleeding involves exclusion of a colorectal neoplasm and finding the cause of the bleeding.

Classification and causes of chronic rectal bleeding are given in Table 61.1.

History

A detailed history should be taken. The nature of the rectal bleeding must be determined (duration, colour and amount of blood). Macroscopic bleeding recognised by the patient usually arises from the left side of the colon or rectum. Right-sided colonic bleeding usually presents with anaemia but without overt bleeding. The presence of anal pain should be inquired about. This occurs with anal fissure, strangulated haemorrhoids and anorectal cancer. Prolapse occurs with second- and third-degree haemorrhoids and with mucosal or full-thickness rectal prolapse. Other symptoms that may be seen are mixture of blood with stool, alteration in bowel habit, abdominal pain or distension and weight loss. These suggest that the source of bleeding is more proximally located in the colon or rectum. Anaemia is also indicative of a colonic or upper rectal lesion.

A past and family history of colorectal neoplasm must be gained from the patient, as well as a past history of colonic diseases such as inflammatory bowel disease.

Anorectal examination

Anorectal examination is essential in any patient presenting with rectal bleeding. Inspection should determine the presence of anal fissure, strangulated haemorrhoids or anal canal cancer. During straining, look for prolapsing haemorrhoids or rectal prolapse. Digital examination is used to feel for a rectal polyp or cancer. This may not be possible in the presence of an acute anal fissure because of anal sphincter spasm and pain.

Proctoscopy can be used to visualise any anal canal lesion and haemorrhoids. On rigid sigmoidoscopy the

Table 61.1 Classification and causes of chronic rectal bleeding

Classification	Causes
Anal outlet bleeding	Haemorrhoids
Bright blood per rectum, separate from the stool and often present as a smear of bright blood on the toilet paper	Anal fissure
Bleeding associated with defecation	Anorectal cancer
No change in bowel habits	Rectal prolapse
No past or family history of colorectal neoplasm	Proctitis
Suspicious bleeding	Colorectal neoplasm
Dark blood or blood mixed with stool	Diverticular disease
Change in bowel habit or passage of mucus	Inflammatory bowel disease
Past or family history of colorectal neoplasm	Angiodysplasia

level of the rectum visualised should be recorded together with the level of any abnormality seen. Any suspicious lesion seen should be biopsied. The presence of blood clots or blood-stained faeces beyond the reach of the sigmoidoscope indicate a more proximal pathological process. Fibre-optic flexible sigmoidoscopy allows for an easier examination of the rectum and a variable length of the sigmoid and descending colon. In many specialist colorectal practices, this has replaced rigid sigmoidoscopy.

Special investigations

These include colonoscopy and air-contrast barium enema. Either of these tests may be performed to evaluate the colon. They are necessary only if the source of the bleeding is not clearly established and if there is doubt that a more proximal cause in the colon may be present. Colonoscopy has the advantage that small tumours and lesions that are bleeding may be more readily detected than by an air-contrast barium enema; as well as being therapeutic in that polyps may be removed endoscopically and angio-dysplasia may be treated with argon plasma coagulation or cautery. Capsule endoscopy is a newer investigation to identify a bleeding source in the small bowel.

Massive rectal bleeding

Clinical evaluation

A detailed history is important. The nature and amount of bleeding give an indication of the cause of the bleeding (Box 61.1). Massive colonic haemorrhage is dark red or plum coloured and is to be differentiated from melaena, which is black. Melaena almost invariably arises from the stomach or small bowel. A rapidly bleeding peptic ulcer may occasionally present with bright red rectal bleeding. The haemodynamic condition of the patient will also reflect the severity of bleeding. Massive bleeding indicates bleeding of more than 1500 mL in 24 hours. In these circumstances, the patient has signs of shock on admission that demand urgent management with transfusion. Massive rectal bleeding will cease spontaneously in 80% of cases.

A prior history of a bowel disorder such as inflammatory bowel disease or haemorrhoids is ascertained. Use of anticoagulant therapy or non-steroidal anti-inflammatory drugs may contribute to bleeding. Liver disorders with impaired coagulation are also noted. A rectal examination with rigid proctosigmoidoscopy is performed to exclude bleeding haemorrhoids or rectal tumours.

Box 61.1 Causes of massive rectal bleeding

- Diverticular disease
- Angiodysplasia/angioma
- Ulcerated cancer
- Rare colonic causes (e.g. radiation colitis, inflammatory bowel disease, ischaemic colitis)
- Upper gastrointestinal lesions

Resuscitation

Resuscitation should be immediately initiated with massive rectal bleeding while diagnostic tests are performed.

Investigations

Upper gastrointestinal endoscopy

In cases of severe rectal bleeding with shock, an upper gastrointestinal endoscopy should be performed as soon as clinically feasible to exclude an upper gastrointestinal lesion, such as a bleeding peptic ulcer, oesophageal varices or aorto-enteric fistula. Alternatively a nasogastric tube is passed to exclude blood in the stomach.

Colonoscopy

Colonoscopy is performed as soon as feasible the following day with a full bowel preparation to locate the site of colonic bleeding, even if the bleeding continues. Emergency colonoscopy is difficult with active bleeding and requires a great deal of experience.

Enteroclysis

If the bleeding has ceased and the source of bleeding is yet to be identified, an enteroclysis is performed to exclude a gross small bowel lesion.

Capsule endoscopy

This involves patient swallowing a small videocapsule (Pillcam) which will capture digitised images of the small bowel. The duration of test is limited by the battery life of the videocapsule, which is eight hours. This is best done in a patient who is haemodynamically stable and has had recurrent gastrointestinal bleeding of unknown origin despite being previously investigated with upper gastrointestinal endoscopy, colonoscopy and barium small bowel follow-through.

Radionuclide scan

If bleeding continues and the site of haemorrhage is not located by colonoscopy, a radionuclide scan is done using technetium-99m sulphur colloid or technetium-99m-labelled autologous red cells. A bleeding rate of 0.1–0.5 mL/min can be detected. The accuracy of these scans is variable, ranging from 40% to 90%. If the scan is positive and bleeding continues, mesenteric angiogram is performed to confirm the bleeding site.

Mesenteric angiogram

Selective angiogram of the inferior mesenteric, superior mesenteric and coeliac arteries is performed if bleeding continues and the rate is greater than 0.5 mL/min. Angiography is likely to be positive if there is active bleeding at the time of injection of contrast. If the site of bleeding is identified and the patient is elderly and frail, haemostasis with intra-arterial infusion of vasopressin through selective arterial cannulation should be considered. If effective, this is continued for 24 hours.

Surgery

If bleeding continues, laparotomy is performed. If the site of bleeding is not clearly localised pre- or intra-operatively, intra-operative enteroscopy using a colonoscope inserted transorally is performed. The most distal part of the ileum may be examined using a colonoscope passed transanally. The bowel is transilluminated during intra-operative enteroscopy in a darkened room to detect angiodysplasias or small bowel angiomas. If the site of bleeding remains unclear, a subtotal abdominal colectomy is performed.

Review

If the diagnosis is unresolved despite a full investigation, the patient is observed. If bleeding recurs, a full investigation is repeated as in a new case of active bleeding. Laparotomy and intra-operative enteroscopy may be necessary if these re-bleeding episodes are moderately severe.

MCQs

Select the single correct answer to each question.

1 Most patients presenting with massive rectal bleeding:
- a will bleed to death unless they have surgery
- b usually were found to have colon cancer
- c usually were found to have rectal cancer
- d should have a capsule endoscopy performed immediately
- e should have a proctosigmoidoscopy performed before a colonoscopy

2 Patients with massive rectal bleeding:
- a should never have surgery until the precise site and cause of rectal bleeding is identified
- b should have a nasogastric tube inserted before any other investigation to exclude an upper gastrointestinal source of bleeding
- c should proceed directly to a mesenteric angiogram
- d should be appropriately resuscitated
- e should have radionuclide scan performed immediately, regardless of the amount of bleeding

62 Haematemesis and melaena

Robert J. S. Thomas

Introduction

Definition

Haematemesis is the vomiting of blood, either bright or altered blood (so-called 'coffee grounds' vomitus), due to the action of acid on the blood. Melaena is the passage of black tarry stools. The tarriness is characteristic and distinguishes melaena from the passage of black stools due to dietary agents, including the ingestion of iron. Haematemesis occurs from a point that is usually not distal to the duodenum but melaena may occur not only from a proximal bleeding site, but rarely from a small intestinal cause.

Incidence

Haematemesis and melaena is a common and important symptom complex presenting either as an acute catastrophic illness or more electively with prolonged minor bleeding. Patients with this condition make a major demand on hospital beds.

Significance

Patients with haematemesis and melaena require admission to hospital. The condition has a high mortality and demands a systematic approach to the initial resuscitation process, the diagnostic method and the therapeutic program. The overall management of this condition has been revolutionised by the introduction of new endoscopic techniques to control bleeding.

Causes of haematemesis

Swallowed blood from, for example, a bleeding site in the post-nasal space, must be excluded as a cause for haematemesis.

Table 62.1 Common causes of haematemesis and melaena

Oesophageal	Reflux oesophagitis – other associated hiatus hernia Oesophageal varices (portal hypertension) Oesophaeal tumours Mallory–Weiss mucosal tear
Gastric	Gastric ulcer – usually benign Haemorrhagic gastritis Gastric varices Gastric cancer Delafoy lesion
Duodenum	Duodenal ulcer Duodenitis

The list of causes of haematemesis and melaena is long (Table 62.1). The common causes are:
- peptic ulcer (i.e. gastric or duodenal ulceration)
- oesophageal varices
- gastritis or duodenitis.

The site of bleeding usually lies in the oesophagus, stomach or duodenum.

Oesophagus

The most common cause of bleeding in the oesophagus is from oesophageal varices secondary to portal hypertension. Oesophageal varices are the cause of some 10–30% of major haematemesis episodes in most Western countries. Less commonly, oesophagitis secondary to gastro-oesophageal reflux is associated with haemorrhage. Oesophageal cancer rarely presents with bleeding.

Stomach

Gastric ulcer is one of the most common causes of haematemesis and melaena. The ulcer may be in the body or the antrum of the stomach. The pre-pyloric position is the most common. Gastric ulcer may be the site of torrential haemorrhage because of the invasion of a major vessel (e.g. the splenic artery). Gastritis is also a common cause of gastric bleeding.

The common use of non-steroidal anti-flammatory drugs (NSAID) are associated with haematemesis and melaena due to gastric ulceration in many elderly patients. Despite the use of Cox2 inhibitor anti-arthiritic agents, ulceration can still occur, particularly when these drugs are prescribed in conjunction with aspirin. A Mallory–Weiss tear is a tear of the gastro-oesophageal junction as a result of retching, with differential intra-abdominal and thoracic pressures leading to the tear. Characteristically the haematemesis appears after initial blood-free vomit.

Gastric varices may be associated with portal hypertension and coexist with oesophageal varices. Gastric cancer is not a common cause of haematemesis and melaena but a gastric ulcer may bleed and prove to be malignant on biopsy.

Duodenum

Duodenal ulcer is traditionally the most common cause of haematemesis and melaena. The ulcer is usually on the posterior wall of the duodenum and characteristically invades the gastroduodenal artery. Haemorrhage may be profuse but is usually self-limited.

In Western societies the number of patients presenting with duodenal ulcers is decreasing. However, there is an increasing number of patients presenting with gastric ulceration, particularly elderly patients on NSAID.

Management

Initial assessment

In most hospitals, patients with haematemesis and melaena are managed in a special unit and along a clinical pathway or algorithm to systemise management (Fig. 62.1).

The circulatory state of the patient is assessed. The extent of blood loss can be estimated on the basis of the patient's clinical status. Apprehension, air hunger, cerebral changes, marked pallor, thready pulse and hypotension indicate significant blood loss (up to 50% of blood volume). Maintenance of normal peripheral circulation without cerebral findings but with mild tachycardia and postural drop in blood pressure is consistent with 10–20% blood volume loss. This estimation of circulatory status gives an indication of the urgency of fluid replacement.

The cause of bleeding must then be diagnosed. This is often not obvious. However, the presence of a previous history of peptic ulceration or evidence of hepatic cirrhosis may indicate a likely site of blood loss.

Management of the patient

Optimal management of the patient with haematemesis and melaena involves vigorous resuscitation and early diagnosis.

Resuscitation

Intravenous therapy is started with normal saline and/or colloid (Haemaccel or 5% albumin solution). Blood is then taken for cross-matching. Depending on the clinical state of the patient, urgent cross-match can be performed and blood given immediately. Rarely, O-negative blood is required for a patient *in extremis*.

Monitoring is essential to estimate the effectiveness of blood replacement. Successful resuscitation can be observed by noting improvement in the clinical state of the patient, return of blood pressure and pulse rate towards normal, and the presence of a satisfactory urine output.

Diagnosis

Early endoscopy has been shown to be a safe and effective way of making a diagnosis. Once the patient's clinical condition is stabilised, this procedure is carried out either urgently if there is concern about continuing bleeding, or on the next elective endoscopy list if there is no indication for urgent intervention.

The patient is sedated with intravenous medication and the gastroscope is passed. The oesophagus, stomach and duodenum are carefully examined. There may be some difficulty in this examination process with the presence of either old blood, blood clot or fresh bleeding. Adequate suction and irrigation is required in order to define the bleeding point. Rarely the bleeding point is not identifiable. Throughout this procedure the patient requires adequate monitoring, the airway must be controlled and oxygen administered.

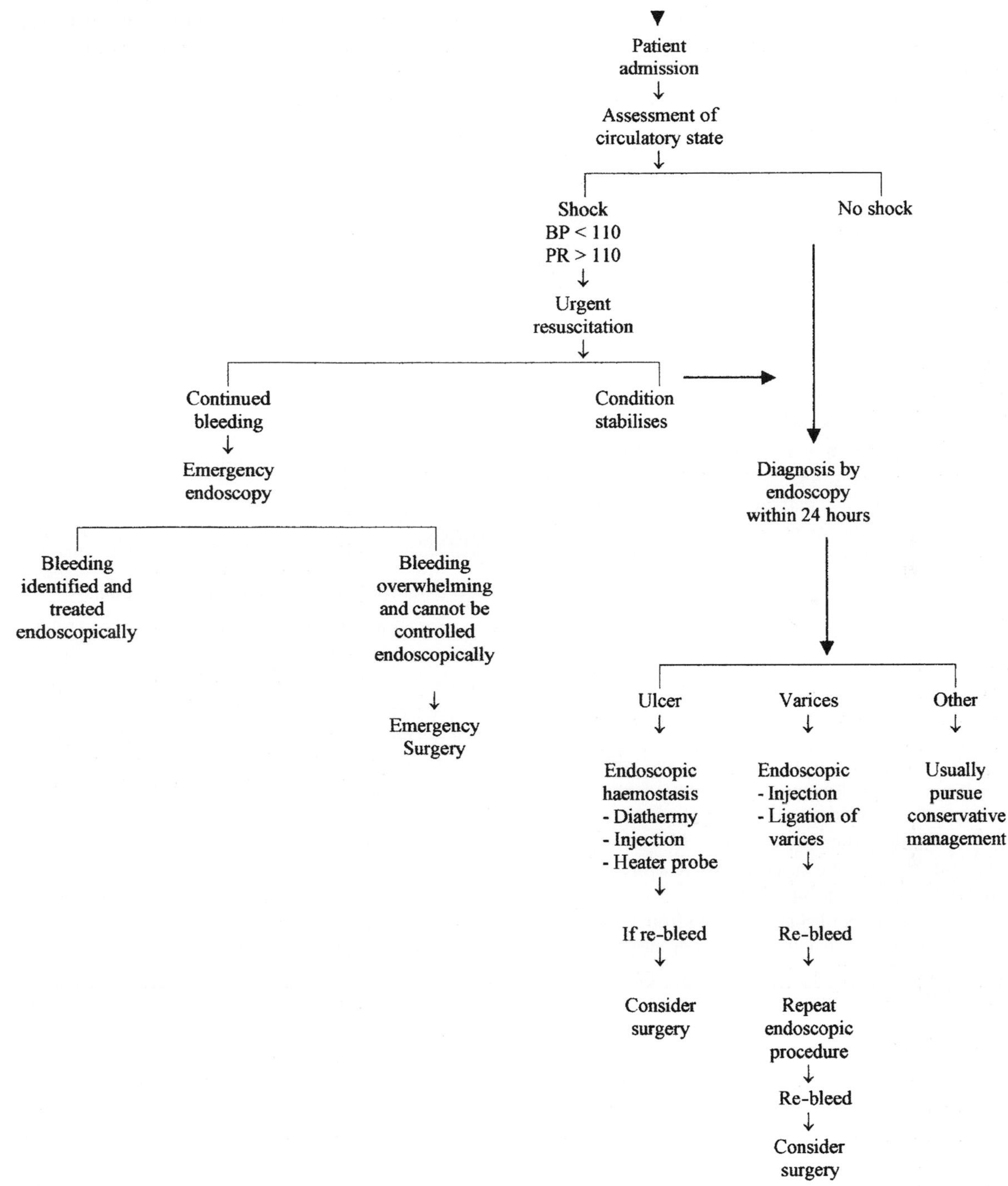

Fig. 62.1 Algorithm for management of haematemesis and melaena.

Therapy

Usually a therapeutic procedure can be carried out at the time of endoscopy. Injection of alcohol or adrenaline close to the bleeding point will usually result in cessation of bleeding. If oesophageal varices are present, these may be injected or banded. If it is evident that a major problem exists, such as a large gastric ulcer or persistent bleeding from a large duodenal ulcer, or bleeding from oesophageal varices, then immediate consultation with the surgical team is mandatory and combined management is implemented.

Indications for surgical intervention

The indications for surgical intervention include massive haemorrhage not responding to conservative means, patients requiring more than six units of blood, and elderly patients, particularly if a large ulcer is present, because they tolerate blood loss poorly.

Where a second haemorrhage occurs in hospital or there is concern about persistent ongoing bleeding, surgery is necessary.

Results of treatment

Most bleeding sites causing haematemesis and melaena stop bleeding spontaneously or with interventional endoscopy. The modern medical management of peptic ulcers, including the eradication of *Helicobacter pylori*, is so effective that surgery is to be avoided unless absolutely indicated to save life.

The results of treatment of bleeding from varices due to portal hypertension will depend on the degree of liver disease and the extent of the varices. These patients usually require an intensive care unit program of therapy. In the short term, injection or banding of varices is usually effective in stopping the bleeding. If bleeding persists then the use of a Sengstaken–Blakemore tube or Linton balloon to apply direct pressure to the cardia will usually result in tamponade of the bleeding point and control the haemorrhage. Occasionally emergency surgery is required, with some form of direct ligation of varices or gastric disconnection in order to control bleeding. Direct ligation of varices involves opening the stomach or oesophagus and directly suturing the varices. A gastric disconnection procedure involves devascularising the stomach completely in order to interrupt the venous channels supplying the varices.

Prognosis

Prognosis from this condition will depend upon the underlying cause and the clinical state of the patient. Overall, haematemesis and melaena patients have a high mortality and morbidity rate, varying from 5% to 20% in most series. This is because most patients with haematemesis and melaena are elderly, often with cardiac and pulmonary disease. These patients tolerate surgery poorly. Thus, the balance between surgical intervention and persisting with medical management in the face of continuing haemorrhage is often very fine and the best results are obtained in dedicated units for the management of this condition.

MCQs

Select the single correct answer to each question.

1 The INCORRECT statement regarding passage of black, tarry stools is:
- **a** it is usually an indication of bleeding from the upper gastrointestinal tract
- **b** it can be mimicked by the ingestion of iron medication
- **c** it is commonly a symptom of a cancer of the colon
- **d** It can be present without other symptoms
- **e** it is often but not universally associated with haematemesis

2 The causes of haematemesis and melaena include the following EXCEPT:
- **a** oesophageal varices
- **b** gastric ulceration
- **c** epistaxis with swallowed blood
- **d** beetroot ingestion
- **e** gastritis
- **f** Mallory–Weiss tear

3 The following statements apply to the patient who has suffered a GI bleed EXCEPT:
- **a** be pale and sweaty
- **b** be faint and have a bradycardia
- **c** be faint and have a tachycardia
- **d** require urgent resuscitation with normal saline initially
- **e** appear quite well with normal supine blood pressure

4 Which of the following is the INCORRECT statement on the diagnosis of the cause of the bleeding episode?
  a is the most urgent requirement in patient management
  b may be suspected from a history of NSAID (non steroidal inflammatory drug) intake
  c can made by early endoscopy of upper GI tract
  d can often be combined with treatment at the initial endoscopy
  e surgical intervention is required for ongoing blood loss

5 INCORRECT statement on haematemesis and melaena:
  a is a serious condition with a high mortality and morbidity rate?
  b now occurs in an older age group of patients.
  c has been eliminated with the advent of Cox2 inhibitor anti-inflammatory drugs.
  d when associated with oesophageal varices may require repeated interventions for control.
  e is best managed in a dedicated specialist treatment unit.

63 Obstructive jaundice

David Fletcher

Introduction

This chapter will discuss the clinical, diagnostic and therapeutic approach to a patient presenting with obstructive jaundice, as demonstrated by Fig. 63.1.

History and examination

The first step is a detailed history. If pain is present, and that pain is consistent and of a biliary origin, then a history of repeated episodes, associated nausea, radiation to the back and symptoms of fever should be elicited. Pain may also be due to malignancy and is then more constant and is usually associated with weight loss. The patient should be asked if they have noted pale stools or dark urine. Generalised itch in more chronic obstruction is also a symptom that may not be volunteered spontaneously. A history of intermittent fever suggests the potentially serious consequences of unrelieved cholangitis.

A history of prior surgery should be obtained both in relation to anaesthetic agents such as halothane and to surgery for biliary disease, which may result in early or late complications of bile duct surgery. A history of previous endoscopic retrograde cholangiopancreatography (ERCP) and sphincterotomy should be elicited, because sphincter stenosis due to the diathermy damage may occur months to years after the procedure.

The history should determine whether the patient is at risk for hepatitis, either from sexual contact or intravenous drug use, and whether any family members have been affected by hepatitis recently or in the past. A full drug history should also be obtained because of the risk of hepatotoxic drug reactions, which are of various types and include antibiotics such as flucloxacillin, sulphas, erythromycin, nitrofurantoin and other agents such as oestrogens and paracetamol. Excess vitamin A intake, an occasional feature of health food fanatics, may lead to hypercarotenaemia, which gives the skin a jaundiced appearance with normal sclera and liver function tests (LFT).

On examination, once the bilirubin is more than double the normal level, icterus should be evident in the sclera. On examining the abdomen, a palpable mass, either a pancreas, which is fixed and that the palpating hand may get above, or a gall-bladder, which the palpating hand will not get above and that moves down on respiration, may be elicited. If malignancy is suspected, other masses in the abdomen (particularly the liver) and the left prescalene (Virchow) node should be looked for. Evidence of skin scratching as a response to pruritus should be noted.

Investigations

Liver function tests

A ward test of the urine in obstructive jaundice will demonstrate the presence of bilirubin and the absence of urobilinogen. The plasma bilirubin will be elevated and will be principally in the conjugated form. Small changes only should occur in the alanine aminotransferase (ALT) and the aspartate aminotransferase (AST), which are indicative of hepatocyte injury. Alkaline phosphatase will be more markedly elevated with levels more than double those of the transaminases. The alkaline phosphatase is normally higher in children and will also be elevated in bony disease, the latter being differentiated either by alkaline phosphatase isoenzymes or by the gamma glutamyl transpeptidase (γ-GT). If the bilirubin is elevated but the alkaline phosphatase, γ-GT and transaminases are normal, one of the congenital hyperbilirubinaemias should be considered. Examples are Gilbert's syndrome, a conjugated hyperbilirubinaemia due to a deficiency in glucuronyl transferase

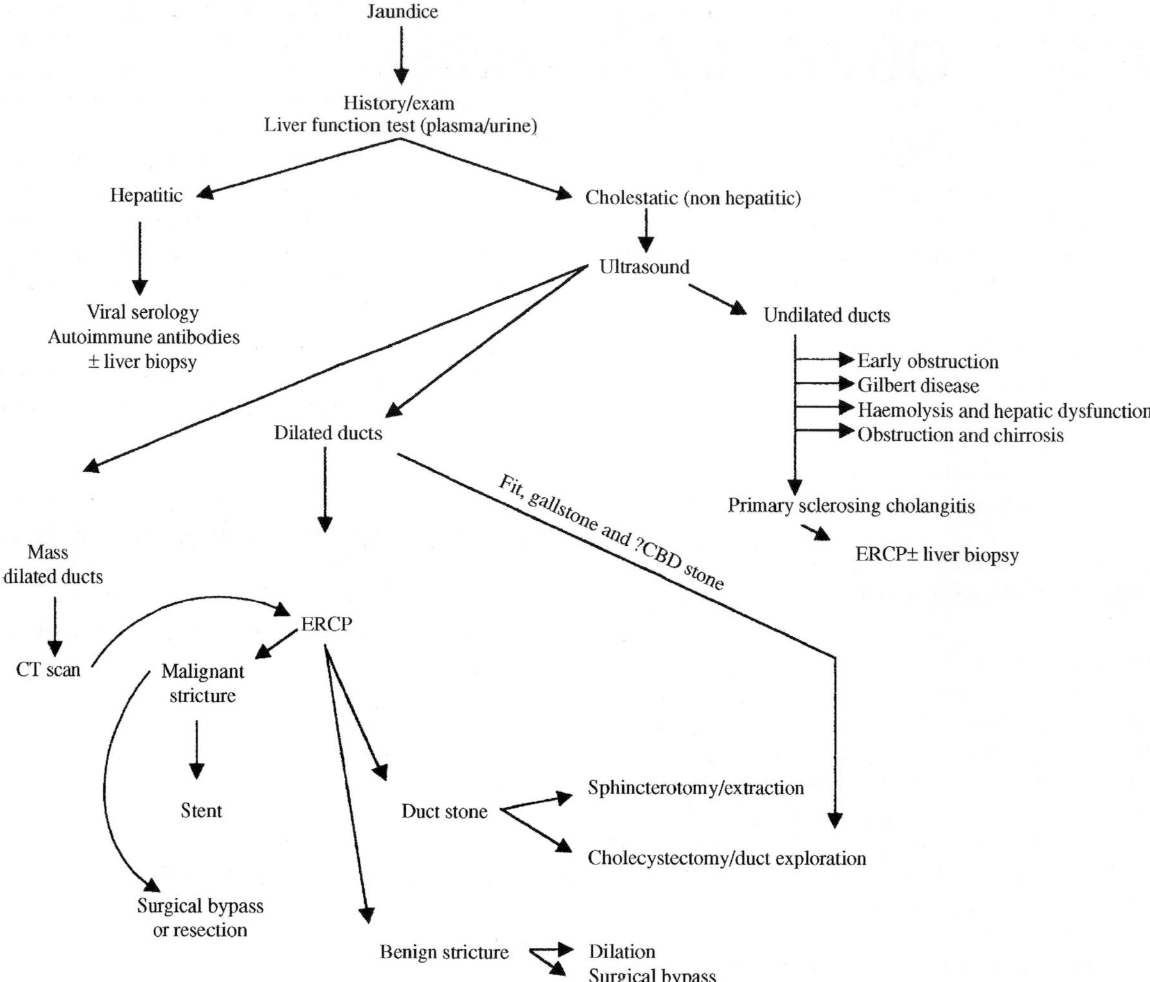

Fig. 63.1 Diagnostic and therapeutic approach to a patient with jaundice. CBD, common bile duct; ERCP, endoscopic retrograde cholangiopancreatography; PTC, percutaneous transhepatic cholangiography; CT, computed tomography.

activity, or Dubin Johnson syndrome, also a conjugated hyperbilirubinaemia, but due to a defect in the transport of bilirubin. Neither requires treatment. The abnormalities in bilirubin become more evident during infective or traumatic episodes.

Coagulation studies should be performed. If abnormal, and particularly if surgical, intervention is likely, vitamin K should be given.

If LFT suggests that the process is hepatitic, viral serology and autoimmune antibodies should be investigated. Liver biopsy may be required for confirmation, but only after obstructive causes have been ruled out first by ultrasound, to prevent the potential problem of bile fistula if a major duct is punctured by the biopsy needle.

Ultrasound and computed tomography scans

Ultrasound is the key technique in distinguishing medical from surgical jaundice, and should be performed on all cases of jaundice if LFT are not absolutely confirmatory of a hepatitic picture.

If the LFT are obstructive, but ultrasound shows non-dilated ducts, then there are four possibilities. First, the ultrasound may have been performed so early that the ducts have not yet dilated, in which case the scan should be repeated after 24–48 hours. Second, in the presence of defective liver function, a sudden bilirubin load from haemolysis or absorption of a large haematoma may produce jaundice. Third, the patient has cirrhosis, preventing dilation of the ducts (the extrahepatic ducts, however, will still dilate if the obstruction is outside the liver). Fourth, primary sclerosing cholangitis produces multiple strictures with segmental duct dilation occurring late. The diagnosis is usually indicated on ERCP, but liver biopsy may be required to confirm the diagnosis and the extent of hepatic damage secondary to the obstruction.

If the ultrasound shows a mass, usually in conjunction with dilated ducts, then the next step is a computed tomography (CT) scan to determine whether the lesion will be surgically resectable. This is then followed by ERCP to determine the nature of the obstruction.

Endoscopic retrograde cholangiopancreatography

This may demonstrate that a duct stone is the cause of the jaundice. If the patient is unfit for surgery, has cholangitis as a result of the stone or has already had a cholecystectomy, then the ideal treatment is ERCP/sphincterotomy and stone extraction. If the patient has an intact gall bladder containing stones, the history is typical of stone disease and he or she is fit (the majority), then it is best to treat by a laparoscopic cholecystectomy with intraoperative cholangiography, followed by laparoscopic duct exploration if a stone is still present in the duct. If the latter is unsuccessful, the duct can be explored by open operation immediately or by performing a post-operative ERCP and sphincterotomy to remove the stone.

If ERCP demonstrates a benign stricture, it should be dilated to improve the patient's clinical condition and then a decision can be made as to whether repeated dilations should be performed, or whether surgical bypass should be undertaken.

If ERCP demonstrates a malignant stricture and CT shows the lesion is not resectable or the patient is not fit for surgery, a stent is inserted, as definitive palliative treatment. Because stents obstruct and have to be replaced in 3–4 months, if the patient is fit enough, likely to live long enough, surgical bypass provides better palliation. Curative resection is uncommon. If ERCP fails to define the ductal system adequately, so surgery cannot be appropriately planned, then a percutaneous transhepatic cholangiogram may need to be performed. Such failure may be due to technical difficulties in accessing the papilla (prior gastrectomy, duodenal diverticulum) or because the stricture is so tight that contrast cannot be made to pass into the upper duct system.

MCQs

Select the single correct answer to each question:

1 Which of the following conditions may *not* be a cause of obstructive jaundice?
a choledochal cyst
b ulcerative colitis
c hydatid disease
d scleroderma
e chronic pancreatitis

2 Drugs which may cause hepatotoxic drug reactions do *not* include:
a paracetamol
b vitamin A
c nitrofurantoin
d flucloxacillin
e oestrogen

64 The acute abdomen

Michael Levitt

Introduction

The aim of this chapter is to provide a broad set of guidelines for the management of patients presenting with acute abdominal pain. The detailed clinical, laboratory and radiological features of the numerous causative conditions are provided elsewhere in this text book.

The management of patients with acute abdominal pain comprises two concurrent processes – diagnostic and therapeutic – culminating in the decision to operate or to observe (Box 64.1).

Diagnostic

Regardless of the severity of the presenting illness, management of patients with acute abdominal pain depends heavily upon early and accurate establishment of the clinical diagnosis or, at least, a workable differential diagnosis. This is an important discipline to develop and the label 'acute abdomen, for surgical review' should be regarded as unsatisfactory.

Box 64.1 Management of the acute abdomen

Diagnostic	Therapeutic
• History and examination – Establish and explore the differential diagnosis • Investigations – Assess severity – Specific diagnoses – Pre-operative investigations – General investigations	• Resuscitation • Symptom control – Analgesia – Anti-emesis – Nasogastric tube • Monitoring the patient – Urinary catheter – Central venous catheter • Non-surgical treatment – Blood transfusion – Intravenous antibiotics
Operate or observe	

History and examination

The process of making a diagnosis on the basis of history and examination is achieved by a combination of pattern recognition (drawn from clinical experience) and probability (based on theoretical knowledge).

The pattern of pain (its site, periodicity, radiation, aggravating and relieving factors, etc.) immediately establishes a 'shortlist' of diagnostic possibilities (or differential diagnosis). Each of these options can then be explored in more detail. The age and sex of the patient along with any history of causative, aggravating or precipitating factors make certain diagnostic alternatives more or less probable.

In this manner, clinical assessment can be abbreviated, permitting the focus to fall quickly upon the realistic alternatives. More detailed history and examination can then be used to select the most likely diagnosis (see clinical example, Box 64.2).

Some examples of clinical patterns in patients with acute abdominal pain are:

I. Pain that commences *instantaneously* suggests either hollow organ perforation (e.g. perforated peptic ulcer) or a vascular accident (e.g. mesenteric occlusion, ruptured intra-abdominal aneurysm)
II. *Syncope* associated with abdominal pain suggests acute blood loss (e.g. ruptured abdominal aortic aneurysm, ruptured ectopic pregnancy)
III. The combination of vomiting and diarrhoea suggests gastroenteritis
IV. Colicky abdominal pain suggests hollow organ obstruction (e.g. ureteric calculus, small bowel obstruction) or excessive peristalsis (gastroenteritis)
V. Pain made worse by movement suggests peritoneal irritation (e.g. appendicitis) or muscular strain.

Box 64.2 Clinical scenario: a 65-year-old man presents with the sudden onset of generalised abdominal pain and collapse. On examination, he is pale, sweaty and distressed, with pulse rate = 110 beats per minute, blood pressure = 90/50 mm Hg and temperature = 36.0°C

Diagnostic

1. **History and examination** (establish and explore the likely differential diagnosis)
   - Ruptured abdominal aortic aneurysm
     - pain radiating to back or groin
     - history of smoking, other vascular diseases
     - palpate abdomen for pulsatile mass
   - Mesenteric infarction
     - history of palpitations, arrhythmia, digitalis therapy
     - palpate pulse for atrial fibrillation
   - Perforated peptic ulcer
     - history of dyspepsia, antacid therapy, NSAID ingestion
     - board-like abdominal rigidity
   - Acute pancreatitis
     - prominent vomiting, pain referred to back
     - alcoholic aetiology
   - Acute myocardial infarction
     - past history of ischaemic heart disease
2. **Investigations**
   - Full blood count – low haemoglobin points to haemorrhage, high white cell count suggests mesenteric ischaemia
   - Urea and electrolytes – to guide resuscitation
   - 12-lead ECG – changes of acute ischaemia
   - Abdominal X-ray, supine and erect
     - free intraperitoneal gas, loss of psoas shadow, calcification of abdominal aortic aneurysm, dilated loops of small intestine.
   - Serum amylase/lipase – >1000 U/L diagnostic of acute pancreatitis
   - Cross-match – if haemoglobin <10 and/or major surgery anticipated
   - Ultrasound scan – to confirm ruptured abdominal aortic aneurysm

Therapeutic

1. **Resuscitation**
   - Intravenous access (beware of overtransfusion in acute myocardial infarction)
   - Oxygen mask (plus airway support if appropriate)
   - MAST suit if in hypovolaemic shock
   - Transfuse if haemoglobin <8
   - Consider transfusing if haemoglobin <10 and further bleeding or major surgery is planned
2. **Symptom control**
   - Intravenous or intramuscular opiate analgesics
   - Antiemetic therapy
   - Nasogastric tube if vomiting
3. **Monitoring the patient**
   - Indwelling urinary catheter
   - Central venous catheter
4. **Non-surgical treatment**
   - Intravenous gentamicin, amoxycillin, (suspected perforated peptic ulcer, mesenteric ischaemia)
   - Subcutaneous octreotide in severe pancreatitis

Operate or observe?

- **Ruptured abdominal aortic aneurysm** – immediate laparotomy.
- **Perforated peptic ulcer** – immediate operation if abdominal signs are generalised (occasionally may be treated by antibiotics and observation if abdominal signs are localised).
- **Mesenteric infarction** – immediate operation to exclude closed-loop small-bowel obstruction.
- **Acute pancreatitis** – intravenous fluid replacement, oxygen mask, +/– antibiotics, +/– octreotide. Observe for progressive abdominal signs, features of intra-abdominal sepsis. Monitor full blood count, liver function tests, blood glucose level, arterial blood gases.
- **Acute myocardial infarction** – monitor patient in critical care facility, specific therapy according to local protocols.

Some examples of the application of probability in the clinical setting are:

I. Recent onset of abdominal pain and anorexia in a previously well young man (acute appendicitis)
II. Left iliac fossa pain and tenderness in a 60-year-old (sigmoid diverticulitis)
III. Upper abdominal pain and vomiting in a known alcoholic (acute pancreatitis).

It is beyond the scope of this chapter to cover all of the possible clinical scenarios that account for patients who present with acute abdominal pain. At the heart of their management, however, is a determination on the part of the clinician to establish an accurate clinical diagnosis on the basis of history and examination.

Investigations

It is not possible, at the outset, to anticipate all of the investigations that might ultimately prove helpful in patient diagnosis and management. In the event of a confident clinical diagnosis – e.g. acute appendicitis – in a fit individual, no confirmatory or diagnostic investigations may be deemed necessary. Numerous factors affect the choice of initial diagnostic investigations.

I. The severity of the presenting illness
   - urea and electrolytes if the patient is clinically dehydrated
   - full blood count and cross-match if haemorrhage is suspected
II. Specific diagnostic possibilities
   - serum beta HCG in suspected ruptured ectopic pregnancy
   - serum amylase or lipase in suspected acute pancreatitis
   - abdominal ultrasound in cases of suspected biliary disease, obstructive uropathy, ruptured abdominal aortic aneurysm.
   - 12-lead ECG in suspected acute myocardial infarction.
III. If surgery is anticipated
   - prior to undergoing a general anaesthesia, certain investigations may be obtained, particularly in older patients, as a routine. This will vary from centre to centre; these tests include urea and electrolytes, full blood count, ECG, chest X-ray as well as cross-match in appropriate cases.
IV. General investigations in patients with acute abdominal pain of uncertain origin
   - even before a clinical diagnosis is formulated, certain diagnostic investigations may have been instigated in anticipation of subsequent need. Amongst these, the two most frequently of value are:
   - **full blood count:** an elevation of the white cell count is a cardinal sign of sepsis but it may also be raised by the 'stress' of pain alone; it is also mildly elevated during normal pregnancy. In general, an elevation of white cell count should never be dismissed and a very high white cell count (>30) in the context of a patient with acute abdominal pain raises the possibility of intestinal ischaemia (mesenteric infarction, closed-loop small-bowel obstruction).
   - **abdominal X-rays:** a supine abdominal X-ray reveals distension of intra-abdominal gas (intestinal obstruction), thickness of intestinal wall (mesenteric ischaemia), abnormal calcification (ureteric colic, chronic pancreatitis) and outlines the psoas shadows (possibly obscured in ruptured abdominal aortic aneurysm). The erect abdominal X-ray reveals fluid levels (confirmation of intestinal obstruction). Decubitus films are used to detect free intraperitoneal gas (perforated hollow viscus) although this may be better demonstrated by an erect chest X-ray.

Therapeutic

At the same time as these diagnostic steps are being taken, it is often appropriate – and not infrequently essential – to initiate treatment.

Resuscitation

Unwell patients may require preliminary resuscitation before any practical diagnostic steps can be taken. Tachycardia, hypotension, pallor, sweating and cool extremities all suggest a more severe clinical presentation and the possibility of sepsis or hypovolemia. Immediate *intravenous access* should be established and *fluid replacement* appropriate to the clinical setting commenced. An *oxygen mask* to maximise vital organ oxygenation is usually appropriate. A *MAST suit* is occasionally required in cases of profound haemorrhagic shock (e.g. ruptured abdominal aortic aneurysm).

In cases of haemorrhagic shock, a *blood transfusion* should commence as soon as practicable. Transfusion should not, however, be allowed to delay the commencement of urgently needed surgery (e.g. ruptured abdominal aortic aneurysm) where the need to control the bleeding point outweighs the desire to restore intravascular volume by transfusion.

Symptom control

In the acute setting it is easy to overlook the need to provide basic symptom control. *Analgesia* should not be withheld pending 'surgical review'. *Anti-emetic therapy* usually accompanies opiate analgesics; for repeated vomiting (e.g. intestinal obstruction, acute pancreatitis) and a *nasogastric tube* should be passed. This will relieve the symptoms, permit more accurate measurement of fluid loss and protect the patient from the risks of aspiration of gastric content.

Monitoring the patient

In the unwell patient, it is important to monitor the outcome of resuscitation and fluid replacement. Apart from the standard vital signs (pulse rate, blood pressure, temperature), additional information can be obtained by measuring urine output (*indwelling urinary catheter*) or central venous pressure (*central venous catheter*). These tools are more sensitive to changes in intravascular fluid status than are the pulse rate and blood pressure.

Non-surgical therapy

Broad-spectrum *antibiotics* should be administered according to the likely clinical diagnosis. This may precede the formulation of an accurate clinical diagnosis especially in unwell patients. Agents active against Gram-negative bacilli (aminoglycosides, third-generation cephalosporins) and anaerobic organisms (metronidazole) are generally preferred in patients presenting with acute abdominal pain.

In cases of acute pancreatitis, *subcutaneous octreotide* (a somatostatin analogue) may be instituted in an attempt to moderate the course of the pancreatitis.

Surgery vs. observation

Ultimately, an assessment needs to be made about the need for surgery. This may be clear-cut where a confident diagnosis has been made (e.g. appendicitis appendicectomy, ureteric colic analgesia and initial observation).

In some cases, advanced age or infirmity might caution against surgery even where a confident diagnosis points to a surgical remedy (e.g. ruptured abdominal aortic aneurysm in a frail 90-year-old).

Often, however, the precise diagnosis is uncertain and the need for urgent surgery is made obvious by virtue either of the clinical features of generalised peritonitis (e.g. perforated hollow viscus, mesenteric infarction, closed-loop small bowel-obstruction) or the severity of the presenting illness (e.g. associated shock). In this situation, clinical experience (pattern recognition) enables early identification of the need for prompt surgical intervention.

Where the need for surgery is unclear – e.g. some cases of right iliac fossa pain or small intestinal obstruction – observation rather than exploratory surgery is appropriate. This involves regular clinical review conducted at a frequency appropriate to the severity of the illness (e.g. review in 12 hours for a 20-year-old woman with mild right iliac fossa pain and tenderness or 1–2-hourly review in a 75-year-old with small bowel obstruction and associated abdominal tenderness). At times, such review may be augmented by further laboratory or radiological investigations. Of these, the *white cell count* is most often of practical value; a rising white cell count generally indicates progression of the underlying pathological process.

Clinical example

The following clinical scenario (Box 64.2) serves as a demonstration of the dual processes – diagnostic and therapeutic – in the management of a patient with acute abdominal pain. Note especially the rapid construction of a workable differential diagnosis to permit subsequent history and examination to focus on identifying the most likely diagnosis.

MCQs

Select the single correct answer to each question.

1 Which of the following clinical features is found in a patient presenting with acute abdominal pain who has generalised peritonitis?
 a slow pulse rate
 b extreme restlessness and writhing around in agony

c motionless with pain, worse with movement
d normal bowel sounds
e deep palpation of most abdominal organs is possible

2 Acute epigastric pain is unusual in which of the following conditions?
a acute pancreatitis
b acute cholecystitis
c perforated peptic ulcer
d acute diverticulitis
e ruptured abdominal aortic aneurysm

3 Immediate laparotomy would not be recommended in a patient diagnosed as having which of the following conditions?
a mesenteric infarction
b perforated peptic ulcer with generalised peritonitis
c acute pancreatitis
d acute cholecystitis
e ruptured abdominal aortic aneurysm

4 Which of the following parameters is the most practical for monitoring the progression of the underlying pathological process responsible for acute abdominal pain in a patient being initially managed non-operatively?
a erythrocyte sedimentation rate (ESR)
b C-reactive protein (CRP)
c white cell count
d white cell scan
e serum phosphate

65 Peritonitis and intra-abdominal abscesses

Joe J. Tjandra

Peritonitis

Peritonitis is inflammation of the peritoneum, which lines the peritoneal cavity. Initially, peritonitis is localised and contained by a wrapping of greater omentum, adjacent bowel and fibrinous adhesions. With ongoing inflammation, localised peritonitis may progress to a generalised peritonitis, associated with massive exudation of fluid, with resultant hypovolaemia, toxaemia and septicaemia if sepsis is present. Paralytic ileus is invariably present with generalised peritonitis.

The principal signs of peritonitis include tenderness, guarding, rigidity and rebound tenderness. With generalised peritonitis, the patient is very unwell, with marked fever, tachycardia and dehydration. There is diffuse abdominal pain, exacerbated by even the slightest movement.

Causes of peritonitis

Acute primary peritonitis

Acute primary peritonitis is rare and usually occurs in association with immunosuppression, such as post-splenectomy, nephrotic syndrome or in cirrhosis, where the proteinaceous ascitic fluid provides a good culture medium for bacteria. Sometimes it affects young girls following pelvic inflammatory disease. Common organisms are haemolytic streptococci, *Escherichia coli* and *Klebsiella* species. Acute primary peritonitis is often a diagnosis of exclusion and requires aggressive antibiotic therapy. (Box 65.1)

Secondary peritonitis

Secondary peritonitis may be suppurative, chemical or chronic sclerosing.

Box 65.1 Common varieties of peritonitis

- Acute peritonitis
  - Primary (spontaneous)
  - Secondary
  - Acute suppurative (e.g. perforated viscus)
  - Chemical-induced
- Chronic (sclerosing) peritonitis
  - Infections (e.g. tuberculosis, *Candida albicans*)
  - Chemical-induced (e.g. surgical talc in the gloves, chlorhexidine)
  - Carcinomatosis

Acute suppurative peritonitis may occur secondary to a disease process of an intra-abdominal organ; that is, perforation (e.g. peptic ulcer, diverticular disease, Crohn's disease, appendix or gall bladder), infection (e.g. appendix abscess, pyosalpinx) or ischaemia (volvulus, mesenteric ischaemia or strangulated hernia). Most of these cases will require urgent surgical intervention. Erect chest X-ray may show free gas beneath the diaphragm, indicating a perforated viscus (Fig. 65.1).

Chemical peritonitis may occur secondary to bile (displaced T-tube from common bile duct, unrecognised division of accessory bile duct) or blood (post-operative bleeding, abdominal trauma). Less commonly urine (ureteric injury in pelvic surgery or intraperitoneal rupture of bladder) may also be the cause. Bacterial contamination and overgrowth may develop.

Intra-abdominal abscesses

Intra-abdominal abscesses are one extreme in the spectrum of bacterial peritonitis. They require drainage in addition to antibiotic therapy. The pathogenesis requires a polymicrobial infection, with the presence of

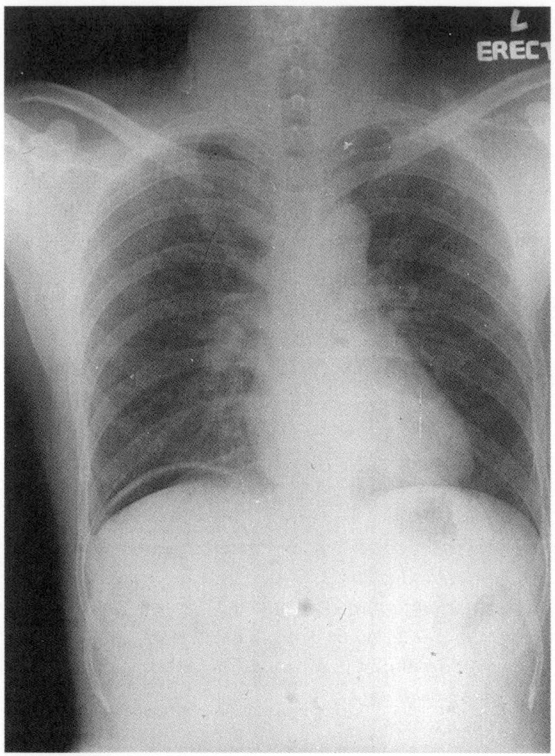

Fig. 65.1 Erect chest X-ray showing free gas beneath the right hemidiaphragm.

foreign matter facilitating the development of progressive infection. The bacterial flora of the gastrointestinal tract varies from small numbers of aerobic streptococci and facultative Gram-negative bacilli in the stomach and proximal small bowel, to larger numbers of these species with an increasing number of anaerobic Gram-negative bacilli (*Bacteroides* spp.) and anaerobic Gram-positive flora (streptococci and clostridia) in the distal ileum and colon. In patients who have received prolonged antibiotic therapy and in those with extended hospital stay, colonisation by yeasts such as *Candida* species or a variety of nosocomial pathogens may occur. Skin flora may be responsible following penetrating abdominal injuries. Pelvic abscesses in women may occur as part of pelvic inflammatory disease. Common organisms include *Neisseria gonorrhoeae* and *Chlamydia trachomatis*.

There are four functional compartments within the peritoneal cavity: pelvis, right and left paracolic gutters and the subdiaphragmatic spaces. In the recumbent patient, diffuse intraperitoneal fluid collects under the diaphragm and in the pelvis. These are the common sites for abscess formation. More localised abscesses may develop in relation to the affected viscus (e.g. abscesses in the lesser sac secondary to severe pancreatitis or a perforated peptic ulcer, or a peri-appendiceal abscess).

Clinical features

The clinical presentation of an intra-abdominal abscess is highly variable. In a patient with a predisposing primary intra-abdominal disease or following abdominal surgery, persistent abdominal pain, focal tenderness, swinging fever, persistent paralytic ileus and leucocytosis suggest an intra-abdominal purulent collection. The patient may simply fail to thrive and may have mildly abnormal liver function.

With a pelvic abscess, there may be urinary frequency, dysuria, diarrhoea or tenesmus due to irritation of the anatomically related organs. With a subphrenic collection, there may be shoulder tip pain, hiccups and unexplained pulmonary symptoms (pleural effusion, basal atelectasis).

Investigations

Investigations in patients with suspected intra-abdominal abscess include full blood examination, urea and electrolytes and liver function test. Blood cultures and other appropriate cultures (urine, sputum, catheter) may also be performed.

Computed tomography (CT) scan with iodinated soluble oral contrast is useful. Serial images are obtained from the diaphragm to the pelvis. It is particularly useful for localising small or deep intra-abdominal abscesses (Fig. 65.2). Interpretation in post-operative patients can be particularly difficult, as loculated, non-infected serous collections are common physiological events.

Ultrasound equipment is mobile and examinations may be readily performed in a critically ill patient in the intensive care unit. However, the quality of such studies is not as good as a CT scan and is vastly operator-dependent. Endovaginal ultrasound is particularly useful to detect tubo-ovarian abscess complicating pelvic inflammatory disease in women.

Laparoscopy is occasionally used if there is diagnostic uncertainty between a tubo-ovarian abscess and a phlegmon.

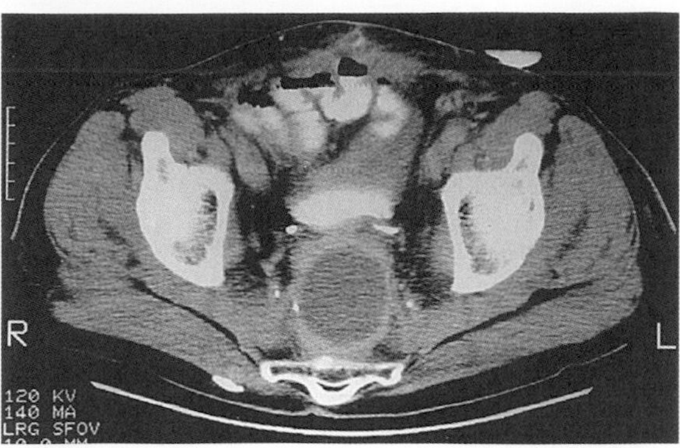

Fig. 65.2 Computed tomography scan showing a pelvic abscess.

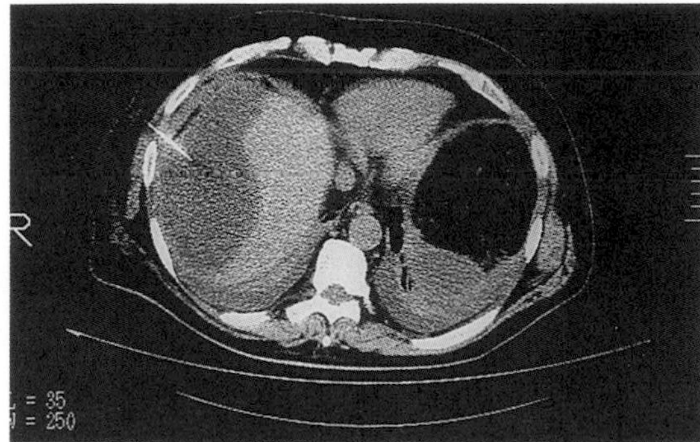

Fig. 65.3 Computed tomography (CT) scan of the abdomen showing a large subphrenic abscess that was aspirated percutaneously under CT guidance.

Therapy

Parenteral antibiotics

Parenteral antibiotics should be administered prior to drainage of the abscess. Initial choice of antibiotics is empirical but should provide a broad-spectrum activity against Gram-negative bacilli and anaerobes. Specific therapy is guided by the results of cultures. With adequate drainage of the abscess, it may not be necessary to treat each component of the polymicrobial flora. Commonly used antibiotics include metronidazole with a second- or third-generation cephalosporin or imipenem alone. Alternatively, combinations of amoxycillin, gentamicin and metronidazole provide additional cover against enterococci as well. In immunosuppressed patients, *Candida* species may have an important pathogenic role, and treatment with amphotericin B is indicated.

Percutaneous drainage

Computed tomography scan or ultrasound localises the abscess cavity and guides safe access for percutaneous drainage (Fig. 65.3), avoiding adjacent viscera and blood vessels. A diagnostic needle aspiration is initially performed to confirm the presence of the abscess and to obtain pus for Gram stain and culture. A large-bore drainage catheter is then placed in the most dependent position. While percutaneous drainage is effective in a single, unilocular abscess, it is more limited in a multiloculated abscess, especially if the contents are tenacious.

Preliminary percutaneous drainage is useful in improving and reducing the sepsis, prior to definitive surgical treatment. In some cases, as for complicated diverticular disease or Crohn's disease, it may facilitate subsequent single-stage resection and primary anastomosis, rather than traditional multi-stage procedures with diversion. Repeat imaging with sinography or CT scan will estimate the size of the residual cavity and any enteric communication.

Surgical drainage

Surgical drainage is mainly undertaken in patients who have not improved with percutaneous drainage or in whom the collections are not appropriate for percutaneous drainage, as in multiple abscesses, severe necrotising pancreatitis or interloop abscesses with Crohn's disease. An extraperitoneal approach, if possible, is generally preferred because it limits the risk of further contamination of the peritoneal cavity. With a distally located pelvic abscess that is bulging, the drainage may be performed through the rectum or vagina. The loculae are gently broken down digitally and soft drains are placed in the most dependent position.

Definitive surgery

Definitive surgery is generally deferred after preliminary drainage of the abscess. In some situations, surgery on the offending organ is performed, for example, appendicectomy for appendiceal abscess, unilateral salpingo-oophorectomy for tubo-ovarian abscess, omental patch of a perforated duodenal ulcer.

MCQs

Select the single correct answer to each question.

1 Pelvic abscess that occurred 5 days after an anterior resection of rectum:
  a is usually due to anastomotic leak
  b usually requires surgery and a Hartmann's procedure
  c will usually settle with intravenous antibiotics
  d is best detected by MRI
  e is best detected by endorectal ultrasound

2 Common causes of post-surgical pelvic abscess include:
  a cholecystectomy
  b appendicectomy
  c laparoscopic but not conventional open anterior resection
  d rectovaginal fistula
  e use of powdered surgical gloves

66 Ascites

David M. A. Francis and David A. K. Watters

Introduction

Ascites is an abnormal accumulation of free fluid within the peritoneal cavity. Ascites is due to either increased portal venous pressure, low plasma proteins (hypoproteinaemia), chronic peritoneal irritation, leakage of lymphatic fluid into the peritoneal cavity, or fluid overload (Box 66.1).

Box 66.1 Causes of ascites

Increased portal venous pressure
- Pre-hepatic: portal vein compression or thrombosis; schistosomiasis
- Hepatic: cirrhosis; acute hepatic necrosis; viral hepatitis
- Post-hepatic: Budd–Chiari syndrome, myeloproliferative disorders, constrictive pericarditis; right heart failure, hypercoagulable states

Hypoproteinaemia
- Renal-disease–causing severe proteinuria
- Malnutrition and malabsorption
- Protein-losing enteropathy
- Acute or chronic liver disease
- Severe acute or chronic illness

Chronic peritoneal inflammation and infection
- Chronic infection: tuberculosis; fungal infection
- Secondary malignant infiltration (carcinomatosis peritonei)
- Post-irradiation

Leakage of lymphatic fluid (chylous ascites)
- Congenital
- Surgical trauma
- Primary and secondary lymphatic malignancy

Other fluids
- Pancreatic ascites
- Bilious ascites
- Urinary ascites

Ascites needs to be differentiated from other causes of abdominal distension including bowel obstruction, bleeding and huge intra-abdominal masses or cysts.

Pathophysiology of ascites

Increased portal venous pressure (Fig. 66.1)

Any cause of increased resistance to hepatic or portal venous blood flow can lead to ascites. Gross ascites occurs when increased pressure within the hepatic veins or at the post-sinusoidal level dramatically increases hydrostatic pressure within the hepatic sinusoids in the liver, and within the portal venous system. Collateral vein formation, shunting of blood to the systemic circulation and splanchnic vasodilatation (due in part to the local production of nitric oxide) develop particularly in the later stages of cirrhosis. Systemic arterial pressure is maintained by vasoconstriction and antinatriuretic factors resulting in sodium and water retention. The increased portal pressure combined with splanchnic vasodilation alters the capillary pressure and permeability, enabling intravascular fluid to move through pores between the vascular endothelial cells of the portal system into the extravascular space of the liver and intestine. Lymphatic flow is increased proximal to the point of vascular obstruction and, when the capacity of the lymphatic system is surpassed, the transudate moves across the surfaces of the liver, mesentery and intestine into the peritoneal cavity. Cirrhosis and schistosomal periportal fibrosis are the commonest causes of portal hypertension.

Any cause of hepatic venous outflow obstruction may cause ascites by increasing portal venous pressure (Budd–Chiari syndrome). The site of obstruction may be at the hepatic venules (haematological or liver disease), large hepatic veins, inferior vena cava or right atrium (right heart diseases).

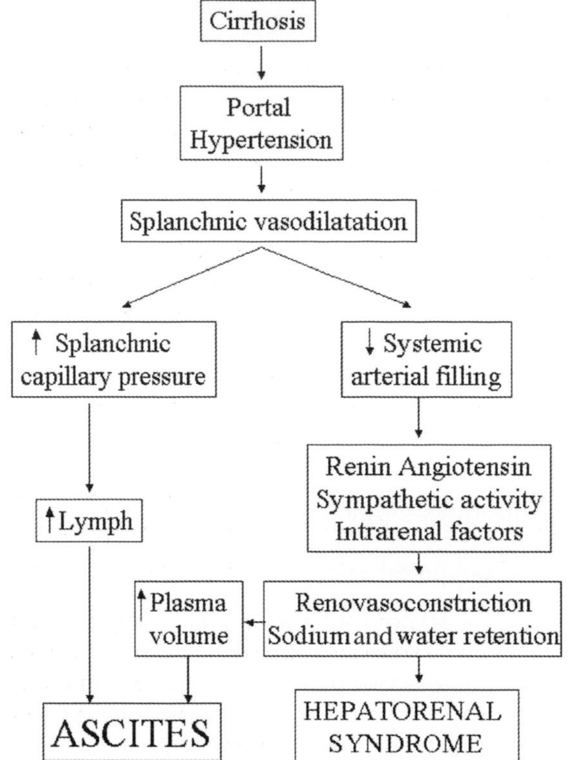

Fig. 66.1 The pathophysiology of ascites due to cirrhosis.

Hypoproteinaemia

Low concentrations of plasma proteins, particularly albumin, reduce the osmotic pressure of plasma. In health, the relatively high osmotic pressure of intravascular plasma tends to draw extravascular fluid back into the intravascular space. The osmotic gradient is reduced in hypoproteinaemic states so that less fluid is removed from extravascular sites. When the capacity of the hepatic and intestinal lymphatics to remove fluid from the extravascular interstitial space is exceeded, ascites develops.

Sodium and water retention

Reduced circulating plasma volume, as a result of loss of intravascular fluid into the peritoneal cavity and interstitial spaces (third-space fluid loss) and pooling of blood in the splanchnic vascular space secondary to portal venous outflow obstruction, reduces renal blood flow and glomerular filtration. Decreased renal perfusion stimulates increased renin secretion from the juxtaglomerular apparatus in the ascending limb of the loop of Henle of the kidney. The resultant secondary aldosteronism causes retention of sodium and water. Impairment of renal excretion of water and renal vasoconstriction lead to dilutional hyponatraemia and increase the risk of hepatorenal syndrome.

Chronic peritoneal inflammation

Any chronic inflammatory process within the peritoneal cavity results in considerable increases in flow within peritoneal blood and lymphatic vessels. Peritoneal microvascular permeability increases markedly with consequent exudation of plasma proteins and fluid into extravascular spaces. When the capacity of the lymphatics to reabsorb the fluid is exceeded, it accumulates within the peritoneal cavity. The high protein concentration of this peritoneal fluid further retards fluid reabsorption. As the inflammatory process resolves, and microvascular permeability returns to normal, less peritoneal fluid is formed and fluid is removed by absorption. The commonest cause of chronic peritoneal inflammation worldwide is abdominal tuberculosis but other peritoneal infections and foreign matter may also induce ascites.

Malignant infiltration

Metastatic deposits cause ascites by a combination of inflammation, shedding of cells, exudation and sometimes bleeding. Gross ascites does not usually occur until late. Gastric and ovarian cancers are the most notorious for causing ascites due to their ease of transperitoneal spread, but any peritoneal malignant process may be responsible.

Leakage of fluid

Leakage of fluid directly into the peritoneal cavity occurs when intra-abdominal lymphatics are transected (e.g. abdominal surgery, trauma) or obstructed (e.g. primary or secondary lymphatic malignancy, surgical ligation). Ascites forms when the rate of leakage into the peritoneal cavity exceeds the rate of absorption by peritoneal lymphatics.

Exudation of pancreatic fluid from an inflammed pancreas may occur in acute pancreatitis. If the pancreatic duct ruptures due to inflammation or surgical damage, pancreatic ascites may persist as an internally draining pancreatic fistula.

Bile leaks may be termed bilious ascites although the bile is normally very irritant to the peritoneal cavity and normally induces more of a peritonitis/acute abdomen type reaction.

Urine may leak into the peritoneal cavity either from damage to a ureter, the bladder or an obstructed hydronephrotic kidney.

Clinical features

Ascites should be suspected from a history of abdominal distension. Ascites can be detected clinically on examination of the abdomen when the volume reaches approximately 1 L. Inspection of the abdomen reveals distension, which may vary from slight fullness laterally in the flanks to gross distension predominantly in the centre of the abdomen. Sometimes a hernial sac protrudes as it becomes full of ascitic fluid, particularly at the umbilicus. Other abnormal findings on inspection may include signs of liver disease (jaundice, scratch marks because of pruritus, spider naevi, caput medusae and dilated veins on the anterior abdominal wall, hepatomegaly), para-umbilical and other abdominal hernias, pitting oedema and surgical scars.

On palpation the abdomen may feel thicker owing to the fluid asserting more than the expected degree of resistance. In cases of chronic inflammation, particularly tuberculosis, the abdomen may feel 'doughy'. Gross ascites causes tense abdominal distension that is unyielding to the examining hand. Ascites is confirmed by the presence of a fluid thrill and shifting dullness on percussion.

Fluid thrill

Large amounts of intraperitoneal fluid, either free or encysted, may give rise to a fluid thrill. The abdomen is flicked on one side and the transmitted shock wave is palpated by the examiner's other hand, which has been placed flat on the far side of the abdomen (Fig. 66.2A). An accessory hand prevents transmission of the shock wave through the subcutaneous fat of the anterior abdominal wall. A fluid thrill may also be elicited by tapping in the loin and palpating at the front (Fig. 66.2B). To detect a fluid thrill in an abdomen with smaller volumes of ascitic fluid, the area of stony dullness is first determined by percussion.

Shifting dullness

Free intraperitoneal fluid gravitates to the most dependent parts of the peritoneal cavity, namely the pelvis and paracolic regions, while the gas-filled intestine tends to 'float' uppermost. Fluid-filled structures have a stony dull percussion note, while gas-filled structures are resonant or hyper-resonant on percussion. Thus, when a patient with ascites lies supine, the flanks or lateral parts of the abdomen are stony dull to percussion while the peri-umbilical area is resonant. When the patient lies on one or other side, ascitic fluid gravitates to that side because it is then the most dependent part of the abdomen, and so the percussion note over that area becomes stony dull, while the other side becomes resonant.

Shifting dullness is elicited by percussing the abdomen and determining the point at which the percussion note changes from resonant to dull. The patient is then asked to roll about 45° to one side, and percussion is repeated after waiting for a few seconds. Shifting dullness is confirmed by a significant change in position of the area of stony dullness. It should be noted that slight changes in the percussion note may be caused by positional changes in the small intestine.

Investigation of ascites

Investigation of a patient with ascites aims to detect the cause of the fluid accumulation. This is usually evident from the history and clinical examination, including habits and previous travel or domicile. Specific investigations depend on the likely cause of the ascites (Box 66.1). Ascites is a multisystem disease and the probable cause will determine which systems require investigation. The choice includes urinalysis, serum concentrations of electrolytes, urea and creatinine, total proteins and albumin, liver function tests, serology, abdominal ultrasonography (Fig. 66.3A), computed tomography (CT) scan (Fig. 66.3B), portal vein Doppler scan and echocardiography. Diagnostic aspiration of a small volume of ascitic fluid for biochemical (protein and amylase estimation), microbiological (microscopy and culture) and cytological assessment may be necessary. Laparoscopy or minilaparotomy may be required to perform a peritoneal biopsy to diagnose abdominal tuberculosis and other inflammatory conditions. Schistosomiasis may be suspected from a history of swimming or living in endemic areas and confirmed by rectal or liver biopsy, ultrasound or serology. Plain abdominal

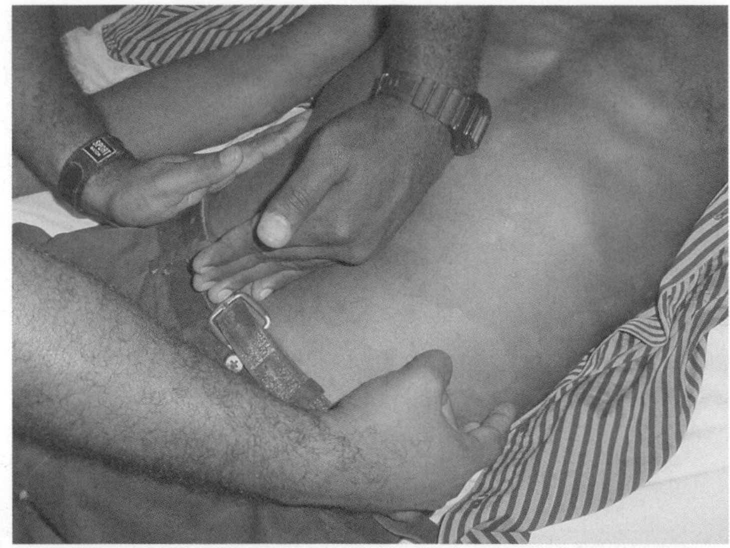

(A)

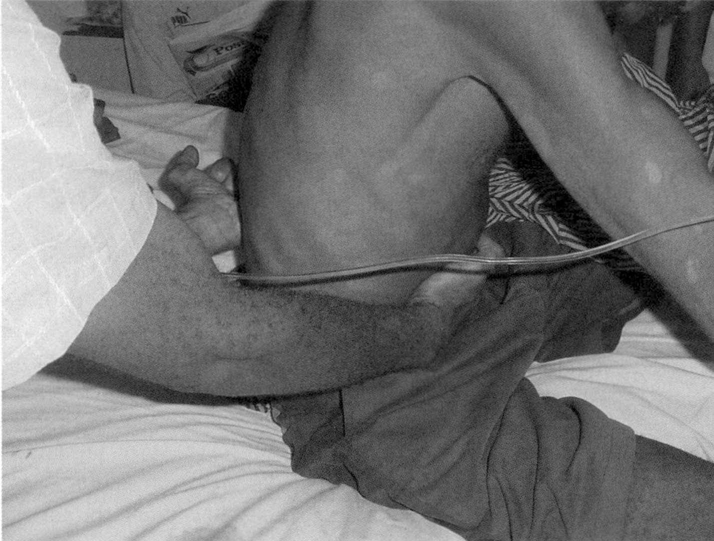

(B)

Fig. 66.2 (A&B) Clinical examination: palpating for ascites.

films are not a method of diagnosing ascites but sometimes gross ascites give an appearance of ground glass.

Clinical outcome

Mild to moderate ascites may cause few symptoms. Large-volume ascites (more than 3–4 L) is very unpleasant for patients because it produces a constant feeling of abdominal fullness and discomfort, nausea and anorexia, limitation of movement and leg swelling. Respiratory difficulty and shortness of breath is due to elevation of the diaphragm, atelectasis and pleural effusions. Ascites may be complicated by previously unrecognised abdominal hernias and rarely by primary bacterial peritonitis. Primary or spontaneous bacterial peritonitis may be difficult to diagnose, does not always cause a lot of guarding or rigidity and patients'

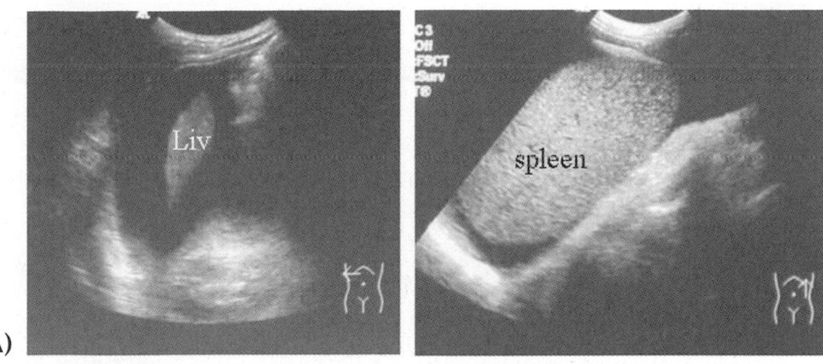

(A)

Ultrasound showing ascitic fluid (black) around liver on right and around spleen on left.

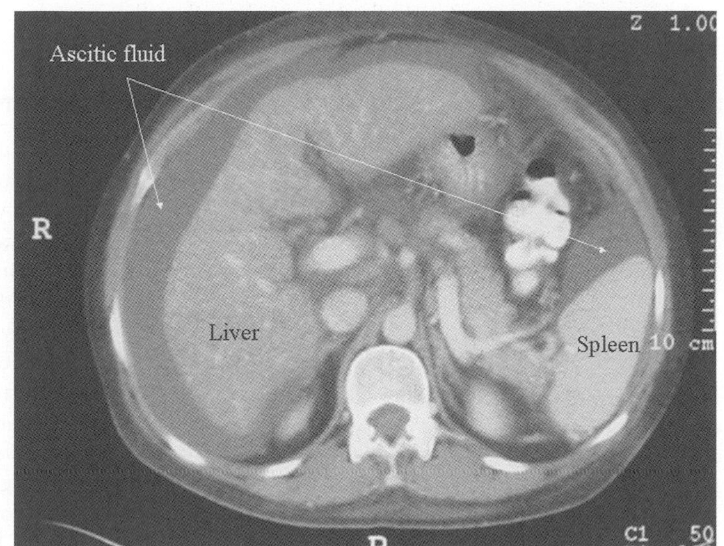

(B)

Fig. 66.3 (**A**) Ultrasound showing fluid (black) around the liver. (**B**) CT scan showing ascitic fluid, anterior abdominal distension and there is contrast in the loops of the bowel.

immune response to the infection may be impaired owing to their underlying disease, for example liver, renal or malignancy. Sometimes the peritonitis presents with general deterioration (e.g. development of hepatic encephalopathy or renal failure) rather than abdominal signs. Reduced renal blood flow and glomerular filtration, poor urine output, and low urinary sodium excretion cause pre-renal renal impairment with increased urea and creatinine, which may progress to acute renal failure (hepato-renal syndrome). Development of ascites in patients with chronic liver disease indicates severe liver impairment, and 1-year survival of such patients with intractable ascites is approximately 50%. Malignant ascites is most commonly due to intraperitoneal metastatic deposits of cancer originating in the ovary, stomach, breast and colon. Survival of these patients is poor, with a median survival of about 3 months.

Treatment

Most patients with ascites are treated non-operatively. Ascites can be classified as moderate-volume, high-volume and refractory with regard to the approach to treatment. By definition, refractory ascites does not respond to high doses of diuretics (spironolactone and furosemide). Moderate-volume ascites does not require paracentesis and large-volume ascites is controlled by a combination of medical treatment and paracentesis.

Medical management

Dietary sodium is restricted to approximately one-third of the normal daily intake (i.e. to about 60–90 mEq/day). Diuretic therapy commences with an aldosterone antagonist, such as spironolactone or amiloride. These two measures are successful in controlling ascites in about 60–70% of patients. In addition, a thiazide diuretic may be required. Diuretic therapy must be monitored closely to ensure that progressive renal failure and electrolyte imbalance (potassium, sodium, calcium and magnesium) do not occur.

Prophylactic antibiotics are not given. Primary or spontaneous peritonitis-complicating ascites is treated with appropriate antibiotics, although sometimes a laparotomy is required either for diagnosis or to wash out the peritoneal cavity. Specific causes of ascites such as tuberculosis are treated with appropriate anti-tuberculous chemotherapy according to national guidelines. Surgical intervention is reserved for diagnosis and to treat complications such as acute bowel obstruction, bleeding or perforation due to intestinal tuberculosis.

Paracentesis

Paracentesis, or drainage of ascitic fluid, brings immediate though temporary relief to patients with symptomatic tense ascites. Paracentesis is performed under local anaesthetic and with a strict aseptic technique by inserting a cannula through the anterolateral abdominal wall, avoiding the inferior epigastric artery and the colon. It can often be performed under ultrasound or CT control. Fluid is drained into a sterile collecting system and the cannula is either removed immediately or left *in situ* for 24–48 hours. Rapid removal of large amounts of ascites may lead to serious hypovolaemia because the underlying reason for formation of ascites has not been eliminated and ascites re-forms rapidly with fluid from the extracellular space (interstitial and intravascular fluid). Volume replacement may be required during paracentesis and is undertaken cautiously with concentrated or normal serum albumin, to avoid hypovolaemia on one hand, and fluid overload and rapid reaccumulation of ascites on the other. The complications of infection, intestinal perforation and bleeding are rare when performed with an appropriate technique and an appropriate cannula.

Relief of acute hepatic venous obstruction

When the cause is due to an acute thrombus, thrombolytic therapy or angioplasty may be performed. Where these are unsuccessful a portosystemic shunt should be considered.

Transjugular intrahepatic portosystemic shunts

A shunt is placed between the portal and systemic circulations in the liver using the transjugular route for venous access. It may stabilise the patient while consideration is being given to liver transplantation. The shunts have a fairly high rate of blockage or stenosis (up to 75% after 6–12 months) and the shunt may induce hepatic encephalopathy.

Portosystemic shunts

If ascites is due to portal hypertension, portosystemic shunting may be performed in selected patients to reduce portal venous pressure. This may be using transjugular intrahepatic portosystemic shunts (TIPS) or by making a formal anastomosis between the splenic and renal veins (lienorenal shunt) or portal vein and inferior vena cava (portocaval shunt). These shunts do not adress the problem of the underlying liver disease, nor the accompanying oesophageal varices. Shunt surgery may be complicated by hepatic encephalopathy and hepatorenal syndrome. The presence of ascites in patients undergoing shunt surgery for portal hypertension is a poor prognostic sign.

Peritoneovenous shunts

Symptomatic relief by draining ascitic fluid from the peritoneal cavity into the systemic venous system can be achieved by way of a peritoneovenous shunt (PVS). A PVS (Denver shunt, LeVeen shunt) consists of a silastic tube, with multiple side holes at each end and a one-way valve situated in the middle. The PVS is placed entirely subcutaneously, with one end inserted into the peritoneal cavity and the other into the superior vena cava (SVC) via a jugular or subclavian vein, so that the valve allows flow of ascites from the peritoneal cavity to the venous system. A PVS is indicated when medical therapy has failed to control ascites in patients with (i) intractable ascites in the presence of reasonably good liver function, or (ii) rapidly accumulating ascites secondary to abdominal carcinomatosis. Concern about infusing ascitic fluid laden with malignant cells into the circulation is theoretical because these patients have widely disseminated malignant disease before insertion of the PVS.

The post-operative mortality of PVS is 10–20%, reflecting the serious underlying disorder of patients requiring the procedure. However, most patients obtain useful palliation. A minor coagulopathy is common postoperatively but can be partly prevented by completely aspirating the ascites and replacing it with warmed normal saline or Hartmann's solution when inserting the PVS. Long-term complications include occlusion of the PVS (particularly with bloody or highly proteinacious or mucoid ascites), SVC thrombosis, bacteraemia and shunt infection, which may lead to subacute bacterial endocarditis.

Surgery on patients with ascites

Surgery is prone to complications in patients with ascites. Abdominal surgery is prone to infection and there is a potential for poor wound/anastomotic healing. The underlying liver disease may cause a coagulopathy. Renal failure complicating liver disease (hepatorenal syndrome) is a major risk which can be minimised by ensuring optimal renal perfusion. Patients who have obstructive jaundice are often surgical candidates, at least for some form of bypass procedure. The presence of ascites in these patients increases the mortality, particularly from hepatorenal syndrome, and thus less invasive procedures such as biliary stenting are preferred.

MCQs

Select the single correct answer to each question.

1 In portal hypertension:
- **a** there is increased portal blood volume
- **b** there is a decrease in portal blood pressure
- **c** there is increased splanchnic vasoconstriction
- **d** there is hypoproteinaemia due to increased renal protein losses
- **e** there is reduced splanchnic lymphatic flow

2 The following conditions are typically associated with ascites:
- **a** filiariasis
- **b** Gilbert's disease
- **c** abdominal tuberculosis
- **d** large uterine fibroids
- **e** ectopic pregnancy

3 In patients with ascites:
- **a** bacterial peritonitis can be prevented by prophylactic antibiotics
- **b** leveen shunts may alleviate ascites associated with portal hypertension
- **c** pancreatitis may develop
- **d** may be relieved by spironolactone
- **e** paracentesis gives long periods of relief, often lasting several months

4 In jaundiced patients with ascites:
- **a** there is a low risk for hepatorenal syndrome because of splanchnic vasodilatation
- **b** coagulation profiles are usually normal
- **c** the systemic blood volume is increased
- **d** the renal blood flow is increased
- **e** there is a poor prognosis when operating for malignant disease

5 The following cancers are commonly associated with the development of ascites:
- **a** lymphoma
- **b** endometrial
- **c** GIST tumours
- **d** mucus-secreting villous adenoma
- **e** ovarian

67 Neck swellings

Christoper J. O'Brien

Introduction

Swellings or lumps in the neck are a common clinical problem. Patients presenting with neck lumps are likely to be fearful that they have cancer. Neck lumps in children are common although rarely malignant, but the situation is quite different in adults. The following rule should apply: an adult with a lump in the lateral neck has cancer until proven otherwise. Adults with lateral neck swellings should not be subjected to lengthy trials of observation or antibiotic therapy; instead, diagnostic efforts should be aimed at excluding malignancy.

Basic knowledge

Most neck lumps can, with a little experience, be diagnosed clinically. It is important to have some knowledge of head and neck anatomy to assist with clinical diagnosis (see Chapter 38). In Fig. 67.1 the triangles of the neck and the distribution of lymph nodes are shown. The lymph nodes can be grouped into levels and these are shown in roman numerals. Level I consists of the submandibular and submental lymph nodes. Levels II, III and IV are respectively the upper, middle and lower jugular chain nodes. Level II also contains the jugulodigastric lymph node. Level V has the lymph nodes of the posterior triangle. The following facts should be remembered:

- The jugulodigastric lymph node is commonly enlarged in both inflammatory and malignant conditions. Children with tonsillitis, young adults with glandular fever or Hodgkin's disease and middle-aged adults with cancers of the oral cavity and oropharynx can all present with lymphadenopathy at this site.
- The lymph nodes in the posterior triangle are all distributed along the spinal accessory nerve. These nodes are most commonly involved in benign

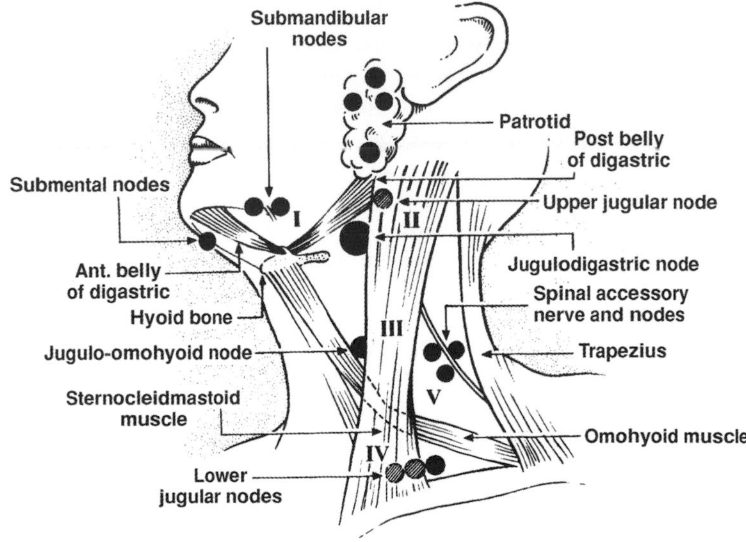

Fig. 67.1 The triangles, lymph node levels and normal lymph nodes in the neck. It shows the main muscular anatomy of the neck with the sites of normal, named lymph node groups. In addition, the lymph nodes are subdivided into levels as follows: level I, submandibular and submental triangle; level II, upper jugular chain lymph nodes (including the jugulodigastric lymph node); level III, mid-jugular chain nodes (including the jugulo omohyoid node); level IV, lower jugular chain lymph nodes (including lymph nodes overlying scalenus anterior muscle and those in the supraclavicular fossa); level V, lymph nodes of the posterior triangle, lying along the course of the spinal accessory nerve.

infective conditions (usually viral) in children and young adults.

- Metastatic involvement of posterior triangle (spinal accessory) nodes may occur with naso-pharyngeal cancer and skin cancers arising on the posterior scalp, neck and shoulder region.
- Skin cancer is common in Australia and both melanoma and squamous carcinoma can metastasise to the lymph nodes in the parotid gland, those in the submandibular triangle and those in the posterior triangle.
- Approximately 80% of lateral neck lumps in adults will be due to metastatic cancer. It is important to examine the possible anatomical primary sites that may lead to metastatic disease in the neck. They are the skin of the head and neck (including the scalp), the lip, the oral cavity, the oropharynx, the post-nasal space (especially in Asian patients), the larynx and hypopharynx.
- A solitary lump, low in the neck, deep to the sternomastoid muscle in the supraclavicular fossa (level IV) is likely to be a metastasis from a primary cancer below the clavicles, that is, the lung, the oesophagus, the stomach or the pancreas.

Clinical assessment

Evaluation of the patient in the office or clinic begins with a careful history, taking into account first the age of the patient and second whether the swelling is in the lateral or anterior compartment of the neck.

Children are likely to present with a short history of either enlarged tender lymph nodes, suggesting an infective or inflammatory process, or multiple small non-tender nodes, particularly in the posterior triangle, suggesting a subclinical viral infection. Long-standing cystic swellings in children suggest a congenital problem, possibly cystic hygroma (also called lymphangioma). Thyroid swellings in children are very uncommon, but 50% of them are malignant when they do occur.

Adolescents can also present with acute inflammatory lymphadenopathy in the jugulodigastric region and occasionally also in the posterior triangle. Glandular fever and viral conditions should be considered. The presence of multiple enlarged lymph nodes is more suggestive of infection. Adolescents, however, can develop lymphomas, particularly Hodgkin's disease and prominent lymph nodes. Those larger than 2 cm should be evaluated to exclude malignancy, especially where the history suggests that there has been progressive slow enlargement. Skin cancers are rare in children and uncommon in adolescents. Young adults can develop melanoma and a history of previous removal of a pigmented skin lesion could be highly relevant.

Other common clinical conditions in adolescents and young adults are:

- thyroglossal cyst, presenting as a painless swelling at or below the level of the hyoid bone, which elevates on tongue protrusion
- branchial cyst, presenting at the anterior border of the sternomastoid muscle below the jaw (level II); there is usually rapid painless development of the swelling although secondary infection and inflammation may occur
- plunging ranula, a cystic swelling in the submandibular region due to extravasation through the mylohyoid muscle of mucoid saliva from a disrupted sublingual gland in the floor of the mouth.

The clinical evaluation of adults with lateral neck lumps is aimed more specifically at the exclusion of malignancy. The history is usually one of painless progressive enlargement of a lymph node. There may be a pre-existing history of skin cancer (squamous carcinoma or melanoma) or treatment for some other malignancy involving the lip, oral cavity, oropharynx or some other mucosal site. Neck lymphadenopathy in an Asian patient should raise the possibility of nasopharyngeal carcinoma; however, tuberculosis is also relatively common among Asian patients who have recently immigrated. The smoking history is important. Mucosal cancers, which are nearly always squamous carcinoma, occur rarely among non-smokers and so a history of heavy tobacco and alcohol use raises the possibility that cervical lymphadenopathy represents metastatic cancer from a mucosal primary squamous carcinoma.

Physical examination

The usual evaluation of lumps involves clarification of the following features: site, size, shape, consistency, deep and superficial attachments, the nature of the surface and the edge of the lump, the presence of fluctuation, pulsation and translumination. In the neck the following issues apply:

- Which triangle of the neck is involved? (Is the lump in the lateral or anterior compartment of the neck?)

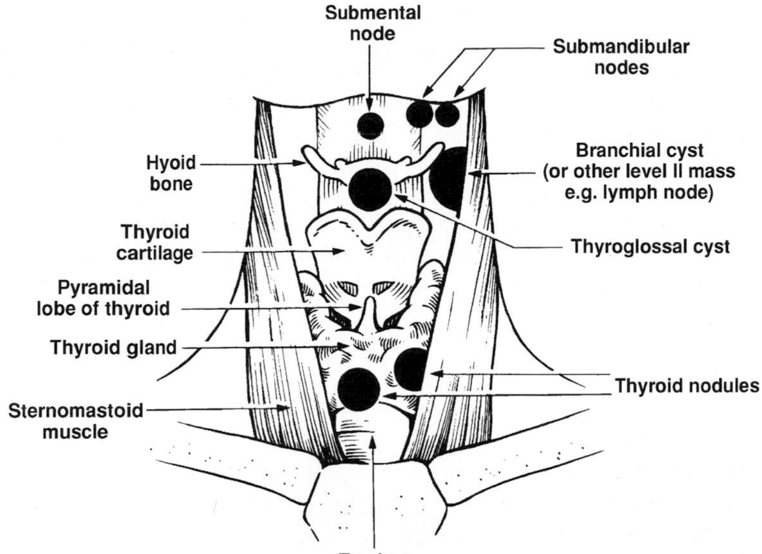

Fig. 67.2 The anterior compartment of the neck showing the trachea, thyroid gland and laryngeal framework consisting of the thyroid cartilage and hyoid bone. This area is made up of the two anterior triangles of the neck, each consisting of the area bounded by the jaw superiorly, the anterior board of the sternomastoid muscle posteriorly and the midline medially. The sites of various anterior and anterolateral neck lumps are shown.

- Does it move with swallowing? This indicates it is deep to the pretracheal fascia and likely to be thyroid.
- Does it move with protrusion of the tongue? This applies to upper anterior neck lumps, and the physical sign refers to thyroglossal cysts.
- What is the relationship to the sternomastoid muscle? This final point is important for differentiating lumps in the upper neck. Tumours in the tail of the parotid gland will lie superficial to the sternomastoid muscle and, when the muscle is contracted by turning the head to the opposite side, the lump will remain easily palpable. By contrast, an upper jugular chain (level II) lymph node, lying deep to the sternomastoid muscle, will become less obvious and more difficult to palpate when the head is turned to the opposite side.
- Where the neck lump appears to be an enlarged lymph node, either benign or malignant, the possible sources of infection or malignancy should be searched for.

Sites of common anterior compartment swellings are shown in Fig. 67.2.

Fine-needle aspiration biopsy

Fine-needle aspiration biopsy is the single most important test in the evaluation of neck lumps, particularly in adults who may have malignancy. It is usually necessary to carry out needle biopsy of tender lymph nodes in children; however, non-tender swellings in the central and lateral compartments of the neck in adolescents and adults should be evaluated by needle biopsy as the initial investigation. Metastatic malignancy can usually be diagnosed with a very high degree of accuracy. In general, reactive lymphadenopathy can be distinguished from lymphoma on needle biopsy; however, occasionally atypical lymphocytes are identified and it is necessary to carry out an excision biopsy of the node to clarify the diagnosis. Branchial cysts mainly occur in young adults and when they are aspirated thick creamy fluid is removed along with benign squamous cells. Under the microscope cholesterol crystals and cellular debris are visible. Branchial cysts occasionally occur in middle-aged adults, otherwise at risk of metastatic cancer, and it can sometimes be difficult to distinguish between metastatic squamous carcinoma with central necrosis and a benign branchial cyst on cytology. Excision of the lump may be necessary.

Fine-needle biopsy is also the best initial investigation of the thyroid swellings. The presence of colloid, normal follicle cells and haemosiderin-laden macrophages is consistent with the presence of a colloid nodule. The presence of papillary structures raises the possibility of papillary carcinoma, while a finding of multiple follicle cells in a microfollicular pattern with very little colloid indicates that the nodule is a

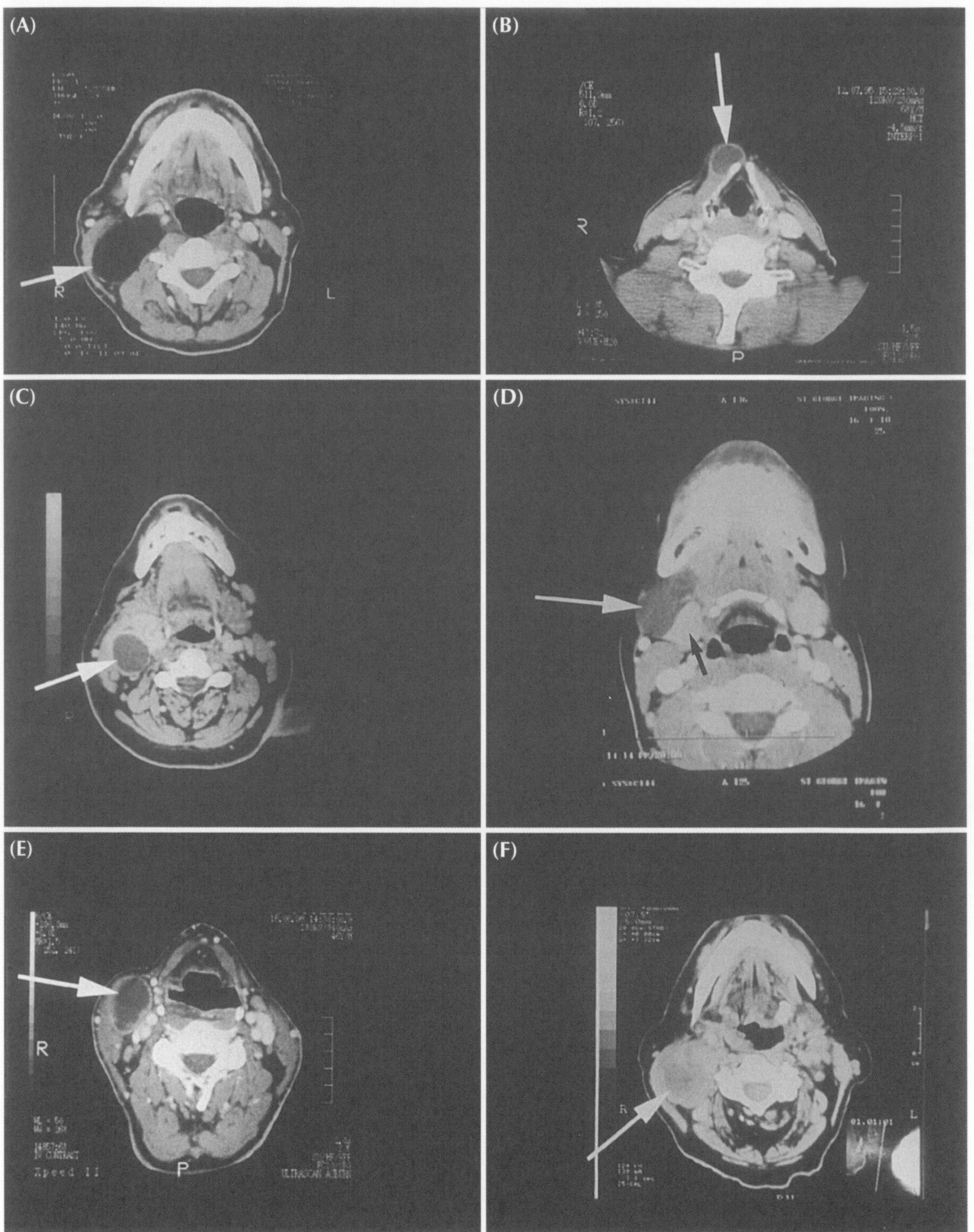

Continued

solid follicular lesion. In this setting it is necessary to completely remove the lump (by thyroid lobectomy) to differentiate between follicular adenoma and follicular carcinoma.

Fine-needle aspiration biopsy is very safe and the risk of tumour implantation along the needle tract is negligible.

Ultrasound

In general, ultrasound is not particularly useful in the evaluation of head and neck lumps. Ultrasound can differentiate between solid and cystic masses and can indicate whether or not there are multiple enlarged lymph nodes or the presence of multiple nodules in the thyroid gland. Ultrasound, however, rarely assists in clarifying the diagnosis.

Computed tomography

Computed tomography (CT) scans are far more helpful than ultrasound in assisting with the diagnosis of neck swellings, especially when they are larger than 2 cm. Computed tomography scanning can provide an idea of the consistency of a lump along with its size and anatomical relations. Figure 67.3 shows a series of CT scans of common neck lumps, demonstrating the typical radiological appearance.

Excision biopsy

If a diagnosis cannot be confirmed on fine-needle aspiration biopsy, an excision biopsy may be necessary to confirm or exclude malignancy. Care should be taken not to spill tissue or break up a lymph node in the course of biopsy because malignant cells may be implanted into the surrounding tissue. The biopsy incision should be oriented in a natural skin crease in such a way that the biopsy scar can be excised in a subsequent operation. Furthermore, care must be taken not to damage related anatomical structures, for example, the spinal accessory nerve in the posterior triangle and the marginal mandibular nerve in the submandibular triangle, during excision biopsy procedures.

Chest X-ray

Chest radiology is important in young adults, when lymphoma is the possibility, and in all adults. It may demonstrate mediastinal widening or primary or secondary lung neoplasms. It should be remembered that lung cancers are more common than mouth and throat cancers and that smokers, who are at risk for head and neck cancers, are also at risk of having lung cancer.

Treatment

The management algorithm for neck lumps is summarised in the decision-making flow chart (Fig. 67.4). Following the history, physical examination and investigations, a diagnosis can usually be made. Excision of the lump may be necessary and if the lump proves to be benign, the excision biopsy is likely to be curative. Some benign lumps (e.g. reactive lymph nodes, lipomas and sebaceous cysts) may be simply observed and left untreated. Other benign lumps require removal either for patient comfort, cosmesis, or to avoid future problems. Branchial cysts, thyroglossal cysts, plunging ranulas, dermoid cysts, some lipomas and sebacous cysts, and benign salivary and thyroid swellings fall into this category.

Fig. 67.3 Computed tomography scans showing common pathological processes in the neck. Each has a typical appearance. **(A)** Large lipoma neck deep to sternomastoid muscle and impinging on the parapharyngeal region. Note that the lesion is black, the same as the subcutaneous fat. **(B)** Thyroglossal cyst. Note the smooth-walled, well-circumscribed cystic mass closely attached to the anterior part of the right thyroid cartilage lamina. **(C)** Branchial cyst. This is a smooth-walled, well-circumscribed cyst deep to the sternomastoid muscle in the right neck in a young patient. It must be differentiated from metastatic squamous carcinoma with cystic degeneration (see (E)). **(D)** Plunging ranula. This cystic swelling is more dense than subcutaneous fat but less dense than the soft tissue of the adjacent submandibular salivary gland (small black arrow). It is due to extravasation of mucoid saliva from the sublingual gland into the submandibular space and through the mylohoid muscle. **(E)** Metastatic squamous carcinoma of the neck with cystic degeneration. Note that this is also cystic but, unlike the branchial cyst (see (C)), the wall of the lesion is irregular. **(F)** Large mass of metastatic squamous carcinoma in the right neck. This is a predominantly solid mass with little cystic degeneration.

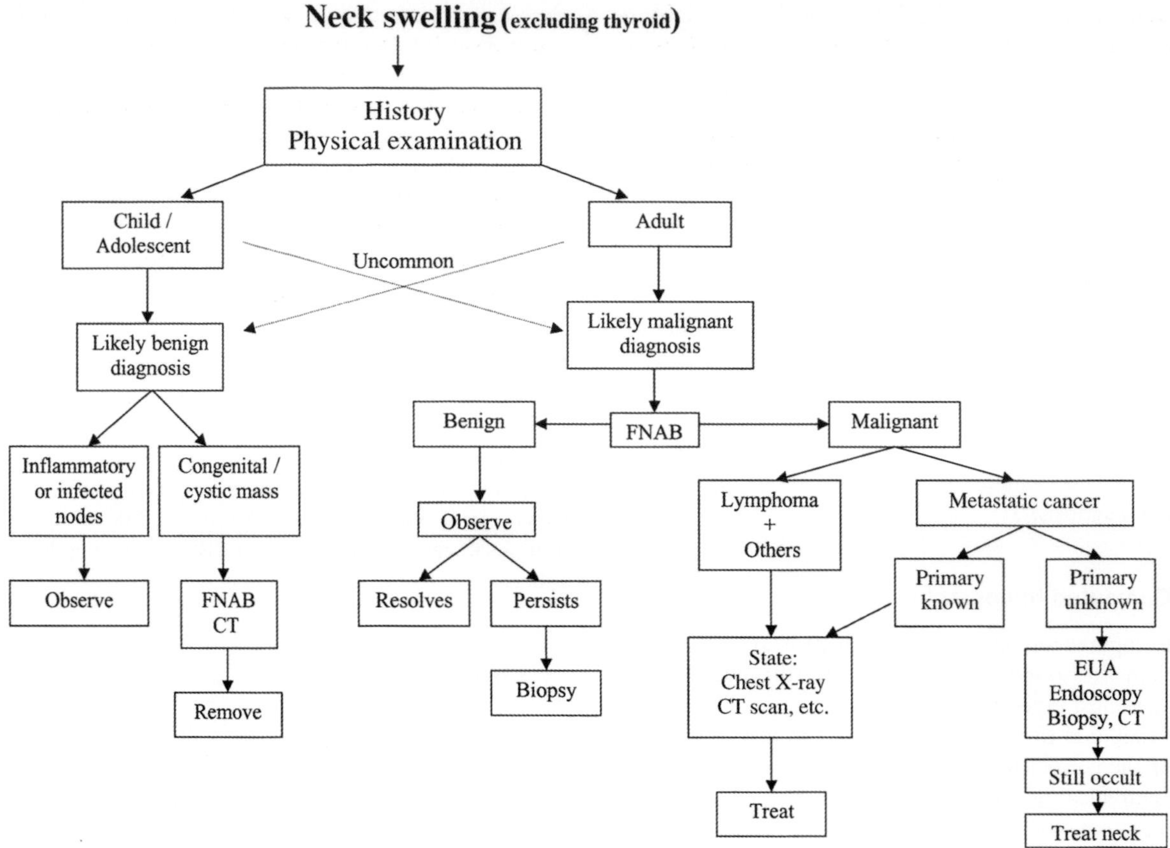

Fig. 67.4 Management algorithm for neck lumps.

Once a diagnosis of malignancy is made, definitive treatment is necessary. Lymphoma requires further staging investigations and treatment by chemotherapy, radiotherapy or both.

The treatment of metastatic cancer depends on the type of cancer and whether or not the primary site can be identified.

If the primary cancer is found (skin or mucosa of the upper aerodigestive tract), it should be treated definitively with the metastatic neck disease. If a primary cancer cannot be found and the fine-needle aspiration biopsy shows metastatic squamous carcinoma, a thorough investigation of the upper aerodigestive tract should be carried out with biopsies of potential occult primary sites. These include the nasopharynx, tonsil and tongue base. When the primary site is still not identified, the metastatic disease in the neck requires treatment by surgery, with or without post-operative radiotherapy.

When metastatic adenocarcinoma is identified by fine-needle aspiration biopsy an attempt should be made to determine whether there is a treatable primary cancer; for example, in the thyroid gland or a salivary gland. Adenocarcinomas from the prostate, breast or abdomen that metastasise to the neck lymph nodes, are not curable and so radical treatment to the neck is not warranted. Also, an extensive work-up in an asymptomatic patient should not be carried out when metastatic adenocarcinoma is diagnosed, as cure is unlikely.

The operation used to treat cancer in the neck is called neck dissection. Neck dissections can vary in their extent and according to which anatomical structures are preserved (see Chapter 38). Radiotherapy is given after surgery when multiple lymph nodes are involved with metastatic disease or when there is evidence of spread outside the lymph node capsule (extracapsular spread).

MCQs

Select the single correct answer to each question.

1 The most common cause of enlargement of the jugulodigastric lymph node in a child 9 years of age is:
- **a** Hodgkin's disease
- **b** glandular fever
- **c** tonsillitis
- **d** non-Hodgkin's lymphoma
- **e** metastatic Wilm's tumour

2 Metastatic involvement of the posterior triangle nodes in the neck is most likely to be due to:
- **a** nasopharyngeal carcinoma
- **b** basal cell carcinoma of the shoulder region
- **c** laryngeal carcinoma
- **d** squamous cell carcinoma of the posterior scalp
- **e** carcinoma of the oesophagus

68 Dysphagia

Robert J. S. Thomas

Introduction

Definition

Dysphagia is defined as difficulty in swallowing. It is a common and important symptom. Two types are recognised:

- Oropharyngeal: involving the transfer of food from the mouth into the upper oesophagus.
- Oesophageal: involving the transport of food down the oesophagus and into the stomach.

Significance

The significance of this condition relates to its multitude of causes. Dysphagia may be caused by mild muscular spasm or incoordination due to psychological causes or, at the other end of the spectrum, may be progressive, associated with loss of weight and due to a malignant obstruction of the oesophagus. Consequently any patient complaining of the symptom of dysphagia requires full investigation to exclude malignancy, and to effectively treat the condition.

Incidence

Dysphagia is a common symptom affecting most individuals transiently at some time in life. One of the important causes of dysphagia is adenocarcinoma of the lower oesophagus. This is a tumour that is increasing in incidence throughout the Western World and often occurs in middle-aged males. It is associated with long-standing gastro-oesophageal reflux and the development of Barrett's mucosa in the oesophagus (see Chapter 10).

Box 68.1 Symptoms associated with dysphagia

- Chest pain due to reflux oesophagitis.
- Odynophagia or pain on swallowing. May be associated with oesophagitis or oesophageal spasm.
- Physical reflux of food or bile into the mouth, associated with severe gastro-oesophageal reflux.
- Coughing and aspiration of food, indicating possible recurrent laryngeal nerve or bulbar palsy.
- Palatal incompetence, with food being regurgitated through the nose on attempted swallowing. This is associated with bulbar palsy following cerebrovascular accident.
- Loss of weight and anorexia. This often indicates a malignant obstruction.
- Hoarseness of voice due to malignant involvement of the larynx or recurrent laryngeal nerve compression.

Associated symptoms

There are a variety of other symptoms that may accompany the presence of dysphagia (Box 68.1). The presence of these symptoms helps in making a clinical diagnosis.

Causes of dysphagia

Problems within the mouth may cause difficulties in swallowing food. Simple examples include painful ulceration or abscesses, severe tonsillitis, lack of teeth, or deformity after head and neck surgery. Many of these problems can easily be excluded, and the causes of dysphagia that raise concern relate to the pharyngo-oesophageal area and the oesophagus itself (Box 68.2).

Box 68.2 Causes of dysphagia

Pharyngo-oesophageal disorders
- Diminished pharyngeal propulsion: motor neurone disease; myasthenia gravis; cerebrovascular accident with dysfunction of ninth, tenth and twelfth cranial nerves.
- Relaxation anomalies: upper oesophageal achalasia or cricopharyngeal spasm; cricopharyngeal bar.
- Incoordination: cerebrovascular accident resulting in ninth, tenth and twelfth cranial nerve palsy; gastro-oesophageal reflux with cricopharyngeal spasm; pharyngeal diverticulum with cricopharyngeal spasm.

Oesophageal causes
- Motor disorders: achalasia of the oesophagus; diffuse oesophageal spasm; scleroderma.
- Mechanical causes: luminal obstruction due to a large food bolus or bone impaction; mucosal strictures; webs (e.g. Patterson-Brown-Kelly syndrome, Schatzki ring); fibrous strictures (which result from inflammation and scarring from long-standing gastro-oesophageal reflux); ingestion of caustics (which causes fibrous scarring and predisposes to malignancy); squamous cell carcinoma; adenocarcinoma; rare tumours including lymphoma and metastatic tumours; benign tumours (rarely).

Extrinsic pressure on the oesophagus
- Retrosternal goitre.
- Pharyngeal diverticulum.
- Vascular abnormalities (right subclavian artery and right-sided aortic arteries).
- Any mediastinal mass may cause oesophageal compression.

Diagnosis of the causes of dysphagia

Clinical features

The clinical history can give a major lead to the diagnosis of the cause of dysphagia. For example, difficulty in swallowing fluids rather than solids suggests a muscular incoordination problem. Progressive dysphagia for solids suggests a malignant cause. Dysphagia in the presence of retrosternal pain, associated with regurgitation of fluids may indicate the stricture or carcinoma associated with reflux. Coughing or the aspiration of fluid into the larynx will give a guide to lesions such as cranial nerve palsies. Loss of weight is one of the most important accompanying symptoms of dysphagia, and indicates malignancy. Lymph node and other masses may be palpable in the neck. However, physical signs are usually absent.

Investigations

Not all investigations need to be carried out in all cases of dysphagia, but in those cases where the diagnosis is difficult or obscure, the whole gamut of investigations may be needed (Fig. 68.1).

Radiological examination

The barium swallow examination provides good views of the upper oesophagus and helps makes the diagnosis of pharyngeal pouch, webs and strictures. However, a negative barium swallow examination in the presence of persistent dysphagia demands further investigation by endoscopy.

Oesophagoscopy and gastroscopy

This is usually the first investigation for dysphagia and is done using flexible endoscopes under intravenous sedation. Care has to be taken to avoid perforation, particularly if there is suspicion of a pharyngeal pouch or if a stricture is present. The oesophagus is carefully examined for abnormalities such as inflammation and stricture. A stricture can usually be easily determined as being benign or malignant. In the absence of stricture, features such as oesophageal dilatation with food residue may suggest achalasia. Rarely, rigid oesophagoscopy is necessary if flexible endoscopy is unsuccessful.

Radiological staging

Radiological staging includes computed tomography (CT) examination and, less commonly, magnetic resonance imaging. This can help make the diagnosis in obscure cases, but its major role is helping to stage the extent of malignant disease.

Endoscopic ultrasound

Endoscopic ultrasound is a very effective way of diagnosing abnormalities within the oesophageal wall. It is not useful if there is a tight narrowing in the proximal oesophagus preventing the passage of the instrument. It is the most precise method for detecting the depth of penetration of a cancer into or through the wall of the oesophagus.

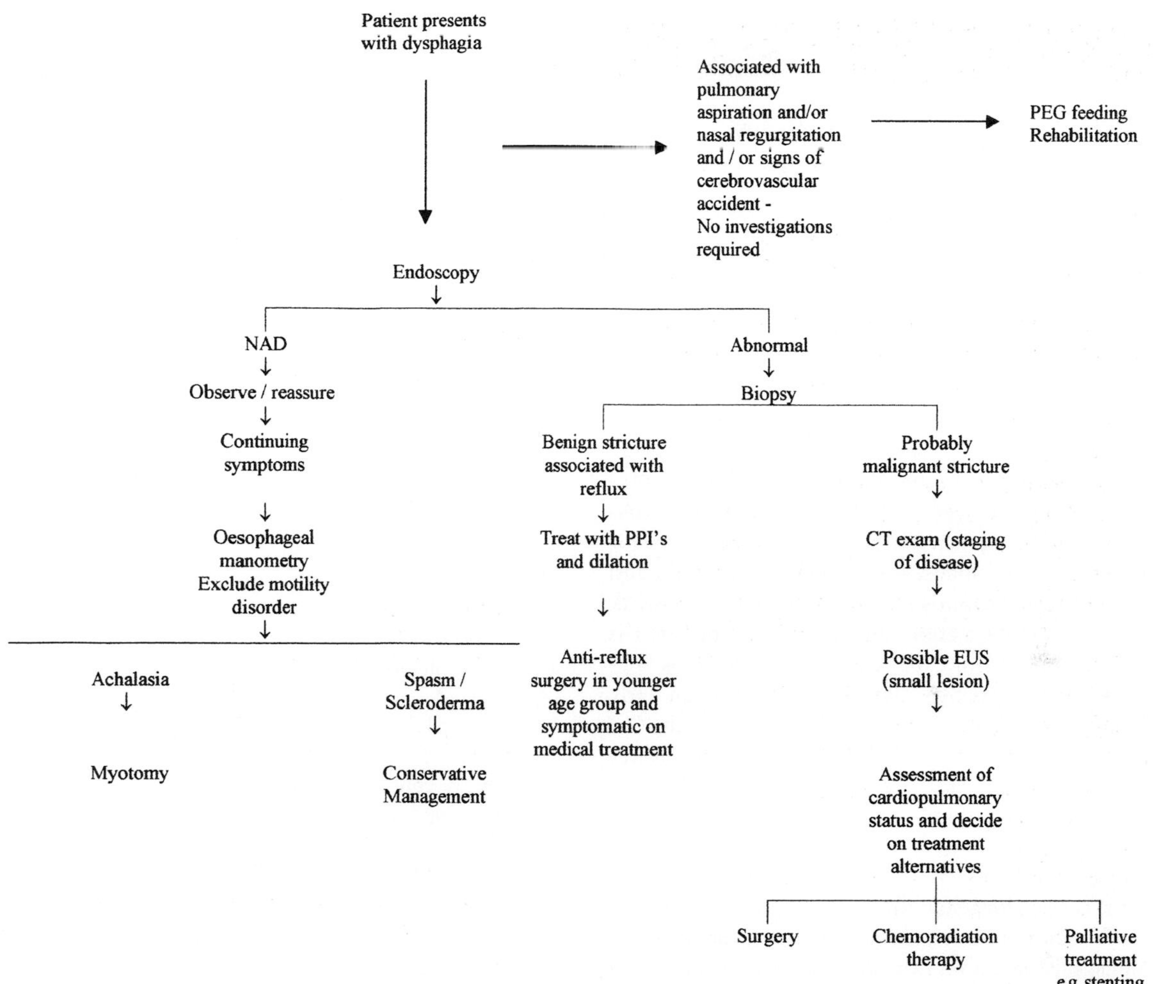

Fig. 68.1 Management of dysphagia.

Oesophageal motility studies

These are done via a multilumen catheter inserted into the oesophagus via the nose. Propulsive waves in the oesophagus can easily be measured and the response to a swallowing effort detected. Abnormalities can be identified in achalasia, scleroderma and oesophageal spasm.

Other investigations

Twenty-four-hour pH monitoring will help document the degree of oesophageal reflux. Gastro-oesophageal reflux studies using nuclear scan techniques can be helpful in difficult cases. Reflux may be associated with fibrous stricture or oesophageal spasm, thereby causing dysphagia.

Specific causes of dysphagia

Transfer or pharyngo-oesophageal dysphagia

More correctly this is an inability to swallow and is associated with aspiration, coughing and nasal regurgitation. The common cause of this type of problem is a cerebrovascular accident. It produces major problems in attempting to rehabilitate a stroke patient with a bulbar palsy. Feeding via nasogastric tubes or gastrotomy tubes (percutaneous endoscopic gastrostomy [PEG]) may be necessary to provide nourishment.

Motility disorders of the oesophagus

See Chapter 10.

Achalasia

Achalasia of the oesophagus is also known as cardiospasm and is often associated with the presence of a so-called mega-oesophagus. It occurs most commonly in the young to middle-aged (30–60 years). The incidence is 1 in 100 000 people. There are associated neural abnormalities in the ganglia but the exact cause is not known. The dysphagia is intermittent, but progressive in the longer term. It is detected by the patient as being suprasternal in position and occurs for both liquids and solids. Regurgitation is postural and aspiration pneumonitis may occur. Usually only weak oesophageal contractions occur and the condition is painless. In 10% of cases a condition known as 'vigorous achalasia' exists. This is regarded as an early stage of the disease and is associated with pain. Oesophageal manometry reveals markedly elevated lower oesophageal sphincter pressures and diminished oesophageal contractions.

COMPLICATIONS

In the chronic long-standing case, weight loss and chest pain occur. Pulmonary disease from aspiration of oesophageal content and the development of carcinoma within the dilated oesophagus are significant complications.

DIAGNOSIS AND TREATMENT

Chest X-ray, barium meal and manometry examinations help to confirm the diagnosis, which may be difficult to determine. Treatment is by surgical division (myotomy) of the hyperactive lower oesophageal sphincter, usually approached laparoscopically. A thoracoscopic approach can also be used. Reflux is a complication after myotomy and an anti-reflux procedure at the time of surgery is commonly performed. An alternative treatment is by manometric dilatation using a balloon placed across the hypertensive lower oesophageal sphincter, which is then expanded causing disruption of the sphincter. The results of both methods of treatment are good in about 90% of cases.

Diffuse oesophageal spasm

This is usually a primary disorder but may be secondary and associated with:

- peptic oesophageal reflux
- ingestion of irritants
- emotion and tension
- possibly an underlying carcinoma.

SYMPTOMS

The patient complains of dysphagia that is often worse for liquids, is intermittent and is noted in the midsternal region. Pain, which is retrosternal and severe, is also common, is sometimes misdiagnosed as being cardiac in origin, and is worse under emotional stress. There is rarely any weight loss. There is marked belching and other indigestion-type symptoms.

DIAGNOSIS

The diagnosis is made on X-ray, which shows tertiary contractions in the oesophagus, and motility studies, which show simultaneous, vigorous, repetitive waves in the oesophageal body when the lower oesophageal sphincter relaxes.

THERAPY

Therapy is generally simple, using simple bougienage without rupturing oesophageal muscle, and medication.

Scleroderma

This systemic connective tissue disorder is characterised by muscle atrophy, dilatation of the oesophagus and smooth muscle fibrosis. It is diagnosed by motility studies that show a non-contractile oesophagus. Oesophageal reflux is often a contributing and secondary factor causing strictures. No satisfactory therapy exists.

Chagas' disease

This is a parasitic infection, common in South America. It produces destruction of the ganglia of the oesophagus and an achalasia-type stricture.

Mechanical causes of dysphagia

The mechanical causes of dysphagia are those that are most commonly the province of the surgeon. The diagnosis depends upon taking a clinical history and often requires a full investigation (see 'Investigations') to make the diagnosis. The difficult diagnosis is often between a benign and a malignant stricture in the oesophagus (see Chapter 10). Repeated biopsies may be necessary to make this distinction. Malignant obstruction in the lower oesophagus demands either extensive surgery or combined surgery and chemoradiation therapy if curative therapy is indicated. However, in about 30% of patients with malignancy, palliative treatment only is indicated. Intubation of the tumour or laser ablation are two effective methods of palliation.

MCQs

Select the single correct answer to each question.

1 The symptoms of dysphagia include the following EXCEPT:
- **a** very common and thus can be ignored in most cases
- **b** may be associated with reflux symptoms
- **c** may be associated with significant pain
- **d** can present acutely with total obstruction of the oesophagus
- **e** may be associated with diminished pharyngeal propulsion

2 The causes of dysphagia may be the following EXCEPT:
- **a** classified as pharyngo-oesophageal and oesophageal
- **b** pharyngo-oesophageal causes are often neurological in origin, e.g. CVA
- **c** associated with altered motility of the oesophagus
- **d** achalasia is a disease primarily of the oesophageal musculature and is coexistent with gastro-oesophageal reflux
- **e** be associated with an adenocarcinoma of the mucosal lining

3 The cause of dysphagia can often be identified by the following EXCEPT:
- **a** upper GI endoscopy
- **b** barium swallow examination
- **c** upper abdominal ultrasound examination
- **d** CT examination of the chest
- **e** oesophageal manometry

4 Patients with dysphagia may complain of the following EXCEPT:
- **a** regurgitation of fluid and food when recumbent at night
- **b** difficulty with swallowing fluids more than solid food
- **c** difficulty with swallowing solid food more than liquids
- **d** may have significant weight loss
- **e** may have no weight loss
- **f** their partner may complain of snoring

5 dysphagia can be caused by the following EXCEPT:
- **a** benign strictures in the oesophagus
- **b** squamous carcinoma of the oesophagus
- **c** pharyngeal diverticulum
- **d** oesophageal spasm
- **e** uncomplicated sliding hiatus hernia

69 Leg ulcers

John Harris

Introduction

Epidemiological studies have shown that leg ulcers are present in 3–4% of the population aged more than 65. Management of such ulcers is often not optimal and recurrence is common. Consequently, ulcers result in considerable disability and expense. Improved results will follow a rigorous diagnostic approach, more specialized medical care and critical application of compression to facilitate healing.

Aetiology and pathogenesis

Impaired venous return

Musculo-venous pumps, the most important of which is the calf muscle pump, augment venous return to the heart. The pumps work best when the veins are patent, the valves competent and the pump used by regular exercise.

Venous insufficiency results from failure of the normal mechanisms returning venous blood from the lower limb, particularly incompetence of valves. Incompetence of the deep venous system may follow deep vein thrombosis (DVT) or occur spontaneously. Incompetence of the venous values causes a reduction in the volume of blood expelled by the calf-muscle pump. The calf muscle pump may also be impaired by limited ankle joint mobility caused by arthritis. With increasing obesity and a sedentary lifestyle in an ageing population, the calf-muscle pump may be simply not used.

The common pathway is ambulatory venous hypertension, which leads to soft tissue damage in the leg and eventually ulceration.

Oedema

Raised venous pressure alters the fluxes across the wall of the capillaries so that fluid accumulates in the tissues. Lack of mobility and prolonged standing add a gravitational component so patients often describe the swelling worsening during the day.

Development of collateral pathways

Small venules and veins dilate and attempt to develop alternative connections to the deep venous system. The walls of these veins are fragile and the veins are exposed to high pressure, so they may bleed externally or rupture in the subcutaneous tissue, leading to skin pigmentation.

Impaired nutrition of the skin and subcutaneous tissue

With sustained ambulatory venous hypertension in the lower extremity, there is impaired tissue perfusion. Atrophy and fibrosis results in the thinning of the subcutaneous tissue of the lower one-third of the leg, giving an 'inverted champagne bottle' appearance.

Ulcers

Minor injury, which may be unrecognised, can initiate leg ulceration. Healing is poor because of the impaired nutrition of the tissues and tissue breakdown follows. Ulceration can be compounded by infection, particularly streptococcal cellulitis.

Arterial disease

This is the predominant cause of about 20% of leg ulcer cases and a contributing factor, with venous disease, in a further 20%. As arterial insufficiency can often be corrected, it is important that arterial perfusion is checked even if the clinical appearance of an ulcer is typically venous.

Other causes

There is a miscellaneous group that comprises only 10% of patients with ulcers. Ulcers associated with hypertension (Martorell's ulcers) occur predominantly on the anterior and lateral aspects of the calf. The ulcers are distinguished from arterial ulcers by their site. Multiple ulcers may occur and may be painful. Treatment is conservative with healing often delayed.

A common injury is a fall that lifts a distally based skin flap which can leave a post-traumatic ulcer.

Several systemic diseases are associated with leg ulceration including rheumatoid arthritis, inflammatory bowel disease and vasculitis.

Finally, but most important, malignant change (Marjolin's ulcer), usually squamous cell carcinoma, should be suspected in any long-standing ulcer or one with an atypical appearance or that fails to heal despite adequate management. Biopsy of the ulcer edge is then indicated.

Clinical presentation

Chronic venous insufficiency

The patient presents with ulcers, often recurrent, and the history may extend over many years. The ulcers may be painful in the early stages, relieved by elevation of the leg. The most common site is on the medial side of the lower third of the calf. On examination, the ulcer is usually irregular in outline and surrounded by eczematous and/or pigmented skin with a base of granulation tissue. Careful serial measurement of the size of the ulcer will help determine if healing or progressive ulceration is occurring.

Arterial disease

The ulcer may be anywhere on the lower leg, characteristically over bony prominences such as the malleoli. The pain is worse when the leg is elevated and relieved when the leg is hanging down. The ankle pulses are absent.

Investigations

General investigations should include a full blood examination, fasting blood glucose and serum albumin estimation. With atypical ulcers or non-healing ulcers, markers for connective tissue disorders such as rheumatoid serology should be considered and a biopsy is mandatory.

Local investigations

Measurement of ankle blood pressure

Measurement of the ankle/brachial pressure index (ABI) should be performed to check the arterial circulation with a Duplex ultrasound scan if the ABI is abnormal to determine the site and severity of any arterial disease present. Angiography can then be performed on an intention-to-treat basis, aiming to restore arterial perfusion to normality by angioplasty or bypass surgery.

Venous duplex ultrasound

This test has supplanted venography in the assessment of chronic venous insufficiency. The veins are examined to determine the venous anatomy, patency and valvular competence. It is important to determine if there is superficial venous insufficiency present as this can be corrected surgically more easily than deep venous insufficiency.

Venous haemodynamics

Normally venous blood is emptied from the calf with muscular contraction and then slowly refills. Measurement of venous pressure or venous recovery time (the time taken for venous refilling) can quantitate the degree of venous insufficiency present and help differentiate between superficial and deep venous incompetence. These tests are generally performed only in specialised centres and include non-invasive tests such as strain gauge, photo-plethysmography and air plethysmography. The refilling time measured using these methods correlates well with that determined by direct venous pressure measurement. Air plethysmography provides more sophisticated indices of lower extremity venous function. These parameters complement the anatomic information demonstrated with venous ultrasound scanning.

Treatment

The principles of treatment have come to be applied more aggressively in recent years (Box 69.1). Such treatment should be directed to correct the underlying cause of the ulcer, to optimise healing and to prevent recurrence.

Treatment of the underlying cause

Venous insufficiency

An immediate concern is to control oedema of the subcutaneous tissue and to minimise the sequelae. This is best done by keeping the patient ambulatory by wearing elastic stockings or using compression bandaging although occasionally bedrest with elevation of the leg is required. Neglected or inadequate lower extremity compression is the commonest reason for failed healing or early ulcer recurrence. Elderly patients need considerable physical and emotional support to help them persevere with stockings, particularly for those with arthritis or limited mobility.

Surgery has a limited place in relieving venous obstruction, restoring valvular competence or dealing with superficial venous insufficiency or perforating veins. Superficial varicose veins should be treated, unless they are forming important collateral around obstructed deep veins. Patients with only superficial incompetence and normal deep veins are an important group to identify as they can be cured of the tendency to ulceration. Incompetent calf perforating veins, communicating between the deep and superficial venous systems, can be treated by sclerotherapy or by endoscopic surgery.

Attempts have been made to relieve venous obstruction or restore valve function by surgical means. The most successful procedure has been femoro-femoral vein bypass to relieve unilateral iliac venous obstruction. Procedures to restore valve function by applying cuffs to restore valvular competence or autotransplantion of vein segments containing competent valves into an incompetent deep vein have met with limited success. These measures are applicable to only about 1–2% of patients with venous ulceration.

Skin grafting can hasten healing, but in almost all patients it is unnecessary. Performance of a skin graft does not remove the need for the other measures described; in particular, the need to wear supporting stockings remains an essential component of the post-operative care.

The most important therapeutic measure to heal venous ulcers, supported by Level 1 evidence, is external compression preferably by stockings or alternatively, well applied elastic bandaging. The choice of dressing is far less important, other than to cover the ulcer and protect the skin. A variety of elastic stockings are now available with application devices to make it easier for patients to put them on. These stocking are designed to provide graduated compression, greatest around the ankle, less proximally. Graduated compression should be applied with a 40 mm Hg pressure gradient at the ankle level, tapering to 20 mm Hg at the knee. The ankle arterial pressure should be measured before compression bandaging is applied to ensure that there will

Box 69.1 Management algorithm for leg ulcers

1. **Define and treat cause**
   - **Measure ABI**
   - If ABI < 0.5
   - Do not apply compression bandaging
   - Arterial duplex scan
   - Improve arterial inflow
   - Angioplasty ± bypass surgery
   - If ABI > 0.9
   - Apply compression
     - Class I-II surgical stocking or four-layered banding
2. **Determine venous patency and competence**
   - **Venous duplex scan**
     - Check deep vein patency and competence
     - Check saphenofemoral and short-saphenopopliteal competence
       - If saphenofemoral and/or short-saphenopopliteal veins incompetent, and the deep veins are patent, consider surgery to correct superficial venous incompetence
       - If iliac vein stenosed/occluded, consider stenting or venous bypass
3. **Biopsy**
   - Long-standing ulcers
   - Ulcers with atypical appearance
   - Ulcers that recur despite adequate initial management
   - Remember, a leg ulcer may be malignant *de novo*
4. **Prevent recurrence**
   - Nutritional support
   - Perseverance with surgical stocking support

be no compromise of arterial inflow. In most cases a below-knee stocking provides adequate support.

Provide conditions to allow healing

Careful attention should be given to nutrition as elderly, immobile patients with painful ulcers may neglect themselves.

Treat infection

In addition to these general measures, local skin care and antibiotic therapy for any associated cellulitis will help control infection and provide optimal local conditions for healing. It is important to distinguish between invasive infection and contamination of the wound. Prolonged courses of antibiotics should not be given because this will usually result in colonisation of the wound by strains of bacteria resistant to the antibiotics.

Provide and maintain optimum conditions for healing

The two major elements of this are to remove dead tissue and to apply appropriate dressings. Dead tissue can be removed enzymatically or surgically. Although correct application of external compression is the most important therapeutic measure, dressings are important as wounds heal best in warm, moist conditions. There are now a large number of products available to provide and maintain optimum conditions for healing. The choice of dressing will depend on the depth of the wound and the amount of exudate.

Prevention of recurrence

Treatment that results in healing of an ulcer is not sufficient. The next objective is to prevent recurrence, by general measures such as life-style change encouraging greater mobility and weight loss and local measures, the most important of which is perseverance with surgical stocking support.

MCQs

Select the single correct answer to each question.

1 A 65-year-old woman has a chronic leg ulcer. Which of the following is the least likely case?
a squamous cell carcinoma
b giant cell arteritis
c superficial venous valvular incompetence
d deep venous valvular incompetence
e trauma

2 The most important measure to get a chronic venous ulcer to heal is:
a apply a dressing
b stop smoking
c apply compression bandaging/stockings
d surgery to excise the ulcer
e counselling

3 Which of the following is true regarding chronic leg ulcers?
a they are generally well managed
b 80% are due to superficial venous insufficiency
c a biopsy is best done of the ulcer edge
d basal cell carcinoma is the commonest malignancy in the leg
e arterial and venous ulcers are easily distinguished

4 Which of the following is true regarding the calf-muscle pump?
a it plays no part in venous return to the heart
b it cannot work if the valves are incompetent
c it is the only musculo-venous pump
d it depends on good ankle movement
e it cannot work if arterial disease is present

70 Leg swelling

Steven T. F. Chan and David M. A. Francis

Introduction

Leg swelling generally occurs because of an abnormal accumulation of interstitial fluid – oedema – of the lower extremity and it may be bilateral or unilateral. The commoner causes of leg swelling are summarised in Box 70.1. Lesions that result in discrete leg swellings are not discussed in this chapter. Systemic causes include cardiac failure, renal failure and hypoproteinaemia, and patients who present with bilateral leg swelling should have these causes excluded. Localised causes may result in either unilateral or bilaterial swelling depending on the site of the 'localised problem'. The most common localised cause of a unilateral leg swelling is venous disease. Lymphoedema is almost always secondary to a disorder of lymph nodes since primary lymphoedema is a rarity.

Box 70.1 Commoner causes of leg swelling

Systemic causes
- Congestive cardiac failure
- Renal disease
- Hypoproteinaemia

Venous causes
- Occlusion or compression: deep vein thrombosis; abdominal or pelvic tumour; trauma; ligation; IVC plication; retroperitoneal fibrosis; ascites
- Stagnation: dependent position
- Valve incompetence
- Arterialisation: arteriovenous fistula

Lymphatic causes
- Primary: congenital lymphoedema; lymphoedema praecox; lymphoedema tarda
- Secondary: neoplastic obstruction; irradiation damage; surgical excision; insect bite

Inflammatory causes
- Acute infections (streptococci, staphylococci)
- Chronic infections (fungi, filariasis, mycobacterium)

Pathophysiology of leg swelling

There is normally a balance between the inflow and outflow of extracellular fluid as blood flows through capillaries. Figure 70.1 shows the four basic forces that determine the rate of accumulation of interstitial fluid:
- capillary pressure
- interstitial fluid pressure
- plasma colloid osmotic pressure
- interstitial fluid colloid osmotic pressure

The capillary and interstitial fluid pressure are opposed by an oncotic gradient that is determined by the different protein concentrations of the interstitial and intravascular fluid compartments. About 90% of the fluid that leaks from the capillaries is estimated to return into the post-capillary venules, while the remaining 10% enters the lymphatic system.

Oedema can be caused by:
- increased filtration pressure as a result of
  - arteriole dilatation
  - venule constriction
  - raised venous pressure
- reduced oncotic pressure
  - hyproproteinaemia
  - accumulation in interstitial space
- increased capillary permeability
- reduced lymphatic removal of exudate

Systemic causes of leg swelling

Congestive cardiac failure

Congestive cardiac failure (right heart failure) is a common cause of bilateral leg swelling. Venous pressure

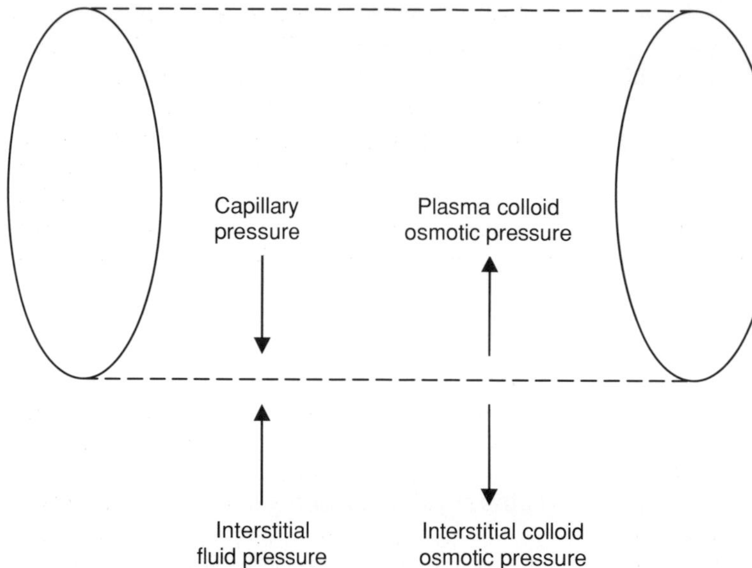

Fig. 70.1 Pressures influencing net movement of fluid in and out of capillaries (Reproduced with permission from A G Guyton and J E Hall, *Textbook of Medical Physiology*. 10th ed. Philadelphia: W B Saunders Company; 2000).

is increased proximal to the failing right heart, as demonstrated clinically by raised jugular and central venous pressures. Post-capillary venous pressure and intravascular hydrostatic pressure are increased consequently. Also, fluid may be retained because of reduced glomerular filtration and secondary aldosteronism. Excessive fluid intake, which may be iatrogenic, and hypoproteinaemia also contribute to leg swelling.

Renal disease

Renal failure results in the inability to excrete water and expansion of the extracellular fluid compartment, unless fluid restriction is instituted. If renal disease is complicated by the nephrotic syndrome, hypoproteinaemia is an additional factor contributing to leg swelling.

Hypoproteinaemia

A low concentration of plasma proteins, particularly albumin, is a common cause of leg swelling in hospitalised patients. Hypoproteinaemia reduces plasma osmotic pressure and so alters the balance of opposing forces across the capillary wall in favour of fluid leaking out of capillaries into the interstitial space. Hypoproteinaemia causes a generalised oedema, but is more apparent in regions of increased hydrostatic pressure, especially gravity-dependent limbs. Hypoproteinaemia is due to either increased protein loss (extensive burns, tissue catabolism, proteinuria, protein-losing enteropathy, gastrointestinal fistulas, paracentesis), decreased synthesis by the liver (acute or chronic liver disease, malnutrition, malabsorption), or fluid overload.

Localised causes of leg swelling

Venous disorders

Venous hypertension or obstruction increases intravascular hydrostatic pressure and reduces movement of fluid into the venous end of capillaries, with subsequent rapid accumulation of dilute interstitial fluid. Varicose veins secondary to saphenofemoral incompetence alone are associated only rarely with marked oedema. However, failure of the normal calf muscle pump, due to valvular incompetence or deep vein obstruction, results in failure of the normal reduction of hydrostatic pressure within superficial veins, which occurs with exercise. Incompetence of several perforating veins leads to only mild oedema because the calf pump mechanism can still lower superficial venous pressures to some extent. Gross unilateral oedema results from occlusion or stenosis of the femoral or iliac veins. Bilateral swelling results from occlusion or extrinsic pressure on the inferior vena cava or major pelvic veins. Deep vein thrombosis is discussed in Chapter 54.

Lymphatic disorders

Lymphatic obstruction reduces the clearance of fluid and protein from the interstitial space, resulting in an increased amount of interstitial fluid with a relatively high protein concentration (lymphoedema). Lymphoedema usually develops slowly. The high protein content of lymphoedema eventually leads to subcutaneous fibrosis. Movement of fluid and protein in and out of capillaries is essentially normal. Lymphatic disorders are discussed in Chapter 54.

Inflammatory disorders

As part of the inflammatory response to injury, vasoactive amines and peptides are released from damaged cells and produce vasodilatation and increased capillary permeability. Fluid and plasma proteins, in addition to cells, leak out of capillaries into the interstitial space and cause swelling. Oedema may be limited to the inflamed area but may drain by gravity to the dependent part of the limb, often causing circumferential swelling of the leg and swelling of the dorsum of the foot. Repeated acute infections (cellulitis, lymphangitis) or chronic infections (fungal infections, filariasis, tuberculosis) produce secondary lymphoedema because of lymphatic obstruction. Lymphoedema and chronic leg swelling may be complicated by infection, which increases swelling of the limb.

Assessment of the swollen leg

As with all medical problems, assessment relies on the history, examination and appropriate investigations.

History

Specific inquiry is made for symptoms suggesting disorders of the heart (chest pain, dyspnoea, paroxysmal nocturnal dyspnoea, palpitations, haemoptysis, hypertension), gastrointestinal tract (abdominal pain and distension, indigestion, vomiting, haematemesis, diarrhoea, rectal bleeding, alcohol intake, drug ingestion, jaundice) and kidneys (back pain, dysuria, haematuria, nocturia, urine volume, frothy urine, tiredness, lethargy). Recent nutritional intake must be considered, especially in hospitalised patients who may become malnourished because of long periods of anorexia, nausea, vomiting, gastrointestinal dysfunction, or fasting for investigations and treatment. Similarly, in hospitalised patients, the volume of intravenous fluid infusions must be reviewed. The duration and rapidity of onset of leg swelling must be ascertained. Family history of similar problems may be relevant. Past history of varicose veins, malignant disease, radiotherapy, surgery, previous episodes of leg swelling or infection, or deep vein thrombosis (perhaps complicating surgery or childbirth) must be identified.

Examination

A full physical examination must be performed. General points of examination include the patient's nutritional status, and abnormal pigmentation of the skin, sclera and mucous membranes. Look at the abdomen and lower limbs for the presence of suspicious skin lesions and vascular abnormalities, surgical scars, and signs suggestive of radiotherapy (skin atrophy, telangiectasia, scaly skin).

Swelling of one or both legs is confirmed by inspection and measurement at a designated point. Remember that the swollen limb may be tender to touch. Pitting oedema is determined by slow, gentle pressure over the medial malleolus or the shaft of the tibia. Lymphoedema is characterised by non-pitting swelling of the leg and the foot, as well as swelling of the toes. Intradermal vesicles, weeping of the skin, dry and scaly skin, and an 'elephant skin' appearance occur in longstanding cases. The legs are examined for signs of venous disease (varicose veins, venous flares, pigmentation, liposclerosis, eczema, venous ulceration). The Trendelenburg test is performed (Chapter 54). An arteriovenous fistula is characterised by a pulse, thrill and bruit over dilated veins. The hip, knee and ankle joints should be examined, together with the popliteal fossa. Regional lymph node groups must be examined. Rectal and pelvic examinations may be indicated.

Signs of inflammation (erythema, heat, tenderness, swelling, reduced movement) with or without infection (pus) should be noted. Tinea pedis between the toes and on the soles of the feet leads to cracking and breakdown of the skin, and may produce the portal of entry for bacteria causing cellulitis of the legs and feet (see Chapter 7).

Investigations

A full blood examination; erythrocyte sedimentation rate; levels of serum creatinine, urea and electrolytes;

liver function tests and levels of plasma proteins and albumin are measured. An electrocardiograph and chest X-ray are performed. Urinalysis for blood and protein is performed. Abdominal ultrasound scan or computed axial tomography is required to define organomegaly or tumour mass.

If venous disease is suspected, a Doppler study of the deep veins is performed to detect patency. Venography demonstrates the deep veins, the extent of stenosis or obstruction, and the presence of collateral circulation.

Lymphangiography may be attempted when venous and other diseases have been excluded. It may fail to demonstrate any lymphatics, or may show a reduced number of lymphatics, lymphatic dilatation proximal to obstruction, lymphatic valve incompetence, or lymph node disease.

Treatment

The treatment of leg swelling depends on the cause. Cardiac, hepatic and renal disorders are treated along medical lines. Protein deficiency is treated by nutritional supplementation, either orally, enterally or intravenously (see Chapter 5). Infective conditions are treated with antibiotics with or without surgical drainage. Specific treatments of venous and lymphatic diseases are discussed in Chapter 54. Non-specific measures that help in the treatment of the swollen leg include wearing elastic support stockings, elevation and massage.

Elastic stockings

The use of elastic stockings is described in Chapter 54.

Elevation

Simple elevation of the leg relieves oedema by reducing intravascular hydrostatic pressure. The principle is to avoid having the swollen leg in a dependent position and to avoid having it still. First, patients must keep off their feet as much as possible, and elevate the affected limb above the level of the hip whenever sitting. The limb should be raised above the horizontal whenever possible and, ideally, the patient should lie on the floor with the legs vertically against a wall for 15–20 minutes several times each day. This may not be practical for many patients but should be advised and encouraged. Second, when patients are standing, they should avoid standing still and should be encouraged to exercise the calf muscles and to walk with a support stocking. Third, the foot of the bed should be elevated by at least 10 cm.

Massage

Massage of the limb towards the hip, using a surface skin oil, reduces subcutaneous tissue swelling and helps keep the skin and subcutaneous tissues soft and supple.

Diuretic therapy and fluid restriction

Diuretic therapy and fluid restriction are indicated in congestive heart failure and in some renal and hepatic diseases, and may be of value in some cases of limb swelling due to local causes. However, care must be taken not to induce significant electrolyte abnormalities or dehydration.

MCQs

Select the single correct answer to each question.

1 Bilateral leg swelling with pitting oedema may be caused by the following EXCEPT:
- **a** reduced lymphatic removal of exudate
- **b** increased capillary permeability
- **c** decreased filtration pressure at the arteriolar end
- **d** reduced oncotic pressure
- **e** excessive fluid intake

2 A 75-year-old female underwent a right-sided total hip replacement. On post-operative day 10, she complained of discomfort and swelling over her right thigh and calf. She has been ambulating satisfactorily. Which of the following statements is true?
- **a** bed rest and diuretic therapy should be prescribed
- **b** a CT scan of the lower pelvis and right hip should be done
- **c** a Doppler study of the lower limb deep venous system should be performed
- **d** local complications of surgery is the most likely cause for the swelling
- **e** a plain X-ray of the right hip is most informative

3 The following statements on acute lymphangitis of the lower limb are correct EXCEPT:
- **a** improperly managed, it may lead to lymphadenitis
- **b** lymphangiography is the investigation of choice in the management
- **c** rest and elevation of the affected limb is appropriate

d cellulitis may be the initiating cause
e appropriate antibiotics should include cover for streptococcal infection

4 Eight days following a low anterior resection for carcinoma of the rectum, a 65-year-old man developed unilateral gross swelling of his right lower limb. Select the correct statement:
a a diagnosis of deep venous thrombosis can confidently be made on the basis of clinical signs
b deep venous thrombosis is unlikely as the patient had received peri-operative prophylactic subcutaneous heparin
c a past history of superficial thrombophlebitis in this patient is almost certainly related to deep venous thrombosis
d the short saphenous vein is usually the site of origin of deep venous thrombosis
e ilio-femoral thrombosis is likely as it commonly follows pelvic surgery

71 Haematuria

Dean Lenz

Introduction

Definition

Haematuria refers to the presence of red blood cells in the urine. The source of bleeding may be anywhere along the genitourinary tract. When visible to the naked eye, it is termed 'gross'. When evident only with magnification, it is termed 'microscopic'.

Significance

The presence of blood in the urine, regardless of the quantity, warrants further investigation. A small percentage of people may lose several red blood cells per high-power field via 'leaking' glomeruli. Likewise, many benign conditions and anti-coagulant use may cause haematuria. No matter the circumstance, however, haematuria may be the only sign of serious underlying pathology and should not be deemed acceptable until a thorough evaluation has been completed.

Presentation

Patient history is a key in identifying the cause of bleeding. Haematuria can be total throughout the urine stream, and has a source from the bladder or higher in the urinary tract. It can be terminal, or only at the end of voiding, and usually originates from the prostate in males. Initial haematuria, which clears as voiding continues, often originates in the urethra, prostate, or external genitalia. A history of trauma or other symptoms, such as loin pain or dysuria, can also help identify the cause. Likewise, other items in the history may point to a diagnosis. These may include smoking or a family history of urologic disease to name a few. Microscopic haematuria is usually asymptomatic and found by urinalysis alone.

Physical examination

A proper evaluation for haematuria begins with a thorough physical examination. The loins should be assessed for haematoma and palpated to elicit costovertebral angle tenderness. External genitalia in both males and females should be inspected for lesions. A bimanual examination in the female patient and assessment of the prostate in the male by rectal examination completes the examination.

Investigation

Urinalysis

Urine dipstick indicators are frequently used to identify the presence of blood. Unfortunately, false positives can occur with these colour indicators by the presence of items such as myoglobin or povidone iodine. Therefore, microscopy following centrifugation is the best tool to analyse the urine. In addition to the character and number of red blood cells seen, white blood cells, bacteria, yeast, and crystals can help make a diagnosis.

Urine cytology is another helpful tool for identifying malignant cells in the urine. Dysplastic, suspicious, and overtly malignant cells are frequently seen, with high-grade urothelial cancers and carcinoma *in situ*, but not with lower-grade lesions.

Many new urine markers are currently under investigation and may prove to be more useful than cytology in identifying urothelial carcinoma.

Serum chemistry

Serum electrolytes, creatinine, haemoglobin, and white cell count provide objective insight into the degree of haematuria, renal function, and the presence of infection. If calculus disease is suspected, serum uric acid

Box 71.1 Representative glomerular diseases

Minimal change disease
Thin basement membrane disease
Membranous glomerulonephropathy
IgA nephropathy
Focal segmental glomerulosclerosis
Post-infectious glomerulonephropathy
Membranoproliferative glomerulonephropathy
Systemic disease
- Henoch–Schönlein purpura
- Systemic lupus erythematosus
- Goodpasture's disease

and calcium are also indicated. Prostate specific antigen (PSA) is useful if there is suspicion of prostate cancer.

Aetiology and diagnosis

Nephrogenic

Many authorities accept between two and five red blood cells per high-power field as normal filtration through the glomerular basement membrane. A host of glomerulopathies also allow increased loss of erythrocytes into the urine (Box 71.1). Nephrogenic causes of haematuria should be more actively pursued when associated with a negative urologic evaluation, proteinuria, and hypertension. Dysmorphic red blood cells and red cell casts on urinalysis support the diagnosis of nephrogenic haematuria. If glomerular disease is suspected, creatinine clearance and 24-hour urine measurements of protein excretion should be obtained in addition to the serum chemistry discussed earlier.

Upper urinary tract

The upper urinary tract includes the kidneys and ureters. Sources of haematuria in these structures are listed in Box 71.2. They can include neoplasms (renal cell carcinoma, urothelial carcinoma), calculi, infection, and vascular malformations.

Renal ultrasound is an adequate screening modality for the upper tracts. It can identify a renal mass, stones, and give supporting evidence for obstruction (hydronephrosis). Renal ultrasound clearly differentiates solid from cystic renal lesions. Ultrasound is also useful when radiation exposure must be limited as in, for example, the pregnant patient. Non-contrast CT scan of the abdomen and pelvis is also useful as a screening study for haematuria. It can demonstrate almost every type of urinary calculus (stones from protease inhibitors, such as indinavir, are invisible to all imaging modalities) and renal masses and identify hydronephrosis. CT scan has the added benefit of evaluating structures outside the urinary tract. A triple-phase CT scan, one taken before contrast, with contrast, and following contrast provides complete evaluation of the upper urinary tracts. The contrast image, or nephrogram phase, evaluates and characterizes suspicious renal lesions. The delayed image, or pyelogram phase, evaluates the renal collecting system and ureters for obstruction and filling defects (which could represent urothelial tumours). Measuring the attenuation of suspicious renal

Box 71.2 General causes of haematuria

Kidney
- Infection
- Calculi
- Neoplasm
- Trauma
- Vascular malformation
- Congenital malformations
- Cystic diseases

Ureter
- Calculi
- Neoplasm

Bladder
- Infection
- Neoplasm
- Calculus
- Trauma
- Radiation

Prostate
- Benign neoplasm
- Malignant neoplasm

Urethra
- Infection
- Stricture
- Trauma
- Neoplasm
- Diverticulum
- Calculi

lesions, in Hounsfields units, aids in the diagnosis of neoplasms.

The intravenous pyelogram (IVP) is a valuable imaging study to evaluate the upper urinary tract. It clearly demonstrates the presence of and level of an obstruction. Although the IVP is often used for identifying filling defects throughout the collecting system, it can also demonstrate the presence of and the level of an obstruction. Causes of filling defects include blood clots, stones, tumours, sloughed renal papilla, and infectious debris including fungus balls. The IVP is also useful for visualizing the anatomy of the renal units.

Both the contrasted CT scan and the IVP require injection of intravenous contrast medium that can cause acute renal failure and should not be used in patients with impaired renal function (creatinine > 170μmol/L). The contrast medium can also incite anaphylaxis in allergic individuals. A steroid preparation can be given prior to the study in those with minor allergic reactions, but contrast should be avoided in anyone with a more pronounced reaction. MRI with and without gallidinium is an alternative to these studies. Like the CT scan, it can identify and characterize obstruction, filling defects, and renal lesions, but avoids the use of contrast.

Retrograde ureteropyelogram, or direct visual injection of contrast into the ureteral orifice during cystoscopy, is another means to evaluate the upper urinary tract. It is more invasive, but can be used in cases of contrast allergy. Retrograde ureteropyelograms are quite useful when an obstruction limits visualisation of the lower segment of a ureter. Ureteroscopy allows direct visualisation of the ureter and renal collecting system. In addition, biopsies of suspicious areas can be taken through the ureteroscope.

Lower urinary tract

The lower urinary tract includes the bladder and urethra. It also includes the prostate in males. Some causes of haematuria in these structures are listed in Box 71.2. The only way to completely visualise the bladder and urethral mucosa is with cystourethroscopy. It involves placing a lighted endoscope directly through the urethra and into the bladder for inspection. Cystourethroscopy can be performed under local anaesthesia, but spinal or general anaesthesia is often required if biopsies or other intervention is to be performed.

External source

Occasionally, conditions of the male and female genitalia can cause haematuria and must be considered when all other investigations are normal. A repeat urine specimen or catheterised specimen is recommended in menstruating women to exclude contamination.

Overview

Baseline studies for the evaluation of haematuria should include urine culture and cytology, renal ultrasound, and cystourethroscopy. Additional studies are tailored to each patient and the most likely disease process. Haematuria should never be attributed to benign processes until a complete evaluation has been performed. Although relatively infrequent, urologic neoplasms such as urothelial carcinoma can be quite aggressive and must be excluded. Should microscopic haematuria persist without an attributable cause, a limited reassessment should be performed in 6 months time with consideration given to a full nephrogenic workup.

MCQs

Select the single correct answer to each question.

1 A 24-year-old female at 32 weeks' gestation presents with loin pain and haematuria. The best initial radiologic study is:

a IVP
b non-contrast CT scan
c renal ultrasound
d cystourethroscopy
e PET scan

2 The best evaluation of the lower urinary tract is with:

a bladder ultrasound
b cystourethroscopy
c voiding cystourethrogram
d triple-phase CT scan
e MRI

72 Post-operative complications

Peter Devitt

Introduction

The management of post-operative complications can be approached in a number of ways. Perhaps the most practical way is to consider the frequency in which various complications may occur (Box 72.1). Another strategy is to consider the problems that relate directly to the procedure and those that are more general and patient-related (Box 72.2).

This chapter will take the former approach, but obviously it is sensible that in managing any patient with a post-operative problem, the doctor considers:

- the procedure
- the general state of health of the patient before the illness/operation
- progress since the procedure.

Thus, the questions to be asked should include:

- what procedure was done, when was it done and why was it done
- is there any coexisting illness (i.e. is there a past medical history of note [e.g. chronic respiratory disease])
- is the patient on any medication
- what has now happened to the patient to demand your attention
- what investigations have been done (both pre- and post-procedure)?

These will then be followed by:

- is the cause of the problem clear-cut
- if yes, how should I proceed with management
- if no, what will I need to do to make a clear diagnosis?

This chapter contains a number of examples of post-operative complications. A model answer is provided for each scenario. As a learning exercise, cover each model answer (in italics) and provide your own answer. Put yourself in the position of the intern.

Box 72.1 Common and important post-operative problems

Cardiorespiratory
- Atelectasis
- Pneumonia
- Congestive failure
- Arrhythmias

Infection
- Chest
- Operative site and wound
- Urinary
- Catheters and other lines

Venous thromboembolism
- Deep vein thrombosis
- Pulmonary embolism

Box 72.2 Categorisation of potential post-operative complications

a. Those related to the procedure:
   e.g. laparoscopy: air embolism
   pancreatic leak after pancreaticoduodenectomy
   sympathetic ophthalmia after eye surgery (very rare)
b. Those related to specific patients:
   e.g. increased risk of infection in the immunocompromised individual
   consequence of infection in a patient with a synthetic heart valve
   bleeding in a patient with a coagulation disorder
c. General problems:
   e.g. cardiorespiratory
   venous thromboembolism
   infection

Confusion

A 67-year-old man becomes confused 2 days after a laparotomy for a perforated peptic ulcer. The operation was uneventful and 2 litres of gastric contents were evacuated from the peritoneal cavity. Lavage was performed and the perforation closed. What critical piece of information would help you determine the cause of the confusion? How would you approach the problem?

Hypoxia is the most important and common cause of confusion. If this patient has a chest infection, you may have the quick explanation for his confusion.

To approach the problem, gain all the information you can about the patient's pre-operative state of health, the details of the procedure and progress since the operation. From the case notes you will hopefully glean information on the patient's past medical history, medications, examination findings and general fitness. From the past history, look for evidence of chronic respiratory disease and sustained alcohol consumption. Various investigations may have been undertaken (e.g. blood biochemistry) that may give clues as to the current problem. Any problems associated with the operation (the procedure itself or the anaesthetic) should be noted. The case records and the nursing observations since the procedure may help determine the cause of the current problem. Note any investigations that have been performed since the procedure.

Take a history from the patient, if his state of confusion allows. Examine the patient, looking particularly for evidence of hypoxia. A chest infection may explain the confusion. There may be other causes of hypoxia to consider (e.g. opiate toxicity, cardiac failure). If the patient is not obviously hypoxic, he may be septic, have a fluid and electrolyte disturbance, be suffering a drug complication or be in alcohol withdrawal.

To test some of these hypotheses, several investigations may be required. These may include arterial blood gas analysis, serum biochemistry, blood culture, an electrocardiogram (ECG) and a chest X-ray.

Before you start the investigations, some simple measures can be adopted. Ensure that the patient is given supplemental oxygen through a face mask and that intravenous fluids are being given. If sepsis is likely, you may want to start the patient on a broad-spectrum antibiotic. Ideally, you would like pulse oximetry performed and may even want to consider further management on a high-dependency unit.

You have excluded hypoxia as a cause for the confusion and the patient does not appear to be septic. There is no apparent electrolyte disturbance and you are reasonably confident that the patient is suffering alcohol withdrawal symptoms (delerium tremens). Describe your plan of management.

Move the patient to a quiet, well-lit room. Arrange continuous nursing care, preferably with a nurse familiar to the patient. Institute an alcohol withdrawal program. The protocol for this program will stipulate regular observations of the patient's symptoms, allocating a score to various symptom grouping and correlating the amount of sedation (if any) that needs to be given according to the score. Symptoms to be scored include nausea, anxiety, visual disturbances and agitation. The preferred sedative is oral diazepam.

Pulmonary embolism

Five days after a bilateral salpingo-oophorectomy and total abdominal hysterectomy, your 62-year-old patient complains of breathlessness and right-sided chest pain. You suspect she might have suffered a pulmonary embolism. Describe your initial plan of management.

If she has had a major pulmonary embolism, the patient may have circulatory collapse and require resuscitation. Your priority will be an assessment of her cardiovascular system. Provided the patient is stable, you can proceed with your investigations. These will include an ECG, arterial blood gas analysis, a chest X-ray and either a CT pulmonary angiogram (CTPA) or a ventilation-perfusion (V/Q) isotope scan performed The CTPA will allow accurate definition of the major pulmonary vasculature and can detect filling defects and obstruction. The scans are undertaken after rapid bolus administration of 100–140 mL of non-ionic contrast. This technique can be used to detect 3–4-mm clots in the second-, third- and fourth-order branches of the pulmonary vasculature. The V/Q scan (looking for mismatch defects) is better in the definition of peripheral lung lesions.

Once the diagnosis of pulmonary embolism has been confirmed, the patient should be given intravenous heparin.

Clinical examination of a patient with suspected deep venous thrombosis (DVT) or pulmonary embolism is relatively inaccurate and should not be relied on to determine diagnosis or treatment.

Fever

Six days after an open appendicectomy and removal of a perforated appendix, your 45-year-old patient develops a fever. He has a temperature of 38.5°C and a tachycardia of 100 beats per minute. Describe your actions at the bedside.

The temperature is almost certainly the result of sepsis, and the timing of the fever in relation to the date of the procedure suggests that the infection probably originates at the site of the operation (rather than the chest).

First, make an overall assessment of the general state of health of the patient. Is he relatively well, or is he about to slip into septic shock? Establish the progress since the operation. Inquire if there is anything that may predispose the patient to infection; for example, he might be a diabetic. Look at the nursing observation chart and observe the pattern of the fever and pulse rate. This may give a clue as to the likely cause. A spiking fever over several days could be due to an intra-abdominal abscess.

Although a chest infection may not be the cause of the fever, the chest must be examined carefully. After that, the abdomen should be inspected and the wound examined. Cannula and drain sites should also be examined for evidence of infection. Occasionally, a DVT will be accompanied by a low-grade fever, and the legs should be examined.

The patient has only recently spiked the fever and prior to this had been making an uneventful recovery from his operation. He was otherwise in good health before developing appendicitis. The only abnormal finding is a 2-cm tender and red swelling in the middle of the wound, with a narrow margin of surrounding erythema. What would you do?

This problem may be solved relatively easily by an incision into the abscess. It is possible to do this at the bedside. Explain to the patient the problem and what you propose to do. Provided the incision is kept within the previous incision, it should be relatively pain-free. A small nick with a scalpel could be all that is required to relieve the problem. Otherwise, the patient could be provided with some analgesia and then the abscess drained more formally under local anaesthetic. This would enable the wound to be probed and opened somewhat more than might have been achieved with a scalpel blade alone.

There is no need for investigation or antibiotics; the problem is one of localised superficial infection.

Initial assessment of a patient with suspected sepsis must include an appreciation of the type of procedure undertaken and the risk of infection from that procedure. Also to be considered are the consequences, should infection in that particular patient occur, for example, reduced resistance to infection in an immunocompromised individual. The type of procedure and the pattern of fever will give important clues as to the site of sepsis and the causative organism. Investigations to be considered include those to:

- identify the site of infection
- diagnose the type of infection.

Oliguria

You have received a telephone call from the nurse who is looking after your 68-year-old patient. He informs you that the patient has only voided 50 mL of urine in the 6 hours since he returned from the operating suite after a sigmoid colectomy for perforated diverticular disease. The nurse wants to give a bolus of frusemide to increase the urine output. What do you do?

While it is possible that this man's problem may be fluid retention and pump failure, it is more likely that he has received inadequate fluid replacement, either during or immediately after the operation and you are dealing with an under-filled patient.

There are many causes of oliguria in the post-operative period and a diuretic may be the worse way of managing the patient if appropriate assessment has not been made. You must go and see the patient. Given the scenario, this patient may have lost a considerable amount of fluid as a result of the peritonitis and may still be losing fluid into the peritoneal cavity. Remember that not all fluid lost by a patient may be readily evident. Patients with paralytic ileus and/or peritonitis can accumulate many litres of fluid within the peritoneal cavity – so-called 'third space' loses.

At the bedside you will look at the charts, note the details of the surgical procedure, calculate how much fluid was lost during the operation and how much was given. The amount of fluid given since the time of the operation should be noted. Any discharge from drains or a nasogastric tube should be measured.

The pre-operative state of health must be noted. A history of cardiac disease and heart failure will alert you to the possibility of pump failure.

In most instances it will be relatively safe to manage the problem at the bedside. Run in 500 mL of isotonic saline rapidly and observe the effect on urine output over the next few hours. Further boluses of fluid may be required and a diuretic should only be given once you are confident that the patient has had adequate fluid replacement. In more complex cases, the resources of an intensive care unit may be required to help determine the nature of the underlying problem.

In summary, the oliguria may be due to:

- inadequate filling
- inadequate output (pump failure)
- renal tract obstruction.

In other words, all the alternative explanations for oliguria must be considered; the problem may be something as simple as a blocked urinary catheter.

Wound discharge

Five days after undergoing a laparotomy for ischaemic small bowel (and bowel resection), your 73-year-old patient develops a pinkish discharge from the wound. What action do you take and why?

While there are a number of causes of discharge, the most urgent to consider is the possibility that this discharge is the harbinger of disruption of the deep layers of the wound, with the consequent risk of complete wound failure. Alert the nursing staff to provide some sterile dressings to cover the wound, should it suddenly burst.

Look to see if the patient has any risk factors for wound failure. What was his pre-operative nutritional status and have his serum proteins been measured? Find out what has happened to the patient since the operation. Has there been any process that could have led to an untoward increase in intra-abdominal pressure, such as a chest infection or paralytic ileus.

Explain to the patient what you fear and that he may need to be taken back to the operating theatre (for the wound to be resutured). The wound must be inspected. A non-inflamed wound with seepage of pink fluid is highly suggestive of acute failure of the wound. Extensive bruising around the wound might suggest discharge of a seroma, while a red, angry wound might make you think of infection.

If there is any doubt as to the nature of the problem, the wound should be gently probed (with sterile instruments). If you see the intestine, go no further. Be prepared to cover a dehisced wound with a sterile drape and call for help.

If the patient has suffered a deep wound dehiscence, why might it have happened?

The reasons for acute wound failure may be classified as follows:

- local factors: poor suturing techniques; poor tissue healing (infection, necrosis, malignancy, foreign bodies); increased intra-abdominal pressure
- general factors: malnutrition, diabetes mellitus.

In most instances, acute wound failure is due to a local factor.

Bleeding

You have been asked to review a 27-year-old man who has recently undergone a splenectomy for trauma. The nursing staff report fresh blood in the drain. How would you approach this problem?

You need further information. The bleeding may be localised or generalised. It may be reactionary, primary or secondary. How long ago was the operation and how much blood is in the drain? A small amount of fresh blood a few hours after the operation may be of little consequence. Is the bleeding confined to the drain or is there evidence of bleeding at other sites (wound, intravenous cannula)? If the former, the problem may be haemorrhage from the operative site, and if the latter, the patient may have a disorder of coagulation.

Your initial assessment must include a review of the charts. In what circumstances was the operation performed? If the patient had a massive and rapid transfusion to maintain his circulatory state, then the problem may be one of a coagulation defect. What has happened since the operation? A rising pulse and falling blood pressure would suggest that the patient is still bleeding, and what is seen in the drain may only be the tip of the iceberg. In other words, there could be a considerable volume of blood collecting at the operative site, with only a little escaping into the drain. Remember that when a drain drains, positive information may be gleaned; however, an empty drain means little.

Examine the patient and look for evidence of circulatory insufficiency. The material in the drain tube and drainage bag may be fresh and not clotted, or it may be serosanguinous. A normotensive patient with old clot in the drain is probably a stable patient.

It is more important to pay attention to the general state of the patient, rather than the contents of the drainage bag.

In summary, your clinical assessment of this case should include:
- the severity of the bleed
- the site of the bleed
- the cause of the bleed
- the need for further action (e.g. coagulation studies, cross-matching blood, contacting senior staff).

Shock

You are on your way to the ward to review a 66-year-old man who collapsed 3 hours after a transurethral prostatectomy. He is hypotensive and confused. What are your thoughts?

Your priority will be on resuscitation. However, to do this effectively you must have a clear idea of the probable cause of his collapse. The important causes of shock to consider in these circumstances are:
- pump failure (cardiogenic)
- haemorrhage (hypovolaemia)
- sepsis (septicaemia)
- anaphylaxis (drug reaction).

What will you do at the patient's bedside?

Make a rapid assessment of the state of the patient. How profound is the hypotension? If he is connected to a monitor, see if you can determine any changes in the ECG that would suggest an acute myocardial problem.

Ensure that the patient has an oxygen mask in place and run oxygen at 6 L/min. Attach a pulse oximeter. On the assumption that the cause of the problem is not cardiac failure, run in 500 mL of isotonic saline rapidly. While this is happening, take blood samples for assay of cardiac enzymes (creatine kinase), myocardial breakdown proteins (troponin), haematological and biochemical screen, blood cross-match and culture. Arterial blood gas analysis should be considered.

Once these things have been done, stand back and review the situation. Look at the charts. Is there a history of ischaemic heart disease or other cardiac problems? Did the patient come in with urinary retention and could he have infected urine. How major was the procedure that was performed and how much fluid was used during the procedure, both intravenous administration and as irrigation? What is in the urine drainage bag? A large volume of fresh blood would suggest hypovolaemia as the cause of the collapse. Were there any complications during the procedure? How has been the patient's progress since the operation? It is important to know if this has been a sudden collapse or a steady deterioration since the procedure.

There is nothing of significance from the past medical history and the operation was uneventful and associated with minimal blood loss. The fluid in the bladder irrigation system is tinged with blood and there are no blood clots. The patient's vital signs were within normal limits until about 15 minutes before you were alerted to the problem. The ECG monitor does not show any acute changes. How are you going to further the management of this case?

The cause of the problem appears not to be hypovolaemia. It is either septicaemia or a cardiac event. A normal ECG does not exclude an acute myocardial problem and you must await the enzyme assays and troponin levels.

Work on the assumption that the patient is in septic shock. In addition to the oxygen by face mask and fluid loading, antibiotics should be given. The choice of antibiotics will depend on the likely organisms. Gram-negative aerobes are an important and common cause of urinary infection, and working on the assumption that the presumed sepsis has originated from the urinary tract, concentrate on these organisms. The trio of an aminoglycoside (gentamicin), metronidazole and amoxycillin remains perhaps the most effective antibiotic combination in the management of patients with Gram-negative septic shock.

Leg swelling

Five days after major surgery, your patient complains of pain and swelling in the right leg. Discuss your initial assessment of the problem.

Of prime concern is whether this patient has a DVT. Before you examine the patient, determine if there is a past history of venous thromboembolic disorders and establish the risk factors for DVT. See exactly what type of surgery was performed and what, if any, prophylactic measures were taken to minimise the risk of clot formation. Remembering Virchow's triad, consider the changes that may bring about DVT:
- change in flow
- change in the vessel wall
- change in the constituents of the blood.

Apart from DVT, other conditions to consider include congestive cardiac failure, dependent oedema and cellulitis. Remember that clinical assessment for the presence of DVT is, at best, unreliable. A tender, swollen calf suggests that the patient may have a DVT.

The patient is 63 years old and had an unremarkable past history. In particular, he had no history of thromboembolic problems or cardiac disease. He was not overweight and had been mobile before the operation. The patient had been classified as having a low risk for DVT and immediately before the operation had been given a dose of an unfractionated heparin preparation. A calf vein compression device had been used during the procedure. He had undergone an anterior resection of the rectum for carcinoma. The procedure had been uncomplicated.

From your assessment you suspect the patient may have a DVT. What do you do next?

An ultrasonographic examination of the deep veins of the thigh and leg should confirm or refute the diagnosis. If the patient has a DVT, it will be important to document the extent of the clot and the degree of luminal occlusion. Extension of the clot into the femoral vein increases the risk of detachment and pulmonary embolism.

If clot is present and extends into the popliteal vein or beyond, heparin should be started and graded compression stockings applied. If conventional heparin is to be used, a typical regimen is a loading dose of 5000 IU followed by 1000 IU per hour. The patient will require monitoring with serial activated partial thromboplastin time (APTT) measurements. Alternatively, a low-molecular-weight heparin can be given. This does not require APTT estimations and can therefore be used on an outpatient basis.

The patient will probably be anticoagulated with warfarin for 3–6 months.

MCQs

Select the single correct answer to each question.

1 You are asked to see a 65-year-old man who 3 days previously underwent a laparotomy for a perforated duodenal ulcer. He has become confused and is causing a disturbance in the ward. You see from the notes that he suffers with chronic obstructive pulmonary disease and normally drinks three glasses of wine a day. The only medication he was taking prior to admission was atenolol. To this stage his post-operative recovery has been uneventful and he has been given morphine regularly. Your first action should be to:

a start on an alcohol withdrawal protocol and give diazepam
b attach a face mask and administer oxygen
c examine his chest and start antibiotics
d increase intravenous fluids and give 1 L isotonic saline over 4 hours
e substitute pethidine for morphine on the drug chart

2 You are called to see a 56-year-old man with dyspoea and pleuritic chest pain. Five days earlier he underwent a laparotomy and gastric resection. On examination he has a temperature of 37.5°C, a tachypnoea of 25, a pulse rate of 90 and a blood pressure of 130/95 mm Hg. His heart sounds are normal and there are no added sounds or murmurs. There is good air entry to both bases and the percussion note is resonant in all areas. A chest X-ray and a ventilation-perfusion scan are performed. Which one of the following combinations of test results indicates a high probability of a pulmonary embolus in a particular zone of the lung:

	chest X-ray	ventilation scan	perfusion scan
a	normal	normal	reduced
b	normal	abnormal	normal
c	consolidation	normal	reduced
d	consolidation	abnormal	normal
e	normal	abnormal	reduced

3 You are asked to see a 65-year-old woman who feels unwell and faint. Seven days previously she underwent an elective sigmoid colectomy for carcinoma. The procedure was uncomplicated and until now, she had been making an uneventful recovery. On examination she has a temperature of 39.5°C, a pulse rate of 100 beats per minute and a blood pressure of 90/60 mm Hg. Her respiratory rate is 15 breaths per minute. She has cool clammy peripheries. Her abdomen is tender in the left iliac fossa, around the wound site. Which of the following is the most reasonable explanation for her current problem?

a myocardial infarction
b pneumonia
c secondary haemorrhage

d pulmonary embolus
e septic shock

4 A 72-year-old diabetic develops a discharge from his midline abdominal wound 7 days after surgery for perforated diverticular disease. The most likely cause of the discharge is:
a a faecal fistula
b wound haematoma
c wound infection
d deep wound dehiscence
e small-bowel fistula

5 An otherwise fit 57-year-old man spikes a temperature of 39°C 5 days after an open appendicectomy for acute appendicitis. There is a tender, reddened and fluctuant swelling at the medial end of the wound. What is the most appropriate initial action to take?
a arrange a CT scan of the abdomen
b arrange an ultrasound scan of the wound and anterior abdominal wall
c start the patient on oral antibiotics
d open the wound to allow free drainage
e send off blood samples for a white cell count and culture

terossei adduct. Loss of function of intrinsics leads to

73 Claw hand

Wayne Morrison

Introduction

A common clinical deformity is 'claw hand', also known as the 'intrinsic minus' hand. This is characterised by hyperextension of the metacarpophalangeal joints and flexion of the proximal and distal interphalangeal joints. Any functional deformity of this type results from an imbalance of the actions of the tendons acting in this region. The intrinsic tendons of the fingers, namely lumbricals and interossei, span the metacarpophalangeal joints palmar to their axis of rotation and function to flex these joints. The lumbricals act more powerfully than the interossei because they attach more distally and have a greater moment of force. Beyond the metacarpophalangeal joints these tendons continue on as the lateral bands of the extensor tendons linking with the extensor mechanism and pass dorsal to the axis of the proximal and distal interphalangeal joints thus extending these joints. The interosseous muscles also insert into the bases of the proximal phalanges, such that the dorsal interossei abduct the fingers from each other while the palmar interossei adduct. Loss of function of intrinsics leads to an imbalance of the tensions between the long extrinsic (extensor and flexors) and the short intrinsic muscles. The resting tone of the intrinsics is lost leading to unopposed long extensors across the metacarpophalangeal joints and unopposed long flexors across the interphalangeal joints, resulting in this characteristic deformity of the hand.

Causes

Ulnar nerve palsy

In this condition all interossei are paralysed as well as the ulnar-sided lumbricals, but the median nerve innervated lumbricals to the index and middle fingers are preserved. As a consequence the clawing is confined to the ring and little fingers and the thumb. The most common cause of ulnar nerve palsy is wrist laceration. At this level the proximally innervated long flexors to the ring and little fingers are intact, compared to high ulnar nerve injuries where the long flexors are also paralysed, making finger flexion and the claw deformity less obvious. Ulnar nerve compression at the elbow will cause ulnar claw and ulnar sensory loss. Spontaneous ulnar clawing with no sensory loss is most likely due to compression of the motor branch by a ganglion in the region of the piso-hamate joint.

Paralysis of the ulna and median nerves

This produces a full claw hand. This deformity will also result from C8 and T1 nerve root lesions.

Nerve palsy due to leprosy

On a worldwide basis, leprosy still remains the most common cause of the claw hand.

Differential diagnosis

Certain conditions mimic the claw hand.

Volkmann's contracture

This deep flexor compartment compression syndrome results in ischaemic necrosis of the profundus tendons in the forearm causing flexion contracture of the fingers. The superficialis tendons are usually spared, but the intrinsic tendons may also be contracted. This produces flexion of all joints of the fingers, rather than hyperextension of the metacarpophalangeal joints. The flexor tendons are tight.

Intrinsic muscle contracture

This can be of ischaemic origin, due to crush injuries and produces the opposite deformity to the claw hand, namely tight intrinsics, or intrinsic plus hand, rather than the loose intrinsic minus claw hand. The metacarpophalangeal joints are flexed and the interphalangeal joints extended. This condition spontaneously occurs in rheumatoid arthritis and may lead to Swan neck deformity. The Bunnell test for intrinsic tightness involves passive extension of the metacarpophalangeal joint followed by assessment of the passive flexibility of the interphalangeal joints. In the normal hand when the metacarpophalangeal joint is maximally extended the interphalangeal joints can be fully flexed passively. When the intrinsics are tight and the metacarpophalangeal joints are stretched into extension, thereby further tightening the intrinsics, there will be secondary tightening of the extensor mechanism distally in the fingers, which will limit passive flexion of the interphalangeal joints. By individually manipulating the fingers into either ulnar or radial angulation and applying the Bunnell test, tightness of the radial or ulnar intrinsics can be selectively examined.

Dupuytren's contracture

This typically involves the little and ring fingers and can mimic a claw hand, but the metacarpophalangeal joint is flexed and the contracted fingers cannot passively be extended. Palpation of the Dupuytren's tissue in the palm confirms the diagnosis.

Congenital flexion contracture (camptodactyly)

This condition usually involves only the little finger, it is often bilateral and is hereditary. It is present at birth. The finger is flexed at the proximal interphalangeal joint and often cannot be passively fully straightened.

Spastic hand

This results from an upper motor neuron palsy and usually involves a clasping deformity of the thumb in the palm and tightening of the flexor tendons that cannot be easily passively extended. The wrist is also characteristically flexed.

Neuropathies

Various muscular dystrophies present as bizarre hand deformities of an atypical type.

Signs

The classic claw hand involves hyperextension of the metacarpophalangeal joints and flexion of the interphalangeal joints. The ulnar nerve paralysis results in ulnar claw, where the clawing is confined to the little and ring fingers. The high ulnar palsy has less obvious clawing than the low ulnar palsy.

There is loss of abduction/adduction of the fingers and wasting of the interosseous muscles, most obvious in the first web space and the hypothenar eminence.

There will be numbness in the distribution of the involved nerve or nerves.

Frequently in ulnar paralysis, the little finger remains permanently abducted from the ring finger (Wartenberg's sign). The basis of this deformity is unclear, but in some way relates to an imbalance between the intrinsic muscles either side of the little finger metacarpophalangeal joint and the long extensor mechanism.

Median nerve thenar muscle paralysis results in the 'simian palm' deformity where the thumb metacarpal moves dorsally into the plane of the finger metacarpals due to the unopposed extension of the pollicis longus tendon. Abduction and opposition of the thumb are now impossible. Although the claw hand is most obviously a deformity of the fingers, the thumb is inextricably involved and disturbance of thumb function is frequently the major disability.

Functional disability

Weakness, especially in turning doorknobs, keys in locks and taking tops off jars is a common complaint due to the lack of abduction/adduction of the fingers. Pickup is clumsy especially in the full claw hand where the pulps of the fingers cannot be presented to the object because of inability to fully extend the interphalangeal joints. This results in the nails pushing the object away during attempts at pick-up. Thumb pinch grip is also greatly weakened and clumsy due to adductor paralysis and the collapsing interphalangeal joint converting the pulp pinch of the thumb into nail pinch. Thumb disability is further magnified in the full claw hand where median innervated thenar muscles are also paralysed. Strong power grip of the fingers into the palm, however, is retained, except where the long flexors are involved in high nerve injuries. Fixed flexion contractures of the proximal interphalangeal joints of the clawed fingers can develop as a secondary phenomenon due to lack of active extension and trophic changes may occur due to numbness. Wartenberg's abducted little finger is a frequent source of nuisance.

Treatment

Nerve repair or decompression where possible is the treatment of choice. If the nerves are unrepairable or repairs have failed, tendon transfers can be considered. Tendon transfers at best correct the claw deformity and thumb collapse, but do little to restore the functional disability of loss of abduction/adduction of the fingers or thumb collapse. Various techniques have been described. Most have been designed for the management of the sequelae of leprosy.

If surgical treatment cannot be offered, rehabilitation with physiotherapy and splintage may help the patient.

MCQs

Select the single correct answer to the following question.

1 The claw hand:

- **a** is sometimes called an intrinsic plus hand
- **b** occurs following a median nerve injury
- **c** results in loss of power grip of the fingers into the palm
- **d** is more obvious in a proximal, ulnar palsy than a distal palsy
- **e** includes metacarpophalangeal joint extension of the involved fingers

74 Massive haemoptysis

Julian A. Smith

Introduction

Massive haemoptysis is rare but carries with it a high mortality. Any amount of blood loss in excess of 100 mL in 24 hours may constitute massive haemoptysis. Some patients may expectorate several litres of blood per day. The risk to life is from respiratory compromise due to the tracheobronchial tree filling with blood rather than from hypovolaemia and haemodynamic deterioration.

Aetiology of massive haemoptysis

The causes of massive haemoptysis are listed in Box 74.1. The majority are benign inflammatory or infective lung disorders. Malignancy seldom presents with massive bleeding.

Box 74.1 Causes of massive haemoptysis

Infective lung conditions
- Tuberculosis
- Bronchiectasis
- Lung abscess
- Aspergillosis
- Cystic fibrosis

Pulmonary neoplasms

Pulmonary embolus

Trauma
- Pulmonary artery catheter
- Penetrating or blunt external

Arteriovenous malformation

Cardiac valve disease
- Mitral stenosis
- Infective endocarditis

Surgical pathology

The source of bleeding is nearly always the high pressure bronchial circulation. These vessels are often enlarged in response to the primary pathology (e.g. bronchiectasis) or are involved in the inflammatory or necrotic process (e.g. tuberculosis). The pulmonary arterial circulation is the source of bleeding from arteriovenous malformations.

Clinical evaluation

A thorough history and examination is required bearing the possible causes in mind. Epistaxis and haematemesis must be excluded. Any anticoagulant intake should be established. A history of fever, night sweats, weight loss, previous tuberculosis or an exposure to tuberculosis may suggest active tuberculosis. Recurrent pulmonary infections may point to bronchiectasis. Helpful physical signs may include finger clubbing, peripheral or cervical lymphadenopathy and localised wheeze, crepitations, or consolidation. Abnormal respiratory signs may be absent if the blood is effectively expectorated.

Investigations

The investigations for massive haemoptysis are listed in Box 74.2. A chest X-ray may be completely normal if little blood is retained within the airway. Infection or tumour may be localised but shadows of aspiration may be confusing. Serial chest X-rays may be helpful. Bronchoscopy, performed while bleeding is occurring, is the best way to localise the source. The rigid instrument provides a superior view and facilitates airway suction and bronchial toilet. Occasionally the flexible

Box 74.2 Investigations of massive haemoptysis

Haemoglobin level
Arterial blood gases
Coagulation studies
Sputum microscopy and culture
Chest X-ray
Bronchoscopy
Computed tomography
Radionuclide perfusion scanning
Angiography

instrument may be passed through the rigid bronchoscope to visualise more peripheral lung lesions. If the patient is fit enough to tolerate computed tomography scanning, the majority of causes of massive haemoptysis will be demonstrated. Bronchial angiography and possible embolisation may have a role in high-risk surgical patients where initial bronchoscopy has been unhelpful.

Management plan

The key principles in the management of this potentially fatal condition are:
- prompt early resuscitation
- precise localisation of the bleeding source
- definitive therapy.

The patient requires intensive care monitoring of vital signs and oxygen saturation. The patient should be positioned head down and bleeding side down (if known). Adequate amounts of blood should be available for administration via a large-bore intravenous line based on haemodynamic parameters rather than the amount of blood lost (notoriously unreliable). Broad-spectrum antibiotics should be given pending results of sputum cultures. Specific antituberculosis therapy is added in the presence of active tuberculosis.

Rigid bronchoscopy is vital to maintain the airway, aspirate blood and secretions from the airway and for ventilation. After localising the source of bleeding, control may be obtained by ice-cold saline lavage (leading to vasospasm) or placement of an endobronchial balloon blocker and endotracheal intubation. Patients are ventilated (with positive end-expiratory pressure) and bronchoscopy is repeated 12 to 24 hours later to assess ongoing bleeding prior to definitive therapy.

Definitive therapy may include one or more of the following:
- medical therapy: antibiotics, reversal of anticoagulation
- surgical resection (immediate or after initial control of bleeding source)
- angiography and arterial embolisation (for arteriovenous malformations; up to 20% incidence of rebleeding, so should be followed with surgical resection)
- radiotherapy (for non-resectable tumours or if patient is unfit for surgery).

Massive re-bleeding can occur following the initial establishment of control. Surgical resection of the lesion, therefore, offers the best hope of cure. All endobronchial and angiographic therapies should be considered temporary answers to this problem. Surgical resection is contraindicated in patients with severe cardiorespiratory dysfunction, uncorrectable coagulopathy, unresectable cancer and in those in whom the bleeding site is impossible to localise by any method.

Further reading

Dweik RA, Stoller JK. Role of bronchoscopy in massive hemoptysis. *Clin Chest Med.* 1999;20:89–105.

Jean-Baptiste E. Clinical assessment and management of massive hemoptysis. *Crit Care Med.* 2000;28:1642–1647.

Corder R. Haemoptysis. *Emerg Med Clin North Am.* 2003;21:421–435.

Jougon J, Ballester M, Decambre F, et al. Massive haemoptysis: What place for medical and surgical treatment. *Eur J Cardiothoracic Surg.* 2002;22:345–351.

MCQs

Select the single correct answer to each question.

1 From which of the following blood vessels does the bleeding in a patient with massive haemopytsis usually occur?

a pulmonary artery
b pulmonary vein
c bronchial artery
d bronchial vein
e thoracic aorta

2 Which of the following lung conditions is NOT a common cause of massive haemoptysis?
a carcinoma of the lung
b pulmonary arteriovenous malformation
c tuberculosis
d lung abscess
e aspergillosis

3 The investigation which will most reliably determine the site of bleeding in a patient with massive haemoptysis is:
a chest X-ray
b CT scan of the chest
c radionuclide lung scan
d bronchoscopy
e pulmonary angiogram

4 Definitive therapy in a patient with massive haemoptysis may include:
a broad-spectrum antiobiotics
b surgical resection of the bleeding source
c pulmonary arterial embolisation
d radiotherapy
e all of the above

75 Epistaxis

Neil Vallance

Epistaxis is best considered in two settings, the paediatric and the adult patient.

Paediatric epistaxis

Minor epistaxis

This is a common problem in the paediatric population and is usually more of a nuisance than a health risk. It can usually be treated in the office situation. Bleeding almost always occurs from vessels on the anterior nasal septum (Little's area). This site is an area of anastamosis of blood vessels supplying the anterior nasal septum and is commonly quite vascular. The site of bleeding can frequently be cauterised with local anaesthetic in the cooperative child. In situations of non-cooperation, cauterisation under general anaesthetic may be resorted to if the problem is troublesome enough.

Severe epistaxis

This is a rare event in the paediatric population. It is so unusual that it requires the exclusion of conditions causing abnormal bleeding. Tests include the exclusion of blood conditions such as acute leukaemia, clotting factor deficiencies, platelet abnormalities and thrombocytopaenia and unsuspected disorders such as von Willebrand's disease.

Rare conditions such as tumours need to be considered. Rhabdomyosarcoma is a malignant tumour that affects the paediatric population and sometimes occurs at the back of the nose or in the nasopharynx. Angiofibroma is an unusual tumour usually affecting adolescent males. It is benign, but highly vascular, and usually presents with severe epistaxis. The diagnosis must be suspected because biopsy is contraindicated due to the potential for severe life-threatening haemorrhage. The appearance on CT scanning and angiography is diagnostic.

Adult epistaxis

Minor epistaxis

Minor nosebleeds in the adult population are very common. It is worthwhile remembering that many adults take aspirin as a preventive for heart disease or stroke and they do not regard this as a medication. It must, therefore, be specifically asked about, as it may not be mentioned when enquiries are made about medication history. The epistaxis can usually be controlled without the need to withdraw aspirin.

In young adults, the usual site is again the anterior nasal septum, and cauterisation under local anaesthesia usually controls the problem. In the older adult, particularly those with hypertension, the bleeding may be further back in the nasal cavity and more difficult to reach. Cauterisation under local anaesthetic is usually sufficient.

Cauterisation usually involves the application of silver nitrate or alternatively electrocautery if available.

Severe epistaxis

Severe epistaxis is more commonly seen in the older adult population. It can, on occasion, be a life-threatening situation. The following steps should be taken in the assessment and management of an adult with severe epistaxis:

Make an assessment of the general condition of the patient, the degree of blood loss and whether there is a need for immediate resuscitation and blood volume replacement.

Take a brief history and enquire as to the following:

- Medications and, in particular, anticoagulants and aspirin
- Hypertension, and whether it is well controlled
- Other illnesses/conditions which may affect blood

clotting, such as alcoholism, liver disease, blood disorders

- The presence of a heart condition which may be aggravated by blood loss and may require treatment as well as epistaxis
- Whether epistaxis is recurrent. This may suggest abnormalities such as Osler's Disease (hereditary haemorrhagic telangiectasia). In this condition, multiple small arteriovenous malformations in the nose can cause frequent recurrent severe epistaxis.

Thorough examination of the nose with adequate light and instrumentation is necessary. Often the bleeding source can be seen and dealt with. Packing the nasal cavity usually provides control. Most emergency departments have specialised packing devices, inflatable balloons or packing material for this purpose. Thorough topical anaesthesia is required for nasal packing as the procedure can be very uncomfortable and/or painful. The pack is usually left in for 2 days and antibiotics given to prevent nasal infection.

If packing fails to control the epistaxis, a firmer pack may need to be inserted under general anaesthetic. Better examination of the nasal cavity can be done at this time and the nose examined further back for the possible presence of a bleeding vessel that could be cauterised.

During examination, unusual conditions such as tumours are obvious and are dealt with after the acute bleeding is controlled.

Special investigations and techniques are usually not required. Contrast angiography to determine the bleeding vessel is almost always unsuccessful. Balloon occlusion of main vessels supplying the nose, such as the internal maxillary artery, have occasionally been resorted to for severe life-threatening epistaxis. Surgical ligation of the internal maxillary artery and, occasionally, ligation of the external carotid artery have been resorted to for severe epistaxis.

MCQs

Select the single correct answer to the following question.

1 Severe epistaxis in the elderly patient is most likely to be due to:
 a cardiac failure
 b hypertension
 c nasal tumour
 d alcoholism
 e Osler's Disease

76 Leg pain

Bhadrakant Kavar

Introduction

Leg pain is a common problem, which in most patients is benign and self-limiting. Anatomically the leg refers to that part of the lower limb below the knee, athough when discussing leg pain, it commonly refers to any part of the lower limb – the buttock, thigh, leg and foot.

There are a few terms that are regularly used when discussing leg pain: sciatica, claudication and antalgic gait being the important ones.

- Sciatica – is a symptom not a disease. It is a syndrome characterized by pain radiating from the back into the buttock and into the lower extremity along its posterior or lateral aspect; the term is also used to describe pain in the distribution of the sciatic nerve
- Claudication – lower limb pain on walking, possibly associated with lameness or limping
- Antalgic gait – a limping gait as a result of a painful lower limb

Aetiology

Leg pain will result from an injury or compression of any neural structure supplying the leg; reduction in blood flow or disturbance of venous return; injury to the soft tissue structures of the leg; injury, inflammation or neoplasm involving the bony structures of the leg and pain referred to the leg from the abdomen and pelvis.

Pathology

Table 76.1 presents the common clinical problems, their presentation, level and type of pathology.

Clinical presentation

Neural compression of spinal origin

Presentation

Sciatica is a common clinical problem and the commonest cause is entrapment of the nerve root in the lumbar spinal canal or the exiting foramen by a disc prolapse or foraminal stenosis (see Table 76.1 for possible causes).

The pain is often unilateral and involves one or more of the nerves from L4 to S1. Patients complain of sharp shooting pain, often originating in the buttock and radiating down the leg in the distribution of the nerve root under pressure (the sciatic nerve is not under pressure – rather a nerve root that contributes to the formation of the sciatic nerve). The pain is often associated with numbness, pins and needles and tingling, typically in a dermatomal pattern (see Fig. 76.1A for dermatomal patterns). Patients can go on to develop weakness (see Fig. 76.1B for myotomal patterns) in the distribution of the nerve root. Patients may occasionally develop leg pain as a result of pressure on the L3 and rarely L2 nerve root, and will radiate to the anterior thigh and knee.

The patient presents with an antalgic gait, a tilt of the torso away from the affected side, avoids sitting or does so with the leg straightened at the hip and flexed at the knee. This posture tends to relieve the stretch on the nerve and help with pain control.

Examination reveals limitation of straight leg raising, limited back movements, altered sensation, numbness or weakness in the distribution of the nerve root. An absent reflex aids significantly in confirming the root involved.

Be wary of the patient whose pain has resolved but still has numbness or weakness or has bilateral leg pain. Alarm bells must ring if the patient has any sense of numbness of the saddle area or has any suggestion of

Table 76.1 Causes of leg pain

Clinical problem	Presentation	Region of pathology	Pathology
Neural – spinal			
Sciatica	Radiating leg pain (Table 76.2)	Nerve root compression in spinal canal or exit foramen	Disc prolapse (Fig. 76.2) Lateral recess stenosis Osteophyte (Fig. 76.3B) Synovial cyst Spondylolisthesis (Fig. 76.3A) Foraminal stenosis Tumour
Neurogenic claudication	Bilateral leg pain, pins and needles, heaviness	Multiple roots under compression in the spinal canal	Lumbar canal stenosis Facet hypertrophy Ligamentum flavum hypertrophy Diffuse disc bulge Spondylolisthesis
		Venous hypertension or ischaemia of the spinal cord	Dural arterio-venous fistula
Neural – peripheral nerve			
Meralgia parasthetica	Burning pain, numbness anterolateral thigh	Lateral cutaneous nerve of thigh	Entrapment under inguinal ligament medial to anterior superior iliac spine
Piriformis syndrome	Pain in sciatic distribution	Sciatic nerve	Entrapment by piriformis muscle
Common peroneal nerve entrapment	Weak ankle dorsiflexion and anterolateral leg pain	Common peroneal nerve	Trapped as it winds around the head of fibula
Tarsal tunnel syndrome	Burning pain in the plantar surface of foot	Posterior tibial nerve	Flexor retinaculum from medial malleolus to calcaneus
Morton's neuralgia	Pain in third web space of foot and adjacent toes	Digital nerve in foot	Compression between metatarsal heads
Vascular			
	Acute vascular compromise Vascular claudication Varicose vein/Venous insufficiency Deep vein thrombosis		
Joint/bony			
	Degenerative arthritis Rheumatoid arthritis Bony pathology – fracture, infection, malignancy Soft tissue – muscle Ligament Joints – facet, sacroiliac, symphysis pubis, hip, knee, ankle, foot		
Referred			
	Retroperitoneal pathology Appendicitis Inguinal hernia Aortic dissection Renal colic		

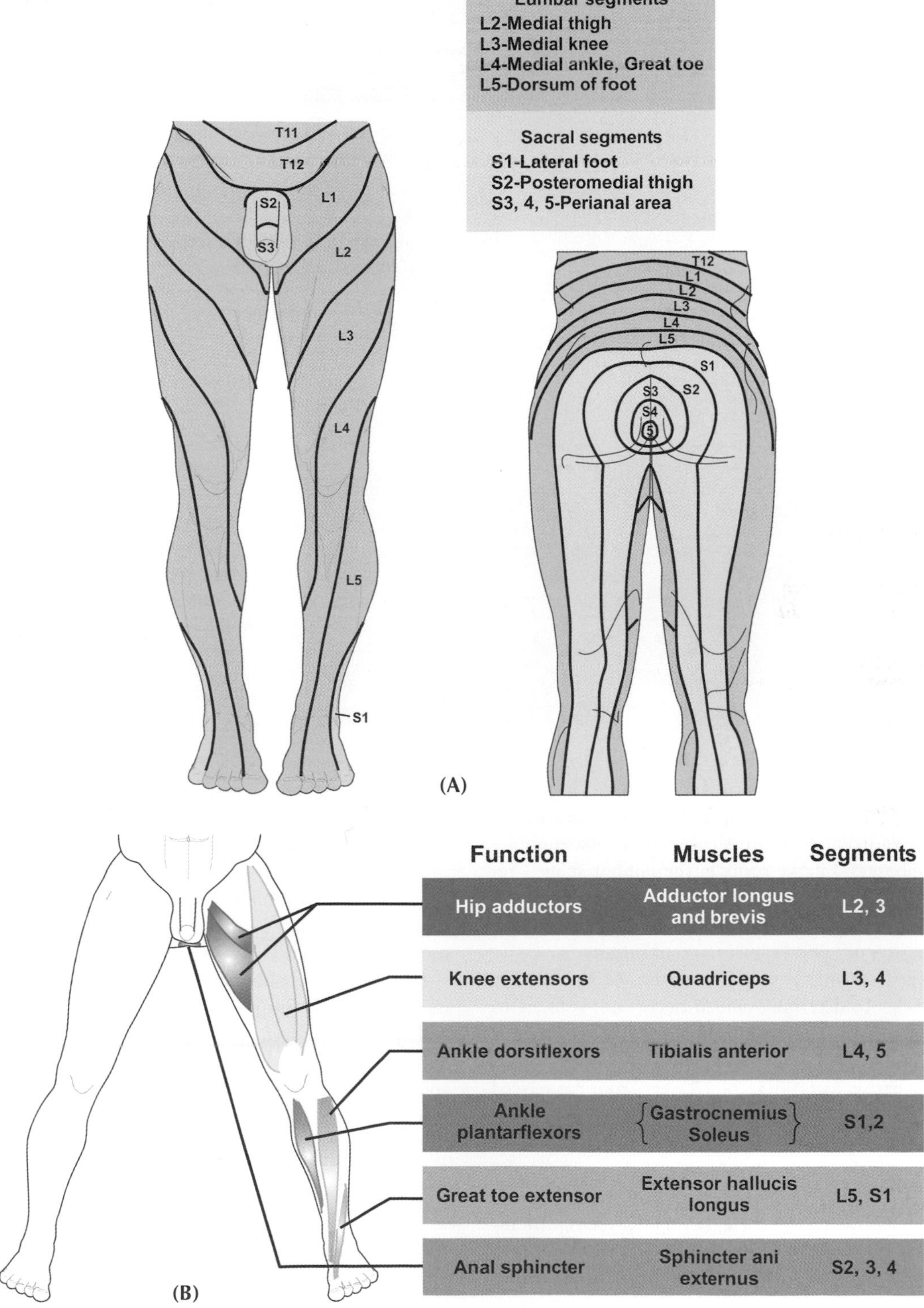

Fig. 76.1 (**A**) Dermatomal pattern of sensory supply. Adapted from *The CIBA Collection of Medical Illustrations*, Vol 1. Nervous System, Part II: Neurologic and Neuromuscular Disorders, p. 183, by Frank H. Netter. (**B**) Nerve root supply of muscles. Adapted from *The CIBA Collection of Medical Illustrations*, Vol 1. Nervous System, Part II: Neurologic and Neuromuscular Disorders, p. 182, by Frank H. Netter.

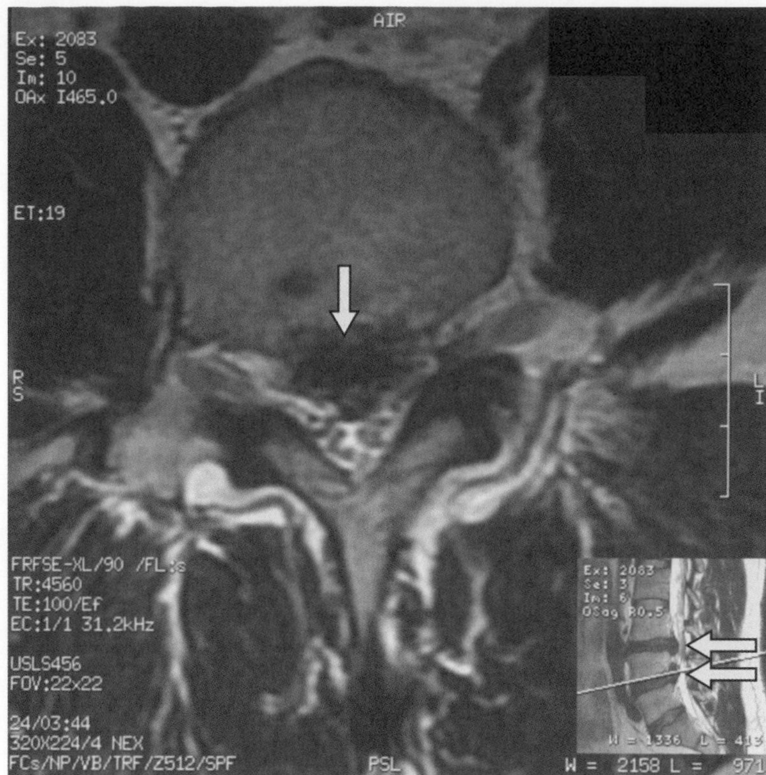

Fig. 76.2 Axial T2 MRI of the lumbar spine – the arrow points to a large central L4–L5 disc prolapse causing secondary canal stenosis and nerve root entrapment. The smaller sagittal view confirms the L4–L5 disc prolapse and a large L3–L4 disc prolapse.

difficulty with micturition or incontinence. The patient may have a large disc prolapse that can cause a cauda equina syndrome (compression of the cauda equina – the lumbosacral nerve roots in the lumbar spine – resulting in sacral anaesthesia plus bowel and bladder disturbance). A cauda equina syndrome is a neurosurgical emergency and requires urgent surgery.

An understanding of the anatomy of the lumbar spine helps to determine which nerve root is likely to be compressed. The most frequent clinical picture is a posterolateral L4–L5 disc prolapse causing an L5 radiculopathy. At L4–L5, the L4 nerve root has passed inferior to the pedicle to pass through the L4–L5 foramen and is superior to the L4–L5 disc. Thus an L4–L5 posterolateral disc prolapse will trap/compress the nerve crossing the disc (L5 root) and exiting via the foramen below (L5–S1 foramen). However, in rare instances a foraminal disc prolapse will affect the nerve exiting through its foramen (an L4–L5 forminal disc compressing L4 nerve root).

Neurogenic claudication is characterised by bilateral leg pain, worse with walking but can be present when upright and standing still and improves with a change in posture (as compared to vascular claudication, which resolves with rest, irrespective of the posture of the patient). The pain is an ache-like discomfort, often with pins and needles, heaviness, and tiredness of the legs, with variable numbness and a sense of weakness with walking. Lumbar canal stenosis is the commonest cause (see Table 76.1 for other causes).

Examination is often unremarkable and hyporeflexia may be the only finding.

Thoracic or cervical myelopathy is a rare cause of leg pain. Occasionally compression or pathology in the spinal cord in the thoracic or cervical spine can result in a syringomyelia (a cavity in the spinal cord) that can cause leg pain.

Investigation

A lumbar spine X-ray is important as it will exclude any obvious fracture, slip/malalignment or destructive lesion involving the vertebra. A computed tomography (CT) scan of the lumbar spine will provide greater information regards the vertebral bodies, discs, facet joints, spinal canal and intervetebral foramina. In most

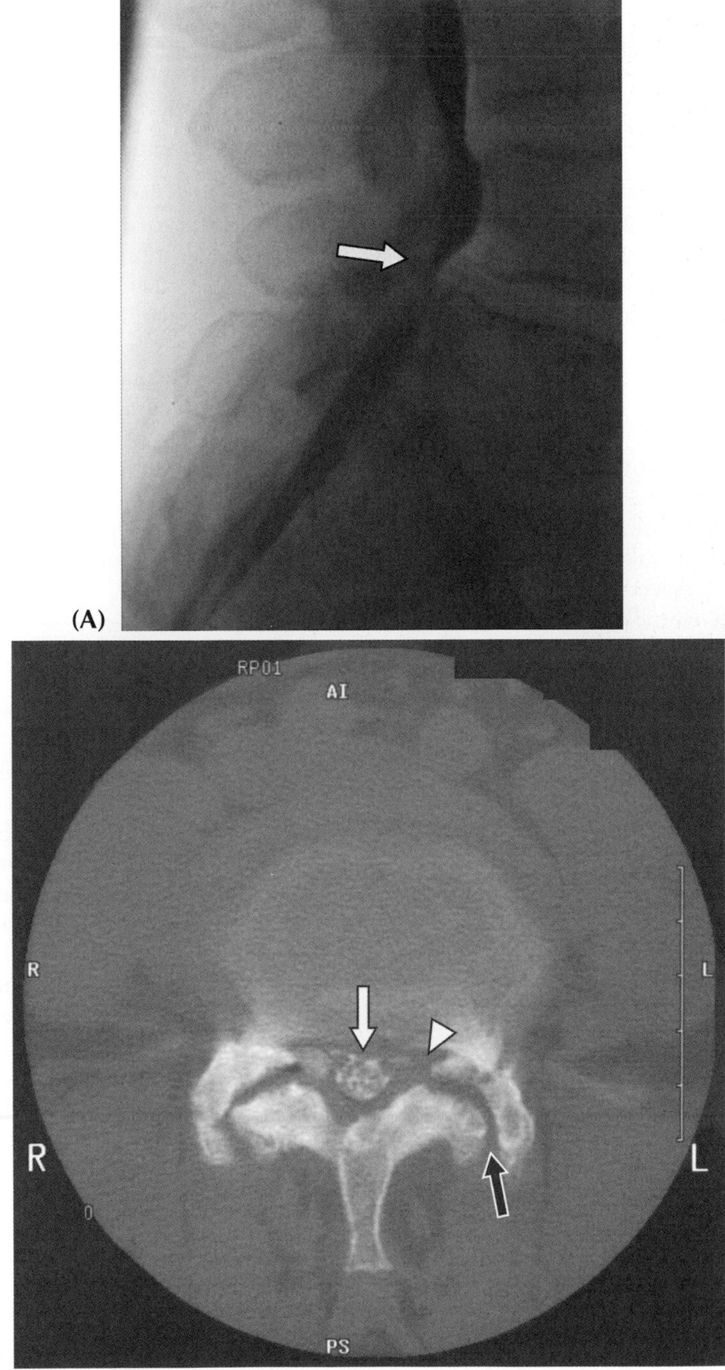

Fig. 76.3 (A) Sagittal lumbar myelogram – grade I L4–L5 spondylolisthesis with secondary canal stenosis. L3–L4 lumbar canal stenosis. (B) Post-myelogram CT scan of lumbar spine – marked facetal degeneration and hypertrophy (black arrow), lumbar canal stenosis (white arrow) and lateral recess stenosis (white arrowhead).

instances a good quality CT scan of the lumbar spine will reveal the presence of a disc prolapse. The other pathologies to be excluded are lateral recess stenosis, foraminal stenosis, and synovial cysts. Beware that occasionally a very large sequestrated disc prolapse can occupy most of the spinal canal and thus be missed when interpreting the CT scan.

The investigation of choice is an MRI of the lumbar spine, as it provides better visualization of the thecal sac and nerve roots. If an MRI is contraindicated a myelogram and post-myelogram CT scan can provide the necessary information.

Management

More than 80% of the patients with sciatic respond to non-operative treatment – being a combination on analgesia, anti-inflammatories, judicious rest balanced with exercise – especially walking. Patients also need to avoid factors that will exacerbate the pain – thus avoid heavy lifting, repetitive bending and twisting. The role of physiotherapy is to re-educate the patient in terms of posture, exercises to strengthen back, abdominal and pelvic muscles and stretches.

The role of warm/cold therapy, massage, acupuncture, hydrotherapy in the acute stage is uncertain and unpredictable. The patient must be cautioned against manipulation as it may precipitate a larger disc prolapse and a cauda equina syndrome.

In the acute setting the benefit from epidural steroids or foraminal steroids is not predictable and more likely to succeed in patients that have a small disc bulge or a foraminal disc prolapse.

The role of non-surgical treatment for neurogenic claudication is limited in patients with significant symptoms. They may have some benefit from analgesia, anti-inflammatories, physiotherapy and hydrotherapy; however, in view of the mechanical compression, decompression offers the best long-term result.

Surgical intervention is indicated in the patient with intractable pain, failure to respond to medical therapy, and those that have a neurologic deficit. Most surgical patients have a better than 90% success rate of control of the leg pain provided the clinical picture matches the imaging.

Patients that have a disc prolapse and have failed non-operative treatment would benefit from a microdiscectomy and neurolysis. Those with lumbar canal stenosis require a decompressive laminectomy, lateral recess decompression and neurolysis. In either situation, the presence of instability will require an instrumented fusion.

Entrapment neuropathies

The pain is restricted to the distribution of the nerve root and thus a good history and examination can often provide the diagnosis.

These syndromes (meralgia parasthetica, piriformis syndrome, tarsal tunnel syndrome, Morton's neuralgia) present primarily with pain restricted to the distribution of the nerve under pressure (Table 76.1). Medical therapies with an anticonvulsant (carbamazepine) or antidepressant (amitriptyline) can provide good control of their symptoms. The alternative is a diagnostic and therapeutic block with local anaesthesia and steroids. Should this fail, surgical decompression of the nerve should be considered.

Vascular

The vascular causes are described in greater details in Chapters 52 and 54.

- Acute arterial vascular compromise. It is caused by trauma or acute arterial occlusion of a diseased artery by a thrombotic or embolic event. The patient presents with leg pain and parasthesia with coldness and pallor. Acute intervention to restore circulation is vital to preserve limb function.
- Vascular claudication – It is a well-recognized and common problem of leg pain, often calf pain. The pain is worse with walking and improves with rest. The pain is often a cramp-like pain in the muscles of the legs with a sense of tiredness and fatigue. Pain at rest is present with very severe disease. This is a result of progressive arteriosclerotic disease and the distribution of the pain reflects the site of arterial disease. Patients may benefit from bypass surgery.
- Venous disease – Incompetence of the valves of the veins of the lower limb result in progressive gravitational congestion of the leg. This results in a painful, achy swollen leg that improves with rest and elevation of the leg. A major associated complication is thrombophlebitis and consequent risk of deep vein thrombosis. Surgery is only indicated in major vascular incompetence.

Joint/bone pain

- Joint pain as a result of acute inflammation as seen in rheumatoid disease, connective tissue disease, gout or septic arthritis is often acute, associated with swelling, redness and tenderness of the joint with radiation up or down the leg.
- Gout is a metabolic disorder characterised by an excess of uric acid in the blood. It usually presents in middle-aged men with rapid-onset painful swelling of a joint – usually the first metacarpophalangeal joint – which is red, hot and associated with proximal and distal pain. It must be differentiated from septic arthritis and other causes of leg pain discussed above.
- Septic arthritis is often bacterial in origin, presents with pain, swelling, redness and tenderness of a joint with radiation. Inflammatory markers are abnormal and patients require antibiotics and possibly aspiration or irrigation of the joint.
- Pain from wearing down of the cartilage of the articular surface is a progressive event and thus the pain has an insidious nature and progresses over a long period.
- An injury or inflammation of the joint capsule, tendon and muscle around a joint can also simulate joint pathology with secondary leg pain. Both muscle and joint pain can occur from metabolic and connective tissue disorder; thus these patients may require a blood screen looking at ESR, RhF, ANF and a rheumatology review.
- Sacroiliitis, arthritic changes in the hip, knee, ankle or arch of foot will cause local and radiating pain.

Referred

Pathology of any of the structures in the abdomen, retroperitoneum and pelvis can result in this. In most of these patients the pain is likely to be non-radiculopathic, with no dermatomal pattern unless there is involvement of the lumbosacral plexus.

MCQs

Select the single correct answer to each question.

1 An L4–5 disc prolapse is most likely to cause:
- **a** pain from the buttock across the thigh, but not beyond the knee
- **b** an L4 radiculopathy
- **c** weakness of ankle plantar flexion
- **d** weakness of extensor hallucis longus
- **e** an absent ankle jerk

2 A cauda equina syndrome:
- **a** is a benign clinical problem
- **b** requires urgent decompression
- **c** has no influence on bladder function
- **d** can only be present if the patient has severe leg pain
- **e** can be managed best with manipulation

77 Acute scrotal pain

Anthony J. Costello

Introduction

The scrotum is the bag-like structure which contains the male reproductive organs, the testes, and adjacent structures. The nerve supply to the scrotum is usually from the ilio-inguinal nerve and the genital branch of the genito-femoral nerve, as well as sympathetic supply brought with the testis into the scrotum, originating in the deep neural plexuses in the renal and aortic area. The testes are richly innervated, and thus even minor trauma can be followed by severe pain in the testes, which is often felt as a more generalised systemic appreciation of deep-rooted pain.

Acute scrotal pain can be the presenting symptom of a wide range of surgical and non-surgical conditions as diverse as organ-threatening testicular torsion and more rarely conditions as life-threatening as a ruptured aortic aneurysm. The diagnosis can usually be made via a careful history and examination with judicious use of investigations.

The management of the various conditions varies greatly and rapid speed of intervention is often the key to a good outcome. The diagnosis is strongly suggested by many factors in the presentation, especially age of the patient, the onset of the pain and presence of associated symptoms.

The most serious and common causes are outlined below.

Testicular torsion

Pathology

Testicular torsion is a surgical emergency and the salvage of the testicle is dependant on the time between onset of symptoms and surgical intervention.

It is caused by the testis rotating on the axis of the spermatic cord. This can lead to complete occlusion of the testicular artery with interruption of testicular blood flow causing testicular ischaemia and necrosis. In the case of the less significant torsion, the testicular vein can become occluded causing an increase in intra-testicular venous pressure and subsequent cessation of local supply of oxygen-rich arterial blood to the testis.

Clinical features

Torsion occurs in two main age groups and for different anatomical reasons. In the neonatal type the torsion occurs before the posterior aspect of the testicle has had time to fuse to the inner layers of the scrotal wall. In these cases this can occur before or after birth and consists of an extra-vaginal torsion (the whole cord and its investing layers twist). It is notoriously hard to diagnose due to the lack of localisation of symptoms in a baby and therefore has a low rate of testicular salvage, around one third of acute presentations. In many the diagnosis is missed and the testicle atrophies either in the scrotum or along the line of testicular descent.

The other main type of testicular torsion is intra-vaginal caused by an abnormally high investment of spermatic cord by the tunica vaginalis. This anatomical variant is frequently bilateral and allows testicle to lie transversely, the so called 'bell clapper' testicle. Torsion of this type can occur at any age but is most common during adolescence perhaps due to differential growth rates between the testicle and adjacent structures. The prevalence has been estimated to be 1 in 4000 males less than 25 yrs old and in males presenting with an acute scrotum this is the diagnosis in 16.0–39.5%.

Presentation is typically with a sudden onset of severe scrotal pain often associated with other symptoms particularly nausea and vomiting due to the common innervation of the testicle and the gastrointestinal tract by fibres from the coeliac ganglion. The presentation is usually rapid due to the severity of the symptoms and may be preceded by milder self-limiting episodes due to spontaneous detorsion.

Atypical presentations however do occur and has been reported in the context of trauma. Urinalysis can also be positive, leading to a misdiagnosis of epididymo-orchitis so a high index of suspicion should be applied.

On examination the boy is usually in severe pain and may refuse examination. If examination is possible the testicle is tense, tender and is usually high in the scrotum ('high-riding'). If early in the course of the condition the twist in the spermatic cord may be felt as a tight 'knot' as the cord exits the external inguinal ring. The pain may persist on elevation of the scrotum, whereas the pain of epididymo-orchitis often resolves on elevation of the scrotum.

Investigations

Various imaging modalities have been used to reduce the need for surgical exploration. Colour Doppler ultrasound can show decreased or absent blood flow in many cases of testicular torsion but is not sensitive enough to be relied on to avoid exploration in someone with a strong history. There have also been reports of normal blood flow on Doppler ultrasound in cases of proven testicular torsion. A detorted testicle and epididymis can also be hyperaemic and thus a false diagnosis of epididymo-orchitis can be made.

Radio-nucleotide scintigraphy can also be used to evaluate testicular blood flow and whilst more accurate than sonography it suffers from lack of rapid and widespread availability. Both imaging modalities should be reserved for ambiguous cases and should not delay the transfer of the patient to theatre.

Magnetic resonance imaging has been used in an experimental setting and may become a clinical imaging modality in the future.

Treatment

Management of suspected testicular torsion consists of surgical detorsion and fixation (orchidopexy) of both testicles due to the chance of contralateral torsion in the future. Under general anaesthesia, the scrotum is explored via a midline incision through the median raphe. The affected testis is delivered from the scrotum and the cord is detorted and the testis is wrapped in warm swabs. The opposite testis is also delivered and fixed in place to the muscular wall of the scrotum, often with non-absorbable sutures, although the use of absorbable sutures is probably to be advised in the paediatric population.

If the testicle is necrotic on detorsion it should be removed. The rate of testicular loss is dependent on the time from onset of pain. Long-term follow-up has shown that up to 67% suffer testicular atrophy and infertility after prolonged torsion whilst others have reported that semen quality and fertility should remain within normal limits if detorsion is performed promptly prior to irreversible damage to the germinal epithelium.

If there is a delay in availability of theatre, manual detorsion has been recommended. The torsion usually occurs by the anterior surface of the testicle rotating medially, the method of detorsion has therefore been described as 'opening a book' after adequate analgesia. Of concern however is a series which reported finding at least some degree of torsion in 28% of those who had undergone successful detorsion, and therefore theatre should not be delayed after this manoeuvre.

Other modalities of treatment that have been used in an attempt to increase salvage rates include hyper-baric oxygen and (in animal studies) scrotal cooling with ice-packs post-operatively.

Initial studies showing that the contralateral testicle can be affected by 'sympathetic atrophy', possibly due to an immunological insult, by the torsion of its neighbour appear to be unfounded.

Torsion of appendages

Appendages of the structures within the scrotum represent remnants of embryological structures which have undergone regression during development. They have been described in various sites on both the testicle and epididymis but the most important clinical appendage is found at the superior pole of testicle, a remnant of the mesonephric duct called the hydatid of Morgagni. It is involved in 92% of appendage torsions. The other appendage that accounts for most (7%) of the other appendage torsions is found on the head (superior) of the epididymis with other appendages, making up a minority.

The mean age of presentation is 9–10 which is younger than for testicular torsion and the presentation is often with milder pain and fewer associated symptoms compared to testicular torsion. The patient often will present later in the course of the condition and

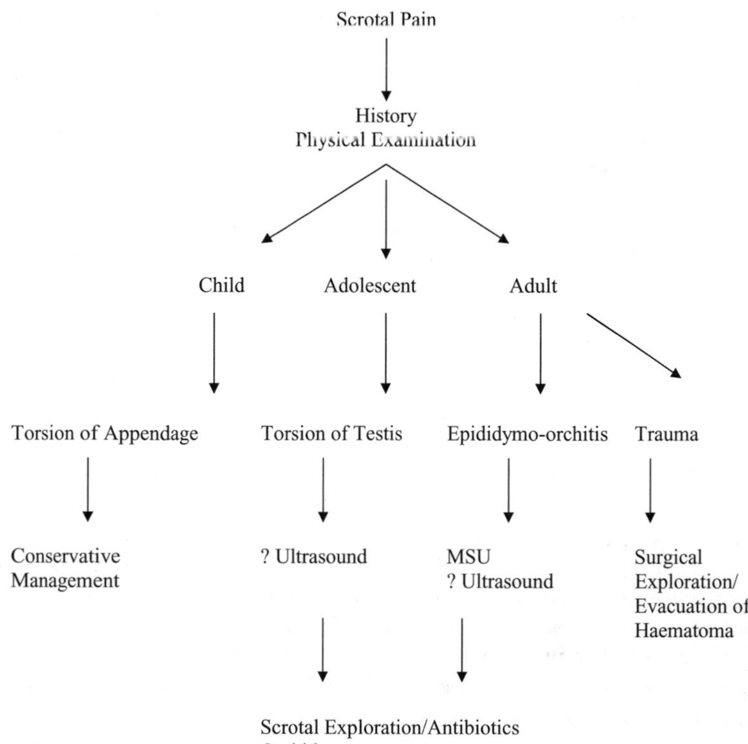

Fig. 77.1 Management of Acute Scrotal Pain.

classically has a small tender 'blue dot' on scrotal examination; this is particularly obvious in children due to their thin scrotal skin. The cremasteric reflex is usually still present and the torted appendage is often able to be identified on ultrasound examination or radionucleotide scintigraphy (68% after 5 hours).

Management of this condition is usually conservative, if the diagnosis can be made with certainty preoperatively, with rest, analgesia and scrotal support. Surgical excision can be reserved for those whose pain is slow to settle.

Epididymo-orchitis

Pathology

This is an inflammatory condition usually infective in nature and thus has a more gradual onset of symptoms. Infective processes usually tracking down from the genito-urinary tract can infect the epididymis and the testis itself. This leads to swelling and severe testicular pain, as the testis swells within the taut tunica albuginea. There may be a history of dysuria and urethral discharge due to urethritis, and systemic symptoms and signs such as fever are common. A history of previous surgery, urinary tract infections and a full sexual history should be obtained as appropriate.

Clinical features

The patient presents with swelling of the hemiscrotum, often of gradual onset, and erythema of the overlying scrotal skin. The testis is swollen and tender, and the epididymis is engorged, swollen and tender. This sign is extremely important in the differentiation between epididymo-orchitis and testicular torsion. The patient will often also experience an acute leucocytosis, and pyrexia.

Management

Treatment is with antibiotics, which may have to be administered intravenously, non-steroidal anti-inflammatories and scrotal support. Urinalysis with culture and sensitivity and blood cultures are also important.

Epididymo-orchitis can occur at any age although the organisms involved vary depending on the aetiology.

Infantile epididymitis has a high incidence of associated urogenital abnormalities, particularly in those with coliform organism isolated from their urine and thus these children require full urological evaluation after treatment of the infection. In children presenting with an acute scrotum, the diagnosis of infection is made in 20–30%. In older children there is a lower association with these structural abnormalities and a lower rate of positive urine cultures. Dysfunctional voiding has been proposed as an aetiological factor in these older children.

In sexually active adolescents and adults the organisms involved are commonly *Chlamydia trachomatis* and *Neisseria gonorrhoeae* although penetrative anal intercourse can lead to coliform infection. Older men with epididymo-orchitis will often have coliform infections owing to bladder outlet obstruction, instrumentation, surgery and catherisation.

More exotic organisms such as *Brucella, Candida* and tuberculosis are occasionally involved in the immuno-compromised and those who have been exposed during overseas travel.

Testicular trauma

Pathogenesis

The testis can survive extremely great forces before being damaged. The testicle can be injured by direct trauma, assaults, sporting injuries and less commonly road traffic accidents and other major trauma.

Clinical features

The scrotum is usually very swollen, with significant ecchymosis if presenting after a period of time. The testis itself is often impalpable as result of the extensive swelling and the common occurrence of a haematocoele. If the testis itself is palpable, and the tunica albuginea is intact, with little to no significant haematocoele, then the patient may be managed conservatively. However, if there is any evidence of the tunica albuginea being breached or if there is significant haematocoele present, surgical exploration is mandatory if the patient's overall condition allows it.

Management

The ruptured testis is exposed and the devascularised portion is excised. The tunica is then closed and the scrotum closed in layers. The aim of testicular exploration in this trauma situation is to preserve as much testicular tissue as possible to allow for testosterone production and spermatogenesis which may be important if the other testis is compromised in any way at this time or in the future.

Testicular neoplasms

Testicular cancers can cause acute pian if there is haemorrhage or infarction in the neoplasm. The presence or history of an abnormal swelling in conjunction with acute pain should alert the examining physician to this. Ultrasound can be used to further evaluate this.

Hydrocoele

A hydrocoele is a collection of fluid between the tunica albuginea and the testis itself. If rapidly forming, it can cause pain in the scrotum. The most effective way of dealing with this situation is to surgically repair the hydrocoele. In the paediatric patients, it often involves the presence of a patent processes vaginalis, which must be repaired. It is unusual to get acute pain from a hydrocoele.

Varicocoele

A varicocoele is a dilatation of the veins of the pampiniform plexus around the testis. This is almost always on the left hand side, the swelling feels like a 'bag of worms' surrounding the testis. This can lead to a dragging sensation, and, if thrombosed, can cause acute pain. Repair is surgical or radiological, and should be considered in patients with large varicocoeles, with asymmetric or small testes, if discovered during the pubertal years or with subfertility, as varicocoeles are associated with reduced production of viable spermatozoa. Again, this situation does not commonly cause acute pain.

Epididymal cyst/spermatocoele

Epididymal cysts or spermatocoeles can both enlarge quickly or have haemorrhage into them which can cause acute pain. These can be surgically excised at a later date if deemed appropriate.

Hernia

Incarcerated or strangulated inguinal hernias can often be found having travelled into the scrotum. The inability to palpate above a scrotal mass is a significant sign of a hernia. A history of a pre-existing hernia or the presence of bowel sounds in the scrotal lump aids in the diagnosis. This distinction can be difficult in the paediatric age group.

Other causes

Pain can be referred from extra-scrotal sites and organs, and can be confused with scrotal pathology. A clear history and examination usually differentiates the cause. For example, the pain from ureteric colic often radiates down to the ipsilateral hemiscrotum and testis, but is of a different nature from most scrotal pains. This is especially common if the stone is low down in the course of the ureter, for example at the vesico-ureteric junction. Pain from a ruptured abdominal aortic aneurysm has been misdiagnosed as scrotal pain, and this diagnosis should be entertained in the older patient.

Conclusions

In summary, acute scrotal pain can be from many causes. The most common of these are testicular torsion, epididymo-orchitis and testicular trauma. Because of the vital nature of the testes as the site of germ cells, nature has caused the testis to be highly innervated by nerves, causing a large pain response to any noxious stimuli, alerting to potential damaging problems. Acute scrotal pain can often present diagnostic difficulties, but the performance of a clear history and examination, aided by appropriate investigations, will make the diagnosis much clearer. Surgical intervention, if warranted, is usually required early, and may have to be undertaken in an exploratory manner to first confirm the diagnosis, and then fix the underlying problem. In general, especially with testicular torsion, it is better to err on the side of caution and offer surgical intervention early, than to agonise over an unclear diagnosis and risk testicular damage and possible loss.

MCQs

Select the single correct answer to each question.

1 Which of the following features is *not* true of complete testicular torison?

- **a** most common between puberty and the age of 25 years
- **b** is not associated with tenderness of the cord
- **c** pain is relieved by elevation of the scrotum
- **d** usually shows changes on colour Doppler ultrasound
- **e** requires urgent surgical treatment

2 Torsion of a testicular appendage:

- **a** occurs most commonly after puberty
- **b** involves the head of the epididymis
- **c** involves the hydatid of Morgagni
- **d** causes severe scrotal pain
- **e** requires urgent surgery

3 Acute epididymo-orchitis is characterised by the following features *except*:

- **a** history of urinary tract infection
- **b** rapid onset of pain
- **c** swollen tender testes
- **d** tenderness of the cord
- **e** pyrexia and leucocytosis

78 Acute back pain

Jeffrey V. Rosenfeld

Introduction

Back pain is one of the commonest ailments suffered by humans, probably because our erect posture places excess mechanical strain on the spine. In addition, acute stressors of the spine may be cumulative and accelerate a natural tendency to osteoarthritic degeneration. Genetic factors, underlying structural anomalies, occupation, pain tolerance, psychological factors and social circumstances all contribute to the origin and persistence of back pain.

There are many possible pain generators in the back, including discs, ligaments, facet (zygapophysial) joints, nerve roots, paraspinal muscles and extraspinal structures. It is difficult to identify the exact cause of back pain in many cases, particularly as the pain is often emanating from multiple structures at multiple segmental levels in the spine. This makes the treatment of back pain problematic, particularly as much of the treatment available for back pain is not founded on a strong evidence base. Back pain results in a large financial cost to the community and is therefore an important public health issue. Prevention of back injury is an important strategy to reduce the prevalence of back pain.

Applied anatomy

There are seven cervical vertebrae, twelve thoracic vertebrae, five lumbar vertebrae and five sacral vertebrae. The spinal cord terminates in the adult at the LI–L2 disc level, where it becomes the filum terminale. The nerve roots of the cauda equina arise from the conus and pass through the lumbar and sacral canal.

The spinal nerve roots exit through the intervertebral foramina, and in the lumbar spine each nerve root passes under the pedicle of its numbered level; for example, the L5 nerve root passes inferiorly across the back of L4–L5 intervertebral disc to exit below the L5 pedicle. Therefore, a posterolateral disc prolapse at L4–L5 will compress the L5 nerve root. A posterolateral disc prolapse at L5–S1 will compress the S1 nerve root. A 'far' lateral disc prolapse may compress the lumbar root passing beneath the pedicle above; for example, a far lateral disc prolapse at L4–L5 may compress the L4 nerve root. There are 8 cervical spinal nerve roots, and the pattern is similar to the lumbar spine; for example, C7 passes across the C6–C7 disc and exits the C6–C7 intervertebral foramen. Posterolateral C6–C7 disc prolapse will therefore compress the C7 nerve root.

Pain generators in the back

Pain arising from the bones of the spine, ligaments, muscles, or intervertebral discs is often called *mechanical back pain*. There is a lot of crossover in segmental nerve supply in the lumbar spine between different structures. The annulus of the intervertebral disc and the facet joints are supplied with nerve fibres. Pain from the disc (*discogenic pain*) or facet joints is felt in the back centrally (*somatic pain*) but may radiate to the buttock and upper thigh (*somatic referred pain*). Somatic back pain may also emanate from musculoskeletal structures, bone and extra- or paraspinal structures.

Nerve root compression or irritation results in *radicular pain*, which is sharp lancinating pain radiating down the lower limb and may pass into the foot or down the arm into the hand. It may not follow an exact dermatomal pattern. It is often difficult to distinguish somatic referred pain from radicular pain. The overall clinical assessment and correlation with the radiological findings is important. Local anaesthetic facet joint blocks which suppresses facet joint pain, and discograms which evoke discogenic pain, have also been used to identify the principal pain generators in patients with chronic back pain (see below).

Box 78.1 Differential diagnosis of back pain.

- Pancreatic disease, e.g. pancreatitis
- Renal disease, e.g. hydronephrosis (usually lateral loin pain)
- Abdominal aortic aneurysm
- Pelvic disease
- Rectum, bladder, gynaecological
- Hip disease – there is pain on moving the hip. The pain may radiate to the buttock and posterior or lateral thigh down to the knee.
- Sacroiliitis
- Lumbo-sacral plexus pathology
- Peripheral nerve pathology, e.g. schwannoma, entrapment, inflammation

The history

A detailed history will provide a likely cause of the patient's back pain and should help to distinguish mechanical, radicular and long tract symptoms. If the patient has limb pain or paraesthesia, a nerve root may be compressed by whatever pathology is causing the back pain. The site of limb pain and paraesthesia will help localize the site of the pathology in the spine. The age of the patient is an important factor in the analysis of cause of back pain. Back pain can be caused by disordres of organs that are not part of the musculo-skeletal system (see Box 78.1).

Examination of the spine

The examination is done in the erect, prone and supine positions. It is important to differentiate between upper and lower motor neuron lesions and to identify the level of spinal pathology.

Spine and joints

Standing

Inspection for midline skin lesions such as a pit, sinus, hairy patch, lipoma, naevus or angioma over the spine. These may indicate underlying occult spinal bifida, spinal dysraphism or tethering of the spinal cord.

Assess general posture and spinal alignment, particularly for scoliosis or kyphosis. Are both feet planted symmetrically on the ground? The cervical spine and the lumbar spine normally have a lordosis (forward curve).

Range of movement includes forward flexion, lateral flexion, rotation and extension. Examine the shoulders and upper limbs if the patient has neck pain.

Supine

Examine the movements of the hips and knees. Examine the sacroiliac joint by adduction and internal rotation of the flexed hip.

Prone

Palpate the back for tenderness, paraspinal mass, paraspinal muscle spasm. Percuss the spine for tenderness. Complete the examination of the hip joint with extension.

Motor function

Neurological examination

Even in the absence of limb pain a careful examination must be made of the limbs, as the neurological signs that may be detected will often lead you to the precise site of pathology in or around the spine.

Gait

Observe for limping, rate of movement, length of stride, and need for walking aid. This will give many clues as to what is wrong and the severity.

Muscles

Muscle wasting and fasciculation imply denervation of muscles – examine all of the muscle groups including the shoulder girdle and gluteal region.

Muscle tone, power and reflexes including the plantars, are measured to determine whether it is an upper or lower motor neurone problem, or a mixed picture (Table 78.1).

Sensation

If you suspect a spinal cord lesion then full sensory testing should be performed. Test pain with pinprick (spinothalamic tracts), and light touch and proprioception (dorsal columns). Do not forget to test sacral,

Table 78.1 Myotomes and deep tendon reflexes

	Muscle weakness	Tendon reflex
C5	Deltoid, supraspinatus, infraspinatus	Biceps
C6	Biceps, brachioradialis (± wrist extension)	Brachioradialis
C7	Triceps (± wrist extension)	Triceps
C8	Finger flexion	–
T1	Interossei	–
L2–L3	Iliopsoas	–
L4	Quadriceps, tibialis anterior	Patella
L5	Extensor hallucis, extensor digitorum	–
S1	Gastrocnemius, toe flexors (± hamstrings)	Achilles
S2	Glutei, hamstrings	

perianal and scrotal/vulval sensation. Establish a sensory level on the trunk for a suspected case of spinal cord compression. This will help with the localisation of the pathology.

Special tests

Straight leg raising is normally to 90 degrees with the patient in the supine position. Lift the whole lower limb passively whilst it is straight, flexing at the hip joint. This stretches sciatic nerve roots. Record the angle at which sciatica stops the movement.

Lesegue's stretch test is a test of pressure on the sciatic nerve.

The ankle is dorsiflexed with the lower limb outstretched and flexed at the hip, placing extra stress on the sciatic nerve, which, if it is already tethered by some pathology such as a disc prolapse, will cause a sharp jab of pain.

Femoral stretch test is a test of pressure on the upper lumbar nerve roots.

The patient is *prone* and the lower limb is extended at the hip, placing tension on the upper lumbar roots.

Rectal examination includes prostate and pelvis, anal tone, external sphincter contraction (the patient tightens the anus with the gloved finger in the rectum), perianal and perineal sensation. Assess the abdomen for bladder fullness.

Anal reflex (S4.5) involves contraction of the subcutaneous portion of the external sphincter in response to scratching the perianal skin.

Sacral sparing may occur within a widespread area of sensory loss caused by an intramedullary spinal cord lesion, and is due to the laminar arrangement of the fibres in the spinothalamic tract. The sacral segments are lateral in the tract. It thus means there is an incomplete spinal cord problem and may be the only sign of this.

General examination

The examination includes chest, abdomen and lymph nodes. Rectal and internal pelvic examinations are done when relevant. In a patient with back or radicular pain always consider intra-abdominal and other pathologies as a cause for pain.

Assess the adequacy of the arterial circulation in the lower limbs in the older patient.

Causes of acute back or neck pain (Box 78.2)

Musculo-ligamentous strain

This is the commonest cause of acute back or neck pain. Usually there is an acute event such as a twisting, bending or lifting motion. The pain is localised but may spread to the trapezius, shoulder, occiput, or interscapular region if from the neck, or the buttock and upper thigh if from the lumbar region. There is spinal stiffness, local paraspinal muscle tenderness but no abnormal neurological signs.

Intervertebral disc prolapse

This is a common problem. The fibrous annulus of the disc tears, allowing the softer nucleus of the

Box 78.2 Key points and pitfalls

- Most back pain is benign in nature and cause, and usually resolves, even without treatment, in 3 to 4 weeks.
- It is important to try and differentiate radicular pain from musculoskeletal spinal pain and spinal cord compression
- Hip pain may mimic sciatica due to compression of a spinal nerve root
- Back pain in children should not be ignored as it often has a serious underlying cause.
- Negative plain radiographs or CT scans do not exclude the presence of serious spinal pathology.
- Make sure adequate investigation of back pain is undertaken at an early stage so that serious pathology is not missed.
- In patients with signs of spinal cord compression, do not forget to examine perineal sensation or to percuss the bladder.

disc to herniate or *prolapse*. If the prolapsed nucleus separates from the disc it becomes a *sequestrated* fragment and may not resolve with expectant treatment. The intervertebral disc usually prolapses posterolaterally and may compress the exiting spinal nerve root which is adjacent to it and cause sciatica or brachialgia. In the acute phase the back pain is usually a minor component. Much less common is the central disc prolapse, which compresses the spinal cord or the cauda equina nerve roots depending on the spinal level.

Disc prolapse is most frequent in the lower cervical spine (C5–C6, C6–C7) and the lower lumbar spine (L4–L5, L5–S1). These are also the levels where degenerative changes are most common. *Disc bulging* (protrusion) occurs where the there is no prolapse (or extrusion) of nucleus. This is a common finding on CT or MR imaging and is not necessarily the cause of back pain and sciatica.

Thoracic disc prolapse may compress an intercostal nerve laterally and cause radiating pain in the distribution of that nerve or may cause spinal cord compression when central.

Infection

Osteomyelitis may be due to pyogenic infection usually by haematogenous spread, or due to tuberculosis. This will cause acute back pain and may cause neurological deficit due to vertebral deformity, bony instability or secondary epidural abscess.

Primary epidural abscess may occur without osteomyelitis particularly if bacteria are introduced into the spinal epidural space by a needle puncture or placement of an epidural catheter for analgesia. The problem has been reported following childbirth, with the mother developing severe back pain and possibly neurological deficit in the weeks following the placement of an epidural catheter for analgesia during labour. Discitis caused by a bacterial infection may also cause acute (and chronic) back pain.

Trauma

Trauma to the spine may cause vertebral fractures which may be unstable and may cause neurological injury. These injuries cause acute and often severe local pain and tenderness.

Vertebral collapse

Crushing of the anterior portion of the vertebral body in the thoracic or lumbar region is common following a hyperflexion injury to the spine. This causes a wedging of the affected vertebral bodies and acute pain. Wedging and vertebral collapse is also common in elderly patients and may be due to neoplastic infiltration, osteoporosis or, less commonly, infection.

Haematoma

An acute subdural or epidural haematoma in the thoracic spinal canal may cause acute cord compression with severe back pain and paraparesis. The cause of the bleed may be a ruptured vascular malformation or a spontaneous bleed in a patient on anticoagulants such as warfarin.

Spinal stroke

Thrombotic occlusion of the anterior spinal artery usually in a patient with diffuse atherosclerotic vascular disease causes an acute paraplegia, with severe acute back pain in the thoracic region. Myelogram does not show any compressive lesion but MRI may show cord signal hyperintensity, which indicates oedema or developing infarction.

Investigation of back pain

Plain X-rays

Plain X-rays are often done as an initial screen for patients with back pain but have a low sensitivity. Plain cervical X-rays are also used as a routine screen in multiple trauma patients and other regions of the spine if clinically indicated.

Computed tomography

Computed tomography (CT) scan is often ordered as the initial investigation for back pain. It shows the bony anatomy and the facet joints very clearly but is of variable and often inferior quality at showing the soft tissues, including the discs and intraspinal pathology.

Magnetic resonance

Magnetic resonance (MR) is now the main modality for spinal imaging and has virtually replaced CT myelography because it is non-invasive and because of the extensive information provided in different projections including the sagittal.

Myelography

The introduction of intrathecal contrast produces a myelogram which outlines the spinal roots and cord and is a dynamic study which can demonstrate a spinal block of the subarachnoid space by a mass lesion. Myelography is often followed by CT (CT myelography) which shows the contrast on the axial (horizontal) CT images.

Discography

Discography involves the injection of the intervertebral disc with contrast which may show internal derangement of the disc and may be used as a provocative test to identify the origin of back pain. It may not be reliable.

Dynamic (flexion–extension) views

These are plain radiographs, fluoroscopy, or MR scans used to demonstrate mechanical instability of spinal segments.

Biopsy and needle aspirate of vertebral or paraspinal disease

Biopsy and needle aspirate under CT guidance is a useful diagnostic technique which may be used when open surgery is not indicated and provides specimens for histopathology and microbiology analysis.

Blood tests

Blood tests, including blood cultures, full blood examination and inflammatory markers are performed selectively.

Treatment

Nonoperative treatment

Most back pain is benign in nature and cause, and usually resolves in 3 to 4 weeks even with no treatment. Degenerative disease and disc prolapse are initially managed conservatively and surgery should be considered a last resort unless there is spinal cord or cauda equina compression, when urgent surgery may be required (see below). Conservative treatments may include rest, and physiotherapy, which may include cervical collar, massage, traction, interferential heat treatment, and manipulation. Chiropractic treatment and acupuncture offer alternatives. Drugs include non-steroidal inflammatory drugs, analgesics, muscle relaxants, and steroids. Acute sciatica or brachialgia may require opiates to control the pain. Exercises are not useful in treating acute back pain, but have a role once it has largely settled so as to strengthen the paraspinal and abdominal muscles (e.g. Pilates program) which are often weakened in patients with degenerative spinal disease and disc prolapse.

Spinal surgery

A patient with disc prolapse and unremitting sciatica or brachialgia and neurological deficit despite conservative measures and who has radiology correlating with the clinical picture should be considered for surgery. Lumbar disc prolapse can be treated with minimally invasive microdiscectomy via an interlaminar approach. Cervical disc prolapse is usually treated with an anterior cervical discectomy and interbody fusion.

Acute or subacute spinal cord compression and cauda equina syndrome are urgent problems which require urgent referral to a neurosurgeon. Emergency decompressive surgery may be required to preserve neurological function and reverse neurological deficit. Whether the decompression of the spinal canal is done via a posterior approach (laminectomy or costotransversectomy) or via an anterior approach (anterior cervical, thoracotomy or transabdominal) depends upon the nature and site of the pathology and the experience of the surgeon. A diseased vertebral body may require excision and replacement by a prosthesis and the stability of the spine may need to be restored with metallic internal fixation using rods, plates, screws and bone grafts. Following such spinal surgery the patient may require radiotherapy or chemotherapy for a neoplasm or prolonged antibiotic therapy for an infection.

An osteoporotic vertebral collapse can be treated with an injection of acrylic cement into the affected vertebral body under radiological guidance to restore the volume and strength of the bone and relieve pain.

MCQs

Select the single correct answer to each question.

1 A 30-year-old man presents with 1 week of right sciatica and has numbness on the dorsum of his right foot and weak dorsiflexion at the ankle. Which of the following is true?

a he probably has an L4–L5 disc prolapse, with compression of the L4 nerve root
b he needs an urgent CT myelogram
c he can be managed initially with rest and analgesics
d he is likely to require surgery
e he should be encouraged to undertake spinal extension exercises

2 A 35-year-old woman presents with acute lumbar back pain, bilateral sciatica, difficulty in voiding and on examination has weakness in the ankles and feet, absent ankle reflexes and decreased sensation in the soles of both feet. Which of the following statements is false?

a she has developed an acute cauda equina compression
b she has developed an acute spinal cord compression
c central disc prolapse at L5–S1 is a likely cause
d urgent magnetic resonance imaging is required
e urgent surgery will be required

3 A 30-year-old diabetic presents with a severe mid and lower thoracic pain, radiation of the pain to the mid-abdomen, and on examination he is tender in the thoracic spine at the level of T10, has weak lower limbs and finds it difficult to walk. Which of the following statements is false?

a CT scan will be helpful as an initial investigation
b he should have an FBE and ESR
c he may have a dissecting aneursym of the aorta
d a needle biopsy is indicated initially
e an MRI is indicated and urgent surgery should be considered

79 Post-traumatic confusion

John David Laidlaw

Introduction

Although confusion is particularly common after significant head injuries, it is also not an uncommon occurrence after other types of trauma. It affects patients of any age, very young and elderly patients being particularly prone. The clinical finding of post-traumatic confusion should not be considered a diagnosis in itself, and requires appropriate clinical assessment and investigation to diagnose the causative pathology before the institution of a management regime appropriate to that particular pathology.

Aetiology and pathogenesis

Relatively minor head trauma is not infrequently overlooked in cases where there are significant other injuries. Although minor head injuries in themselves do not typically cause significant confusion, the effects of secondary brain injury in the post-traumatic period can rapidly develop into a relatively dangerous condition which often has confusion as its presenting symptom. Therefore, any post-traumatic confusion warrants specific clinical assessment and investigation to rule out potentially dangerous intracranial pathology.

However, it must be stressed that the exclusion of significant intracranial pathology is, in itself, insufficient investigation in a patient with post-traumatic confusion. Respiratory problems, metabolic derangements, infections and drugs can all be significant and potentially dangerous causes of post-traumatic confusion, and must be recognized and appropriately managed (Box 79.1).

Management of patient with post-traumatic confusion

Clinical assessment

All patients with post-traumatic confusion require a full physical examination, including full neurological examination. Any suggestion of a reduction in conscious state of 2 or more GCS points (Table 79.1), any focal neurological deficit, or any symptoms of meningism indicate a potential intracranial emergency. Particular attention must also be given to examination of respiratory system and for clinical evidence of sepsis.

Investigation

Investigation is dictated by the clinical history and examination findings. However, most cases of post-traumatic confusion require the following (Box 79.2):

- CT scan brain (urgent if GCS drop >2, or focal neurological signs)
- Arterial blood gas analysis ($Pa\text{O}_2$, $Pa\text{CO}_2$, Bicarbonate, pH, base excess). Note that any patient with confusion must be suspected of having disturbances in respiratory function, and this must be excluded with arterial blood gas analysis. Skin oxygen saturation monitoring (pulse-oximetry) is a useful adjunct to monitor trends in patients with known ventilatory parameters, but is not an alternative to initial ABG analysis.
- Full blood examination (haemoglobin, RCC, WCC, platelets)
- Urea and electrolytes
- Calcium/phosphate
- Consideration of septic work-up (if indicated clinically, and which may include wound swabs, blood cultures, urine analysis and culture, chest X-ray, lumbar puncture for CSF analysis).

Box 79.1 Causes of post-traumatic confusion

Head injury

- Primary brain injury
  - Diffuse axonal injury
  - Cerebral contusions
- Secondary brain injury
  - Hypoxia
    - Hypoxaemia due to respiratory causes
      - Aspiration
      - Pulmonary contusions
      - Pulmonary oedema
      - Pulmonary thromboembolism
      - Pulmonary fat embolism
    - Hypoxaemia due to anaemia
  - Cerebral ischaemia
    - Shock
    - Vascular injury (particularly arterial dissection)
    - Thromboembolism
      - Thromboembolic
      - Cerebral fat emboli
      - Disseminated intravascular coagulation
    - Raised ICP (CPP = MAP – ICP)
      - Intracranial haemaotoma
        - EDH
        - Acute SDH
        - Intracerebral haematoma and enlarging contusions
        - Chronic SDH
      - Hydrocephalus
        - Obstructive
        - Communicating
      - Brain swelling
        - Vascular
          - Vasodilatation
            - Post-traumatic (usually children)
            - Hypercapnia
          - Venous engorgement
            - Jugular compression or obstruction
            - Sinus thrombosis or obstruction
        - Oedema
          - Vasogenic
          - Cytotoxic
          - Hyponatraemia
  - Infection
    - Meningitis
    - Epidural abscess
    - Subdural empyema
    - Intracerebral abscess
    - Septic venous sinus thrombosis

General/Metabolic

- Hypoxia
- Hypercapnia
- Acid–base problems (particularly acidosis)
  - Metabolic
    - Renal failure
    - Lactic acidosis
    - Diabetic ketoacidosis
  - Respiratory
- Electrolyte imbalance
  - Sodium
    - Hyponatraemia
    - Hypernatraemia (unusual to cause confusion)
  - Calcium
    - Hypocalcaemia
- Glucose
  - Diabetic hyperglycaemia/ketoacidosis
  - Hypoglycaemia (usually seen in treated diabetics)
- Infection
  - Septicaemia
    - Primary (iatrogenic, i.v. lines, etc)
    - Secondary (to other infection)
  - Pulmonary
  - Urinary
  - Wound
- Nutritional
  - Vitamin B_{12} deficiency

Drug intoxication/withdrawal

- Medication
  - Sedatives and tranquilizers
  - Analgesics (particularly narcotics)
  - Steroids (although not usually indicated in trauma)
  - Anticonvulsants
  - Hypoglycaemic agents
- Non-medicinal
  - Alcohol
  - Narcotic
  - Hallucinogens
  - Cocaine
  - Solvents

Table 79.1 Glasgow coma score

Score	Best eye opening (E)	Best verbal (V)	Best motor (M)
6			Obeys
5		Orientated	Localizes pain
4	Spontaneous	Confused	Withdraws to pain
3	To speech	Inappropriate words	Abnormal flexion to pain ('decorticate')
2	To pain	Incomprehensible sounds	Extension to pain ('decerebrate')
1	None	None	None

Notes on GCS:
- GCS = E + V + M.
- Worst score is 3, best is 15.
- Use best response if differences between sides for eye opening or motor function.
- GCS measures only conscious state, not neurological deficit.

Box 79.2 Management of post-traumatic confusion

Clinical assessment
- Physical examination
  - Airway, breathing, circulation immediately, then general examination
- Neurological examination
  - Particularly note GCS, papillary inequality or other focal neurological deficit, and meningism

Investigation
- CT scan brain (urgent if GCS drop >2, or focal neurological signs)
- Arterial blood gas analysis ($Pa\text{O}_2$, $Pa\text{CO}_2$, bicarbonate, pH, base excess).
- Full blood examination (haemoglobin, RCC, WCC, platelets)
- Urea and electrolytes
- Calcium/Phosphate
- Septic work-up (wound swabs, blood cultures, urine analysis and culture, chest X-ray, ± CSF analysis)

General management of confused patient
- Environmental
  - Close monitoring and supervision
  - Protection
  - Quiet environment if possible
- Sedation avoided if at all possible
  - If absolutely required, best to use only short-acting parenteral (i.v.) sedatives in small doses titrated to effect, closely supervised
- Analgesia if required
  - If narcotic, only small frequent i.v. doses (e.g. 1–2 mg morphine p.r.n.) titrated carefully, with the patient closely supervised (not intramuscular or subcutaneous)
  - Recognition of legal incompetency
  - Relevancy to consent and refusal of treatment

Specific management of the cause of confusion
- Intracranial Lesions
  - Immediate neurosurgical opinion for all
  - Usually surgical decompression if mass effect, and relatively urgent if a patient is developing lateralising signs or deteriorating GCS
- Hypoxia and respiratory disturbance
  - Oxygen supplementation
  - Immediate intubation if
    - Airway not patent and protected (cough and gag)
    - Respiratory failure
    - Note spinal precautions for all intubations, but do not delay for spinal investigation
- Electrolyte disturbance
  - Appropriate fluid and electrolyte therapy
- Infection
  - Appropriate antibiotic therapy instituted immediately after cultures, and modified when culture and sensitivities known
- Medications and non-medicinal drugs
  - Medications scrutinised
  - Drug and alcohol history determined

General management of confused patient

Environmental

Confused patients are generally best managed in a quiet environment, but need to be closely monitored by experienced nursing and medical staff. Agitated patients need to be protected from falls, etc., and bedsides are therefore essential. Padding to the bedsides, or even nursing on the floor on a thick mattress may provide more protection. On occasions physical restraints may be needed to protect the patient; however these must be checked regularly to ensure they do not cause pressure or pain or subject the patient to a risk for entanglement. It is essential that restraints are not used as a means to avoid close supervision; all confused patients need such supervision and those requiring restraint should be supervised even more diligently.

Familiar faces, such as family or close friends, may help relax a confused patient, although visitors and unfamiliar contacts should be kept to a minimum. Busy wards and noisy areas will often cause a confused patient to become quite agitated and are best avoided if possible.

Sedation

Sedation is best avoided in confused patients if at all possible. The aim is to identify and treat the cause of the confusion rather than sedate the patient. Sedation may rarely be needed in an agitated patient where there is the risk of self-harm or injury. However, very often close supervision in a calm environment will allow sedation to be avoided. Sedation should only be used if significant intracranial and metabolic (particularly hypoxic) problems have been excluded. Sedation should never be used simply to facilitate easier nursing care. On the few occasions where sedation is needed it is most appropriate to use only short-acting parenteral (i.v.) sedatives in small doses titrated to effect. The clinician must constantly be aware of the potential for wrongly attributing decreased conscious state to sedative use, and missing a worsening and dangerous intracranial pathology or metabolic event.

Analgesia

Many patients with post-traumatic confusion have significant pain from other injuries. The pain often causes severe agitation, and the patient can be much better managed if appropriate analgesia is used. Narcotics have the side effects of altering conscious state, causing pupillary constriction and depressing ventilation, all of which are potentially catastrophic in a patient with a significant intracranial pathology. They have therefore historically been shunned by neurosurgeons. However, most modern neurosurgeons and traumatologists recognize the effective analgesic properties and the short and predictable action of narcotics when used by the i.v. route, and are prepared to use them cautiously. It must be stressed that only small, frequent i.v. doses (e.g. 1–2 mg morphine p.r.n.) should be used and these must be titrated carefully, with the patient closely supervised. Intramuscular doses have a more unpredictable and delayed action and should be avoided. The historical anachronism of using codeine instead of narcotics should be discarded; codeine is a narcotic with the same side effects as other narcotics when used in the same analgesic dose, but has the disadvantage of not being available in i.v. preparation. A note should be made that tramadol, which has recently been used increasingly in the management of severe pain, does increase the risk of seizures, and therefore is probably best avoided following head injury.

Legal competency

A confused patient is not competent to make appropriate important decisions. This of course includes giving consent for surgical procedures, and most countries have legal avenues which allow the clinician to undertake emergency medical procedures without consent. It must also be understood that a confused patient cannot competently discharge himself or herself from hospital against medical advice. The clinician must understand that the refusal of a confused patient to follow the clinician's advice is not done from a position of legal competency, and therefore the clinician maintains significant responsibility for consequences of these actions. On occasions, formal declaration of incompetency is required to allow appropriate care or restraint. However, in most cases even very confused patients can be quietly reasoned with and will follow gentle calm advice, particularly if people familiar to them are involved.

Specific management of the cause of confusion

The primary rule in management of a confused patient is to correct the primary cause of the confusion.

Intracranial lesions

Any intracranial mass lesion (haematoma, hydrocephalus, brain swelling) identified on CT scan warrants an immediate neurosurgical opinion. Even patients managed in rural hospitals who are considered to have a relatively small lesion deserve the potential benefits of a telephone consultation between the managing clinician and a neurosurgeon. Whether the lesion requires surgical treatment (craniotomy in the case of an acute haematoma or burr-hole drainage of chronic subdural haematomas or hydrocephalus) depends primarily on the patient's clinical condition and the amount of mass effect of the lesion. Therefore, in a telephone consultation the most important information the neurosurgeon requires is the patient's GCS score, whether this has deteriorated and if so the rapidity of change, any focal neurological signs (e.g. pupillary inequality or unilateral change in motor function) and the amount of midline shift and asymmetry on the CT scan. Teleradiology can be a major benefit in these cases. Most neurosurgeons would generally advise surgical decompression of an accessible intracranial lesion, which causes more than a millimeter or two of midline shift, and would consider this to be relatively urgent if a patient is developing lateralising signs or has a deteriorating conscious state.

Hypoxia and respiratory disturbance

Oxygen supplementation must be used on confused patients until blood gas analysis results are available. Although relatively mild hypoxia or hypercarbia do not usually in themselves cause confusion, following a head injury they can seriously potentiate secondary brain injury and most neurosurgeons would advise maintenance of $Pa\text{O}_2$ of more than 100 mm Hg and $Pa\text{CO}_2$ 30–35 mm Hg. Hyperventilation is not usually recommended now following head injury as it has the potential to exacerbate cerebral ischaemia.

In a confused patient with a deteriorating conscious state it must be determined that not only is the airway patent and the patient has appropriate blood gases, but it needs to be ensured that the airway is protected by an intact and strong gag and cough reflex. If there is any doubt about the adequacy of airway patency or protection then endotracheal intubation becomes an immediate priority. If intubation is required in a trauma patient this must be done immediately, with the head and neck held in a neutral position by an assistant (spinal precautions), and should not be delayed for cervical radiology, brain scans or other investigations.

Electrolyte disturbance

Electrolyte disturbances, particularly sodium anomalies, must be corrected with appropriate fluid and electrolyte therapy. A point of caution is that the rapid correction of long-standing hyponatraemia can cause central pontine myelinosis, and in this case the aim should be to correct slowly over 24–48 hours. More rapid correction of acute hyponatraemia (e.g. that caused by iatrogenic water intoxication) can be safely performed. Similarly, acute hyponatraemia caused by either SIADH or cerebral salt-wasting syndrome can be safely done relatively quickly. It needs to be recognised that while fluid restriction is appropriate for SIADH, salt-wasting syndromes are associated with total body water deficit. Expert endocrinology advice can be invaluable in these cases.

Infection

Infections, particularly pulmonary, urinary, wound or i.v.-line associated, are the most common causes of post-traumatic confusion after the first 24–48 hours. These must be considered in all cases, and a septic work-up performed. Meningitis must be suspected if confusion is associated with decreasing conscious state or meningism. In these cases lumbar puncture is mandatory. However, in a post-traumatic case an urgent cerebral CT is always advisable prior to lumbar puncture; intracranial mass lesions can mimic meningitis and can cause lumbar puncture to be a fatal procedure. If infection is clinically suspected, appropriate antibiotic therapy should be instituted after cultures are collected, and modified when culture and sensitivity results are known.

Medications and non-medicinal drugs

All confused patients must have their current medications scrutinised, and drug and alcohol history determined. Narcotics and sedatives can in themselves cause confusion, particularly in the elderly, and in these cases their use needs to be reconsidered. Anticonvulsant toxicity can also cause an acute confusional state, and their levels should be checked if appropriate. Similarly, withdrawal of chronically ingested substances (sedatives, alcohol, recreational drugs) can cause a potentially dangerous acute confusional state. Usually, in these cases it is not appropriate to reinstitute the drug, and in those cases management is usually supportive with judicious sedative use.

MCQs

Select the single correct answer to each question.

1 Post-traumatic confusion commonly occurs due to the following conditions except:
  - **a** cerebral contusion
  - **b** intracerebral haematoma
  - **c** hypoxia
  - **d** hypernatraemia
  - **e** venous engorgement

2 Post-traumatic confusion may require the following treatments *except:*
  - **a** i.v. sedatives
  - **b** i.v. codeine
  - **c** i.v. morphine
  - **d** physical restraint
  - **e** oxygen supplementation

80 Double vision

J. E. K. Galbraith

Anatomy

The elucidation of double vision depends on knowledge of the anatomy of the extra-ocular muscles and their actions.

The extra-ocular muscles are divided into two groups. The first group arises from the apex of the orbit to attach to the sclera anterior to the equator of the eye. Included in this group are the rectus muscles: medial, lateral, superior and inferior.

The second group consists of the oblique muscles. The superior oblique arises from the apex of the orbit and is deviated through a pulley in the anterior orbit so that it passes backwards and laterally above the globe to attach to the postero-lateral area of the upper surface of the eye. The inferior oblique arises in the anterior orbit and passes backwards and laterally under the globe to attach to the postero-lateral quadrant of the eye inferiorly.

Nerve supply

The extra-ocular muscles are supplied by three cranial nerves. The third cranial nerve passes forward in the lateral wall of the cavernous sinus and divides anteriorly into the superior and inferior divisions, which enter the orbit through the superior orbital fissure. The superior division supplies the levator and superior rectus, while the inferior division supplies the medial and the inferior rectus and the inferior oblique.

The fourth cranial nerve supplies the superior oblique muscle, and the sixth cranial nerve supplies the lateral rectus.

Actions

The medial and lateral rectus pass forward from the apex of the orbit to the globe, and their actions are not influenced by the position of the globe. The medial rectus only adducts the eye, that is turns it towards the nose and the lateral rectus only abducts the eye, turning it outwards away from the nose.

The remaining rectus muscles have three actions depending on the direction of gaze. Clinically one need only consider the action of a muscle when the eye is directed along the axis of that muscle.

Thus, when the eye is abducted, the superior or inferior rectus each has only one action – the superior elevates the eye and the inferior depresses the eye.

When the eye is adducted to look along the line of action of the superior oblique, it has one action, to depress the eye. Its antagonist, the inferior oblique, when the eye is adducted, elevates the eye. The actions can be simply represented diagramatically (see Fig. 80.1).

The superior and the inferior oblique muscles also rotate the eye around an antero-posterior axis. When the 12 o'clock meridian is rotated towards the nose it is called intorsion. Rotation of the 12 o'clock meridian away from the nose is extorsion. The oblique muscles have no torsional effect when the eye is adducted, but when the eye is abducted the torsional effect is maximal. The superior oblique intorts the eye, the inferior oblique extorts the eye.

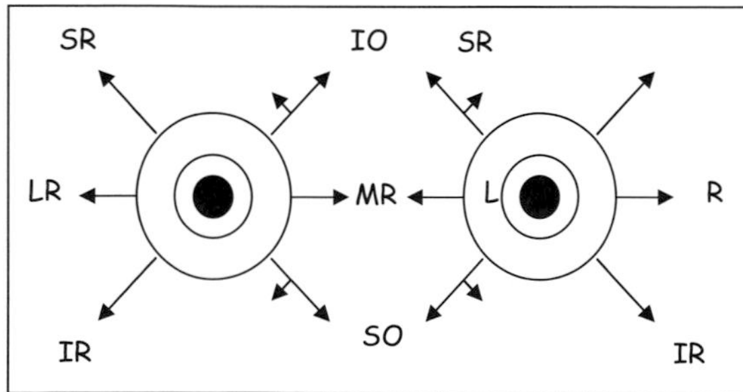

Fig. 80.1 Actions of ocular muscles.

Diplopia

Pathology

Diplopia results when the visual axes are not parallel. Very occasionally, it is due to abnormalities in the refracting surfaces of the eye. The commonest cause of diplopia is palsy of the third, fourth or sixth cranial nerves resulting from vascular accidents, cerebral aneurysm, giant cell arteritis, multiple sclerosis, diabetes or trauma. Muscular causes are myositis, myasthenia gravis, thyroid eye disease and trauma, particularly a blowout fracture of the orbital floor (see Chapter 37).

When a patient complains of sudden onset of painful diplopia, one should always think of cerebral aneurysm or diabetes. Diabetes causes occlusion of the small vessels supplying the fourth or sixth nerve causing pain due to ischaemia.

Diagnosis

The key to the diagnosis of diplopia is the fact that the eye muscles work in pairs (see Fig. 80.1). When the eye turns to the left, the left lateral rectus and the right medial rectus combine to produce the movement. When the eyes look down to the left the movement is produced by the left inferior rectus and the right superior oblique.

When the patient complains of diplopia the first question to ask is, "In which direction is the double vision maximal?" This then isolates the cause to the two muscles involved in turning the eye in that direction.

Because the image in the eye is inverted, the next step is to cover one eye to determine which eye gives rise to the image that is furthest away (image inversion dictates that the eye that moves least has the maximum displacement of the image). This indicates the muscle responsible for the diplopia.

Lateral rectus palsy

If the patient complains of double vision looking to the left, the left lateral rectus or the right medial rectus is responsible for the diplopia. Covering one eye elicits the information that the furthest image comes from the left eye and thus the cause of diplopia is the left lateral rectus – a lesion of the sixth cranial nerve. Furthermore, the medial rectus is one of four muscles supplied by the third nerve, and if the other muscles are acting normally it is unlikely that one of the four would be defective in the presence of three healthy muscles.

Fourth cranial nerve palsy

It is easy to diagnose a fourth nerve palsy because this is the muscle which takes the eye down in adduction. That is it is the muscle used in reading. Thus a person with a fourth nerve palsy will complain of double vision, a line of print will be double, with the second line below the line being read, and that line will be tilted, while the other remains level. Again, covering one eye will enable the diagnosis to be made, as the eye with the tilted image (due to the unopposed action of the inferior oblique) will be the eye at fault.

In unilateral fourth nerve palsy, one line is tilted; in a bilateral fourth nerve palsy both lines of print are tilted in opposite directions.

The sequelae of muscle palsy

The action of the eye muscles is not as simple as detailed here because in every eye movement all the extraocular muscles are involved, some contracting and others relaxing. When one extra-ocular muscle is paretic, changes occur in all the muscles.

The direct antagonist of the paretic muscle undergoes contracture because it is opposed by a weaker muscle. In a right lateral rectus palsy the right medial rectus undergoes contracture. This tends to increase the separation of the two images.

The contralateral synergist of the paretic muscle over-acts. In the case of a right lateral rectus palsy, the left medial rectus will overact, increasing the separation of the images. This is due to the paretic muscle receiving an increased innervation in an attempt to increase its range of movement: because the contralateral synergist, in this case the medial rectus, receives the same innervation it over-acts. Finally, to allow this muscle to overact, there must be an inhibitional palsy of its antagonist (in the example this will be the left lateral rectus).

Another example – a patient with a right superior oblique palsy suffers a contracture of the right inferior oblique, over-action of the left inferior rectus and a secondary palsy of the left superior rectus.

This increases the deviation – this is of value to the sufferer, as the further apart the images, the easier it is for one to be suppressed.

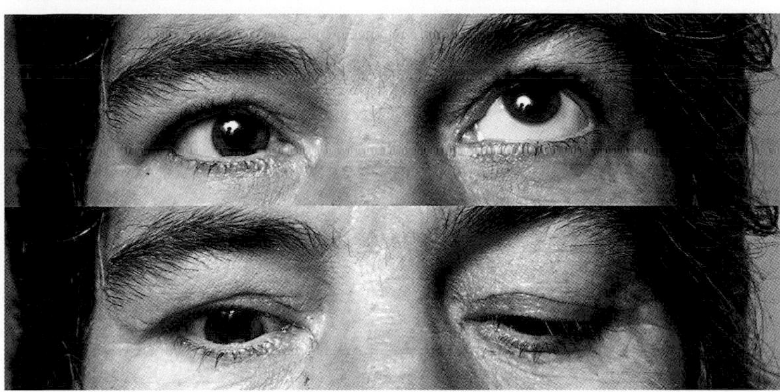

Fig. 80.2 This patient has a right third cranial nerve palsy. In the upper picture he is attempting to look up. The right eye fails to elevate. In the lower picture when he attempts to look down the upper lid elevates owing to misdirection of nerve fibers. In this case fibers intended for the inferior rectus are innervating the levator muscle of the upper lid.

Sometimes the secondary effects of the paretic muscle do not recover when the paresis recovers. Surgery to the overacting, but healthy, muscle may then be necessary to weaken it.

Aberrant regeneration

Aberrant regeneration is commonly seen after a third nerve palsy resulting usually from head trauma. When the nerve recovers, some fibers will be misdirected. Typically, when the patient converges the eyes, the upper eyelid elevates because fibers to the medial rectus have reinnervated the levator of the upper lid. (See Fig. 80.2).

Aberrant regeneration is untreatable.

Surgery of diplopia

The principles of the surgery of double vision are:

- to strengthen weak muscles by lengthening them,
- to weaken overacting muscles by shortening them.

A muscle is strengthened by excising some of the tendon and then resuturing it to its original insertion. A muscle is weakened by removing it from the globe and re-attaching it closer to its origin.

A paretic muscle may be strengthened by excising a small portion (usually 3–6 mm) and its direct antagonist weakened by recessing its attachment to the globe. If this is insufficient to correct the double vision one next proceeds to the contralateral synergist. The patient who has a weak lateral rectus would have an excision of a small length of the tendon of that muscle, a recession of the medial rectus on the same side initially, followed later by recession of the opposite medial rectus if required.

Surgery for diplopia never completely cures the patient because five muscles cannot do the work of six. Rather, the intention is to move the double vision away from the straight-ahead position to the extremes of ocular movement where it is less troublesome.

A patient with a completely paralysed extra-ocular muscle will always have intractable double vision in some direction of gaze. In such cases, surgery is disappointing. Often single vision can be secured in straight-ahead gaze, but not elsewhere.

MCQs

Select the single correct answer to each question.

1 With reference to the actions of the extra-ocular muscles, which of the following is correct?
- **a** in adduction, the superior oblique elevates the eye.
- **b** in abduction, the inferior rectus depresses the eye.
- **c** in adduction, the inferior oblique muscle intorts the eye.
- **d** in abduction, the inferior oblique muscle intorts the eye.

2 The muscle most employed in reading is:
- **a** the medial rectus.
- **b** the lateral rectus.
- **c** the superior oblique.
- **d** the inferior oblique.

3 When investigating a case of diplopia, a helpful sign is:
- **a** the patient prefers to fixate on a target with the eye with the paretic muscle.
- **b** the image from the eye with the paretic muscle is displaced most.
- **c** the paralysis of one extra-ocular muscle has no effect on the other muscles.
- **d** the patient prefers to fixate on a target with the eye with healthy muscles.

Answers to MCQs

Answers to MCQs

Chapter 1

1 (d)
2 (c)
3 (a)

Chapter 2

1 (d)
2 (a)
3 (e)
4 (e)
5 (e)

Chapter 3

1 (b)
2 (c)
3 (a)
4 (d)
5 (d)

Chapter 4

1 (c)
2 (d)
3 (d)
4 (a)

Chapter 5

1 (c)
2 (d)
3 (c)

Chapter 6

1 (c)
2 (e)
3 (a)
4 (d)
5 (b)

Chapter 7

1 (e)
2 (b)
3 (a)
4 (b)
5 (c)

Chapter 8

1 (b)
2 (c)
3 (a)
4 (d)
5 (a)

Chapter 9

1 (e)
2 (b)
3 (c)

Chapter 10

1 (c)
2 (a)

Chapter 11

1 (a)
2 (c)
3 (d)
4 (c)
5 (d)

Chapter 12

1 (b)
2 (d)
3 (c)

Chapter 13

1 (b)
2 (c)
3 (c)
4 (d)

Chapter 14

1 (d)
2 (e)
3 (d)

Chapter 15

1 (a)
2 (e)
3 (c)
4 (e)
5 (d)
6 (d)

Chapter 16

1 (d)
2 (e)
3 (d)
4 (b)
5 (e)

Chapter 17

1 (e)
2 (b)
3 (c)
4 (c)
5 (e)
6 (e)
7 (c)

Chapter 18

1 (b)
2 (e)
3 (b)
4 (c)
5 (e)

Chapter 19

1 (b)
2 (b)
3 (b)
4 (e)
5 (d)

Chapter 20

1 (a)
2 (c)
3 (c)
4 (a)
5 (b)

Chapter 21

1 (b)
2 (b)
3 (e)

Chapter 22

1 (d)
2 (d)
3 (b)

Chapter 23

1 (a)
2 (c)

Chapter 24

1 (e)
2 (b)
3 (e)
4 (a)
5 (d)

Chapter 25

1 (d)
2 (c)
3 (b)
4 (e)

Chapter 26

1 (e)
2 (d)
3 (a)
4 (d)
5 (b)
6 (e)

Chapter 27

1 (e)

Chapter 28

1 (a)
2 (e)

Chapter 29

1 (c)
2 (a)

Chapter 30

1 (e)
2 (d)

Chapter 31

1 (b)
2 (a)
3 (c)
4 (d)
5 (e)

Chapter 32

1 (c)
2 (b)
3 (b)
4 (c)
5 (a)

Chapter 33

1 (d)
2 (a)
3 (c)
4 (b)
5 (e)

Chapter 34

1 (a)
2 (b)
3 (e)
4 (b)
5 (d)

Chapter 35

1 (b)
2 (d)
3 (e)
4 (a)
5 (c)

Chapter 36

1 (b)
2 (a)
3 (d)

Chapter 37

1 (d)
2 (b)
3 (b)

Chapter 38

1 (b)
2 (b)
3 (e)

Chapter 39

1 (d)
2 (d)
3 (c)

Chapter 40

1 (a)
2 (d)
3 (c)
4 (b)

Chapter 41

1 (c)
2 (b)
3 (a)
4 (e)
5 (d)

Chapter 42

1 (c)
2 (d)
3 (a)
4 (b)

Chapter 43

1 (c)
2 (b)
3 (d)
4 (e)

Chapter 44

1 (c)
2 (a)
3 (b)
4 (b)

Chapter 45

1 (d)
2 (b)
3 (e)
4 (a)

Chapter 46

1 (c)
2 (b)
3 (a)
4 (e)

Chapter 47

1 (a)
2 (c)
3 (a)
4 (d)
5 (b)

Chapter 48

1 (a)
2 (b)
3 (a)
4 (a)
5 (c)

Chapter 49

1 (b)
2 (a)
3 (b)
4 (a)

Chapter 50

1 (c)
2 (d)
3 (a)
4 (c)
5 (d)
6 (d)

Chapter 51

1 (d)
2 (c)
3 (c)
4 (c)

Chapter 52

1 (b)
2 (a)
3 (e)
4 (d)

Chapter 53

1 (d)
2 (b)
3 (a)
4 (b)
5 (b)

Chapter 54

1 (d)
2 (a)
3 (e)
4 (d)
5 (b)

Chapter 55

1 (c)
2 (e)
3 (b)
4 (e)
5 (b)

Chapter 56

1 (e)
2 (b)

Chapter 57

1 (a)
2 (b)
3 (e)
4 (e)

Chapter 58

1 (d)
2 (c)
3 (a)
4 (d)

Chapter 59

1 (b)
2 (c)
3 (a)
4 (d)
5 (c)

Chapter 60

1 (d)
2 (c)

Chapter 61

1 (e)
2 (d)

Chapter 62

1 (c)
2 (d)
3 (b)
4 (a)
5 (c)

Chapter 63

1 (b)
2 (b)

Chapter 64

1 (c)
2 (d)
3 (c)
4 (c)

Chapter 65

1 (a)
2 (b)

Chapter 66

1 (a)
2 (c)
3 (d)
4 (e)
5 (e)

Chapter 67

1 (c)
2 (d)

Chapter 68

1 (a)
2 (d)
3 (c)
4 (f)
5 (e)

Chapter 69

1 (b)
2 (c)
3 (c)
4 (d)

Chapter 70

1 (c)
2 (c)
3 (b)
4 (e)

Chapter 71

1 (c)
2 (b)

Chapter 72

1 (b)
2 (a)
3 (e)
4 (c)
5 (d)

Chapter 73

1 (e)

Chapter 74

1 (c)
2 (a)
3 (d)
4 (e)

Chapter 75

1 (b)

Chapter 76

1 (d)
2 (b)

Chapter 77

1 (c)
2 (c)
3 (b)

Chapter 78

1 (c)
2 (b)
3 (d)

Chapter 79

1 (d)
2 (b)

Chapter 80

1 (b)
2 (c)
3 (d)

Index

Page numbers in *italics* refer to figures and those in **bold** to tables or boxes; please note that figures, tables and boxes are only indicated when they are separated from their text references.